W9-CFM-274

PROGRESS IN BIOMEDICAL OPTICS

Proceedings of

Laser-Tissue Interaction IX

Steven L. Jacques
Editor

Abraham Katzir
Biomedical Optics Series Editor

26–28 January 1998
San Jose, California

Sponsored by
Air Force Office of Scientific Research
IBOS—International Biomedical Optics Society
SPIE—The International Society for Optical Engineering

Published by
SPIE—The International Society for Optical Engineering

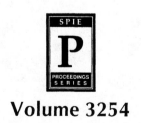

Volume 3254

SPIE is an international technical society dedicated to advancing engineering and scientific applications of optical, photonic, imaging, electronic, and optoelectronic technologies.

The papers appearing in this book comprise the proceedings of the meeting mentioned on the cover and title page. They reflect the authors' opinions and are published as presented and without change, in the interests of timely dissemination. Their inclusion in this publication does not necessarily constitute endorsement by the editors or by SPIE.

Please use the following format to cite material from this book:
   Author(s), "Title of paper," in *Laser-Tissue Interaction IX*, Steven L. Jacques, Editor, Proceedings of SPIE Vol. 3254, page numbers (1998).

ISSN 0277-786X
ISBN 0-8194-2693-8

Published by
SPIE—The International Society for Optical Engineering
P.O. Box 10, Bellingham, Washington 98227-0010 USA
Telephone 360/676-3290 (Pacific Time) • Fax 360/647-1445

Copyright ©1998, The Society of Photo-Optical Instrumentation Engineers.

Copying of material in this book for internal or personal use, or for the internal or personal use of specific clients, beyond the fair use provisions granted by the U.S. Copyright Law is authorized by SPIE subject to payment of copying fees. The Transactional Reporting Service base fee for this volume is $10.00 per article (or portion thereof), which should be paid directly to the Copyright Clearance Center (CCC), 222 Rosewood Drive, Danvers, MA 01923. Payment may also be made electronically through CCC Online at http://www.directory.net/copyright/. Other copying for republication, resale, advertising or promotion, or any form of systematic or multiple reproduction of any material in this book is prohibited except with permission in writing from the publisher. The CCC fee code is 0277-786X/98/$10.00.

Printed in the United States of America.

SESSION 6   OCULAR II: MECHANISMS OF LASER EFFECTS

SESSION 7   ABLATION I

SESSION 8   ABLATION II

Part B *Soft-Tissue Modeling*

Conference Committees

Part A   Laser-Tissue Interaction IX

Conference Chair

> **Steven L. Jacques,** Oregon Medical Laser Center

Program Committee

> **Wei R. Chen,** Oklahoma School of Science and Mathematics and University
> of Oklahoma
> **Robert P. Godwin,** Los Alamos National Laboratory
> **Tayyaba Hasan,** Wellman Laboratories of Photomedicine, Massachusetts General
> Hospital, and Harvard Medical School
> **E. Duco Jansen,** Vanderbilt University
> **Richard A. London,** Lawrence Livermore National Laboratory
> **Alexander A. Oraevsky,** Rice University and University of Texas Medical Branch
> at Galveston
> **Scott A. Prahl,** Oregon Medical Laser Center
> **William P. Roach,** Air Force Office of Scientific Research
> **Rudolf M. Verdaasdonk,** University Hospital Utrecht (Netherlands)
> **Lihong Wang,** Texas A&M University

Session Chairs

1   Immunologic Mechanisms During PDT I
> **Wei R. Chen,** Oklahoma School of Science and Mathematics and University
> of Oklahoma

2   Immunologic Mechanisms During PDT II and Photochemical Mechanisms
> **Tayyaba Hasan,** Wellman Laboratories of Photomedicine, Massachusetts General
> Hospital, and Harvard Medical School

3   Photothermal Mechanisms
> **Steven L. Jacques,** Oregon Medical Laser Center

4   Photoacoustic Mechanisms
> **Richard A. London,** Lawrence Livermore National Laboratory

5   Ocular I: Pulsed Laser Effects on Tissues
> **William P. Roach,** Air Force Office of Scientific Research

6   Ocular II: Mechanisms of Laser Effects
> **Bernard S. Gerstman,** Florida International University

7   Ablation I
> **E. Duco Jansen,** Vanderbilt University

Part B   Soft-Tissue Modeling

Conference Chair

        Jeff Lotz, University of California/San Francisco

Program Committee

        Robert L. Galloway, Jr., Vanderbilt University
        Sharmila Majumdar, University of California/San Francisco
        Robert Sah, University of California/San Diego

Part A

LASER-TISSUE INTERACTION

SESSION 1

Immunologic Mechanisms During PDT I

Cancer treatment by photodynamic therapy combined with NK cell line based adoptive immunotherapy

Mladen Korbelik and Jinghai Sun

Cancer Imaging Department, British Columbia Cancer Agency, Vancouver, B.C., Canada V5Z 1L3

ABSTRACT

Treatment of solid cancers by photodynamic therapy (PDT) triggers a strong acute inflammatory reaction localized to the illuminated malignant tissue. This event is regulated by a massive release of various potent mediators which have a profound effect not only on local host cell populations, but also attract different types of immune cells to the treated tumor. Phagocytosis of PDT-damaged cancerous cells by antigen presenting cells, such as activated tumor associated macrophages, enables the recognition of even poorly immunogenic tumors by specific immune effector cells and the generation of immune memory populations. Because of its inflammatory/immune character, PDT is exceptionally responsive to adjuvant treatments with various types of immunotherapy. Combining PDT with immuneactivators, such as cytokines or other specific or non-specific immune agents, rendered marked improvements in tumor cures with various cancer models. Another clinically attractive strategy is adoptive immunotherapy, and the prospects of its use in conjunction with PDT are outlined.

Keywords: photodynamic therapy, adoptive immunotherapy, tumor draining lymph nodes, NK cell line

1. INTRODUCTION

The insult inflicted by photodynamic therapy (PDT) in treated cancerous tissue is a form of oxidative stress[1-3]. It results in the induction of cellular photooxidative damage occurring mostly in cell membranous structures which are the sites of intracellular localization for the majority of effective photosensitizers. The direct killing of tumor cells is attained when vital cell targets are inactivated by this primary insult. However, considerable damage to PDT treated tumors (ultimately responsible for the successful eradication of targeted lesions) comes from oxidative stress related secondary events. These include: (i) the ischemic death consequent of vascular damage and occlusion of blood supply; (ii) ischemia-reperfusion injury; (iii) killing by activated inflammatory cells; and (iv) tumor sensitized immune reaction. Common to all of these antitumor effects is a strong inflammatory character[2,3].

Photodynamically induced changes in the membranes of cancerous cells elicit two major types of response: (1) the induction/upregulation of early response genes, stress proteins and other genes due to the interaction with early signal transducing elements[3,4]; and (2) initiation of theinflammatory reaction. PDT induced stress proteins may participate in the development of inflammatory/immune processes triggered by this therapy, since they were shown to have a role in cell adhesion and antigen presentation[5,6]. In particular, some of these proteins (known to act as chaperones) have been suggested to serve as carriers for antigenic peptides transferred to MHC molecules to become tumor specific antigens[6].

The inflammatory cellular damage from photooxidative lesions of membrane lipids causes a massive release of lipid degradation products and metabolites of arachidonic acid[2,7]. These products, together with other mediators released from PDT damaged vasculature (e.g. histamine and serotonin), are potent initiators of inflammation, which is the key element responsible for the development of PDT induced tumor immunity. The powerful inflammation associated signaling in PDT treated tumors includes a wide variety of mediators comprising of vasoactive substances, components of the complement and clotting cascades, acute phase proteins, peroxidases, radicals, proteinases, leukocyte chemoattractants, cytokines, growth factors and other immunoregulators[3,7,8]. This signaling is responsible for a rapid and massive invasion of inflammatory cells from the circulation into PDT treated tumors and their activation[9,10]. The activated non-lymphoid immune effector cells (neutrophils, mast cells, monocytes/macrophages) contribute substantially to the destruction of cancerous cells[2,3,11]. In addition, macrophages are likely responsible for mediating the initial critical step in tumor

---

Further author information:-
Dr. Mladen Korbelik (correspondence): Email: mkorbeli@bccancer.bc.ca; Telephone: 604-877-6098, ext. 3044; Fax: 604-877-6077

recognition by lymphoid populations. Prompted to phagocytize large numbers of PDT damaged cancer cells and directed by the generated accessory stimuli, these cells serve as antigen presenting cells by processing tumor specific peptides and presenting them in the context of major histocompatibility complex (MHC) molecules[2,3].

The specific *in vivo* depletion experiments have demonstrated that both CD4 and CD8 T lymphocyte populations participate in PDT induced antitumor immune effects[2]. Thus, as outlined in Fig. 1, the recognition of tumor antigens presented by macrophages may involve helper T lymphocytes. These cells become activated, secrete interleukin-2 (IL-2), and in turn sensitize cytotoxic T cells to tumor specific epitopes. The underlying communication between the macrophages and CD4[+] T cells or between CD4[+] and CD8[+] T cells is established not only through the MHC-TCR/CD3 linkage (stabilized by either the CD4 or CD8 molecule), but requires accessory interaction of other ligand:receptor molecules, as indicated in Fig. 1. These include adhesion pairs such as LFA-1:ICAM-1 and co-stimulatory ligands B7:CD28 or B7:CTLA-4[12,13]. The expression of these molecules in the membranes of immune cells is upregulated under the influence of cytokines and other PDT induced mediators. The formation of clones of tumor-sensitized helper and cytotoxic T lymphocytes is followed by their rapid expansion and maturation. The generation of long lived immune memory cells localized in the spleen of mice cured of subcutaneously growing tumor by PDT was also demonstrated[2]. Thus, although the PDT treatment is localized to the tumor site, due to the induction of the immune reaction its effects can have systemic attributes.

Of a particular relevance to projects of combining PDT with adoptive transfer of NK cells described below are the results of further *in vivo* depletion experiments done in our laboratory which indicate that host NK cells are also activated in killing cells of PDT treated tumors. In these experiments, meth-A fibrosarcomas growing in *scid* mice were treated by PDT, which was followed by the depletion of NK cells in the hosts using anti-Asialo GM1 polyclonal antibody. This treatment resulted in a significant reduction in tumor cures compared to the effect of PDT in the hosts with normal levels of NK cells (Korbelik, unpublished results).

2. PDT AND ADOPTIVE IMMUNOTHERAPY WITH TUMOR DRAINING LYMPH NODE CELLS

The predominant immune response in the rejection of malignant tumors is mediated by T-cells. In most cases, the transfer of activated T lymphocytes, but not specific antisera, can confer cancer immunity to the recipient. Adoptive immunotherapy employing T cell response directed at selective destruction of antigen-containing cancer cells has been demonstrated to result in regression of malignant tumors in humans[14,15]. This strategy for the treatment of malignant lesions is currently under intense investigation both pre-clinically and in clinical trials. Significant advances in this field include defining conditions for the *in vitro* activation and expansion of lymphoid cells and securing their activity upon transfer to the recipients. Tumor draining lymph nodes are considered a most reliable source of autologous lymphoid cells required for clinical adoptive immunotherapy, because they contain the greatest abundance of tumor-reactive T cells[16]. Large numbers of these effector cells needed for clinical therapy ($\geq 10^{11}$, i.e. at least 10^9 per kg body weight) necessitated the development of techniques for their efficient *ex vivo* expansion (1000-fold expansion within several weeks). The techniques that achieve this requirement, while maintaining or increasing specific antitumor activity of effector cells, have been developed. They are based either on the stimulation at the level of the T lymphocyte antigen receptor complex (using anti-CD3 monoclonal antibodies[17,18]) or using compounds which enhance T cell receptor signal transduction pathways[19], both in combination with low dose IL-2.

Although lymphoid cells freshly isolated from cancer patients exhibit poor antitumor reactivity, in many cases the host immune response was triggered and tumor-sensitized pre-effector cells were generated. However, due to the tumor induced suppression and/or immunodeficiency, these pre-effector cells were arrested before maturing into fully functional antitumor effector lymphocytes[20,21]. The functionally deficient pre-effector cells can be induced *in vitro* to differentiate into mature immune cells able to eradicate cancerous lesions upon their adoptive transfer. This was achieved in most studies by using sequential stimulation with anti-CD3 and IL-2[18]. Since antigenic stimulation of T cells involves signal transduction through the antigen receptor complex TCR/CD3, cross-linking these molecules with monoclonal antibodies raised against the CD3 antigen will activate T cells[17,22]. Although these cells will not divide, they will express IL-2 receptors and become capable of reacting to low concentration of IL-2 (e.g. 10 U/ml provided in the growth medium) by vigorous proliferation. The responding populations are both CD4[+] and CD8[+] T cells, although a somewhat preferential expansion of the latter populations can occur[23]. The therapeutic effect of adoptively transferred T cells against established malignancy generally requires both helper and cytotoxic T lymphocytes[24]. Despite the polyclonal nature of anti-CD3 mediated activation, tumor antigen specific lymphocytes are stimulated as one element of this interaction. Importantly, immunosuppression of the host appears to have no influence on the activity of adoptively transferred effector T cells[18,25].

Combining with PDT may help address some critical issues in adoptive immunotherapy:
- The generation of tumor-sensitized pre-effector lymphocytes could be augmented by PDT, which (as indicated above) may stimulate tumor recognition.
- Homing of adoptively transferred cells could be improved by PDT treatment of a malignant tumor growing in the recipient, due to the release of chemotactic factors triggered by PDT.
- De-bulking of tumor mass, also achieved by PDT, could allow T cells to effectively eliminate foci of remaining viable cancer cells.
- Cytokines released by adoptively transferred lymphocytes could stimulate a PDT elicited immune reaction.
- Cytokine release elicited by PDT could secure a prolonged activity of transferred effector T cells, which may permit the adjuvant systemic administration of IL-2 (frequently causing severe side-effects) to be reduced or omitted.
- Pre-clinical studies of adoptive immunotherapy treatment of subcutaneous tumors indicate that positive results are difficult to achieve without additional total body irradiation of the host[18]. It appears that the main underlying effect is the radiation induced release of cytokines which could allow for more active antigen presentation and, consequently, more effective tumor recognition by the effector T cells[18]. It seems reasonable to examine the possibility that PDT can replace total body irradiation as a non-toxic approach to the facilitation of adoptive immunotherapy.

In our studies, we are using mouse tumor models of different antigenicity to investigate combined effects of PDT and adoptive immunotherapy. The source of tumor sensitized pre-effector lymphocytes are the popliteal lymph nodes (PLNs), as they exclusively drain tumors implanted in the footpad of a mouse[18]. The optimal interval for harvesting tumor sensitized lymphocytes is 9-10 days after tumor implant[21]. The PLNs excised at that time are markedly enlarged and contain $2-3 \times 10^7$ cells (>50% of them are T lymphocytes), which is over 100-fold increase compared to the cellular content of PLNs in non-tumor bearing mice. The initial phase of *in vitro* PLN cell culture is the anti-CD3 mediated activation (2 days), followed by the expansion phase (3-4 days) in the presence of mouse IL-2 added to the growth medium (10 U/ml)[16]. These two cycles can be repeated for greater expansion of lymphoid effector cells. Flow cytometry analysis has shown that over 90% of the anti-CD3/IL-2 cultured PLN cells are either $CD4^+$ or $CD8^+$, and the rest are B cells.

In our experiments, activated and expanded tumor draining PLN cells are intravenously administered to tumor bearing mice (at least 2×10^7 per mouse). The tumors are treated by PDT at different time intervals relative to adoptive transfer, and the response (tumor cure or regrowth) is evaluated. The effects of Photofrin and several new generation photosensitizers used for PDT combined with adoptive immunotherapy are being examined. The progress of these studies will be reported elsewhere.

3. PDT AND ADOPTIVE IMMUNOTHERAPY WITH NK CELLS

About 10-15% of human peripheral blood lymphocytes are natural killer (NK) cells. These cells are characterized by the ability to lyse malignant cells (and other targets such as virally infected cells) without prior sensitization in a fashion that is not restricted to MHC antigens, i.e. by a mechanism different from antigen-specific killing mediated by T lymphocytes[26]. The NK cells become activated when exposed to IL-2 or some other cytokines (IL-7, IL-12, or interferons)[27,28], which makes them capable to lyse a variety of target cells by a mechanism still not completely elucidated[29,30]. Human NK cells can be identified by the expression of the CD56 molecule in the absence of CD3 and germline configuration of T-cell receptor genes. Antibodies to mouse NK cell antigens (e.g. NK-1.1, DX5 antigen) are also available.

The ability of activated NK cells to lyse malignant cells has prompted their utilization in clinical trials in cancer patients, with adjuvant IL-2 included in therapy protocols[31,32]. These attempts are confronted with problems of securing high numbers of pure NK cells (not contaminated with T lymphocytes) without compromising their activity. One solution to circumventing these problems is using established human NK cell lines[33,34]. Perhaps the best characterized is the NK-92 cell line, shown to exhibit phenotypical and functional properties of activated NK cells[34,35]. This cell line, isolated from a patient with non-Hodgkin's lymphoma, has the ability of continuous *in vitro* growth in the presence of low dose IL-2[34]. The

NK-92 cells do not express Fcγ receptors (frequently seen with many other NK cell types), but do show a high expression of CD56, a feature characterizing a subpopulation of activated NK cells with high cytotoxic activity[36]. Experiments *in vitro* have shown that NK-92 cells can lyse a broad range of malignant cells at very low effector:target ratios[34,35].

A further step in the development of this cell line was achieved in Dr. Klingemann's laboratory by producing genetically engineered variants. The NK-92MI cells were obtained by introducing a 495 base pair cDNA of the human IL-2 gene using particle-mediated gene transfer. These cells, with the retroviral vector containing IL-2 integrated into the genome, are characterized by a stable production of IL-2 which serves as an autocrine stimulant for their continuous growth (i.e. they do not need IL-2 added to growth medium). Upon transfer into immunodeficient mice, the NK-92MI cells showed a prolonged survival *in vivo*, and the capacity to kill leukemic cells present in these hosts (H.-G. Klingemann, personal communication). The application of the NK-92MI cell line in *ex vivo* purging of leukemia from blood is also being actively investigated in Dr. Klingemann's laboratory[35].

The work in our laboratory is focused on using NK-92MI cells (kindly provided by Dr. Klingemann) for investigating the therapy of solid cancers, particularly in studying the effects of PDT combined with adoptive immunotherapy based on this cell line. There are several important advantages and potential benefits provided by this combination:

- An important plus is the unlimited source of activated NK cells for adoptive transfer provided by the NK-92MI *in vitro* cultures, since for a single treatment at least $2x10^7$ cells need to be injected per mouse.
- Another advantage is the MHC non-restricted activity of NK cells, which eliminates the need for prior sensitization to a particular tumor type. Moreover, restrictions seen with T cell mediated treatment of poorly antigenic tumors are not encountered.
- Although activated NK cells are able to migrate and accumulate in malignant lesions[37], their homing to the target site may be inferior to that seen with effector T cells. The combined PDT treatment could enhance this process due to the release of strong chemoattracting signals, as discussed above.
- The PDT induced immune response may be stimulated by IL-2 and other cytokines (e.g. interferon γ) secreted by adoptively transferred NK-92MI cells.
- An additional improvement in tumor control could be gained from PDT mediated reduction in tumor mass that alleviates the burden left to be eliminated by NK cells.
- As mentioned above, PDT appears to induce the activation of NK cell mediated antitumor activity at least with some tumor types.

In our ongoing studies, we are using either human tumors growing in immunodeficient mice, or mouse tumors implanted in syngeneic immunocompetent or immunodeficient mice. The initial results obtained with SiHa tumors (human cervical squamous cell carcinoma) growing subcutaneously in *scid*/NOD mice are shown in Fig. 2. The mice were administered Photofrin (10 mg/kg i.v.) and tumors treated with 630±10 nm light (150 J/cm^2) 24 hours later. One group of mice received $2x10^7$ NK-92MI cells (i.v.) immediately after light treatment. Although a complete initial tumor ablation was achieved with this PDT dose, all tumors regrew within 18 days post PDT. The combined treatment with adoptivelly transferred NK-92MI cells showed an obvious benefit, manifested as a 10 day delay in regrowth of some tumors. The administration of NK-92MI cells to those mice bearing SiHa tumors of the same size as used for PDT (5-7 mm in largest diameter) was of no obvious effect on tumor growth. However, the tumors became palpable much later in mice that received NK-92MI cells at the time of tumor implant (data not shown). It seems reasonable to expect that the effect of NK-92MI based adoptive immunotherapy (done in conjunction with PDT) can be substantially improved by optimizing the protocols for the delivery of these cells. In this respect, experiments are currently in progress aimed at identifying the most effective route of administration of NK-92MI cells (i.v., i.p., intratumorally), benefits with single or multiple injections of varying cell numbers, and optimized timing of NK-92MI cell delivery relative to PDT treatment.

A potential pitfall with the strategy of using NK-92MI cell line for the adoptive transfer is their immune incompatibility with the recipient. However, even a limited life span (before host rejection) may allow NK-92MI cells to effectively engage in the cytolysis of their targets. Moreover, allografted/xenografted NK-92MI cells may have a prolonged survival in the patient/host who is immunocompromised because of bearing a malignant tumor. The initial results of experiments with mouse tumor models are also very encouraging. Despite the species difference (mouse *vs.* human), NK-92MI cells are apparently not immediately destroyed when injected in immunocompetent BALB/c mice bearing EMT6 mammary sarcoma. This may be related to the known immunosuppressive effect of this tumor[38], which is known to be potentiated by PDT[39].

Since interaction of NK cells with other host immune cells may contribute to the antitumor activity, the ability to investigate the effect of adoptively transferred NK-92MI cells and PDT in immunocompetent mice may provide important information related to the underlying mechanism of tumor eradication. Our preliminary results with the EMT6 sarcoma model indicate that the NK-92MI based adoptive immunotherapy potentiates the antitumor effect of PDT.

4. ACKNOWLEDGMENTS

The research on this project is supported by Grant MT-12165 provided by the Medical Research Council of Canada.

5. REFERENCES

1. A. M. R. Fisher, A. L. Murphree and C. J. Gomer, "Clinical and preclinical photodynamic therapy", *Laser Surg. Med.* **17**, pp. 2-31, 1995.
2. M. Korbelik, "Induction of tumor immunity by photodynamic therapy", *J. Clin. Laser Med. Surg.* **14**, pp. 329-334, 1996.
3. T. J. Dougherty, C. J. Gomer, B. W. Henderson, G. Jori, D. Kessel, M. Korbelik, J. Moan and Q. Peng, "Photochemotherapy of cancer: Basic concepts and clinical applications", *J. Natl. Cancer Inst.* (in press 1998).
4. C. J. Gomer, M. Luna, A. Ferrario, S. Wong, A. M. R. Fisher and N. Rucker, "Cellular targets and molecular responses associated with photodynamic therapy", *J. Clin. Laser Med. Surg.* **14**, pp. 315-321, 1996.
5. G. M. Cuenco, T. Knisely, L. Averboukh, L. Garett, S. Castro and A. H. Cincotta, "Induction of glucose regulatory proteins in tumor cells after treatment with benzophenothiazine analogue", *Photochem. Photobiol.* **65**, pp. 19S, 1997.
6. T. Boon, J.-C. Cerottini, B. Van den Eynde, P. van der Bruggen and A. Van Pel, " Tumor antigens recognized by T lymphocytes", *Annu. Rev. Immunol.* **12**, pp. 337-365, 1994.
7. M. Ochsner, "Photophysical and photobiological processes in the photodynamic therapy", *J. Photochem. Photobiol. B: Biol.* **39**, pp 1-18, 1997.
8. V. H. Fingar, "Vascular effects of photodynamic therapy", *J. Clin. Laser Med. Surg.* **14**, pp. 323-328, 1996.
9. G. Krosl, M. Korbelik and G. J. Dougherty, "Induction of immune cell infiltration into murine SCCVII tumour by Photofrin-based photodynamic therapy", *Br. J. Cancer* **71**, pp. 549-555, 1995.
10. S. O. Gollnick, X. Liu, B. Owczarczak, D. A. Musser and B. W. Henderson, "Altered expression of interleukin 6 and interleukin 10 as a result of photodynamic therapy *in vivo*", *Cancer Res.* **57**, pp. 3904-3909, 1997.
11. M. Korbelik, "Photosensitizer distribution and photosensitized damage of tumor tissues", *The Fundamental Bases of Phototherapy*, H. Hönigsmann, G. Jori and A. R. Young editors, pp. 229-245, OEMF spa, Milan , 1996.
12. T. A. Springer, "Adhesion receptors of the immune system", *Nature* **346**, pp. 425-434, 1990.
13. E. C. Guinan, J. G. Gribben, V. A. Boussiotis, G. J. Freeman and L. M. Nadler, "Pivotal role of the B7:CD28 pathway in transplantation tolerance and tumor immunity", *Blood* **84**, pp.3261-3282, 1994.
14. S. A. Rosenberg, "The immunotherapy and gene therapy of cancer", *J. Clin. Oncol.* **10**, pp. 180-199, 1992.
15. S. A. Rosenberg, J. R. Yannelli, J. C. Yang, S. L. Topalian, D. J. Schwartzentruber, J. S. Weber, D. R. Parkinson, C. A. Seipp, J.H. Einhorn and D.E. White, "Treatment of patients with metastatic melanoma with autologous tumor-infiltrating lymphocytes and interleukin 2", *J. Natl. Cancer Inst.* **86**, pp. 1159-1166, 1994.
16. H. Yoshizawa, A. E. Chang and S. Shu, "Specific adoptive immunotherapy mediated by tumor-draining lymph node cells sequentially activated with anti-CD3 and IL-2", *J. Immunol.* **147**, pp.729-737, 1991.
17. J. A. Ledbetter, P. J. Martin, C. E. Spooner, D. Wofsy, T. T. Tsu, P. G. Beatty and P. Gladstone, "Antibodies to Tp67 and Tp44 augment and sustain proliferative responses of activated T cells", *J. Immunol.* **135**, pp. 2331-2336, 1985.
18. L. Peng, S. Shu and J. C. Krauss, "Treatment of subcutaneous tumor with adoptively transferred T cells", *Cell. Immunol.* **178**, pp. 24-32, 1997.
19. R. E. Merchant, N. G. Baldwin, C. D. Rice and H. D. Bear, "Adoptive immunotherapy of malignant glioma using tumor-sensitized T lymphocytes", *Neurol. Res.* **19**, pp. 145-152, 1997.
20. P. J. Spies, J. C. Yang and S. A. Rosenberg, "*In vivo* antitumor activity of tumor-infiltrating lymphocytes expanded in recombinant interleukin-2", J. Natl. Cancer Inst. **79**, pp.1067-1075, 1987.

21. J. D. Geiger, P. D. Wagner, M. J. Cameron, S. Shu and A. E. Chang, "Generation of T-cells reactive to the poorly immunogenic B16-BL6 melanoma with efficacy in the treatment of spontaneous metastases", *J. Immunother*.**13**, pp. 153-165, 1993.

22. T. D. Geppert and P. E. Lipsky, "Accessory cell independent proliferation of human T4 cells stimulated by immobilized monoclonal antibodies to CD3", *J. Immunol.* **138**, pp. 1660-1666, 1987.

23. S. Shu, J. J. Sussman and A. E. Chang, "*In vivo* antitumor efficacy of tumor-draining lymph node cells activated with nonspecific T-cell reagents", *J. Immunother.* **14**, pp. 279-285, 1993.

24. H. Yoshizawa, A. E. Chung and S. Shu, "Cellular interactions in effector cell generation and tumor regression mediated by anti-CD3/interleukin 2-activated tumor-draining lymph node cells", *Cancer Res.* **52**, pp. 1129-1136, 1992.

25. K. Sakai, A. E. Chung and S. Shu, "Phenotype analyses and cellular mechanism of the pre-effector T-lymphocyte response to a progressive syngeneic murine sarcoma", Cancer Res. 50, pp. 4371-4376, 1990.

26. M.J. Robertson and J. Ritz, "Biology and relevance of human natural killer cells", *Blood* **76**, pp. 2421-2438, 1990.

27. M. R. Alderson, H. M. Sassenfeld and M. B. Widmer, "Interleukin 7 enhances cytolytic T lymphocyte generation and induces lymphokine-activated killer cells from human peripheral blood", *J. Exp. Med.* **175**, pp. 577-587, 1990.

28. M. I. Robertson, R. J. Soiffer, S. F. Wolf, T. I. Manley, C. Donahue, D. Young, S. H. Herrmann and J. Ritz, "Response of human natural killer (NK) cells to NK cell stimulatory factor (NKSF): cytolytic activity and proliferation of NK cells are differentially regulated by NKSF", *J. Exp. Med.* **175**, pp. 779-788, 1992.

29. J. H. Phillips and L. L. Lanier, "Dissection of the lymphokine activated killer phenomenon: relative contribution of peripheral blood natural kiler cell and T lymphocytes to cytolysis", *J. Exp. Med.* **164**, pp. 814-825, 1986.

30. T. L. Whiteside and R. B. Herberman, "Human natural killer cells in health and disease", *Clin. Immunother.* **1**, pp. 56-66, 1994.

31. J. J. Mule, S. Shu, S. L. Schwarz and S. A. Rosenberg, "Adoptive immunotherapy of established pulmonary metastases with LAK cells and recombinant interleukin-2", Science 225, pp. 1487-1489, 1984.

32. B. D. Curti, D. L. Longo, A. C. Ochoa, K. C. Conlon, J. W. Smith, II, W. G. Alvord, S. P. Creekmore, R. G. Fenton, B. L. Gause, J. Holmlund, J. E. Janik, J. Ochoa, P. A. Rice, W. H. Sharfman, M. Sznol and W. J. Urba, "Treatment of cancer patients with *ex vivo* anti-CD3-activated killer cells and interleukin-2", *J. Clin. Oncol.* **11**, pp. 652-660, 1993.

33. J. Yodoi, K. Teshigawara, T. Nikaido, K. Fukui, T. Noma, T. Honjo, M. Takigawa, M. Sasaki, N. Minato, M. Tsudo, T. Uchiyama and T. Maeda, "TCGF (IL2)-receptor inducing factor(s). I. Regulation of IL2 receptor on a natural killer-like cell line (YT cells)", *J. Immunol.* **134**, pp. 1623-1630, 1985.

34. J.-H. Gong, G. Maki and H.-G. Klingemann, "Characterization of a human cell line (NK-92) with phenotypical and functional characteristics of activated natural killer cells", *Leukemia* **8**, pp. 652-658, 1994.

35. H.-G. Klingemann, E. Wong and G. Maki, "A cytotoxic NK-cell line (NK-92) for *ex vivo* purging of leukemia from blood", *Biol. Blood Marrow Transpl.* **2**, pp. 68-75, 1996.

36. T. M. Ellis and R. I. Fisher, "Functional heterogeneity of Leu 19"bright"+ and Leu 19"dim"+ lymphokine-activated killer cells", *J. Immunol.* **142**, pp. 2949-2954, 1989.

37. U. Nannmark, P. Basse, B. R. Johansson, P. Kuppen, J. Kjærgaard and M. Hokland, "Morphological studies of effector cell-microvessel interactions in adoptive immunotherapy in tumor-bearing animals", *Nat. Immun.* **97**, pp. 78-86, 1999-97.

38. A. J. McAdam, A. Felcher, M. L. Woods, B. A. Pulaski, E. K. Hutter, J. G. Frelinger and E. M. Lord, "Transfection of transforming growth factor-β producing tumor EMT6 with interleukin-2 elicits tumor rejection and tumor reactive cytotoxic T-lymphocytes", J. Immunother. 15, pp. 155-164, 1994.

39. M. Korbelik, G. Krosl, J. Krosl and G. J. Dougherty, "The role of host lymphoid populations in the response of mouse EMT6 tumor to photodynamic therapy", *Cancer Res.* **56**, pp.5647-5652, 1996.

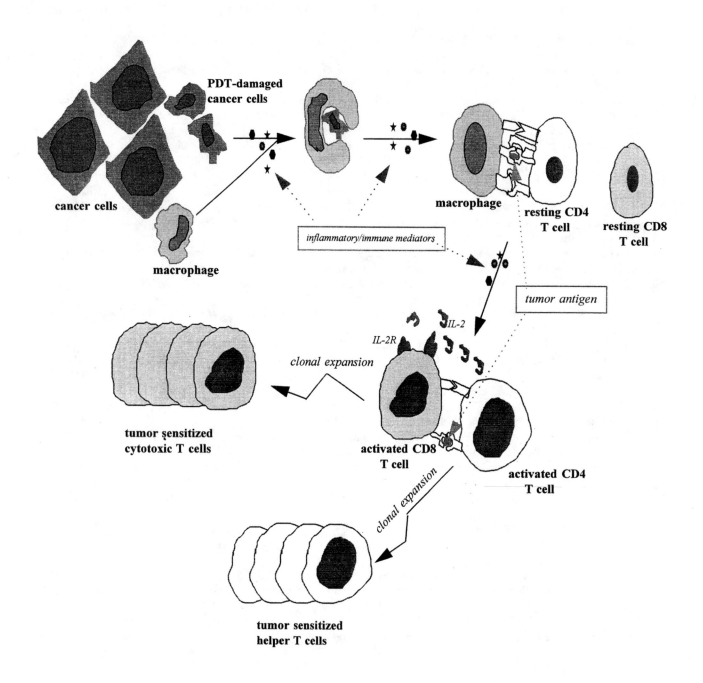

Figure 1: A possible mechanism for PDT-induced development of tumor immunity.

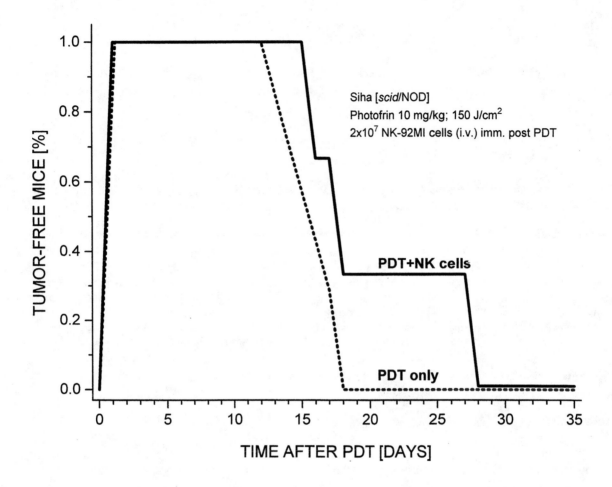

Figure 2: The effect of adoptively transferred NK-92MI cells on the response of SiHa tumors to Photofrin-based photodynamic therapy

Photodynamic therapy with photoactivated Aluminum Disulfonated Phthalocianine and cellular immune response

Gianfranco Canti[a], Rinaldo Cubeddu[b], Paola Taroni[b] and Gianluca Valentini[b]

aDepartment of Pharmacology, School of Medicine,University of Milano,Milano, Italy
bC.E.Q.S.E.,CNR,Milano,Italy

ABSTRACT

Photodynamic therapy (PDT) of cancer is based on the systemic administration of photosensitive drugs followed by exposure of the tumor mass to light of particular wavelength. The combination of drug uptake in malignant tissues and selective delivery of laser-generated light provides for an effective therapy with efficient tumor citotoxicity and minimal normal tissue damage. There are various studies on the effect of photoactivated photosensitizers on host immune response in tumor bearing mice. Since immunity is important in the control of tumor growth and spreading, in our laboratory we examine the effect of PDT on immune compartment. Spleen hyperplasia as well as spleen and marrow hypercellularities were observed in tumor bearing mice treated with Aluminum Disulfonated Phthalocyanine (AlS$_2$Pc) and laser light. Phytohemagglutinine (T lymphocytes mitogen) and Lypolisaccaride (B lymphocytes mitogen), stimulation of spleen lymphocytes caused an increase in blast transformation in tumor bearing mice. Furthermore splenocytes and macrophages collected from mice treated with PDT were cytotoxic in vivo (Winn Assay) parental against tumor cells. The results observed suggest that PDT is able to modulate the immune response and oncological patients treated with PDT could become immune versus a relapse or versus the minimal residual disease.

Keywords: Photodynamic therapy, Phthalocianines, Laser light, Lymphocytes, Macrophages.

2. INTRODUCTION

Photodynamic therapy (PDT) of cancer requires the activation of an administered photosensitizer by light.[1] This treatment has been attractive particularly by its potential for selective tumor destruction.[2] Tumor cell killing in photodynamic therapy is mediated by production of a highly reactive oxygen species by photosensitizers,when excited with light of an appropriate wavelength.[3] Hematoporphyrin derivative (Hpd) or the common available semi-purified preparation called Photofrin II (PhII) are the photosensitizers most commonly used in clinical studies.[4] Toxicological and immunopharmacological properties of Hpd have been investigated by several authors,with and without light exposure.[5,6] In our laboratory we observed various stimulatory effects of Hpd on different functional activities of the immune system.[7,8,9] However, other authors, showed that the combination of Hpd plus light exposure abrogated the ability of peripheral blood mononuclear cells to act as stimulator cells in a mixed lymphocyte reaction.[10] Additionally Hpd was able to decrease dinitrofluorobenzene-induce hypersensitivity.[11] Most recently was published that a complete,thought transitory,suppression of natural killer (NK) cell activity can be achieved by treatment of mice with Hpd and laser light.[12] Thus,in the literature, the effect of Hpd-mediated PDT on the host immune defense mechanism is controversial and not definitevely clear. Many laboratories are studying new photosensitizers,one class of which are the Aluminum Phthalocyanines (AlS$_2$Pc). It was demonstrated that AlS$_2$Pc have photosensitizing activities both in vitro and in vivo,[13] their toxicity is low[14] and they can be useful photosensitizers in PDT.[15]

Aim of this research is to study the effect of PDT with AlS$_2$Pc and laser light on functional activity of lymphocytes and macrophages and their interaction with the antitumor immune mechanism.

3. MATERIAL AND METHODS

3.1 Animals and Tumor

Inbred Balb/c and hybrid DBA/2 x Balb/c male mice,8-10 weeks old,obtained from Charles River,Calco,Italy were used and hereafter called Balb and CDF1 respectively. MS-2 fibrosarcoma,originally induced by the Moloney murine sarcoma virus was maintained in the laboratory by weekly i.m. passage of tumor cell homogenate into the right hind leg of Balb mice.[16]

For the experiments,tumor from mice were removed under sterile conditions. The cell suspension was obtained by Potter homogenization,counted under optical light microscopy and injected intradermally (i.d. 10^6 cells/mouse). Treatment started when the tumor mass measured approximately 1 cm in diameter. The animals were injected i.v. with the drug and irradiated with the laser 24 hrs later. A single light irradiation was done in all experiments.

3.2 Chemicals

Aluminum phthalocyanine with an average degree of sulphonation of 2.1 (hereafter called AlS_2Pc), was kindly provided by Dr. A. McLennan (Paisley College of Technology, Paisley,U.K.). It was dissolved in physiological solution at a concentration of 5 mg/cc.

3.3 Laser source

Irradiation was applied with a continuous wave dye (DCM) laser (Coherent Mod. CR-599,Palo Alto,CA) pumped by an Argon laser (Coherent Mod. Cr-18,Palo Alto, CA) and tuned at 670 nm. The laser output was coupled to a 400 μm plastic-glass optical fiber (Quartz at Silice PCS600,Paris,France). The laser power was monitored at the fiber output.

3.4 Mitogen Stimulation

Spleen cells were checked for viability by trypan blue dye exclusion and counted in a Burker chamber under a light microscope. Cells were then suspended in RPMI 1640 medium supplemented as reported previously,[17] seeded ($5x10^4$cells/200μl) in microplate wells with Phytohemagglutinin or Lipopolysaccharide (Sigma) and incubated 48 hr at 37° in a moist atmosphere of 95% air and 5% CO2. 20 μl containing 0.8 μl of (3H)thymidine (26 Ci/mmol.)were added 18 hr before cultures were harvested onto glass fiber filters with a multiple cell harvester. Experimental results were expressed in cpm $\pm$ S.E. and as

$$\text{Stimulation index} = \frac{\text{cpm in experimental wells}}{\text{cpm in control wells}}$$

3.4 Tumoricidal assay of activated macrophages

Peritoneal cells from CDF1 mice treated with photoactivated AlS_2Pc and untreated were harvested on the 4 th day. The cells were plated on coverglasses in wells and incubated for 1 hour. The non adherent cells were removed and the adherent cells,the macrophages, after intensive washing, were cocultered for 2 hours with target tumor cells. After this incubation the mixtures,macrophages − tumor cells, were injected intradermally,at different concentrations, in syngeneic mice.

3.5 Winn Assay

The in vivo antitumor activiyt of T cells was determined by the Winn tumor neutralization assay.[18] Effector lymphocytes,collected from mice untreated or treated with PDT, were mixed with MS-2 tumor cells in 0.1 ml PBS and then inoculated intradermally in syngeneic mice.

4. RESULTS AND DISCUSSION

Spleens from CDF1 mice bearing MS-2 fibrosarcoma and treated with PDT were weighed and the cell content was counted as were also the femoral bone marrow. Schedules and doses of AlS_2Pc and laser treatment and experimental results are shown in Table 1.

Table 1
PDT induce splenomegaly and hypercellularity in mice bearing MS-2 tumor

Days of treatment		[a]Bone marrow cells x 10^6/femur Mean $\pm$ S.E.	Cells x 10^6/spleen Mean $\pm$ S.E.	[b]Rel.spleen wt (g)
AlS$_2$Pc	Laser			
-	-	3.4 $\pm$ 0.4	95 $\pm$ 7	0.4
-	- 1	4.5 $\pm$ 0.6	111 $\pm$ 9	0.54
- 2	- 1	[c]8.9 $\pm$ 1.4	[c]224 $\pm$ 15	[c]1.02

CDF1 mice challenged i.d. with 10^6 MS-2 fibrosarcoma
AlS$_2$Pc = 5mg/kg i.v.

Laser = 100mW/cm^2 x 10' of exposure
a = Data from 8 mice/group killed at day 0
b = Relative spleen weight = $\dfrac{\text{Mean spleen weight}}{\text{Mean mouse weight}}$ x 100
c = P $\leq$ 0.05 by Student t-test versus untreated mice or treated
   only with laser light

The drug amount and the light dose were the same utilized in other Photodynamic therapy (PDT) experiments carried out in our laboratory (15). Splenomegaly was observed macroscopically in the group of animals treated with AlS$_2$Pc and laser light in respect to untreated control tumor bearing animals. The treatment of the animals only with laser light did not show any appreciable modification of the spleen dimension. Spleen enlargement was correlated with statistically significant increase of number of spleen cells and relative spleen weights. Moreover it was observed in the group treated with AlS$_2$Pc and laser light a significant cellular hyperplasia of femoral bone marrow in respect to untreated animals or animals treated only with laser light.
Functional activity of the T and B lymphocytes from tumor bearing mice previously treated with AlS2Pc at the same doses and schedules mentioned above are reported in Table 2 and 3.

Table 2
Effect of PDT with photoactivated AlS$_2$Pc on PHA stimulated lymphocytes from mice bearing MS-2 tumor

Days of treatment AlS$_2$Pc	Laser	PHA µg/ml	[a]CPM ± S.E.	[b]S.I.
-	-	-	10342 ± 1144	1
		2	73408 ± 6431	7.1
		1	55846 ± 5432	5.4
-	- 1	-	15432 ± 1404	1
		2	123456 ± 10432	8
		1	98765 ± 7346	6.4
- 2	- 1	-	12446 ± 1382	1
		2	[c]186690 ± 16432	[c]15
		1	[c]168021 ± 14324	[c]13.5

CDF1 mice challenged i.d. with 10^6 MS-2 fibrosarcoma
AlS$_2$Pc = 5mg/kg i.v.

Laser = 100mW/cm^2 x 10' of exposure
a   = Data from 8 mice/group killed at day 0
b   = Stimulation Index
c   = P< 0.05 by Dunnet test for multiple comparison on CPM ± S.E.

Table 2 shows the susceptibility to mitogenic stimulation of spleen cells from tumor bearing mice after PDT with photoactivated AlS$_2$Pc compared with the blastogenic response of splenocytes from tumor bearing mice untreated or treated only with laser light. The reactivity to T-lymphocyte mitogen Phytohemagglutinin (PHA),as evaluated by (3H)thymidine incorporation into the nucleus,was significantly increased with a very high stimulation index in respect to the animals untreated. The other group of mice treated only with laser light did not show a significant difference in respect to the control. A similar pattern of responsiveness was shown by spleen cells after stimulation with the B-lymphocyte mitogen Lypopolysaccharide (LPS) (Table 3).

Table 3
Effect of PDT with photoactivated AlS$_2$Pc on LPS stimulated lymphocytes from mice bearing MS-2 tumor

Days of treatment AlS$_2$Pc	Laser	LPS µg/ml	[a]CPM ± S.E.	[b]S.I.
-	-	-	9432 ± 844	1
		10	16977 ± 1232	1.8
		5	19807 ± 1544	2.1
-	- 1	-	11344 ± 1042	1
		10	23822 ± 2056	2.1
		5	21553 ± 2122	1.9
- 2	- 1	-	10322 ± 1056	1
		10	[c]44384 ± 4322	[c]4.3
		5	[c]49545 ± 4564	[c]4.8

CDF1 mice challenged i.d. with 10^6 MS-2 fibrosarcoma
AlS$_2$Pc = 5mg/kg i.v.

Laser = 100mW/cm^2 x 10' of exposure
a = Data from 8 mice/group killed at day 0
b = Stimulation Index
c = P< 0.05 by Dunnet test for multiple comparison on CPM ± S.E.

The value of stimulation index of cells from tumor bearing mice after PDT was significantly higher in respect to control animals untreated or treated only with laser.

Since lymphocytes and macrophages are implicated in the control of tumor development and spread and the results btained show a remarkable increase in lymphocytes blastogenic response after PDT we decide to carry out experiments to study the influence of PDT on antitumor immune response.
Macrophages collected from mice pretreated with AlS$_2$Pc and laser light were cytotoxic against MS-2 tumor cells (table

4). In fact the mixture of PDT activated macrophages and tumor cells (10^4) are unable to grow in 2/3 syngeneic mice while the mixture of normal macrophages and tumor cells are able to kill all the animals like the controls. For 10^5 tumor cells we observed a remarkable increase of survival time.

Table 4
IN VIVO CYTOTOXICITY OF ACTIVATED MACROPHAGES

Groups	MS-2 cells/mouse		MA cells/mouse	MST	D/T
1	10^4	+	0	59	3/3
2	10^4	+	10^7	-	1/3
3	10^5	+	0	49	3/3
4	10^5	+	10^7	80	3/3

MS-2 cells mixed with activated macrophages (MA) collected from mice bearing MS-2, pretreated with PDT, and injected i.d. in CDF1.

Following this experiment we wanted to demonstrate that the lymphocytes of tumor bearing mice treated with PDT with photoactivated AlS_2Pc are immune against the parental line. In a Winn Assay experiment we observed that only spleen lymphocytes from PDT preated animals were cytotoxic against the parental tumor cells while normal lymphocytes collected from virgin mice were not cytotoxic and all the animals injected died with tumor (table 5).

Table 5
IMMUNE LYMPHOCYTES CYTOTOXICITY IN VIVO (WINN ASSAY)

IL	N° of mice with tumors
N	5/5
I_{PDT}	0/5

Immune lymphocytes (20×10^5) mixed with MS-2 cells (10^5) were inoculated i.d. on day 0
N = normal spleen lymphocytes collected from virgin mice
I_{PDT} = spleen lymphocytes collected from MS-2 bearing mice pre treated with PDT

The aim of PDT is to obtain selective destruction of cancer cells. PDT has been use on many patients with encouraging results. Cure requires total elimination of the cancer cells in the targeted tissues as well as in metastasized cancer cells. It would be advantageous if the metastasized cancer cells could be eliminated immunologically rather than through chemotherapy or photodynamic therapy. Our results suggest that PDT with photoactivated AlS_2Pc could modulate the blastogenic response of murine lymphocytes and could induce a potential "Tumor immunity" versus a poor immunogenic murine tumor.

In conclusion the results obtained in the present study could be interesting for the clinical point of view, because oncological patients treated with PDT could become "immune" versus a relapse or versus the minimal residual disease. Additional studies on other murine tumors are required to confirm these results and to identify which lymphocytes subpopulations are involved in this enhancement of the antitumor host immune response.

5. ACKNOWLEDGEMENT

Research supported in part by National Research Coucil (C.N.R.) under the special projects "Applicazioni cliniche della ricerca oncologica" and "Tecnologie Elettroottiche".

6. REFERENCES

1. Doiron D.R. and Keller G.S. "Porphyrin photodynamic therapy: principles and clinical application." Curr.Probl. Derm. 15, 85-93, 1986.

2. Dougherty T.S. " Photosensitisation of malignant tumors."Sem. Surg. Oncol. 2,24-37,1986.

3. Manyak M.,Smith P.D.,Harrigton S.M.,Russo A. "Protection against dihematoporphyrin ether photosensitivity." Photochem. Photobiol. 47,823-830,1988.

4. Wile A.G.,Novotny J.,Mason V.and Berns W. "Photoradiation therapy of head and neck cancer." Prog. Clin. Biol. Res. 170, 681-691,1984.

5. Moan J.,Petterson E.O.,Christensen T. "The mechanism of photodynamic inactivation of human cells in vitro in the presence of hematoporphyrin." Brit. J. Cancer 39,398-407,1979.

6. Yamamoto N.,Homma S.,Sery T.W. and Hoober J.K. "Photodynamic immunopotentiation:in vitro activation of macrophages by treatment of mouse peritoneal cells with Hpd and light." Eur. J. Cancer 27,467-471,1991.

7. Canti G.,Marelli O.,Ricci L.and Nicolin A. " Hematoporphyrin treated murine lymphocytes:in vitro inhibition of DNA synthesis and light-mediated inactivation of cells responsible for GVHR." Photochem. Photobiol. 34,589-594,1981.

8. Franco P.,Nicolin A.,Ricci L.,Trave F. and Canti G. " In vitro hematoporphyrin(Hpd) inhibitory effects on some immunological assays." Int. J. Immunopharmc. 5,533-540,1983.

9. Canti G.,Franco P.,Marelli O.,Ricci L. and Nicolin A. " Hematoporphyrin derivative rescue from toxicity caused by chemotherapy or radiation in a murine leukemia model (L1210)." Cancer Res.44,1551-1556,1984.

10. Gruner S.H.,Meffert H.D.,Volk R. and Jahn S. " The influence of hematoporphyrin derivative and visible light on murine skin graft survival,epidermal Langerhans cells and stimulation of the allogeneic mixed leukocyte reaction." Scand. J. Immunol.21,267-263,1985.

11. Elmetz C.A. and Bowen K.D. " Immunological suppression in mice treated with hematoporphiryn derivative photoradiation." Cancer Res.46,1606-1611,1986.

12. Gomer C.J.,Ferrario A. and Murphree A. " Metastatic potential and natural killer cell activity in mice following porphyrin photodynamic therapy." Photochem. Photobiol.43,635-642,1986.

13. Chan W.S.,Marshall J.F.Grace Y.L. and Hart I.R. " Tissue uptake,distribution and potency of the photoactivated dye chloroaluminum sulfonated phthalocyanine in mice bearing transplantable tumors." Cancer Res.48,3040-3044,1988.

14. Weitraub H.,Abramov A.,Altman A.,Ben Hur E. and Rosenthal I. " Toxicity,tissue distribution and excretion studies for aluminum phthalocyanine tetrasulfonated in normal mice." Laser in Life Science 2,185-195,1988.

15. Canti G.,Franco P.,Marelli O.,Cubeddu R.,Taroni P. and Ramponi R. " Comparative studies of the therapeutic effect of photoactivated hematoporphyrin derivative and Aluminum disulfonated phthalocyanine on tumor bearing mice." Cancer letters 53,123-127,1990.

16. Giuliani F.,Casazza A.M. and Di Marco A. " Virology and immunology properties and response to daunomycin and adryamicin of a non regressing mouse tumor derived from MSV-induced sarcoma." Biomedicine 21,435-440,1974.

17. Furham-Conti A.M.,Marelli O. and Nicolin A. " Immunological and cytogenetic characterization of lymphocytic mouse leukemias after treatment with antineoplastic drugs." Pharmacol. Res.Comunic.10, 867-883,1978.

18. Winn H.J. "Immune mechanism in homotransplantation. II. Quantitative assay of the immunologic activity of lymphoid cells stimulated by tumor homografts." J. Immunol. 146,228-239,1961.

Photodynamic Therapy Affects the Expression of IL-6 and IL-10 *In Vivo*[1]

Sandra O. Gollnick[a], David A. Musser[b] and Barbara W. Henderson[c]

[a]Dept. of Molecular Immunology, [b]Dept of Dermatology and [c]Dept. of Radiation Biology, Roswell Park Cancer Institute, Buffalo, NY 14263

ABSTRACT

Photodynamic therapy (PDT), which can effectively destroy malignant tissue, also induces a complex immune response which potentiates anti-tumor immunity, but also inhibits skin contact hypersensitivity (CHS) and prolongs skin graft survival. The underlying mechanisms responsible for these effects are poorly understood, but are likely to involve mediation by cytokines. We demonstrate in a BALB/c mouse model that PDT delivered to normal and tumor tissue *in vivo* causes marked changes in the expression of cytokines interleukin (IL)-6 and IL-10. IL-6 mRNA and protein are rapidly and strongly enhanced in the PDT treated EMT6 tumor. Previous studies have shown that intratumoral injection of IL-6 or transduction of the IL-6 gene into tumor cells can enhance tumor immunogenicity and inhibit tumor growth in experimental murine tumor systems. Thus, PDT may enhance local anti-tumor immunity by up-regulating IL-6. PDT also results in an increase in IL-10 mRNA and protein in the skin. the same PDT regime which enhances IL-10 production in the skin has been shown to strongly inhibit the CHS response. The kinetics of IL-10 expression coincide with the known kinetics of PDT induced CHS suppression and we propose that the enhanced IL-10 expression plays a role in the observed suppression of cell mediated responses seen following PDT.

Keywords: IL-6, IL-10, PCR, CHS, EMT6

INTRODUCTION

It is widely recognized that the tumor response to PDT involves a complex interplay between primary photodamage to the tumor and tumor microvasculature, and effects mediated by PDT induced inflammatory and immune responses[1,2]. The effects of PDT on the host immune system are complex and multistaged, and the mechanisms underlying these effects, recently reviewed by Korbelik[2], are poorly understood.

Cytokines are pluripotent mediators of the immune response and their expression patterns have been correlated with the type and extent of a given immune response[3]. Cytokines have been classified as either being T_H1 or T_H2 type cytokines. T_H1 cytokines have been shown to promote cell-mediated immunity and include interferon-γ (IFN-γ), IL-2 and IL-12. T_H2 cytokines are known primarily for their ability to enhance the humoral response and include IL-4, IL-5, IL-6 and IL-10.

Very few studies have examined the possible involvement of cytokines in the PDT response. The generation of tumor necrosis factor (TNF)-α and IL-6 from macrophages and/or tumor cells treated *in vitro* has been reported[4,5]. In patients PDT-treated for bladder cancer, high urinary levels of IL-1β, IL-2 and TNF-α have been observed[6]. The significance of these observations for the PDT response is unclear. A recent report[7] shows the up-regulation of TNF-α in keratinocytes treated with phthalocyanine PDT, and also implicates this cytokine in the cutaneous photosensitivity caused by this treatment.

---

[1] This work was supported by NIH Grant CA55791b (to B.W.H.). S.O.G. was supported by NIH Grant HD17013 and a grant from the Elisabeth and Peter Tower foundation. D.A.M. was supported by NIH Grant CA 55791c.

IL-6 (reviewed in[8]), which can be produced by a large variety of cell types, including macrophages, lymphocytes, tumor cells, fibroblasts and endothelial cells, is best known as an inflammatory cytokine causing the release of acute phase proteins by hepatocytes. IL-6 has also been shown to play an important role as a growth factor in late stage B cell differentiation. The effect of IL-6 on B cells and its ability to increase proliferation and differentiation of T cells resulted in it being classified as a T_H2 cytokine.

IL-10, which can be produced by a variety of cell types including T and B cells, monocytes/macrophages, mast cells and keratinocytes, is known to have different effects on the activation and cytokine production of different cell types[9]. IL-10 acts as a stimulator of B cell proliferation and differentiation, increasing major histocompatibility complex (MHC) class II antigen expression. In contrast IL-10 down-regulates MHC class II and costimulatory molecule expression on monocytes and dendritic cells[3,10,11]. Such down-regulation has been observed by Obochi et al.[12] after low dose PDT of skin allografts where surface antigen expression of MHC class II on Langerhans cells (LC) was found to be markedly decreased. IL-10 also inhibits antigen presenting cells (APCs) from stimulating T_H1 cells to produce IFN-γ and IL-2[3,13] and IL-10 pretreatment of LC was found to inhibit the induction of antigen-specific T cell proliferation in T_H1 clones. IL-10 has been shown to inhibit IL-6, IL-8, IL-12 and TNF-α generation in LPS stimulated monocytes[11,14].

The dichotomous effects of IL-6 and IL-10 during the tumor immune response are similar to the effect PDT has on the host immune system. Therefore we have pursued the investigation of the effect of PDT on these cytokines and have explored the molecular mechanisms and functional consequences of PDT altered IL-6 and IL-10 expression.

RESULTS

Localized PDT Induces IL-6 and IL-10 mRNA.

In order to determine the effect of localized PDT on cytokine expression *in vivo* we have examined the effect of PDT on cytokine expression within the EMT6 tumor bed. A tumorgenic dose of EMT6 cells were injected subcutaneously in the shoulder of a BALB/c mouse and allowed to grow for 7 days. Tumor bearing mice were treated with Photofrin® (Pf) PDT and tissue was removed for either total RNA isolation or protein extraction at various times following PDT (for these and all subsequent methods please see[15]). The expression of cytokine mRNA levels were examined using reverse transcriptase-polymerase chain reaction (RT-PCR). Figure 1A shows that PDT induces an increase in the levels of IL-6 mRNA between 1 to 6 h post-treatment and that enhancement persisted for 24 h. There was an absence of IL-6 mRNA in the control, untreated tumor and a slight increase in IL-6 mRNA in drug alone controls.

The effect of Pf-PDT on IL-10 expression in the tumor was more variable. Control tumors were shown to express variable levels of IL-10 prior to treatment and following treatment the levels of IL-10 decreased.

Spleen cell populations isolated from Pf-PDT treated animals also exhibited a transient increase in IL-6 mRNA as well as IL-10 mRNA levels (Fig 1B). The kinetics of the induction of IL-6 are similar to those seen in the tumor bed. IL-6 and IL-10 mRNA was also induced in the spleens of animals after PDT was given to a 1-cm diameter area of skin at the shoulder without the presence of a tumor (data not shown). When a comparable area of skin at the right hind thigh was exposed to PDT, no cytokine induction was observed in the spleen. Therefore it appears as though the cytokine induction seen in the spleen is a result of penetrating light due to the small size of the animal model and that localized PDT does not induce a systemic increase in cytokines.

PDT Induces IL-6 Protein in EMT6 Tumors.

The increase in IL-6 mRNA seen in the tumor bed is accompanied by an increase in IL-6 protein levels (Fig. 2). The control and drug only tumors do not contain detectable levels of IL-6, however a weak signal can be seen in the sample exposed to light treatment only. Strong induction of IL-6 protein was evident by 3 h after PDT and persisted for at least 48 h, but had disappeared by 6 days after PDT.

Large Cutaneous Surface Area PDT Induces IL-10 mRNA and Protein in the Skin

PDT treatment of a large surface area of skin results in the induction of both IL-10 mRNA (Fig. 3A) and protein (Fig. 3B). IL-10 mRNA in control skin samples was absent but was strongly induced at 72 and 96 h after light exposure. IL-10 protein was detectable at 72 h and progressively increased up to at least 120 h after treatment. subsequent studies demonstrated that the levels of protein had returned to baseline by 6 days post-treatment. Induction of IL-10 protein was also evident in the serum of animals which had undergone large cutaneous surface area PDT treatment (data not shown) implying that this type of treatment results in a systemic increase in IL-10 expression. The kinetics of IL-10 induction in the skin mirrors the suppression of CHS seen following PDT (data not shown).

DISCUSSION

We have demonstrated that localized Pf-PDT induces the expression IL-6 in the EMT6 tumor bed *in vivo*. This induction appears to be non-systemic as PDT treatment on the hind leg in the absence of tumor does not lead to the induction of cytokines in the spleen.

The induction of IL-6 mRNA by PDT has been attributed to the induction by PDT of the early-response genes *c-fos* and *c-jun*[5,16,17]. IL-6 transcription appears to be regulated via the AP-1 regulatory element, whose transcription factor is a heterodimer of c-fos and c-jun. IL-10 has been shown to inhibit IL-6, IL-8, IL-12 and TNF-α generation in LPS stimulated[11,14]. IL-10 suppression of IL-6 involved inhibition of AP-1 binding activity[18]. In PDT treated tumors *in vivo* we find that IL-6 and IL-10 expression changes are inversely related which suggests possible effects by IL-10 on the transcriptional regulation of IL-6.

The source of IL-6 in the tumor bed is not yet identified although we have demonstrated that EMT6 tumor cells express IL-6 mRNA in vitro, and that PDT increases the expression of IL-6 mRNA following treatment[15]. Therefore it is likely that the origin of the IL-6 in the tumor bed is due at least in part to the tumor cells themselves. Previous studies of others[19] and ourselves[15] have shown that PDT results in a rapid infiltration of inflammatory cells (macrophages, neutraphils and granulocytes) into the tumor bed. These cells could also be a source of IL-6.

The role of IL-6 in the PDT treated tumor has yet to be defined. IL-6 has been shown to induce anti-tumor immune responses. The systemic administration of rIL-6 to mice results in the regression of pulmonary metastasis from weakly immunogenic tumors. This effect is apparently mediated by IL-6 induced generation of tumor-specific cytolytic T cells (CTLs)[20,21]. Similar results were obtained with IL-6 secreting tumors after transduction of the tumor cells with the IL-6 gene, with some indication that macrophage activation may also occur[22-24]. Intra-tumoral administration of IL-6 also leads to tumor regression, accompanied by the accumulation of large numbers of tumor associated macrophages (TAMs), implying that IL-6 plays a role in the recruitment, proliferation and/or survival of TAMs[25]. The increase in IL-6 in tumors following PDT may therefore have important implications for the PDT response.

Large cutaneous surface area PDT results in the induction of IL-10 mRNA and protein expression in the skin. This induction appears to be systemic and mirrors the known suppression of CHS induced by PDT. T$_H$1 cells are effective inducers of CHS and as mentioned above IL-10 inhibits the ability of APCs to stimulate the T$_H$1 response. These results suggest that IL-10 plays a role in the suppression of CHS by PDT.

UV irradiation induces the release of IL-10 from keratinocytes which was found to be responsible for the observed immunosuppressive effects of UV exposure, including suppression of tumor rejection, APC function and CHS[10,26]. We have recently shown that PDT treatment of a murine keratinocyte cell line, PAM 212, *in vitro*, results in the induction of IL-10 mRNA.

Relatively little is known about IL-10 transcriptional regulation. Both human[27] and mouse[28] IL-10 promoter regions have been isolated and are remarkably similar. The regulatory regions or both contain multiple sequence motifs that have been associated with the regulation of transcription of cytokine genes, including AP-1 and cAMP responsive (CRE) elements. Preliminary data from our laboratory has demonstrated that the increase in IL-10 mRNA in keratinocytes is due at least in part to an increase in promoter activity.

Our results indicate that the type of immune response induced by PDT treatment depends on the nature of the treatment. Localized PDT results in an increase in IL-6 and a strong inflammatory response which may play a role in tumor eradication by PDT. In contrast large cutaneous surface area PDT results in the induction of immuno-suppression, probably mediated via the induction of IL-10. It may be possible to exploit the induction of an immunosuppressive response by PDT in the treatment of autoimmune diseases.

REFERENCES

1. Henderson, B.W. and T.J. Dougherty, "How does photodynamic therapy work?", *Photochem. Photobiol.* **55,** pp. 145-157, 1992.

2. Korbelik, M. "Induction of tumor immunity by photodynamic therapy." , *J. Clin. Laser Med. Surg.,* **14,** pp. 329-334, 1996.

3. Mosmann, T.R. and R.L. Coffman, "T_H1 and T_H2 cells: Different patterns of lymphokine secretion lead to different functional properties.", *Ann. Rev. Immunol.* **7,** pp. 145-173, 1989.

4. Evans, S. Matthews, W. Perry, R. Fraker, D., Norton, J. and H.I. Pass, "Effect of photodynamic therapy on tumor necrosis factor production by murine macrophages.", *J. Natl. Cancer Inst.* **82,** pp 34-39, 1990.

5. Kick, G. Messer, G., Goetz, A., Plewig, G. and P. Kind, "Photodynamic tyerapy induces expression of interleukin 6 by activation of AP-1 but not NF-kB DNA binding." *Cancer Res.* **55,** 2373-2379, 1995.

6. Nseyo, U.O., Whalen, R.K., Duncan, M.R. and B. Berman, "Urinary cytokines following photodynamic therapy for bladder cancer. A preliminary report." *Urology* **36,** pp. 167-171, 1990.

7. Anderson, C., Hrabovsky, S. McKinley, Y. et al., "Phthalocyanine photodynamic therapy: Disparate effects of pharmacologic inhibitors on cutaneous photosensitivity and on tumor regression." *Photochem. Photobiol.* **65,** 895-901, 1997.

8. Kishimoto, T., "The biology of interleukin-6." *Blood,* **74,** pp. 1-10, 1989.

9. Moore, K.W., O'Garra, A., deWaal Malefyt, R., Vieira, P. and T.R. Mosmann, "Interleukin-10." *Ann. Rev. Immunol.,* **11,** pp. 165-109, 1993.

10. Enk, A.H., Angeloni, V.L., Udey, M.C. and S.I. Katz, "Inhibition of Langerhans cell antigen-presenting function by IL-10. A role for IL-10 in induction of tolerance." *J. Immunol.* **151,** pp. 2390-2398, 1993.

11. Strassman, G., Patil-Koota, V., Finkelman, R., Fong, M., and T. Kambayashi, "Evidence for the involvement of interleukin 10 in the differential deactivation of murine peritoneal macrophages by prostaglandin E_2." *J. Exp. Med.* **180** pp. 2365-2370, 1994.

12. Obochi, M.O.K., Ratkay, L.G. and J.G. Levy, "Prolonged murine skin allograft survival after photodynamic therapy (PDT) associated with modification of donor skin antigenicity." *Photochem. Photobiol.* **63S** pp. 64S, 1996.

13. Macatonia, S.E., Doherty, T.M., Knight, S.C. and A. O'Garra. "Differential effect of IL-10 on dendritic cell-induced T cell proliferation and IFN-γ production." *J. Immunol.* **150,** pp. 3755-3765, 1993.

14. Kambayasi, T. Alexander, H.R., Fong, M. and G. Strassman, "Potential involvement of IL-10 in suppressing tumor-associated macrophages. Colon-26-derived prostaglandin E_2 inhibits TNF-α release via a mechanism involving IL-10." *J. Immunol.* **154,** pp. 3383-3390, 1995.

15. Gollnick, S.O., Liu, X., Owczarczak, B., Musser, D.A. and B.W. Henderson, "Altered expression of interleukin 6 and interleukin 10 as a result of photodynamic therapy *in vivo*." *Cancer Res.* **57,** 3904-3909, 1997.

16. Luna, M.C., Wong, S. and C.J. Gomer, "Photodynamic therapy mediated induction of early response genes." *Cancer Res.* **54,** pp. 1374-1380, 1994.

17. Kick, G. Messer, G., Plewig, G., Kind, P. and A.E. Goetz, "Strong and prolonged inductio of *c-jun* and *c-fos* protoncogenes by photodynamic therapy." *Br. J. Cancer* **74,** pp. 30-36, 1996.

18. Dokter, W.H.A., Koopmans, S.B. and Vellenga, E., "Effects of IL-10 and IL-4 on LPS-induced transcription factors (AP-1, NF-IL6 and NF-kB) which are involved in IL-6 regulation." *Leukemia* **10,** pp. 1308-1316, 1996.

19. Krosl, G., Korvelik, M. and G.J. Doughterty, "Induction of immune cell infiltration into murine SCCVII tumour by Photofrim-based photodynamic therapy." *Br. J. Cancer* **71,** pp. 2549-2555, 1995.

20. Mule, J.J., Custer, M.C., Travis, W.D. and S.A. Rosenberg, "Cellular mechanisms of the antitumor activity of recombinant IL-6 on tumor growth *in vivo*." *Cancer Immunol. Immunother.* **38,** pp. 339-345, 1992.

21. Okada, M. and T. Kishimoto. "The potential application and limitation of cytokine/growth factor manipulation in cancer therapy." In *Cell Poliferation in Cancer, Regulatory Mechanisms of Neoplastic Cell Growth.* Osford, UK, Oxford University Press, pp. 218-244, 1996.

22. Porgador, A. Tzehoval, E., Katz, A., et al., "Interleukin 6 gene transfectioninto Lewis lung carcinoma tumor cells suppressed the malignant phenotypeand confers immunotherapeutic competence against parental metastatic cells." *Cancer Res.* **52,** pp. 3679-3686, 1992.

23. Mullern, C.A., Coale, M.M., Levy, A.T. et al., " Fibrosarcoma cells transduced with the IL-6 gene exhibit reduced tumorigenicity, increase immunogenicity, and decreased metastatic potential." *Cancer Res.* **52,** 6020-6024, 1992.

24. Tanaka, R. Abe, M., Akiyoshi, T., et al., "The anti-human tumor effect and generation of human cytotoxic T cells in SCID mice given human peripheral blood lymphocytes by the *in vivo* transfer of the interleukin-6 gene using adenovirus vector." *Cancer Res.* **57,** pp. 1335-1343, 1997.

25. Doughtery, G.J., Thacker, J.D., Lavey, R.S., Belldegrun, A. and W.H. McBride, "Inhibitory effect of locally produced and exogenous interleukin-6 on tumor growth *in vivo*." *Cancer Immuno. Immunother.* **38,** pp. 339-345, 1994.

26. Ullrich, S.E. "Mechanism involved in the systemic suppression of antigen-presenting cell function by UV irradiation. Keratinocyte-derived IL-10 modulates antigen presenting cell function of splenic adherent cells." *J. Immunol.* **152,** pp. 3410-3416, 1994.

27. Kube, D. Platzer, C., vonKnetten, A., et al., "Isolation of the human interleukin 10 promoter. Characterization of the promoter activity in Burkitt's lymphoma cell lines." *Cytokine* **7,** pp. 1-7, 1995.

28. Kim, J.M., Brannan, C.I., Copeland, N.G., Jenkins, N.A., Khan, T.A. and K.W. Moore, "Structure of the mouse IL-10 gene and chromosomal localzation of the mouse and human genes." *J. Immunol.* **148,** pp. 3618-3623, 1992.

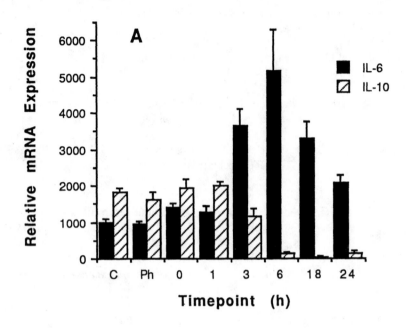

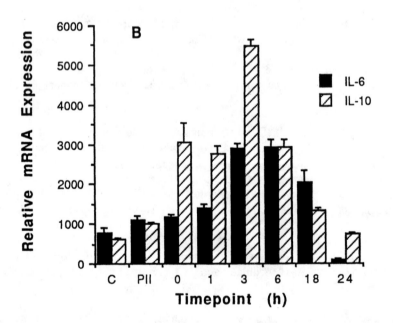

Figure 1. Modulation of IL-6 and IL-10 mRNA expression by PDT. EMT6 tumors were treated *in vivo* at 630 nm with 100J/cm^2 after animals were exposed to 5 mg/kg Pf for 24 h. Total RNA was isolated from the tumor bed (A) or spleen (B) at 0, 1, 3 6 and 24 h after treatment and used in RT-PCR. Graphs represent the average desitometry results of 3 independent experiments. Samples were normalized to the actin. *bars*, SE.

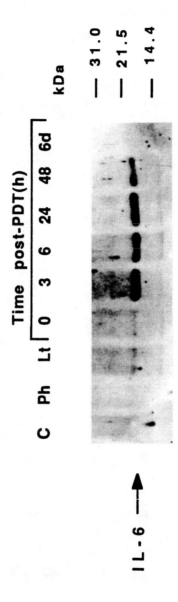

Figure 2. Western analysis of IL-6 in EMT6 tumor by PDT as a function of time after treatment. Tumors were exposed to 5mg/kg Pf and 34 J/cm^2 and excised at 0, 3, 6, 24, 48 h, and 6 days after treatment. Cell suspensions were prepared by enzymatic digestion, and whole-cell lysates were subjected to Western blotting; 2.5μg protein per sample were resolved on 12.5% SDS-PAGE, transferred to a nitrocellulose membrane and probed with a biotinylated anti-mouse IL-6 antibody. Controls included untreated samples (C), samples exposed to Pf alone (Ph), and light alone (Lt; harvested 24 h after exposure).

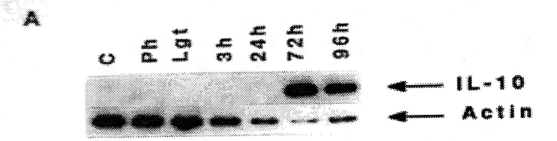

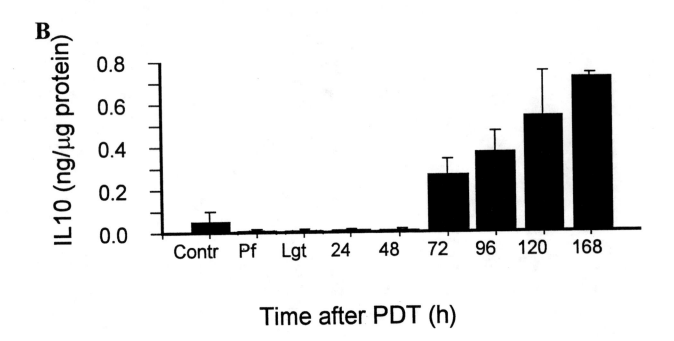

Figure 3. RT-PCR (A) and ELISA (B) analysis of IL-10 in murine skin exposed to PDT (10mg/kg Pf, 6 h later 1.3 J/cm^2 of blue light). In A, 2 μg of total RNA from each sample were subjected to RT-PCR analysis. In B, 10 μg of total protein from each sample or appropriate standards (rIL-10) were analyzed by ELISA. Untreated control samples, samples exposed to Pf only (Ph), and samples exposed to light only (harvested at 72 h after light) were analyzed in parallel. Data are the mean of two independent experiments, each with duplicate wells; *bars*, SE.

Anti-tumor immune responses induced by photodynamic immunotherapy in rats

Wei R. Chen

Oklahoma School of Science and Mathematics, 1141 North Lincoln Boulevard, Oklahoma City, Oklahoma 73104 &
Department of Physics and Astronomy, University of Oklahoma, Norman, Oklahoma 73109

Karen E. Robinson

Oklahoma School of Science and Mathematics, 1141 North Lincoln Boulevard, Oklahoma City, Oklahoma 73104

Robert L. Adams

Dean A. McGee Eye Institute & Dept. of Ophthalmology, Univ. of Oklahoma, 608 Stanton L. Young, Oklahoma City, OK 73104

Anil K. Singhal

Pacific Pharmaceuticals, Inc., 6730 Mesa Ridge Road, Suite A, San Diego, CA 92121

and

Robert E. Nordquist

Wound Healing of Oklahoma, Inc., 3939 N. Walnut Street, Oklahoma City, OK 73105

ABSTRACT

A new laser immunotherapy was used to treat metastatic mammary rat tumors. This new modality consists of three components: a near-infrared diode laser, a photosensitizer, and an immunoadjuvant. The sensitizer-adjuvant solution was injected directly to the tumor, followed by a non-invasive laser application. The new method resulted in total eradication of the treated primary tumors and eradication of untreated metastases at remote sites. Observed was the long-term survival of treated tumor-bearing rats: up to 120 days after tumor inoculation, a 300% increase in survival length compared with untreated control tumor-bearing rats. In addition, the successfully treated rats were refractory to tumor rechallenge with 10 times of the original tumor dose. Fluorescein and peroxidase immunochemical assays were also performed using sera from cured rats as the primary antibody. Strong antibody binding to both live and preserved tumor cells was observed. Western blot analysis, using the cured rat serum as primary antibody also showed distinctive protein binding, suggesting the induction of tumor-specific humoral immune response. These results indicated that an immune response was induced by the treatment of laser, photosensitizer and immunoadjuvant.

Keywords: Laser immunotherapy; Indocyanine green; Immunoadjuvant; Immunochemical assays; Western blotting; Humoral immune response; *In situ* administration; 805 nm diode laser; Cancer treatment

1. INTRODUCTION

Laser immunotherapy was proposed to treat metastatic tumors using an induced tumor-specific immune response. [1-2] It uses a co-injection of a photosensitizer and an immunoadjuvant directly into the tumor, followed by a non-invasive irradiation of a near-infrared laser light. Comparing with the widely used photodynamic therapy (PDT) [3-10], this new laser immunotherapy has several advantages. The laser used in this novel treatment modality emits an 805 nm light, therefore it limits unnecessary damage to normal tissue surrounding the tumor, even at high laser power and long exposure. [11-15] Since at this wavelength, the laser energy can penetrate deeply into tissue with little absorption, it is potentially capable of reaching deep tumors. The direct injection of the photosensitizer, indocyanine green (ICG), can achieve high concentration in tumor and can confine the laser-tissue interaction in and around the tumor. The introduction of an immunoadjuvant adds a new dimension to the treatment -- the stimulation of host immune system. Together with the well-targeted photothermal tumor cell destruction by the 805 nm laser energy and the *in situ* ICG, the immunoadjuvant glycated chitosan functions as a catalyst to induce an immune reaction.

Previous studies using this new method in treatment of DMBA-4 tumor in female rats showed very promising results, including eradication of both treated primary tumors and untreated metastases at remote sites, as well as long-term tumor immunity. [1-2] In this paper, we report further results of its efficacy, and of the immunological search for the induced tumor-specific antibody using fluorescein and peroxidase immunochemical assays as well as using western blot analysis.

2. MATERIALS AND METHODS

2.1 Laser immunotherapy treatment of DMBA-4 metastatic mammary tumor

The animal model used in our experiments was the metastatic rat mammary tumor (DMBA-4) in Wistar Furth female rats. Approximately 100,000 live cancer cells were injected subcutaneously into the inguinal fat pads. Seven to ten days after the tumor implant, the tumors became palpable. When the tumor reached a size of 0.2 to 0.5 cm^3, the tumor was injected with 200 μl ICG/adjuvant solution (0.25% ICG and 1% adjuvant). Totally 1200 J of the 805 nm laser energy (2 watts and 10 minutes) was directly to the tumor by an optical fiber. See Refs. 1 and 2 for detailed animal preparation, immunoadjuvant preparation and laser treatment.

2.2 Tumor rechallenge

The successfully treated tumor-bearing rats, defined as tumor free 120 days after tumor implantation, were rechallenged with 10^6 viable tumor cells, 10 times the original tumor dose. To compare the tumor growth, control rats of the same age were also injected with the same amount of tumor cells. All the rats were observed either until death of the rats in the control group, or until 60 days (tumor free) after tumor rechallenge.

2.3 Fluorescein immunoassay

Serum from the cured rats was collected one month after tumor rechallenge. Then the serum was diluted 1:1000 in phosphate buffered saline as the primary antibody. Freshly collected tumor tissue was dispersed to a single cell suspension in solution. The live cells were incubated with the diluted serum for one hour at 4^0C, then rinsed three times in phosphate buffered saline followed each time by low speed centrifugation at 4^0C. The cells were then incubated in a secondary fluorescein labeled goat anti-rat antiserum for one hour, then rinsed in phosphate buffered saline three times at 4^0C. The cells were then mounted in aqueous mounting medium and viewed immediately with a fluorescence microscope. For comparison, the serum from an untreated tumor-bearing rat was used as the primary antibody in the same assay.

2.4 Peroxidase immunoassay

Tumor tissue was collected from a live untreated tumor-bearing rat and then fixed in 2% paraformaldehyde, followed by dehydrated and embedded in paraffin. Sections were cut and mounted on glass slides then rehydrated. The sections were incubated for one hour with the same primary antibody as in the fluorescein immunoassay. Then, the sections were rinsed three times in phosphate buffered saline. After the final wash, the sections were labeled with peroxidase with the Vector ABC kit and viewed with an optical microscope. For comparison, the serum from an untreated tumor-bearing rat was also used as the primary antibody in the same assay.

2.5 Western blot analysis

Viable tumor tissue was collected from an untreated tumor-bearing rat, and then the tissue was homogenized to a single cell suspension. The tumor cells were solubilized with sodium dodecyl sulfate (SDS) and reducing agent dithiothreitol (DTT). The protein samples were run on a 10% SDS-polyacylamide gel. The proteins on the gels were then electrophoretically transferred to a nitrocellulose membrane. The antigens on the membrane were incubated over night with the serum (1:100) from a tumor-bearing rat successfully treated by laser immunotherapy, one month after tumor rechallenge. The specimens were then incubated for one hour with a 1:5000 solution of Anti-rat Ig, horseradish peroxidase linked whole antibody (Amersham) as the secondary antibody. Finally, Enhanced Chemiluminescence (ECL) (Amersham) was used, followed by x-ray exposure, to visualize the bands on the membrane.

For comparison, sera from a healthy rat and an untreated tumor-bearing control rat were also collected and the same western blotting procedure was performed, using these two different serum solutions as the primary antibody.

3. RESULTS

3.1 Long-term survival of laser immunotherapy treated rats

All the tumors in the treated rats continued to grow, only at a slower rate immediately after the laser immunotherapy. Three to four weeks after treatment, the rats that did not respond would die with multiple tumors. Some treated rats could survive over 45 days after tumor implantation, a 50% increase in survival time comparing with the control rats. A group of treated tumor-bearing rats showed a complete response to the treatment; their metastases would disappear three to five weeks after treatment and their primary tumor would be totally eradicated in six to nine weeks. A recent experiment resulted in a 38% long term survival -- 120 days after tumor implant, a 300% increase in survival time. The results are shown in Table I.

TABLE I

The survival of tumor-bearing rats after laser immunotherapy treatment

Group / Responses	Control Tumor-Bearing Rats N=20	Laser-ICG-GCG Treated Rats N=16
Extended Survival (>45 days)	0%	50%
Cured (>120 days)	0%	38%

3.2 Systemic long-term tumor resistance

Totally 15 cured rats, tumor free 120 days after laser immunotherapy treatment, were rechallenged with 10^6 viable tumor cells. No tumor recurrence was observed in any of the 15 rats up to 60 days after tumor rechallenge. In contrast, all the 18 untreated rats of the same age without previous exposure to tumor died within 40 days of tumor implantation. The results are presented in Table II.

TABLE II

Tumor rechallenge of laser immunotherapy cured tumor-bearing rats

Group	Number of rats	Number of Tumor Cells	Tumor Occurrence	Death rate (in 30 days)	Death rate (in 40 days)	Survival (days)
Cured Rats	15	10^6	0%	0%	0%	>60
Age-Matched Controls	18	10^6	100%	83%	100%	28.2 ± 2.8

3.3 Antibody binding to live and preserved tumor cells

The two histochemical assays showed strong antibody binding to the tumor cells. Figure 1 shows the detection of antibodies that bind to the plasma membrane of isolated live tumor cells. The strong fluorescence in Figure 1A was the

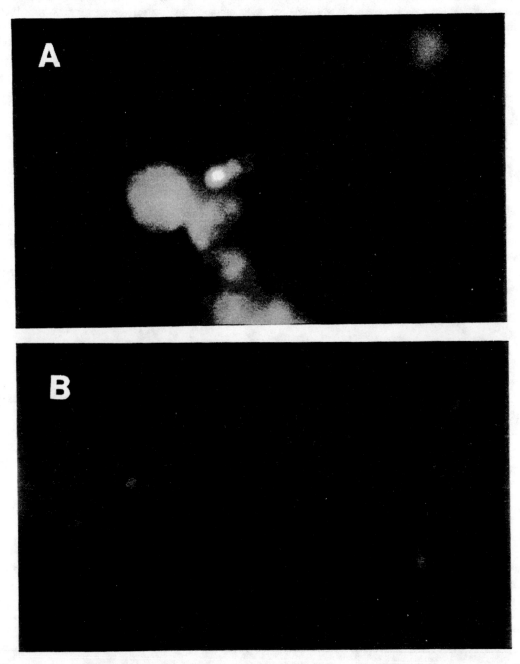

Figure 1.　　　Photomicrographs of living tumor cells (a cluster and a single cell) stained by 1:1000 dilution of serum from a successfully treated tumor-bearing rat one month after tumor rechallenge (A), and by a 1:1000 solution of serum from an untreated tumor-bearing rat (B). There is little, if any, fluorescence in the cell stained by serum from the untreated tumor-bearing rat. In contrast, tumor cells stained with serum from the cured tumor-bearing rat shows high fluorescence and uniform staining over the plasma membrane. Original magnification was 400 x.

result of antibody binding by the serum from a cured rat. In comparison, the serum from an untreated tumor rat resulted in very weak fluorescence as shown in Figure 1B. Figure 2 shows the binding to the plasma membrane and other cellular antigens of preserved tumor cells. Again, the binding, as evidenced by the brown staining around the tumor cells, by the serum from the cured rat was much stronger (Figure 2A) than that by the serum from the untreated tumor-bearing rat (Figure 2B).

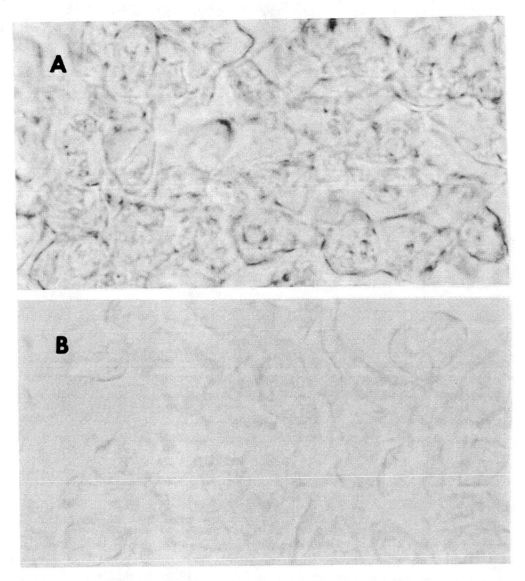

Figure 2.   Photomicrographs of tumor sections incubated with 1:1000 dilution serum from a successfully treated tumor-bearing rat one month after tumor rechallenge (A) and from an untreated tumor-bearing rat (B). Note in (B) the lack of brown reaction product that indicates the peroxidase activity. In contrast, intense staining is shown in (A). Also note the intense staining at the plasma membrane and the lack of staining within the cells. Original magnification was 400 x.

3.4   Antibody binding to tumor protein in the western blotting assay

The western blot results are shown in Figure 3. Serum from a rat successfully treated with the laser immunotherapy stained two heavy bands in 42-56 kD region (Figure 3e) which are absent in the staining by serum from a healthy rat (Figure 3c) and by serum from an untreated tumor-bearing rat (Figure 3d). These two heavy bands may represent specific immunodominant antigens.

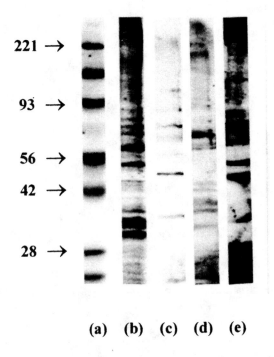

$221 \rightarrow$

$93 \rightarrow$

$56 \rightarrow$

$42 \rightarrow$

$28 \rightarrow$

(a)   (b)   (c)   (d)   (e)

Figure 3. Western blot analysis using sera from different rats as the primary antibodies. (a) Molecular weight markers; (b) Coomassie stained gel of protein from tumor cells of an untreated tumor-bearing rat; (c) Tumor protein stained by antibodies in serum of a healthy rat; (d) Tumor protein recognized by antibodies in serum of an untreated control tumor-bearing rat; and (e) Tumor protein recognized by antibodies in serum of a tumor-bearing rat, cured by the laser immunotherapy and one month after tumor rechallenge. Note that there is very little binding of the antibodies from the healthy rat and the control rat ((c) and (d)). Also note the two heavy bands in (e) between 42 to 56 kD region and the absent of which in (d).

4. DISCUSSION

Immune response has been considered as a possible mechanism in laser-related cancer treatment. [16-20] So far, most work has been concentrated on the cellular immunological reactions. [21-27] The results of laser immunotherapy treatment of the metastatic tumor strongly pointed to an induced immune response, and more importantly a response in the humoral arm. The total tumor eradication and long-term survival of rats that at the time of treatment bore primary tumors and widespread metastases showed the efficacy of this new modality in animal experiments, as shown by the results in Table I, especially considering the aggressive nature of the DMBA-4 cancer which kills almost 100% rats within 35 days on average without this laser immunotherapy treatment. [13] Obviously, the efficacy was not due to the total direct destruction of tumor cells as all the treated tumors would continue to grow and all the treated rats would develop multiple metastases. The crux, as hypothesized earlier, lies in the realm of immunology. Only a systemic reaction can explain the regression and total eradication of the untreated metastases at remote sites. Only the tumor-specific immune response in the host immune system can result in a long-term tumor resistance, as suggested by the results in Table II.

The immunological assays also furnished supporting evidence. The antibodies in the sera from the cured rats, after tumor rechallenge, bound strongly to the same tumor cells, either live or preserved, as evidenced by results in Figures 1 and 2. The western blotting results provided possible molecular evidence that the induced antibodies bound to tumor antigen in

42 to 56 kD region (see Figure 3). The results of animal survival experiments and the immunological assays suggest that the new method has a great potential in treating metastatic tumors.

In conclusion, our current results strongly indicate an induced humoral immune response by the treatment of the laser immunotherapy, although at this stage cellular contributions of the immune system cannot be ruled out. The contribution from combined humoral and cellular immune responses could also be the possible mechanism. Further investigations are currently in progress to test the efficacy of this treatment modality and to search for its mechanism.

5. ACKNOWLEDGMENTS

We thank Scottye Davis for animal preparation. This research was supported in part by grants from Pacific Pharmaceuticals, Inc., and from the Mazie Wilkonson Fund.

6. REFERENCES

1. W. R. Chen, R. L. Adams, R. Carubelli and R. E. Nordquist, "Laser-photosensitizer assisted immunotherapy: a novel modality for cancer treatment," Cancer Letters 115, pp. 25-30, 1997.
2. W. R. Chen, D. A. Okrongly, R. L. Adams and R. E. Nordquist, "Laser-tissue photobiological interaction: a new mechanism for laser-sensitizer-immunoadjuvant treatment of metastatic cancers," SPIE, Vol. 2975, pp. 290-297, 1997.
3. T. J. Dougherty, J. E. Kaufman, A. Goldfarb, K. R. Weishaupt, D. G. Boyle and A. Mlttleman, "Photoradiation therapy for the treatment of malignant tumors," Cancer Research, Vol. 38, pp. 2628-2635, 1978.
4. T. Dougherty, "Photoradiation therapy for cutaneous and subcutaneous malignancies," Journal of Investigative Dermatology, Vol. 77, pp. 122-124, 1981.
5. A. Dahlman, "Laser photoradiation therapy of cancer," Cancer Research, Vol. 43, pp. 430-434, 1983.
6. M. J. Manyak, A. Russo, P. D. Smith, and E. Glatsein, "Photodynamic therapy," Journal of Clinical Oncology, Vol. 6, pp. 380-391, 1988.
7. T. J. Dougherty, "Photodynamic therapy: status and potential," Oncology, Vol. 3, pp. 67-78, 1989.
8. N. A. Buskard, "The use of photodynamic therapy in cancer," Seminars in Oncology, Vol. 21, pp. 1-27, 1994.
9. A. Fisher, L. Murphee, and C. J. Gomer, "Clinical and pre-clinical photodynamic therapy," Lasers in Surgery and Medicine, Vol. 17, pp. 2-31, 1995.
10. J. G. Levy, "Photodynamic therapy," Trends In Biotechnology, Vol. 13, pp. 14-18, 1995.
11. W. R. Chen, R. L. Adams, S. Heaton, D. T. Dickey, K. E. Bartels, and R. E. Nordquist, "Chromophore-enhanced laser-tumor tissue photothermal interaction using an 808-nm diode laser," Cancer Letters, Vol. 88, pp. 15-19, 1995.
12. W. R. Chen, R. L. Adams, K. E. Bartels, and R. E. Nordquist, "Chromophore-enhanced in vivo tumor cell destruction using an 808-nm diode laser," Cancer Letters, Vol. 94, pp. 125-131, 1995.
13. W. R. Chen, R. L. Adams, A. K. Higgins K. E. Bartels, and R. E. Nordquist, "Photothermal effects on murine mammary tumors using indocyanine green and an 808-nm diode laser: an in vivo efficacy study," Cancer Letters, Vol. 98, pp. 169-173, 1995.
14. W. R. Chen, R. L. Adams, C. L. Phillips and R. E. Nordquist, "Indocyanine green in situ administration and photothermal destruction of tumor tissue using an 808 nm diode laser", SPIE Vol. 2681, pp. 94-101 1996
15. W. R. Chen, R. L. Adams, A. K. Higgins and R. E. Nordquist, "Effects of indocyanine green in treatment of murine mammary tumor by an 808 nm diode laser: an in vivo study", SPIE Vol. 2675, pp. 114-121, 1996.
16. G. Canti, O. Marelli, L. Ricci and A. Nicolin, "Hematoporphyrin treated murine lymphocytes: in vitro inhibition of DNA synthesis and light-mediated inactivation of cells responsible for GVHR," Photochemistry and Photobiology, Vol. 34, pp. 589-594, 1981.
17. G. Canti, P. Franco, O. Marelli, L. Ricci and A. Nicolin, "Hematoporphyrin derivative rescue from toxicity caused by chemotherapy or radiation in a murine leukemia model (L1210)," Cancer Research, 44, pp. 1551-1556, 1984.
18. G. J. Dougherty, J. D. Thacker, W. H. McBride, G. Krosl and M. Korbelik, "Effect of immunization with genetically modified tumor cells on recurrence following photodynamic therapy," Lasers Med. Sci. Vol. 7, pp. 226, 1992.
19. G. Canti, D. Lattuada, A. Nicolin, P. Taroni, G. Valentini and R. Cubeddu, "Antitumor immunity induced by photodynamic therapy with aluminum disulfonated phthalocyanines and laser light," Anticancer Drugs, Vol. 5, pp. 443-447, 1994.

20. M. O. Obochi, A. J. Canaan, A. K. Jain, A. M. Richter and J. G. Levy, "Targeting activated lymphocytes with photodynamic therapy: susceptibility of mitogen-stimulated splenic lymphocytes to benzoporphyrin derivative (BPD) photosensitization," Photochemistry and Photobiology, Vol. 62, pp. 169-175, 1995.

21. D. H. Lynch, S. Haddad, K. J. Vernon, M. J. Ott, R. C. Straight and C. J. Jolles, "Systemic immunosuppression induced by photodynamic therapy (PDT) is adoptively transferred by macrophages," Photochemistry and Photobiology, Vol. 49, pp. 453-458, 1989.

22. N. Yamamoto, J. K. Hoober, N. Yamamoto and S. Yamamoto, "Tumoricidal capacities of macrophages photodynamically activated with hematoporphyrin derivative," Photochemistry and Photobiology, Vol. 56, 245-250, 1992.

23. M. Korbelik and G. Krosl, "Enhanced macrophage cytotoxicity against tumor cells treated with photodynamic therapy," Photochemistry and Photobiology, Vol. 60, pp. 497-502, 1994.

24. G. Krosl and M. Korbelik, "Potentiation of photodynamic therapy by immunotherapy: the effect of schizophyllan (SPG)," Cancer Letters, Vol. 84, pp. 43-49, 1994.

25. G. Krosl, M. Korbelik and G. J. Dougherty, "Induction of immune cell infiltration into murine SCCVII tumor by Photofrin based photodynamic therapy," Br. J. Cancer, Vol. 71, pp. 549-555, 1995.

26. M. Korbelik, G. Krosl, V. R. Naraparayu and N. Yamamoto, "The effect of enzymatically generated macrophage activating factor (GCMAF) on the tumor response to photodynamic therapy," Photochemistry and Photobiology, Vol. 61, pp. 97S, 1995.

27. G. Krosl, M. Korbelik, J. Krosl and G. J. Dougherty, "Potentiation of photodynamic therapy-elicited antitumor response by localized treatment with granulocyte-macrophage colony-stimulating factor," Cancer Research, Vol. 56, pp. 3281-3286, 1996.

SESSION 2

Immunologic Mechanisms During PDT II and Photochemical Mechanisms

Morphological studies of metastatic mammary rat tumors after laser immunotherapy treatment

Robert E. Nordquist and John A. Nordquist

Wound Healing of Oklahoma, Inc., 3939 N. Walnut Street, Oklahoma City, OK 73105

James C. Agee and Chad M. Blomquist

Oklahoma School of Science and Mathematics, 1141 North Lincoln Boulevard, Oklahoma City, Oklahoma 73104

and

Wei R. Chen

Oklahoma School of Science and Mathematics, 1141 North Lincoln Boulevard, Oklahoma City, Oklahoma 73104 & Department of Physics and Astronomy, University of Oklahoma, Norman, Oklahoma 73109

ABSTRACT

Laser immunotherapy, using a combination of 805 nm diode laser, photosensitizer indocyanine green and immunoadjuvant glycated chitosan, has shown an induced anti-tumor immune response in treatment of metastatic rat tumors. In additional to an apparent systemic, long-term humoral immunological reaction, there could also be laser induced local cellular immune responses. A morphological study was performed to study the immune cells and their infiltration to tumor tissue after this laser immunotherapy treatment. Tumor-bearing rats were terminated at designated times after the treatment; both the tumor and the surrounding normal tissue were collected. The tissue samples were observed under electron microscope. The number and types of infiltrating cells at the tumor site were studied after treatment to determine the contribution of these cells in the elimination of tumors. The tumor cell structural changes resulted from laser-tissue photothermal interaction was investigated. The morphology of tumor development and activities of immune cells including both lymphocytes and plasma cells could shed light on the mode of action of laser treatment of tumors.

Keywords: Cell-mediated immune response; Humoral immune response; Immune cell infiltration; Morphological cellular structure changes, Indocyanine green; Immunoadjuvant; Photothermal tissue destruction; Cancer treatment

1. INTRODUCTION

With the increasing popularity of laser-photosensitizer treatment of cancers, particularly the photodynamic therapy (PDT) using different new photosensitizers, the host immune responses induced by the laser treatment have attracted more and more attention. Since the complete cure and long-term tumor resistance generally cannot be achieved with photophysical reactions and must rely on the tumor-specific immunity, it is essential to search for the possible immunological effects. Immune responses associated with PDT have been reported, mainly in the cellular domain, such as increased activities of T-cells and local macrophages. [1-8] Some long-term tumor resistance, after PDT treatment, was also reported. [9] Some results also showed negative effects by PDT on host immune system. [10-14]

Because of its importance, it is ideal to actively induce such an immune response in laser treatment of cancer. Laser immunotherapy is a new approach proposed by Chen, et al. [15-16] It uses the laser-dye photothermal tissue destruction and an co-administered immunoadjuvant for immune stimulation. This treatment has yielded certain successes in treatment of a metastatic mammary tumor in rats, including total eradication of primary tumor and untreated metastases, as well as long-tumor immunity. [15-16] The mechanism of this laser immunotherapy has been suggested as an induced humoral immunity, although cellular immune contribution can also play a pivotal role. The objective of this paper is to examine the tissue structure and its cellular components, as well as the activities of immune cells after laser treatment using electron microscopy.

2. MATERIALS AND METHODS

2.1 Tumor model

The animal model used in our experiments was the transplantable, metastatic, rat mammary tumor (DMBA-4) in Wistar Furth female rats. Approximately 100,000 live cancer cells were injected subcutaneously into the right inguinal fat pads. The tumors became palpable five to seven days after tumor transplantation. The metastases started appearing in the unimplanted inguinal and axillary areas about 15 days after tumor transplantation. Without treatment, the control tumor-bearing will die around 30 days after tumor implant.

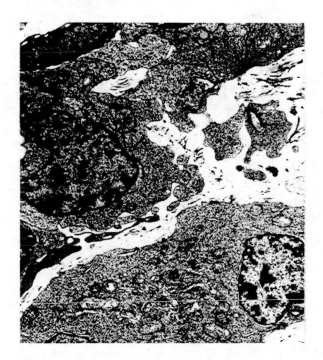

Figure 1. EM image of two tumor cells (4,000 X) with all the normal support structures.

2.2 Laser immunotherapy treatment of rat tumors

The laser used in this experiment was an 805 nm diode laser. The laser energy was delivered through a 1 mm diameter optical fiber. The dye used was indocyanine green (ICG) which has a strong absorption peak around 800 nm. The immunoadjuvant used in our study was glycated chitosan gel (GCG), a chitosan-galactose derivative. The solution of ICG-GCG (200 µl in volume and with 0.25% ICG and 1% GCG) was injected directly into the center of the tumor 2 hours prior to laser treatment. The laser treatment of primary tumor took place seven to ten days after tumor implant. The non-invasive laser application was achieved by maintaining a constant separation between the laser fiber tip and the rat skin overlying the tumor. The fiber tip was smoothly moved over the entire tumor to have a uniform energy delivery from all angles. The laser irradiation was applied at 2 watts for ten minutes.

2.3   Tumor sample preparation for electron microscopy

The tumor samples were collected at designated times: before and immediately after the laser treatment, two weeks as well as one month after the treatment. Tumor tissue was removed and sliced into one millimeter thick slices, following cervical dislocation. These slices were placed in 2% glutaraldehyde and 2% paraformaldehyde in phosphate buffered saline (PBS) for 24 hours. After a brief rinse in PBS, the specimens were post-fixed in 1% osmium tetraoxide for 2 hours, followed by ethanol dehydration and embedding in Epon epoxy resin. Then the samples were examined under a Zeiss electron microscope.

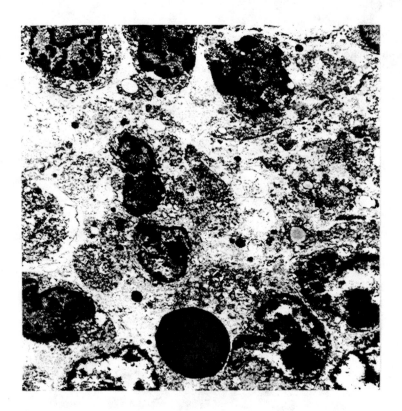

Figure 2. EM image (4,000 X) of a photothermal damage center immediately after the laser immunotherapy. In the center field the cells suffered complete photothermal destruction. The outer field shows the photocoagulated tumor cells with dark nuclei. Further away from the center (not shown) are the less damaged and survivor tumor cells.

3. RESULTS

3.1   Structure of viable tumor cells

The control tumor tissue usually contains large numbers of viable cells with very high mitotic index. Shown in Figure 1 is the EM ultrastructure of two typical live tumor cells. The individual tumor cell is characterized by a large nucleus containing marginated chromatin and prominent nucleoli, as well as a cytoplasm populated with large numbers of polyribosomes. The cytoplasm also contains many mitochondria and a well-developed Golgi apparatus, the endoplasmic reticulum is present but not extensive, as shown in Figure 1. Without any interference, these tumor cells will continue to multiply and metastasize through the lymphatics.

3.2 Photothermal damage to tumor cells

The 805 nm laser, together with indocyanine green *in situ*, resulted in selective photothermal damage to tumor tissue. Depending on ICG distribution and concentration, the thermal damage can have different severity. Shown in Figure 2 is a tumor sample collected immediately after the laser treatment. The damage is characterized by the loss of cellular components and breakage of the plasma membrane and destruction of mitochondria. The nuclear membrane breaks down and the hetrochromatin condenses while the euchromatin is lost. At the center, where tumor cells suffered complete photothermal destruction, there is only a sea of cellular debris. Surrounding this center zone is a second zone of lethality that contains cells that are photocoagulated. Further away from the center are the cells with damaged organelles that are moribund and a number of tumor cells that survived the treatment.

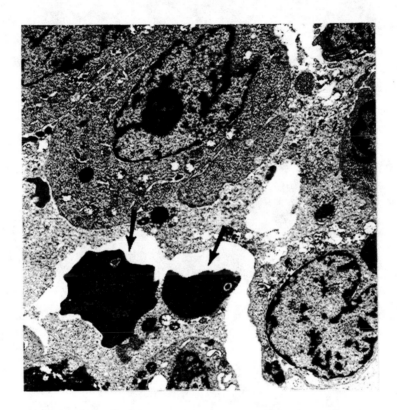

Figure 3. EM image (4,000 X) of tumor tissue two weeks after the laser immunotherapy treatment. It shows an area with incomplete photothermal destruction with several live tumor cells. It also shows small lymphocytes (arrows) adjacent to tumor cells.

3.3 Post-treatment tumor structure and immune cell activities

The survivor tumor cells and tumor cell regeneration are shown in Figure 3 with several tumor cells of different size. These cells began to proliferate and form duct-like nodules two weeks post-treatment. The mitotic index of these tumor cells was as high as the untreated control tumor in Figure 1. However, at this time, the blood vascular component had also begun to proliferate and there were many lymphocytes among the tumor cells as seen in Figure 3. These lymphocytes are characterized by dense cytoplasm and small numbers of mitochondria and very little endoplasmic reticulum; they do however contain large numbers of polyribosomes. Many lymphocytes appeared to be activated, evidenced by their enlarged size and by their close contact with live tumor cells, as shown in Figure 4. Also shown in Figure 4 is a plasma cell with a well-defined Golgi zone and extensive endoplasmic reticulum and moderate numbers of mitochondria.

One month after treatment, if the treatment was successful there are no tumor cells and only a small about of scarring. If the treatment failed to contain the tumor, the field is populated by large numbers of tumor cells exactly like those described in the control specimen (Figure 1).

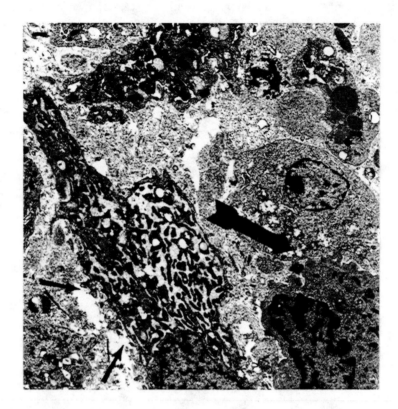

Figure 4. EM image (4,000 X) of tumor tissue two weeks after the laser immunotherapy treatment. Note the enlarged lymphocyte in close contact with a tumor cell (large arrow) and a plasma cell with a distended endoplasmic reticulum in the close vicinity (small arrows).

4. DISCUSSION

The new method for tumor treatment, laser immunotherapy, was used to treat a metastatic mammary tumor in rats and the tumor morphology after treatment was studied. In our experiment, only the primary tumor was treated with injection of photosensitizer-immunoadjuvant solution, followed by a non-invasive local laser irradiation. However, it appears to have induced a systemic anti-tumor effect. Most significant are the eradication of the untreated metastases and long-term tumor immunity. [15-16] This morphological study using electron microscopy is designed to investigate the activities of immune cells after the treatment of tumors.

Our morphological results revealed a selective photothermal tumor destruction depending on the treatment conditions such as the ICG distribution and laser irradiation time. This selectivity can result in different levels of tissue damage ranging from complete photothermal destruction and photocoagulation, as shown in Figure 2. The presence of ICG appeared to be crucial in tissue damage since the 805 nm laser light is not readily absorbed by organized tissue. The survivor tumor cells are common after this laser immunotherapy treatment. These cells could continue to grow and metastasize, as shown in Figures 3 and 4.

In order to control the survivor tumor cells and the metastases, either before or after the treatment, an immune response is required and it is indeed induced by our treatment. In addition to other immunochemical and immunobiological evidence, this morphological study also points to the same conclusion. Two weeks after the treatment, we observed large number of lymphocytes, many of them were apparently activated and had engaged tumor cells (see Figure 4). Similarly, the plasma cells with distended endoplasmic reticulum (see Figure 4) indicate the onset of antibody production. The results suggested that both cellular and humoral immune responses could have been induced. The anti-tumor immunity observed in our experiments may ultimately come from the combined contribution of both immune arms.

5. ACKNOWLEDGMENTS

This research was supported in part by grants from Pacific Pharmaceuticals, Inc., and from the Mazie Wilkonson Fund.

6. REFERENCES

1. G. Canti, O. Marelli, L. Ricci and A. Nicolin, "Hematoporphyrin treated murine lymphocytes: in vitro inhibition of DNA synthesis and light-mediated inactivation of cells responsible for GVHR," Photochemistry and Photobiology, Vol. 34, pp. 589-594, 1981.

2. G. J. Dougherty, J. D. Thacker, W. H. McBride, G. Krosl and M. Korbelik, "Effect of immunization with genetically modified tumor cells on recurrence following photodynamic therapy," Lasers Med. Sci. Vol. 7, pp. 226, 1992.

3. N. Yamamoto, J. K. Hoober, N. Yamamoto and S. Yamamoto, "Tumoricidal capacities of macrophages photodynamically activated with hematoporphyrin derivative," Photochemistry and Photobiology, Vol. 56, 245-250, 1992.

4. M. Korbelik and G. Krosl, "Enhanced macrophage cytotoxicity against tumor cells treated with photodynamic therapy," Photochemistry and Photobiology, Vol. 60, pp. 497-502, 1994.

5. G. Krosl and M. Korbelik, "Potentiation of photodynamic therapy by immunotherapy: the effect of schizophyllan (SPG)," Cancer Letters, Vol. 84, pp. 43-49, 1994.

6. G. Krosl, M. Korbelik and G. J. Dougherty, "Induction of immune cell infiltration into murine SCCVII tumor by Photofrin based photodynamic therapy," Br. J. Cancer, Vol. 71, pp. 549-555, 1995.

7. M. Korbelik, G. Krosl, V. R. Naraparayu and N. Yamamoto, "The effect of enzymatically generated macrophage activating factor (GCMAF) on the tumor response to photodynamic therapy," Photochemistry and Photobiology, Vol. 61, pp. 97S, 1995.

8. G. Krosl, M. Korbelik, J. Krosl and G. J. Dougherty, "Potentiation of photodynamic therapy-elicited antitumor response by localized treatment with granulocyte-macrophage colony-stimulating factor," Cancer Research, Vol. 56, pp. 3281-3286, 1996.

9. G. Canti, D. Lattuada, A. Nicolin, P. Taroni, G. Valentini and R. Cubeddu, "Antitumor immunity induced by photodynamic therapy with aluminum disulfonated phthalocyanines and laser light," Anticancer Drugs, Vol. 5, pp. 443-447, 1994.

10. M. O. Obochi, A. J. Canaan, A. K. Jain, A. M. Richter and J. G. Levy, "Targeting activated lymphocytes with photodynamic therapy: susceptibility of mitogen-stimulated splenic lymphocytes to benzoporphyrin derivative (BPD) photosensitization," Photochemistry and Photobiology, Vol. 62, pp. 169-175, 1995.

11. D. H. Lynch, S. Haddad, K. J. Vernon, M. J. Ott, R. C. Straight and C. J. Jolles, "Systemic immunosuppression induced by photodynamic therapy (PDT) is adoptively transferred by macrophages," Photochemistry and Photobiology, Vol. 49, pp. 453-458, 1989.

12. D. A. Musser, and R. J. Fiel, "Cutaneous photosensitizing and immunosuppressive effects of a series of tumor localizing porphyrins," Photochemistry and Photobiology, Vol. 53, pp 119-123, 1991.

13. C. J. Gomer, A. Ferrario, N. Hayashi, N. Rucher, B. C. Szirth and A. L. Murphree, "Molecular, cellular, and tissue responses following photodynamic therapy," Lasers in Surgery and Medicine Vol. 8, pp 450-463, 1988.

14. C. A. Elmets and K. D. Bowen, "Immunological suppression in mice treated with hematoporphyrin derivative photoradiation," Cancer Research Vol. 46, pp 1608-1611, 1986.

15. W. R. Chen, R. L. Adams, R. Carubelli and R. E. Nordquist, "Laser-photosensitizer assisted immunotherapy: a novel modality for cancer treatment," Cancer Letters 115, pp. 25-30, 1997.

16. W. R. Chen, D. A. Okrongly, R. L. Adams and R. E. Nordquist, "Laser-tissue photobiological interaction: a new mechanism for laser-sensitizer-immunoadjuvant treatment of metastatic cancers," SPIE, Vol. 2975, pp. 290-297, 1997.

Relief of vasospasm by intravascular ultraviolet irradiation

Kanji Nakai, Yuji Morimoto, Hirotaka Ito, Kimito Kominami, Hirotaka Matsuo,

Tsunenori Arai, Makoto Kikuchi

Department of Medical Engineering, National Defense Medical College

ABSTRACT

We investigated the photovasorelaxation with intravascular transluminal irradiation using in vivo model.

A 2.5Fr. catheter was inserted in the femoral artery of a rabbit under anesthesia. A 400 μ m diameter quartz fiber was inserted through the catheter. The catheter was withdrawn from the distal end to the proximal end of the exposed femoral artery without laser irradiation in order to observe the mechanical dilation by the procedure. The femoral artery lumen was irradiated by a Helium-Cadmium(He-Cd) laser (wave length; 325nm) with 8 mW through the fiber during 30 s.

We carried out that the laser irradiation produced vasorelaxation (185% on the average) compared with mechanical vasodilation (150% on the average) with angiography.

The results suggest that intravascular transluminal irradiation with low-power UV laser might be applicable to the relief of acute arterial vasospasm.

Keywords: Helium-Cadmium laser, laser irradiation, photorelaxation, rabbit, femoral artery, nitric oxide

1. INTRODUCTION

Furchgott et al. reported that reversible vasorelaxation can be induced by the exposure of visible and near-ultraviolet light in the range of 310-440nm[1]. Recently, the studies on laser-induced vasorelaxation are motivated by the flexible transluminal light delivery by the optical fiber for possible light treatment of vasospasm. Previous in vitro and in vivo experiments in our laboratory have shown that continuous UV laser to rat femoral artery at low intensity irradiations produces vasorelaxation[2]. All reported in vivo experiments have been performed by the irradiation from the outside of the vessel. In order to treat acute vasospasm, transluminal irradiation with endovascular approach is essential. However, blood existence and blood stream might influence the photovasorelaxation.

We studied the photo-vasorelaxation with intravascular ultraviolet irradiation using in vivo model.

2. METHODS

Four Japanese male rabbits ranging from 2.5 to 3 kg were used. Anesthesia was achieved and continued intravenously with pentobarbital sodium. Mechanical ventilation was not used because of sufficient spontaneous breathing. All surgical procedures were performed under sterile conditions.

The anesthetized rabbits were placed in supine position and fixed by the neck with slight extension. We made midline skin incision, extending from the angle of the mandible to the manubrium sterni. The right common artery was exposed and a 5 Fr. sheath was introduced toward descending aorta. The left femoral artery was exposed by inguinal incision. This artery

---

Further author information -

K. Nakai (correspondence): E-mail:nakai@ndmc.ac.jp; Telephone: +81-42-995-1596; Fax: +81-42-996-5199

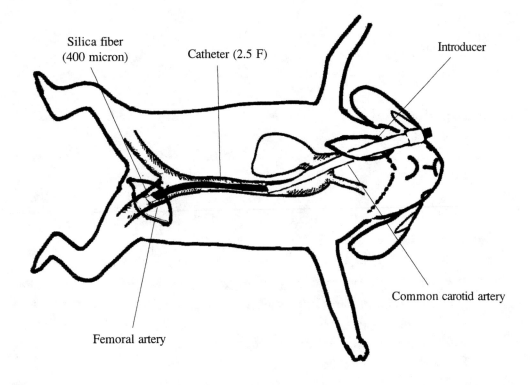

Figure 1. Experimental Set- up

was isolated carefully with a 2cm-long segment. A x-ray opaque markers were placed on both ends of the exposed femoral artery. A coaxial catheter system with a 2.5Fr. catheter was advanced up to the proximal end of the femoral artery. The luminal diameter of the artery was measured angiographically. The obtained angiograms were documented in magnetic videotape. The angiograms were transferred in a personal computer memory. The diameters of three points along the artery were measured from transferred in the computing system with image processing software (NIH image), and the vessel diameter was determined by average of these three points.

The first angiography was performed to measure luminal diameter of the femoral artery. A 0.2mg dose of norepinephrine was infused into perivascular space to contract the artery. A Helium-Cadmium(He-Cd) laser that emitted 325nm UV light with 8mW was employed for the light source. The laser light was delivered through a quartz fiber of which core diameter was 400 μ m. A 2.5Fr.catheter was advanced to the distal marker of the artery, the quartz fiber was inserted through the catheter (Figure 1). To study the mechanical dilation of the catheter with the quartz fiber, the tip of the catheter were gradually withdrawn to the proximal marker of the exposed femoral artery by over 30 s without the laser irradiation. The second angiography was performed to assess the effect of mechanical dilation. After perivascular re-administration of 0.2mg norepinephrine, the femoral artery was irradiated by He-Cd laser through the fiber with the above-mentioned withdrawing motion. The final angiography was performed to evaluate the photovasorelaxation(Figure 2).

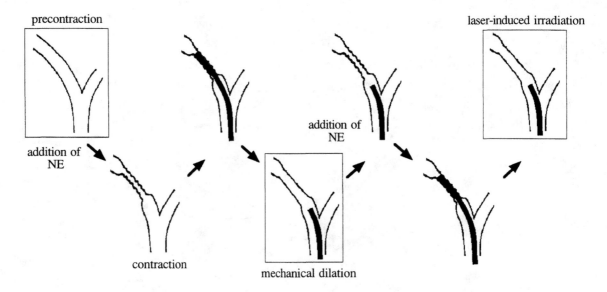

Figure 2. Procedure of transluminal UV irradiation. The arterial diameters
of conditions in boxes were evaluated by angiography. NE; norepinephrine

3. RESULTS

Intravascular application of the UV laser resulted in vessel dilation. The quantitative vasodilation data is presented in
Table 1. We used relative luminal diameter expression normalizing at the precontracted lumen diameter. The UV laser
irradiated luminal diameter was $185\pm55\%$, meanwhile the diameter of mechanical dilation (no laser irradiation) was $145\pm
30\%$. The difference between these conditions was not significant statistically, however in all cases, the UV laser irradiated
diameters were larger than no irradiation.

Table1. The effect in a vessel of UV irradiation

	Angiographic diameter
precontracted state	1
no UV laser irradiation	1.45 ± 0.30
UV laser irradiation	1.85 ± 0.55

The values are mean $\pm$ SD.

4. DISCUSSION

We demonstrated that continuous wave UV-laser irradiation with intravascular approach could produce the vasorelaxation.

Furchgott et al. reported that reversible relaxation of noradrenaline-activated rabbit aortic strips *in vitro* was induced by low-power lamp light exposure[1]. Our studies on photovasorelaxation have demonstrated by laser-induced relaxation, because the laser irradiation could be delivered by the optical fiber. Low-power radiation from a continuous wave visible laser induced relaxation of blood vessels *in vitro* and *in vivo* [3][4].

Photovasorelaxation has been shown to be independent of the intact endothelial layer. The detailed mechanism of photorelaxation in vascular muscles is still not known. However the possible cause of the vasorelaxation may be nitric oxide(NO) / endothelium-derived relaxing factor(EDRF)-like substance releasing by light energy.

Treinin et al. demonstrated that nitric oxide(NO) was produced by the photolysis of nitrite(NO_2^-)[5]. The kinetics of NO production of was proposed below.

$$NO_2^- \quad --\overset{h\nu}{---} \rightarrow \quad NO + O^-$$

Since the serum concentration of NO_2^- is about 10 μ mol/l, the photodissociated NO can be estimated as 10 pmol/l[6][7][8]. The photodissociated NO could have sufficient concentration to induce vasorelaxation because the endogenous NO is about 1pmol/l. If precontracted vascular smooth muscle is irradiated by an UV-laser, NO_2^- containing complex might be photodissociated into NO and cleavage product, then the NO might relax the vessel.

We reported the photovasorelaxation by intravascular transluminal irradiation using *in vivo* model. The results suggest that we might be able to release vasospasm by intravascular transluminal irradiation with low-power UV laser.

REFERENCES

1. R.F.Furchgott, S.J.Ehrreich and E.Greenblatt, "The photoactivated relaxation of smooth muscle of rabbit aorta", *J. Gen.. Physiol.*, **44**, pp499-519, 1961

2. Y.Morimoto, H.Matsuo, T.Arai and M. Kikuchi, "Low-intensity light induces vasorelaxation: a study for possible mechanism", *SPIE*, **2681**, pp126-129, 1996

3. H.Chaudhry, M.Lynch, K.Schomacker, R.Birngruber, K.Gregory and I.Kochevar, "Relaxation of vascular smooth muscle induced by low-power laser radiation", *Photochem. Photobiol.* **58**, pp661-669, 1993

4. Z.F.Gourgouliatos, A.J.Welch, K.R.Diller and S.J.Aggarwal, "Laser-irradiation-induced relaxation of blood vessels in vivo", *Lasers Surg. Med.*, **10**, pp524-532, 1990

5. A.Treinin and E.Hayon, "Absorption spectra and reaction kinetics of NO_2, N_2O_3, and N_2O_4 in aqueous solution", *J .Am. Chem. Soc.* **92**, pp5821-5828, 1970

6. O.C.Zafiriou, M.McFarland, "Determination of trace levels of nitric oxide in aqueous solution", *Anal.Chem*, **52**, pp1662-1667, 1980

7. D.R.Tsikas, R.H.Boger, S.M.Bode-Boger, F.M.Gutzki, J.C.Frolich, "Quantification of nitrite and nitrate in human urine and plasma as pentafluorobenzyl derivatives by gas chromatography-mass spectrometry using their 15N-labeled analogs", *J.Chromatogra.B:Biomed.Appl.*, **661**, pp185-191, 1994

8. K.Kikuchi, H.Hayama, T.Nagano, Y.Hirata, T.Sugimoto, M.Hirobe, "New method of detecting nitric oxide production", *Chem.Pharma. Bull.*, **40**, pp2233-2235, 1992

9. P.G.Steg, D.Gal, A.J.Rongione, S.R.Dejesus, R.J.Clarke, H.J.Levine and J.M.Isner, "Effect of argon laser irradiation on rabbit aortic smooth muscle: evidence for endothelium independent contraction and relaxation", *Cadiovasc.Res.* **22**, pp747-753, 1988

Relative photoreactivity of the pigment inclusions of the retinal pigment epithelium

Randolph D. Glickman[1], Alexander E. Dontsov[2], and Mikhail A Ostrovsky[2]

[1]Department of Ophthalmology, The University of Texas Health Science Center
at San Antonio, San Antonio, TX, USA
[2]Institute of Bio-Chemical Physics of the Russian Academy of Sciences,
Moscow, Russia

ABSTRACT

The cellular pigments of the retinal pigment epithelium are photoactive; that is, they promote free radical oxidative reactions when illuminated with visible or ultraviolet light. This activity is sufficient to cause photo-oxidation of several major cellular components such as antioxidants, dinucleotide cofactors, proteins and fatty acids. The present investigation determined the relative ability of melanin, lipofuscin, and melanolipofuscin granules isolated from human and bovine eyes to oxidize linoleic and docosahexaenoic acids, which are polyunsaturated fatty acids. The dark reactivity as well as the light-stimulated reactions were determined. All RPE pigment granules stimulated fatty acid oxidation when irradiated with the blue-green (488.1 and 514.5 nm) emission of the Argon-ion laser. Only lipofuscin, however, caused peroxidation of fatty acids in the dark. These findings not only suggest that accumulation of lipofuscin in the aging eye may contribute to increased photooxidative stress to the retina and RPE, but also that the photoactive RPE pigments might serve as endogenous photosensitizers for therapeutic applications.

Keywords: RPE, melanin, melanolipofuscin, lipofuscin, polyunsaturated fatty acids, photooxidative stress

1. INTRODUCTION

The retinal pigment epithelium (RPE) of the eye contains several pigments which possess photoactive properties, but are not themselves involved in visual transduction. Melanin, the heteropolymeric product of DOPA or cysteinylDOPA oxidation[1], is a broadband absorber and is generally thought to protect ocular tissues against excess light. The protection presumably offered by melanin could derive from its ability to screen light from sensitive tissues[2], from its ability to sequester heavy metals that might otherwise catalyze oxidative reactions[3], or because it may trap free radicals produced by photochemical or ionizing radiation[4,5]. Melanin, however, has been shown to oxidize physiological substrates such as ascorbic acid, fatty acids, and proteins during visible light irradiation[6-10].

The other noteworthy pigment inclusion in RPE cells is lipofuscin. Long considered an "aging" pigment[11-13], lipofuscin has at least two chromophores, one absorbing maximally at 430 nm and another absorbing at 580 nm[14]. This pigment is capable of promoting photooxidative reactions, including the generation of singlet oxygen[14], superoxide anions[15], and the initiation of lipid hydroperoxides[16]. The decline in melanin content in RPE and choroid with age is often associated with an increase in lipofuscin content[11-13], so that an increase in lipofuscin content in RPE cells has been considered a marker of increased oxidative stress in the eye. In view of these observations, we compared the photoinduced, as well as the constitutive (dark), reactions of isolated RPE melanin, lipofuscin, and complex granules (melanolipofuscin) in a model system with the production of fatty acid hydroperoxides as the endpoint.

SPIE Vol. 3254 ● 0277-786X/98/$10.00

2. MATERIALS AND METHODS

2.1 Pigment Granules

Human eyes were kindly donated by the "Eye Bank" of Moscow, Russia, and were from donors aged from 40 to 65 years who were free of any ophthalmological disorders. The lipofuscin (LF) granules and melanolipofuscin (MLF) granules were obtained only from human eyes. These granules, plus the melanosomes, were obtained from human eyes by a method similar to that described by Boulton and Marshall[17]. Melanosomes (MS) were also obtained from bovine eyes by the method described by Glickman et al.[9]. All of the pigment granules were stored at -20° C until use.

2.2 Measurement of fatty acid peroxidation following visible laser irradiation

The peroxidation of fatty acids was determined by the reaction of NADPH-dependent glutathione peroxidase with the hydroperoxide products and reduced glutathione (GSH)[18]. Linoleic acid (LA) and cis-4,7,10,13,16,19-docosahexaenoic acid (DHA) were obtained from Sigma Chemical, St. Louis, MO. Reactions with LA were carried out with 0.72 mg/ml of linoleic acid in 0.1 M potassium phosphate buffer, pH 7.44, and varying densities of pigment granules. The enzyme assay reagents were added after laser exposure. For DHA reactions, 70-80 µg/ml of the fatty acid were added to 0.1 M potassium phosphate buffer, pH 7.44, 1 mM EDTA, 1mM GSH, 0.7 units glutathione reductase, 0.4 units of glutathione peroxidase (Sigma), 200 µM NADPH (Sigma), and varying densities of pigment granules. With both fatty acids, the sample was divided into two equal parts, one for laser exposure, and one for dark control. Photooxidation was initiated by exposure to the mixed, blue-green output (488.1 and 514.5 nm) of a continuous wave, Argon-ion laser, at various sample irradiances as indicated in the text. After the laser exposure, the loss of absorbance at 340 nm, corresponding to the oxidation of NADPH by the enzyme-catalyzed transfer of peroxide groups

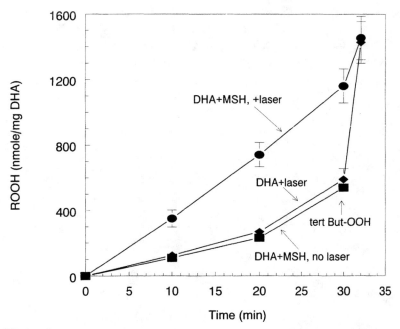

Figure 1
DHA photooxidation by Argon laser exposure (0.8 W/cm^2) in the presence and absence of human melanosomes (MSH) at a density of 2.2 x 10^7 gran/ml. Tert butyl-OOH added at 30 min to test activity of NADPH-dependent GSH peroxidase used to assay fatty acid hydroperoxides.

from the fatty acid to the GSH substrate, was measured in a spectrophotometer and converted into nanomoles of fatty acid hydroperoxides (ROOH) produced during the laser exposure. To confirm the enzymatic activities, 40 - 50 mg tert-butyl hydroperoxide was added at the end of the measurement.

3. RESULTS

3.1 Fatty Acids are Minimally Photooxidized in the Absence of Pigment Granules

The fatty acids, LA and DHA, have negligible optical absorbance in the visible spectrum; therefore, when no pigment granules were present in the reaction mixture and visible wavelengths were used as the photooxidizing source, very little oxidation of the fatty acids occurred (Figure 1). The peroxidation rate of native DHA (without melanosomes), exposed to the blue-green output of the Argon laser, is virtually identical to that of DHA in the presence of MS but kept in the dark for an equal amount of time (Figure 1, curves marked with diamonds and squares, respectively). In contrast, when human melanosomes were present at a density of 2.2×10^7 gran/ml in the reaction mixture, the amount of photooxidized DHA increased linearly with the duration of the laser exposure (Figure 1, curve marked with circles). Linoleic acid was also photooxidized by the laser when melanosomes were present in the reaction mixture, but the extent of the reaction was much less (data not shown).

3.2 Comparison of the Photooxidative Reactivity of the RPE Pigments

The three types of RPE pigment granules, MS, LF, and MLF, were compared with respect to their ability to photooxidize DHA. Reaction mixtures were made up with DHA and either: human MS (1.95×10^7 gran/ml), LF (1.72×10^7 gran/ml), or MLF (1.57×10^8 gran/ml). Aliquots were exposed to the Argon laser for 10 min at 0.8 W/cm^2 for 10 min, or kept in the dark as a control. Following the 10 min exposure or dark control period, the samples were analyzed for hydroperoxides by the NADPH-glutathione peroxidase assay. The results are shown in Figure 2A, with the data expressed as the difference between the laser-exposed and dark control samples. The samples with the MS granules exhibited the largest increase in hydroperoxides after laser exposure, while LF and MLF containing samples had lesser increases in hydroperoxides, in that order. The results of this experiment are also shown as the ratio of laser-induced to dark (i.e. resulting from autoxidation) DHA hydroperoxides (Figure 2B), as well as the total (dark + light) DHA peroxidation (Figure 2C) produced with the three types of RPE pigment granules.

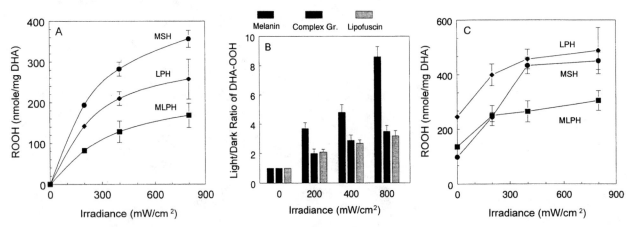

Figure 2
Comparison of DHA peroxidation produced by laser photoactivated human melanosomes (MSH) at a density of 1.95×10^7 gran/ml, lipofuscin (LFH) at a density of 1.72×10^7 gran/ml, and melanolipofuscin (MLFH) at a density of 1.57×10^7 gran/ml. Argon laser exposure was for a duration of 10 m at the indicated irradiances. A: Results expressed as laser-induced hydroperoxides minus dark peroxidation; B: Results expressed as the ratio of laser to dark peroxidation; C: Results expressed as laser plus dark peroxidation, i.e. total DHA peroxidation produced by each pigment granule type.

4. DISCUSSION

The comparison of the photoreactivities towards the fatty acid, DHA, of the three RPE pigment inclusions indicated that MS granules have the highest photooxidative activity. This conclusion may be drawn from the results in Figure 2B, in which the data are expressed as the ratio of light-to dark activity. Two additional conclusions may be drawn from this data set. One is that the photoinduced activity of MS increased markedly with increasing irradiance; while the activities of LF and MLF were much less excited. At a sample irradiance of 800 mW/cm^2, the light activity of MS was nine times its dark level of activity, increasing from a ratio of about 4 at a sample irradiance of 200 mW/cm^2. LF and MLF granules, in comparison, only increased from a ratio of 2 up to about 3.5 (Figure 2C). The second is that, while the activities of LF and MS granules were approximately equal and MLF granules were less reactive during laser irradiation at ≥ 0.4 W/cm^2, the greatest total activity, i.e. the sum of the DHA hydroperoxides produced during dark and light, was measured for LF granules regardless of its light history. In contrast, MS were quiescent in the dark. Thus, LF has the potential to exert the greatest chronic oxidative stress in ocular tissues.

The photochemistry of lipofuscin granules is incompletely understood, and only one of its components has been chemically characterized[19] (Figure 3). It is known that RPE LF granules photogenerate superoxide radicals [Boulton et al., 1993] and singlet state oxygen[14]. However, there is no information about the *in vivo* conditions that cause lipofuscin granules to stimulate free-radical oxidative reactions, namely the wavelength and intensity of light entering the eye, the critical concentration of lipofuscin, the effect of the concentration of oxidizable substrate, pH, temperature, etc. In contrast, the structure of eumelanin is better defined but likely varies throughout the melanin heteropolymer, as evidenced by alternative structures proposed for the melanin polymer[20] (Figure 4). A general reaction mechanism for the photooxidation of fatty acids by melanin is presented below.

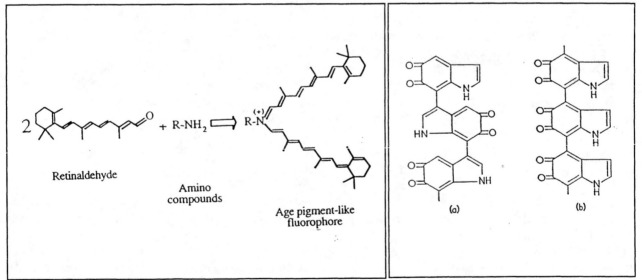

Figure 3. Structure of "orange fluorophore" age pigment in human lipofuscin, characterized by Eldred & Lasky[19]

Figure 4. Proposed structures of eumelanin, from Morton[20].

With the assumption that molecular oxygen is present in excess, and that the reaction of photoexcited melanin proceeds according the mechanism proposed by Rozanowska et al.[10], the primary reactive species in eumelanin are the quinone (MQ), semiquinone radical (MSQ●⁻), and hydroquinone (MQH$_2$) groups of the hydroxyindole subunits of heteropolymer. The effect of visible light is to push the equilibrium between the quinone, hydroquinone, and semiquinone species to the right so that the occurrence of the semiquinone form is favored:

$$hv$$
$$MQ + MQH_2 \rightleftharpoons 2\, MSQ\bullet^- \tag{1}$$

This is presumably the only light-induced reaction. The semiquinones may react directly with DHA in a Type I (free radical) reaction or through a Type II reaction involving an oxygen radical intermediate[21,22] as follows:

$$\text{(Type I)} \qquad MSQ\bullet^- + DHA\text{-}H + H^+ \rightleftharpoons DHA\bullet + MQH_2 \tag{2}$$

where DHA-H represents the polyunsaturated fatty acid, or

$$\text{(Type II)} \qquad MSQ\bullet^- + O_2 \rightleftharpoons MQ + O_2\bullet^- \tag{3}$$

where the reaction of the semiquinone radical with oxygen produces superoxide anion. Following reactions 2 and/or 3, hydroperoxides of the fatty acids may be produced in the following reactions:

$$DHA\text{-}H + O_2\bullet^- + H^+ \rightarrow H_2O_2 + DHA\bullet \tag{4}$$

where $DHA\bullet$ is the alkyl radical formed by abstraction of a hydrogen atom.

$$DHA\bullet + O_2 \rightarrow DHA\text{-}OO\bullet \tag{5}$$

Interaction of the alkyl radical with oxygen forms a peroxyl radical.

$$DHA\text{-}OO\bullet + DHA\text{-}H \rightarrow DHA\text{-}OOH + DHA\bullet \tag{6}$$

Reaction 6 proceeds as a chain reaction between the peroxyl radical and DHA, resulting in accumulation of fatty acid hydroperoxides (DHA-OOH).

Although the relation of these *in vitro* reactions to the generation of oxidative stress in the RPE and choroid *in vivo* is speculative, oxidative reactions between polyunsaturated fatty acids and photochemically-active RPE melanin and lipofuscin granules would likely damage RPE cell membranes, and possibly the photoreceptors with their highly membranous outer segments. The relatively high oxygen tension in the choroidal tissue also increases the risk of lipid peroxidation. In this regard, we have observed that densities of MS granules over $\sim\!10^9$ gran/ml actually reduce the peroxidation of DHA, perhaps because of self-screening or termination of peroxidative chain reactions by melanin at high densities (data to be published elsewhere). This suggests that tissue highly pigmented with melanin may be protected from photooxidative stress. The situation with lipofuscin, however, may be quite different. Although lipofuscin is not as photoexcitable as is melanin, it has a higher dark, or constitutive, reactivity towards fatty acids. Considering the age-related increase of lipofuscin granules in the RPE, it is likely that there is a progressive increase in oxidative stress in the RPE associated with the accumulation of LF granules, and this may be a factor contributing to age-related retinal degenerations. Moreover, the photochemical activity of the RPE pigments may be the basis for another area of clinical interest. Derivatives prepared from some of these pigments, particularly melanin, might have low cellular toxicity, yet their photochemical activity could be activated by exposure to visible wavelengths produced by commonly available lasers. Melanin and hydroxyindolic compounds may therefore represent a useful class of chromophores for the development of novel photosensitizers for photodynamic therapy.

5. ACKNOWLEDGEMENTS

Dr. A.E. Dontsov was an Research to Prevent Blindness International Scholar at the UTHSCSA during the performance of this research. Additional research support was provided by AFOSR grant F49629-95-1-0332 (to RDG), the San Antonio Area Foundation, the Helen Freeborn Kerr Foundation, an Enrichment Subgrant from the Howard Hughes Medical Institute Research Resources Program grant to the UTHSCSA, and an unrestricted grant from Research to Prevent Blindness (RPB) to the Department of Ophthalmology of the UTHSCSA. We thank Ms. Neeru Kumar and Mr. Steven Stubblefield for technical assistance during this project.

6. REFERENCES

1. W. H. Koch and M. R. Chedekel, "Photochemistry and photobiology of melanogenic metabolites: Formation of free radicals", *Photochem. Photobiol.* **46**, pp. 229-238, 1987.
2. M. L. Wolbarsht, A. W. Walsh, and G. George, "Melanin, a unique biological absorber", *Appl. Opt.* **20**, pp. 2184-2186, 1981.
3. T. Sarna, "Properties and function of the ocular melanin - A photobiophysical view", *J. Photochem. Photobiol. B* **12**, pp. 215-258, 1992.

4. M. Porebska-Budny, N. L. Sakina, K. B. Stepien, A. E. Dontsov, and T. Wilczok, "Antioxidative activity of synthetic melanins. Cardiolipin liposome model", *Biochim. Biophys. Acta* **1116**, pp. 11-16, 1992.
5. N. L. Sakina, A. E. Dontsov, G. G. Afanas'ev, M. A. Ostrovski, and I. I. Pelevina, "[The accumulation of lipid peroxidation products in the eye structures of mice under whole-body x-ray irradiation]. [Russian]", *Radiobiologiia* **30**, pp. 28-31, 1990.
6. R. D. Glickman and K.-W. Lam, "Oxidation of ascorbic acid as an indicator of photooxidative stress in the eye", *Photochem. Photobiol.* **55**, pp. 191-196, 1992.
7. R. D. Glickman, R. Sowell, and K.-W. Lam, "Kinetic properties of light-dependent ascorbic acid oxidation by melanin", *Free Rad. Biol. Med.* **15**, pp. 453-457, 1993.
8. R. D. Glickman and K.-W. Lam, "Melanin may promote photooxidation of linoleic acid", in *Laser-Tissue Interaction VI, Proc. SPIE*, S. L. Jacques, ed., **2391**, pp. 254-261, SPIE, Bellingham, WA, 1995.
9. R. D. Glickman, B. A. Rockwell, and S. L. Jacques, "Action spectrum of oxidative reactions mediated by light-activated melanin", *Laser-Tissue Interaction VIII, Proc. SPIE*, S. L. Jacques, ed., **2975**, pp. 138-145, SPIE, Bellingham, WA, 1997.
10. M. Rozanowska, A. Bober, J. M. Burke, and T. Sarna, "The role of retinal pigment epithelium melanin in photoinduced oxidation of ascorbate", *Photochem. Photobiol.* **65**, pp. 472-479, 1997.
11. L. Feeney-Burns, E. S. Hilderbrand, and S. Eldridge, "Aging human RPE: morphometric analysis of macular, equatorial and peripheral cells", *Invest. Ophthalmol. Vis. Sci.* **25**, pp. 195-200, 1984.
12. J. J. Nordlund, "The lives of pigment cells", *Clin. Geriat. Med.* **5**, pp. 91-108, 1989.
13. J. J. Weiter, F. C. Delori, G. L. Wing, and K. A. Fitch, "Retinal pigment epithelial lipofuscin and melanin and choroidal melanin in human eyes", *Invest. Ophthalmol. Vis. Sci.* **27**, pp. 145-152, 1986.
14. E. R. Gaillard, S. J. Atherton, G. Eldred, and J. Dillon, "Photophysical studies on human retinal lipofuscin", *Photochem. Photobiol.* **61**, pp. 448-453, 1995.
15. M. Boulton, A. Dontsov, J. Jarvis-Evans, M. Ostrovsky, and D. Svistunenko, "Lipofuscin is a photoinducible free radical generator", *J. Photochem. Photobiol. B* **19**, pp. 201-204, 1993.
16. M. Rozanowska, J. Jarvis-Evans, W. Korytowski, M. E. Boulton, J. M. Burke, and T. Sarna, "Blue light-induced reactivity of retinal age pigment. In vitro generation of oxygen-reactive species", *J. Biol. Chem.* **270**, pp. 18825-18830, 1995.
17. M. Boulton and J. Marshall, "Repigmentation of human retinal pigment epithelial cells in vitro", *Exp. Eye Res.* **41**, pp. 209-218, 1985.
18. D. T. Organisciak and W. K. Noell, "Hereditary retinal dystrophy in the rat: lipid composition of debris", *Exp. Eye Res.* **22**, pp. 101-113, 1976.
19. G. E. Eldred and M. R. Lasky, "Retinal age pigments generated by self-assembling lysosomotropic detergents", *Nature* **361**, pp. 724-726, 1993.
20. R. A. Morton, "Introductory account of quinones", *Biochemistry of Quinones*, R. A. Morton, ed., pp. 1-21, Academic Press, London, 1965.
21. A. W. Girotti, "Photodynamic lipid peroxidation in biological systems", *Photochem. Photobiol.* **51**, pp 497-509. 1990.
22. L. L. Holte, F. J. G. M. van Kuijk, and E. A. Dratz, "Preparative high-performance liquid chromatograpy purification of polyunsaturated phospholipids and characterization using ultraviolet derivative spectroscopy", *Analyt. Biochem.* **188**, pp. 136-141, 1990.

SESSION 3

Photothermal Mechanisms

Theoretical modelling of heating and structure alterations in cartilage under laser radiation with regard of water evaporation and diffusion dominance

Emil Sobol[a], Moishe Kitai[a], Nicholas Jones[b], Alexander Sviridov[a],
Thomas Milner[c], and Brian Wong[c]

[a]Research Center for Technological Lasers, Troitsk, 142092, Russia,
[b]Queen Medical Center, University of Nottingham, Nottingham, NG7 2UH, UK
[c]Beckman Laser Institute and Medical Clinic, UCI, Irvine, CA, 92612, USA

ABSTRACT

We develop a theoretical model to calculate the temperature field and the size of modified structure area in cartilaginous tissue. The model incorporates both thermal and mass transfer in a tissue regarding bulk absorption of laser radiation, water evaporation from a surface and temperature dependence of diffusion coefficient. It is proposed that due to bound - to free-phase transition of water in cartilage heated to about 70 °C, some parts of cartilage matrix (proteoglycan units) became more mobile. The movement of these units takes place only when temperature exceed 70 °C and results in alteration of tissue structure (denaturation). It is shown that 1) the maximal temperature is reached not on the surface irradiated at some distance from the surface; 2) surface temperature reaches a plateau quicker that the maximal temperature 3) The depth of denatured area strongly depends on laser fluence and wavelength, exposure time and thickness of cartilage. The model allows to predict and control temperature and depth of structure alterations in the course of laser reshaping and treatment of cartilage.

Keywords: cartilage, laser heating, water, diffusion, theoretical modelling, denaturation

1. INTRODUCTION

Non-destructive reshaping of cartilage is one of the new attractive applications of lasers in medicine[1-16]. Cartilage matrix consists of collagen net, proteoglycan aggregates and (up to 80 volume percent) water, A part of water molecules are bound with proteoglycans and taking part in the proteoglycan-collagen interaction, and other water molecules are relatively «free» and could move through cartilage matrix to provide feeding for chondrocytes . It was shown[2,6,14] that the mechanism of laser reshaping is due to bound-to-free phase transition of cartilaginous water taking place at $T_w \cong 70$ °C, but details of this mechanism are still under investigation[14,15].

Various reasons for stress relaxation in cartilage were discussed[2,14,15]: i) local mineralisation of a tissue (neutralisation of negative charged groups of proteoglycans by positive **Na** or **Ca** ions) without any changes in collagen and proteoglycan structure, ii) local depolymerisation of proteoglycans aggregates under short-lived laser heating over 70 °C followed by the formation of new proteoglycan structure without pronounced denaturation (dramatic structural changes) of cartilage matrix, and iii) short-lived break of bonds between collagen and proteoglycan sub-systems allowing decrease stress in cartilage by some alterations in the space structure of proteoglycans. One of the open questions is necessity, degree and scale of structure alterations accompanying the process of laser reshaping of cartilage. It would be of importance to have a theoretical model which allows to describe and predict structure alteration (denaturation) in a biological tissue under laser radiation.

It is well known that phase transformations in a biological tissue and modification of its structure are governed mainly by heat and mass transfer processes. The modeling of non-destructive heating of biological tissues under laser radiation is usually based on a solution of a linear problem of thermoconductivity[6] and does not take into account an effect of low energy phase transformations and mass transfer processes. There are only a limited number of attempts to consider kinetics of laser-induced heating and denaturation of tissues regarding water evaporation and heat of denaturation[6,17].

As it was emphasized in[6], the distance of movement of fragments of biopolymer chains (ones relative others) control reversibility or irreversibility of structure alteration in biotissues. Since the rate of diffusion sharply increases with temperature, and laser treatment may provide short-lived increase in temperature, the processes of laser-induced denaturation and structure alteration have a diffusion-dominated character[6]. It is true also for the process of laser reshaping of cartilage which could be achieved without tissue denaturation, when laser exposure time is short enough[10,16] To the moment we do not know any papers considering the diffusion dominance as one of the main peculiarities of structure alteration in biopolymers under laser radiation.

The aim of this paper is to develop a theoretical model to calculate the temperature field and the size of modified structure area in cartilaginous tissue. We consider both thermal and mass transfer in a tissue regarding bulk absorption of laser radiation, water evaporation from a surface and temperature dependence of diffusion coefficient. Similar approach to the study of mass diffusion dominance was used for the modelling the laser-induced phase transformation in alloys, in particular, for calculation the laser-hardened layer thickness in steel with dominance of carbon diffusion [6].

For laser-induced structural transformations in biopolymers, size distribution of diffusing particles, geometry and mechanism of mass transfer are unknown in details, and could be changed in the course of laser treatment. This makes theoretical analysis of mass transfer difficult. We will present here a very simple, but quite general consideration of mass diffusion in cartilage without identification of geometry of the process, shape and size of diffusant. The possibility of such approach is advocated by experimental data[18] showing that diffusion in proteoglycan solutions increases with temperature, but exhibited no size and molecular mass dependencies, and also by the suggested in[12] mechanism of mass transfer in cartilage as a successive adsorption and desorption of water by proteoglycans.

The developed model illustrates main peculiarities of laser heating and structure alterations in cartilage, allows to examine effect of various parameters and to predict condition as for laser reshaping as for denaturation of cartilage under laser radiation.

2. IDEA OF THE MODEL

Heterogeneous distribution of negative charged groups at proteoglycans polymeric chains is a reason of repulses between them and results in internal stress in cartilage. Stress relaxation in cartilage is due to redistribution of proteoglycan structure to make it more homogeneous. So, to provide stress relaxation, some parts of proteoglycan chains have to diffuse upon the distance comparable with a characteristic size of structure heterogeneity. It is known that water is cartilage is of importance for maintaining its structure[18], and, at a certain temperature $T_w \cong 70$ °C, the bound-to free transition of cartilaginous water increases mutual mobility of parts of the matrix and may lead as to stress relaxation as to denaturation[12.14,15]. The dissociation of proteoglycan aggregates and non-reversible reorganization of the proteoglycan structure under the long heating over 70 °C were documented in[19]. From the other side, liberation of bound water promote a weakness of collagen-proteoglycan interaction[20]. That also may alter cartilage structure and results in stress relaxation and/or denaturation.

When temperature drops, new bonds arise and new configuration could be fixed. So, the degree of structure changes depends on the distance of mass transfer which takes place only during period of time, τ_d, when temperature is higher than T_w. Our aim is to calculate the distance (L) of mass diffusion assuming that the mass transfer takes place only at $T > T_w$. When L is much less that a characteristic size of proteoglycan aggregate L_0, the movement of separate elements will not lead to a dramatic non-reversible structure alteration (denaturation). Denaturation occur when $L > L_0$, Proteoglycan aggregates could be a few micrometers in size[18]. So, the value of $L_0 \cong 5$ μm could be chosen as conventional boundary between two regimes of laser treatment: denaturation and nondestructive stress relaxation in cartilage. Heating and mass transfer problems will be considered following the approach suggested in[6]. We will assume that diffusion coefficient sharply increases with temperature, and that mass transfer processes do not effect on laser heating of a tissue.

3. HEAT TRANSFER PROBLEM

Assuming that laser beam diameter (d) is much more than a thickness of cartilage slab (l), consider one-dimensional equation of thermoconductivity

$$\partial U / \partial t = \chi (\partial^2 U / \partial x^2) + f(x,t,U) \qquad (1)$$

Here $U(x, t)$ is the tissue temperature (in K) depending on time (t) and on distance (x) from the irradiated surface, $f(x, t, U) = (E\alpha / C)\exp(-\alpha x)\,\vartheta(t)+P(U)$, α is the effective coefficient of light absorption by cartilage depending on the laser wavelength; C is heat capacity, χ is thermodiffusivity; E is laser fluence; $\vartheta(t)$ is the step-wise function describing a pulse repetition radiation (assuming the laser pulse intensity is uniform along a pulse duration τ_p). The term $P(U)$ describes the effect of bound-to-free transition of water. This effect depends on the proportion ε between bound and free water in cartilage. Previously we found[12,14] $\varepsilon \cong 0.04$. The numerical calculations based on these data have demonstrated that the contribution of them term $P(U)$ is negligible and we will not take it into consideration.

The initial and boundary conditions for the equation (1) are:

$U(x, 0) = U_0 = 293$ K is the room temperature;

$$-(\partial U / \partial x)_{x=0;\, l} = \pm (v\,QM / \lambda)\,\exp(-V / RU_S) \tag{2}$$

Condition (2) represents water evaporation from both surfaces of a cartilage slab ($x=0$; $x=l$) and makes the thermoconductivity problem nonlinear. Here Q is the evaporation heat of water, R is the gas constant, U_S is the surface temperature, v is the characteristic frequency of oscillation of water molecules, λ is the thermal conductivity, M is the water concentration at cartilage surfaces.

We do not take into consideration any change of water concentration in cartilage during laser treatment. The coefficient of water diffusion is much more than that for heat diffusion[12]. So, the deficit of water in a superficial layer will be compensated very fast in comparison with the characteristic time of heat transfer process. Also It is essential, that the intensity of evaporation depends linearly on M, while exponentially on U_S. Therefore, for small t values, and for not very high temperatures typical for laser reshaping of cartilage, the amount of evaporated water is small and one can neglect alteration of M in the course of laser irradiation.

4. MASS TRANSFER PROBLEM

Consider a transfer of proteoglycan units (or some other parts of proteoglycan structure) during period of time τ_d for which tissue temperature U exceeds $U_w = 343$ K. When diffusion coefficient D is constant, diffusion way could be estimated as $L = \sqrt{D\tau_d}$. When D is a function of temperature and time, the average way of diffusion could be calculated with the use of formula[6]:

$$L = b\sqrt{\int_0^\tau D(t)dt} \tag{3}$$

where b is a coefficient depending on the geometry of diffusion process and on the boundary conditions of respective mass transfer problem[6].

Taking into account that diffusion takes place when $U > U_w$ only, and that diffusion coefficient increases with temperature in accordance with the Arrhenius law[12,19], we can write:

$$D(U) = sgn(U - U_w)\, D_0\, exp(-V_P / R\,U) \tag{4}$$

Here $sgn(U - U_w) = 1$ at $U - U_w > 0$ and $sgn(U - U_w) = 0$ at $U - U_w < 0$, V_P is the activation energy for proteoglycan diffusion, D_0 is a pre-exponential factor.

5. SOLUTION OF THE PROBLEMS

The equation (1) with the nonlinear boundary conditions (2) is a differential equation of parabolic type and can be transformed to the Volterra - type integral equation of the second kind[21]:

$$U(x,t) = \int_0^\ell d\xi\, G(x,\xi, t)\, U(\xi, t-\Delta) + \int_0^\ell \int_0^\Delta d\xi\, d\tau\, G(x,\xi, t)\, f(\xi, t-\tau) \tag{5}$$

The core of this integral equation is connected with the Green's function of the equation of thermoconductivity[21]:

$$G(x, \xi, t - \tau) = [1 / (4 \pi \chi (t - \tau))^{1/2}] *$$

$$* \{ [\exp(-(x - \xi)^2 / (4 \chi (t - \tau))) + \exp(-(x + \xi)^2 / (4 \chi (t - \tau))) +$$

$$+ \exp(-(x + \xi - 2l)^2 / (4 \chi (t - \tau)))] -$$

$$- 2h_0 \int_0^\infty \exp(-h_0 \omega) \exp(-(x + \xi + \omega)^2 / (4 \chi (t - \tau))) d\omega -$$

$$- 2h_l \int_0^\infty \exp(-h_l (l - \omega)) \exp(-(x + \xi + \omega - 3l)^2 / (4 \chi (t - \tau))) d\omega\} \qquad (6)$$

Here $h_0 = (\partial U / \partial x)_{x=0} / U(0, t)$, $h_l = (\partial U / \partial x)_{x=l} / U(l, t)$

The integrals over $d\omega$ in the formula for $G(x, \xi, t - \tau)$ can be calculated, so in place of the terms which are proportional to h_0 and h_l we have relations:

$$h_0 \exp[-(x + \xi)^2 / 4 \chi (t - \tau)] \exp(y^2) \text{Erfc}(y), \quad h_l \exp[-(2l - x - \xi)^2 / 4 \chi (t - \tau)] \exp(z^2) \text{Erfc}(z)$$

where $y = (h_0 + (x + \xi) / (2\chi(t - \tau))) (\chi(t - \tau))^{1/2}$; $z = [-h_l + (2l - x - \xi)] / (2\chi(t - \tau)) (\chi(t - \tau))^{1/2}$, **Erfc** (y) is the Additional Error Function.

So, the Green's function depends on h_0 and h_l and therefore on the temperature field near the sample surfaces. We can write $G = G(x, \xi, t - \tau, U(\xi, \tau))$. The equation (5) has been solved numerically for the values of $U(x, t)$ determined for a sequence (x_i, t_j), where $i, j = 0, 1, 2, 3 \ldots$. The step of this sequence over the co-ordinate was $\alpha^{-1}/40$, and in any case it was not higher than $l/40$. The step of the sequence over the time, Δ, was of 1 ms. Substituting $U(x_i, t_j - \Delta)$ as the «old» value of $U(x_i, t_j)$ into the right hand of the equation (5) we obtain the «new» value $U(x_i, t_j)$ in the left-side hand of this equation. The obtained system of transcendental equations was solved step by step over the time using the method[22] of bisection of the interval between the «new» and the «old» values $U(x_i, t_j)$. We used $U(x_0, t_0) = U_0 = 293$ K as a zero approximation and kept calculating until the maximum of the difference between two last approximations of $U(x, t)$ was less than 0.1 K.

6. CALCULATION RESULTS AND DISCUSSION

When cartilage bent the distance between negative charged groups decreases and this is a reason of repulsive forces and stress. The structure and a shape of cartilage is supported by water molecules promoting interaction between proteoglycan units (to create proteoglycan aggregates) and also between proteoglycan and collagen sub-systems of cartilage matrix. The heat of the bound-to-free transition of water in cartilage is about 27 ± 3 kJ/mole[14] that is close to the activation energy for mutual diffusion of water and proteoglycans[12,19] and to the energy of proteoglycan-collagen interaction estimated in[20]. That is why we can assume that liberation of bound water in cartilage promotes mobility of negative charged chains of proteoglycans and results in stress relaxation but may lead to tissue denaturation. The process of stress relaxation is due to some alteration in cartilage structure, but only when these alteration are significant we say about tissue denaturation.

In this paper, we studied the temperature field $U(x, t)$ and diffusion way L as functions of the following varied parameters: laser fluence (E), exposure time (τ_e), pulse repetition rate (f), cartilage slab thickness (l), absorption coefficient (α). Following characteristics of cartilage were used for calculations: $C = 4.2$ J/cm^3 K; $\chi = 1.4*10^{-3}$ cm^2/s, $\nu = 9*10^{11}$; $\lambda = 3.0*10^{-3}$ W/cm K; $Q = 44$ kJ/mole (all thermophysical properties of cartilage taken equal to these for water[12]); $M = 0.8$ g/cm^3; $V_P = 27$ kJ/mole [12], $D_0 = 4.8*10^{-3}$ cm^2/s [12,19]; $\tau_p = 1$ ms; $b = 1$; $U_0 = 293$ K; $U_w = 343$ K [14].

Some examples of temperature field calculated are shown in the Figures 1-3. Two cases of optically thick (at $l\alpha \gg 1$) and thin (at $l\alpha \ll 1$) samples have been considered for the same bulk density of laser energy $E\alpha \approx 80$ J/cm^3

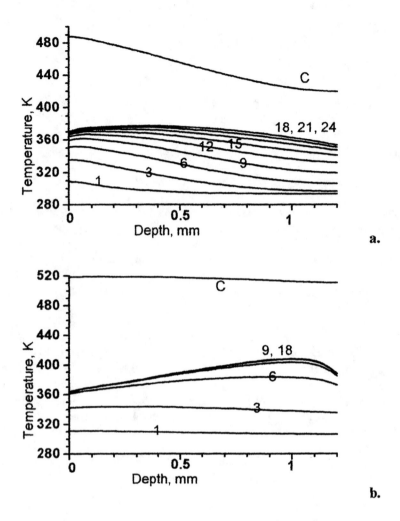

a.

b.

Fig. 1.   Temperature U of a cartilage plate at the end of each laser pulse (the numbers of pulses are dated on the curves) as a function of the distance from irradiated surface, x,
for $l = 1.2$ mm; $f = 5$ Hz;   **(a)** $\alpha = 40$ cm^{-1} , $E = 2$ J/cm^2, and (b) $\alpha = 3$ cm^{-1}, $E = 26.7$ J/cm^2;
C - the curves calculated for the maximal number of pulses without regard of the water evaporation.

The calculation results show that
1) Water evaporation from the cartilage surfaces effect very much on the temperature field,
2) There is a temperature maximum U_m at a some distance x_m from the irradiated surface
3) The values of U_m and x_m increase with τ_e, f and E , and decreases with α.
4) Temperature distribution changes with time only in the beginning of laser irradiation, and after some time becomes a quasi-stationary profile. As sample is thicker, the time to reach quasi-stationary profile of temperature is longer.
5) The quasi-stationary value of the surface temperature (U_s) has been reached faster than that, for the maximal temperature, U_m. It means that a control of the laser heating process by a measurement the surface temperature only, cannot give adequate information about heating level and structure alteration in the bulk of cartilage sample.

6) For various E, l and f, a dependence of stationary surface temperature on laser fluence can be approximated by a relation:

$$U_S = A_S \, (\, 1 - exp(-\beta_S \, E \,)) \; + U_0 \qquad\qquad (7)$$

where $A_S = 120 \pm 5$ K, $\beta_S^{-1} = 1.2 \pm 0.2$ J/cm^2. So, the surface temperature could be used as a signal for a feedback control system[13,17], only if E is not too high compared to β_S^{-1}.

7) Temperature oscillations represent to pulse repetition character of laser radiation (Fig.2). The amplitude of these oscillations increase with laser fluence and always is higher at the front sample surface (x=0) than that at x_m

8) When laser treatment stops, the kinetics of cooling slightly depends on E, f and τ_e

9) Period of time, τ_d, when $U > U_w$ is strongly dependent on parameters α, E, f and τ_e

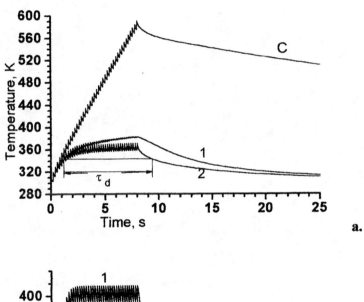

a.

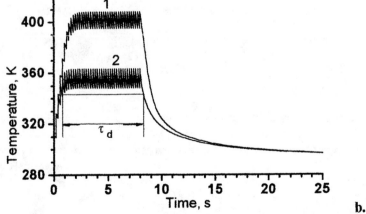

b.

Fig. 2. Time dependence of cartilage temperature for $l = 1.2$ mm; $f = 5$ Hz; $\tau_e = 8$ s; (a) $\alpha = 40$ cm^{-1}, $E = 2$ J/cm^2, and (b) $\alpha = 3$ cm^{-1}, $E = 26.7$ J/cm^2; (1) is the maximal temperature, (2) is the temperature on the irradiated surface, (C) is the surface (maximal) temperature calculated without regard of surface evaporation of water; τ_d is time of diffusion.

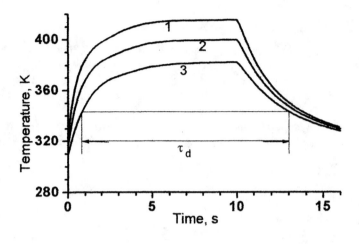

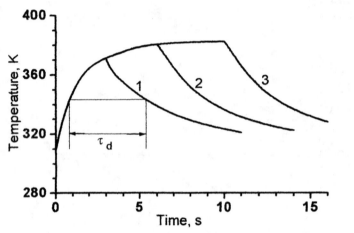

Fig.3. Time dependence of cartilage temperature at the end of laser pulses,
for $l = 1.2$ mm; $f = 5$ Hz; $\alpha = 40$ cm^{-1}
(a) various laser fluences at $\tau_e = 10$ s , (1) $E = 4$ J/cm^2, (2) $E = 3$ J/cm^2, (3) $E = 2$ J/cm^2.
(b) various exposure times at $E = 2$ J/cm^2, (1) $\tau_e = 3$ s, (2) $\tau_e = 6$ s, (3) $\tau_e = 10$ s.

The distance of mass diffusion during a period of time τ_d are calculated for various α, E, f and τ_e (Figs.4,5). These results predict a heterogeneity of structure alteration and denaturation of cartilage irradiated. There is a sharp boundary in the bulk of a sample between areas of altered and non-altered structure, for $\alpha = 40$ 1/cm. For $\alpha = 3$ 1/cm, mass transfer is more homogeneous, but also may give different results at different distances from the irradiated surface. This kind of laminated structure could be easily observed by histological examination of a tissue. Note that the structure can be changed dramatically in the bulk of a sample with very slightly affected at the surfaces. The maximal diffusion way as a function of laser fluence is shown in the Fig.5. There are thresholds of laser-induced structure alteration and denaturation depending on laser exposure time and wavelength. Depth of structure alteration increases with laser fluence and exposure time (Fig.6). For small E and τ_e, when $L < 5$ micrometers, alterations of cartilage structure may lead to stress relaxation without tissue denaturation. For higher E and τ_e, mass transfer leads to non-reversible dramatic changes in structure (tissue denaturation).

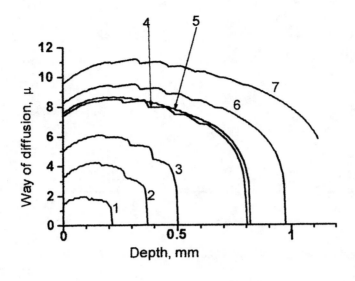

a.

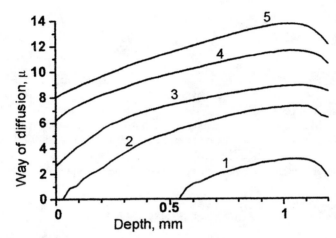

b.

Fig.4. Way of the proteoglycan diffusion, for l =1.2 mm, τ_e = 3 s,
(a) α = 40 1/cm; E = (1) 1.33, (2) 1.50, (3) 1.66, (4) 2.16, (5) 2.16 J/cm^2; f = 20 Hz,
    (6) E = 2.33 J/cm^2, f = 5 Hz, (7) E = 2.5 J/cm^2, f = 5 Hz, for (1-4,6,7);
(b) α = 3 1/cm, f =5 Hz; E = (1) 8.9, (2) 11.1, (3) 13.3, (4) 17.7, and (5) 22.4 J/cm^2

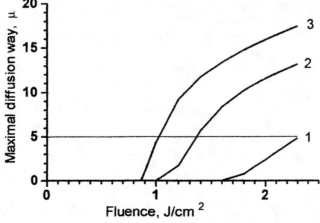

Fig.5. Maximal diffusion way as a function of laser fluence for α = 40 1/cm, f =5 Hz, l = 0.6 mm, and
various exposure times: (1) 1 s; (2) 2 s; (3) 3 s.

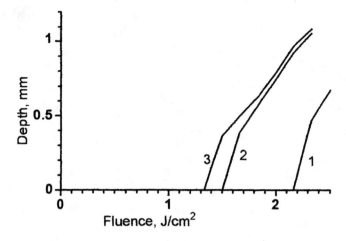

Fig.6. Depth of structure alterations vs laser fluence at various exposure times: (1) 1 s; (2) 2 s; (3) 3 s, for α = 40 1/cm, f =5 Hz, l =1.2 mm.

7. CONCLUSIONS

We develop a theoretical model to calculate the temperature field and the size of modified structure area in cartilaginous tissue. It is shown that: I) the maximal temperature is reached not on the surface irradiated at some distance from the surface; II) surface temperature reaches a plateau quicker than the maximal temperature; III) laser-induced mass transfer in cartilage is heterogeneous along the depth and may results in lamellar structure; IV) the depth of denatured area strongly depends on laser fluence and wavelength, exposure time and thickness of cartilage. The model allows to predict and control temperature and depth of structure alterations in the course of laser reshaping and treatment of cartilage.

8. ACNOWLEDGEMENTS

The authors thank the Russian Foundation of Basic Research (grants No 97-02-17465) and the Coherent Inc. for their support.

9. REFERENCES

1. E. Helidonis, E.N. Sobol. et al. "Laser shaping of composite cartilage grafts", *Amer. J.Otolaryngology*, Vol. 14, pp. 410-412, 1993.
2. E.N. Sobol, V.N. Bagratashvili, A.P Sviridov, et al. "Cartilage shaping under laser radiation", *Proc. SPIE*, Vol. 2128, pp. 43-49, 1994.
3. E.Helidonis, E.N.Sobol, G.Velegrakis, J.Bizakis, "Shaping of Nasal Septal Cartilage with the Carbon Dioxide Laser - Preliminary Report of an Experimental Study", *Lasers in Medical Science*, Vol. 9, pp. 51-54, 1994.
4. E.Helidonis, E.N.Sobol, G.Velegrakis, J.Bizakis, "Shaping of Nasal Septal Cartilage with the Carbon Dioxide Laser - Preliminary Report of an Experimental Study", *Lasers in Medical Science*, Vol. 9, pp. 51-54, 1994.
5. E.Helidonis, M.Volitakis, I. Naumidi, et al. "The histology of laser thermo-chondroplasty", *Amer J. Otolaryngology*, Vol. 15, pp. 423-428, 1994.
6. E.N. Sobol, *Phase Transformations and Ablation in Laser-Treated Solids*, John Wiley &Sons Inc., New York, 1995.
7. G.Velegrakis, M.Volitakis, I.Naumidi, et al. «Thermoplasty of rabbit ear cartilage using the carbon dioxide laser», *Lasers in Medical Science*, Vol.9, pp.265-272, 1994.

8. Z.Wang, M.M.Pankratov, D.F.Perrault, S.M.Shapshay, "Laser-assisted cartilage reshaping: in vitro and in vivo animal studies", *Proc. SPIE*, Vol.2395, pp.296-302, 1995.

9. E.N. Sobol, V.N. Bagratashvili, A.P Sviridov, et al. "Phenomenon of cartilage shaping using moderate laser heating", *Proc. SPIE*, Vol.2623, pp.548-553, 1996.

10. E.N. Sobol, V.N. Bagratashvili, A.P Sviridov., et al. "Stress relaxation and cartilage shaping under laser radiation", *Proc. SPIE*, Vol.2681, pp. 358-363, 1996.

11. Z.Wang, M.M.Pankratov, D.F.Perrault, S.M.Shapshay, "Laser-assisted reshaping of collapsed tracheal cartilage. A laboratory study", *Ann.Otol.Rhinol.Laryngol.*, Vol.105, pp.176-181, 1996.

12. V.N. Bagratashvili, E.N. Sobol, A.P Sviridov, et al. "Thermal and diffusion processes in laser-induced stress relaxation and reshaping of cartilage" *Journal of Biomechanics*, Vol.30, No.8, pp.813-817, 1997

13. B.J.F.Wong, T.E.Milner, B.Anvary, et al "Thermo-optical properties of cartilage during feedback controlled laser-assisted shaping", *Proc SPIE*, Vol. 2970, pp. 380-391, 1977.

14. E.N. Sobol, A.P Sviridov, A.I. Omel'chenko et al. "Mechanism of laser-induced stress relaxation in cartilage", *Proc SPIE*, Vol. 2975, 1997.

15. E.N.Sobol. "Possible mechanisms of cartilage reshaping under laser radiation", *Journ.Techn.Phys Lett.*, 1997 (in press)

16. A.Sviridov, E.Sobol, N.Jones, J.Lowe. " Effect of Holmium laser radiation on stress, temperature and structure alterations in cartilage", *Lasers in Medical Science*, 1997 (in press).

17. G.P.Chebotareva, B.V.Zubov, A.P.Nikitin, S.M.Nikiforov, E.N.Sobol, "Pulsed Photothermal Radiometry of Surgical Laser-Tissue Interaction", *Proc SPIE*, , Vol. 2681, pp. 5-16. 1996.

18. D.Comper. «Physicochemical aspects of cartilage extracellular matrix» in: *Cartilage: Molecular Aspects*, Eds.B.Hall and S.Newman, CRC Press, Boca Raton, 1991.

19. A.M.Jamieson, J.Blackwell, H.Reihanian, et al. «Thermal and solvent stability of proteoglycan aggregates by quasielastic laser light scattering», *Carbohydrate Research*, Vol. 160, pp.329-341, 1987.

20. J.E.Scott. 'Proteoglycan - fibrillar collagen interaction', *Biochem. J.* Vol.252, pp.313-323, 1988.

21. A.N.Tikhonov and A.A.Samarskii, *Equations of mathematical physics*, Nauka, Moscow, 1966.

22. R.W.Hamming, *Numerical methods for scientists and engineers*, Mc Graw-Hill, New York, 1962.

Laser induced heat diffusion limited tissue coagulation. II Effect of random temperature nonuniformities on the form of a spherical and cylindrical necrosis domain

I. A. Lubashevsky, A. V. Priezzhev

Department of Physics, Moscow State University,
Moscow 119899,

ABSTRACT

When heated the living tissue exhibits temperature nonuniformities due to the vessel discreteness. On small scales the particular details of the vessel arraignments are practically unknown, so we regard such nonuniformities as random.

When the tissue region affected directly by laser light is sufficiently small heat diffusion into the surrounding tissue is responsible for the necrosis growth. In this case strong temperature dependence of the thermal coagulation rate gives rise to the substantial perturbations the necrosis boundary due to the random temperature nonuniformities. In the previous papers[1,2] we have analyzed this effect assuming the necrosis boundary quasiplane. In particular, we have found that for typical values of the tissue parameters the correlation length of such perturbations can be comparable with the necrosis size in magnitude.

Therefore, the present paper studies the effect of the random temperature nonuniformities for a necrosis domain of spherical and cylindrical form. In this way we are able to analyze this effect for a more realistic situation, namely, depending on the form of an applicator delivering laser light inside the tissue. In particular, we have shown that for cylindrical applicators the effect of the vessel discreteness can be described by the developed previously model.[1,2] For spherical applicators of small size (about several millimeters) this effect is depressed because in this case blood perfusion does not affect substantially the necrosis growth.

1. INTRODUCTION

In the previous papers[1,2] we have studied the effect of the vessel discreteness on the form of the necrosis domain whose growth is due to local thermal coagulation. By way of example, we have considered the following physical model (Fig. 1). Absorption of laser light delivered into a small internal region of living tissue causes the temperature to attain such high values (about 70 °C) that lead to immediate coagulation of the tissue in this region. Heat diffusion into the surrounding live tissue gives rise to its further thermal coagulation and, subsequently, to the necrosis growth.

Vessels directly controlling the heat exchange between the tissue and blood are separated by distances much greater than their radii, so in the vicinity of the necrosis domain there should be spatial nonuniformities $\delta T(\mathbf{r}, t)$ in the temperature caused by the vessel discreteness.[3] Due to extremely strong dependence of the thermal coagulation rate on temperature these nonuniformities affect substantially the necrosis growth, perturbing the necrosis form.[1,2]

Since the particular details of the vessel arrangement alter in various tissues it is reasonable to use an approach considering the vascular network random.[4] In this way the given temperature nonuniformities should be also treated as random and characterized by the mean amplitude σ and the correlation length λ.

When the tissue is heated by a uniform source to a mean temperature $\overline{T}$ the amplitude σ and the correlation length λ can be estimated as:[5]

$$\sigma \sim \frac{1}{L_n}(\overline{T} - T_a), \qquad \lambda \sim \ell_v \sim \frac{1}{\sqrt{L_n}}\ell_T . \tag{1}$$

Here T_a is the arterial blood temperature in systemic circulation, ℓ_v is the characteristic length of vessels controlling the heat exchange between the tissue and blood,

$$\ell_T \sim \sqrt{\frac{\kappa}{c\rho j f}} \sim 10\,\mathrm{mm} \tag{2}$$

E-mails: lub@moldyn.phys.msu.su (I. A. Lubashevsky); avp@lbp.phys.msu.su (A. V. Priezzhev)

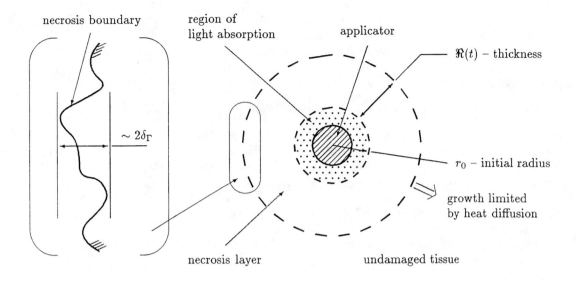

Figure 1. The necrosis growth due to local thermal coagulation limited by heat diffusion. The physical system under consideration.

is the mean penetration length ℓ_T of the temperature into perfused tissue due to heat diffusion and its estimate is given for typical values of thermal conductivity $\kappa \sim 7 \cdot 10^{-3}$ W/cm·K, heat capacity $c \sim 3.5$ J/g·K, and density $\rho \sim 1$ g/cm^3 of the tissue, the perfusion rate $j \sim 0.3$ min^{-1}, and the factor* $f \sim 1/\sqrt{L_n} \sim 0.5$ accounting for the counter-current effect.[6,7] The factor $L_n = \ln(l/a)$, where l/a is the mean ratio of the individual length to radius of blood vessels forming peripheral systems of blood circulation. For the typical value[9] of $l/a \sim 40$ we get $L_n \approx 4$. Taking also into account a numerical factor[5] in the former expression of (1) we get $\sigma \approx (10\text{–}20)\% \, (\overline{T} - T_a)$ and $\sigma \sim 3\text{–}6\,°C$ for the typical value $\overline{T} \sim T^* \sim 65\,°C$ of the temperature in the layer where thermal coagulation is under way.[1,2]

For applicators whose size in not small (about or greater than centimeter) the length ℓ_T also gives the mean thickness $\Re \sim \ell_T$ of the necrosis layer formed during a typical course of local thermal treatment.[10,11] In this case the averaged temperature field $T(\mathbf{r}, t)$ (i.e. the temperature averaged over the vessel arrangement) can be treated as uniform on spatial scales about ℓ_v and formulae (1) give the correct result for the random temperature nonuniformites near the necrosis boundary. In particular, we have shown[1,2] that under such conditions the mean amplitude δ_Γ of the necrosis boundary perturbations is

$$\delta_\Gamma \sim \frac{1}{\sqrt{L_n}} \ell_v \sim \frac{1}{L_n} \Re. \tag{3}$$

It should be noted that the factor $1/L_n$ plays the role of small parameter in the theory of bioheat transfer.[5] So the given estimate enables us to consider the value of δ_Γ small in comparison with the necrosis size $\Re$ and the correlation length λ of the random temperature nonuniformities:

$$\delta_\Gamma \ll \Re, \lambda. \tag{4}$$

However, when the characteristic size of the applicator is sufficiently small (about a few millimeters) the temperature field becomes substantially nonuniform not only due to heat dissipation caused by the blood perfusion but also because of the geometric factor caused by the heat propagation from the applicator into the surrounding tissue. In this case the necrosis growth is depressed by that the temperature at the necrosis boundary has inevitably to drop as the necrosis domain increases in size. Under such conditions the thickness $\Re$ of the necrosis region is less then ℓ_T, namely, can be about ℓ_v[12] and estimates (1) should be modified in order to describe the effect of vessel discreteness on the temperature random nonuniformites near the necrosis boundary and, thus, to describe its perturbations.

---

*It should be noted that a similar numerical estimate for the factor f is presented in Ref. 8

The main purpose of the present paper is to analyze the characteristics of these random perturbations of the necrosis form depending on the form and dimensions of applicators. A theory that can describe the effect of vessel discreteness on the temperature distribution when it is remarkably nonuniform on scales about ℓ_v is far from being developed well. So in the present paper we confine ourselves to a qualitative analysis only and will follow the qualitative approach developed[1] and rigorously justified[2] for a thick necrosis layer ($\Re \sim \ell_T$).

2. RANDOM PERTURBATIONS OF THE NECROSIS BOUNDARY

Due to the strong dependence of the thermal coagulation rate on temperature the layer $\mathbb{L}_\zeta$ where thermal coagulation is under way is sufficiently thin. Namely, its thickness δ_ζ can be treated as the smallest spatial scale in the description of such a local thermal coagulation[13,14,1,2] and, so, we may assume that $\delta_\zeta \ll \delta_\Gamma$. The latter enables us to regard the layer $\mathbb{L}_\zeta$ as an infinitely thin interface Γ of the necrosis region whose motion is governed by the temperature T_c and by its gradient $G = \nabla_n T|_\Gamma$ at this interface.[13,14] By virtue of inequality (4) the perturbations of the necrosis interface Γ (Fig. 1) are well developed,[1,2] i.e. we may ignore transient processes in their evolution and, so, describe them in the steady state approximation. In this way we have shown[1,2] that the form of the interface Γ can be specified by treating the tissue temperature T_c as fixed, $T_c \approx T^* \sim 60\,^\circ\mathrm{C}$.

Therefore, if $\xi(\mathbf{s})$ is the local deviation of the necrosis interface Γ from its averaged position Γ_0 in the vicinity of a point $\mathbf{s}$, G is the unperturbed value of the temperature gradient near Γ, and $\delta T(\mathbf{s}, t)$ is the random nonuniformity of the temperature field at the given point, then we can write

$$G\xi(\mathbf{s}) + \delta T(\mathbf{s}, t) \approx T_c\,. \tag{5}$$

Whence it directly follows the estimate for the amplitude δ_Γ of the necrosis boundary perturbations:

$$\delta_\Gamma \sim \frac{\sigma}{G} \sim \Re \frac{\sigma}{(T_c - T_a)}\,, \tag{6}$$

where σ is the mean amplitude of the random temperature nonuniformties near the necrosis interface and, in addition, we have set $G \sim (T_c - T_a)/\Re$.

In order to find the value of σ let us make use of the generalized bioheat equation[7] for the live tissue:

$$c\rho \frac{\partial T}{\partial t} = \kappa_{\text{eff}} \nabla^2 T - c\rho f(j + \delta j)(T - T_a)\,, \tag{7}$$

where, however, we have singled out the nonuniformity $\delta j(\mathbf{r})$ in the blood perfusion rate caused by the vessel discreteness from the blood perfusion rate $j(\mathbf{r})$ averaged over the vessel arrangement. The effective thermal conductivity κ_{eff} of the perfused tissue is about the thermal conductivity of the cellular tissue,[7,15,5] $\kappa_{\text{eff}} \gtrsim \kappa$, and the amplitude of the random nonuniformities $\delta j(\mathbf{r})$ is of the same order as the averaged perfusion rate,[5] $\delta j(\mathbf{r}) \lesssim j(\mathbf{r})$. In the case under consideration when describing the temperature nonuniformities due to the vessel discreteness we, first, can ignore the transient term. Second, we consider the necrosis region of the cylindrical or spherical shape when the applicator size is sufficiently small and, as a result, the thickness $\Re$ of the necrosis region is less than the characteristic penetration depth ℓ_T of the temperature into perfused tissue due to heat diffusion. Thus, the term $c\rho f j(T - T_a)$ responsible for the temperature variations on scales about ℓ_T can be also ignored. Third, the tissue temperature $\overline{T}(\mathbf{r})$ averaged over the vessel arrangement does not vary substantially on scales about the characteristic length ℓ_v of the vessels controlling directly the heat exchange between the cellular tissue and blood.[5] Whence, in particular, it follows that the minimum of the necrosis thickness can be about ℓ_v, i.e. $\Re > \ell_v$. Besides, the length ℓ_v gives also the correlation length of the nonuniformites $\delta j(\mathbf{r})$ in the perfusion rate due to the vessel discreteness.[5] Therefore in the term $c\rho f \delta j(T - T_a)$ we may set $T \approx T_c$.

In this way for the random temperature nonuniformites we get the following equation:

$$\ell_T^2 \nabla^2 \delta T \approx \frac{\delta j}{j}(T_c - T_a)\,, \tag{8}$$

where, in addition, we have used expression (2). To estimate the amplitude σ of the temperature nonuniformities δT let us set $\delta j/j \sim 1$ and

$$\nabla^2 \delta T \sim \sigma \left(\frac{1}{\ell_v^2} + \frac{1}{\Re^2}\right)\,. \tag{9}$$

The latter term on the right-hand side of (9) qualitatively accounts for the finite thickness of the layer where the temperature drops from $T_c \sim 60\,°C$ to T_a. Then from (1), (6)–(9) we obtain the desirable result

$$\delta_\Gamma \sim \frac{1}{L_n}\Re\left[1 + \frac{\ell_v^2}{\Re^2}\right]^{-1}. \tag{10}$$

The given expression demonstrates the following. First of all, if the applicator size is large (about or greater than centimetre) the thickness of the necrosis domain $\Re \sim \ell_T \gg \ell_v$ and from (10) we again, as it must, obtain expression (3). For an applicator of the spherical form whose size is sufficiently small (about several millimeters) we have found[12] that the thickness $\Re$ of the necrosis region is approximately twice as small as the value of ℓ_T. So taking into account the numeral value of $L_n \approx 4$ and expression (1) we see that in this case $\Re \sim \ell_v$ and the amplitude of the necrosis interface perturbations should be less than one predicted by the model[1,2] for the quasiplane necrosis interface by several times. Moreover, in this case the perturbation amplitude δ_Γ can decrease even down to the thickness δ_ζ of the layer $\mathbb{L}_\zeta$ of partially damaged tissue where thermal coagulation is currently under way. Under such ultimate conditions further analysis of the vessel discreteness is of no physical meaning. In other words, for a necrosis region whose three spatial dimensions are substantially small (about several millimeters) the perturbations of its boundary due to the vessel discreteness are depressed considerably. This property is caused by the fact that in three-dimensional space the temperature field $T(\mathbf{r})$ induced by a small localized source even in a tissue without perfusion will decrease as $1/r$. So under such conditions it is this spatial decrease in temperature that mainly controls the necrosis growth rather than heat diffusion into the surrounding live tissue.

For applicators of the cylindrical form the effect of such a geometric factor is not so pronounced,[12] the thickness $\Re$ of the necrosis layer is not too small, $\Re \gtrsim \ell_v$, and the necrosis interface perturbations can be described with the previously developed model.[1,2] In particular, in this case estimate (3) can be applied to describe the necrosis interface perturbations.

3. CONCLUSION

In the present paper we continue our investigations[1,2] of the effect of the vessel discreteness on the necrosis growth caused by heat diffusion limited thermal coagulation. We have analyzed qualitatively this effect for applicators of the cylindrical and spherical geometry and have shown the following:

- For applicators of cylindrical form perturbations of the necrosis boundary caused by the vessel discreteness can be described by the model[1,2] developed for quasiplane geometry of the necrosis domain. In particular the amplitude of these perturbations is estimated as

$$\delta_\Gamma \sim \frac{1}{L_n}\Re,$$

where $\Re$ is the mean thickness of the necrosis layer (Fig. 1) and the factor $L_n \approx \ln(l/a)$ ($l/a \sim 40$ is the characteristic ratio of the individual length to radius of blood vessels forming peripheral circulation systems).

- For spherical applicators of small size (about several millimeters) the effect of the vessel discreteness is depressed because in this case blood perfusion does not affect the necrosis growth substantially.

ACKNOWLEDGMENTS

This research was supported in part by the Russian Foundation of Basic Researches, Grant 96-02-17576 (I. A. Lubashevsky) and Grant 96-15-97782 (Support of Leading Scientific Schools) (A. V. Priezzhev).

REFERENCES

1. I. A. Lubashevsky and A. V. Priezzhev. "Laser induced heat diffusion limited tissue coagulation. I. Form of the necrosis boundary caused by random temperature nonuniformities", in: *Laser-Tissue Interaction, Tissue Optics, and Laser Welding*, G. Delacrétaz, L. O. Svaasand, R. W. Steiner, R. Pini, and G. Godlewski, Editors, Proc. SPIE **3195**, 1997.

2. I. A. Lubashevsky and A. V. Priezzhev. "Effect of the blood vessel discreteness on the necrosis formation during laser induced thermal coagulation limited by heat diffusion" (submitted to *J. Biomed. Opt.*).

3. Y. W. Baish, P. S. Ayyaswamy, and K. R. Foster. "Small-scale temperature fluctuations in perfused tissue during local hyperthermia", *Trans. ASME J. Biomech. Eng.*, **108**, pp. 246–250, 1986.

4. Y. W. Baish. "Formulation of a statistical model of heat transfer in perfused tissue" *Trans. ASME. J. Biomech. Eng.* **116**, pp. 521–527, 1994.

5. I. A. Lubashevsky, V. V. Gafiychuk, and A. G. Cadjan. *Bioheat Transfer* (monograph, to be published).

6. S. Weinbaum and L. M. Jiji. "A new simplified bioheat equation for the effect of blood flow on local average tissue temperature", *Trans. ASME J. Biomech. Eng.* **107**, pp. 131–139, 1985.

7. COMAC–BME workshop on Modelling and Treatment Planning in Hyperthermia (Lagonissi 1990), Conclusions Subgroup Thermal Modelling. Reported by J. J. W. Lagendijk, *COMAC - BME Hyperthermia Bulletin*, **4**, pp. 47–49, 1990.

8. S. Weinbaum, L. X. Xu, L. Zhu, and A. Ekpene. "A new fundamental bioheat equation for muscle tissue. I. Blood perfusion term" *Trans. ASME. J. Biomech. Eng.*, **119**, pp. 278–288, 1997.

9. G. I. Mchedlishvili. *Microcirculation of Blood. General Principles of Control and Disturbances.* Nauka Publishers, Leningrad, 1989 (in Russian).

10. I. A. Lubashevsky, A. V. Priezzhev, V. V. Gafiychuk, and M. G. Cadjan. "Free-boundary model for local thermal coagulation", in: *Laser-Tissue Interaction VII*, S. L. Jacques, Editor, Proc. SPIE **2681**, pp. 81–91, 1996.

11. I. A. Lubashevsky, A. V. Priezzhev, V. V. Gafiychuk, and M. G. Cadjan. "Local thermal coagulation due to laser–tissue interaction as irreversible phase transition". *J. Biomed. Opt.* **2**(1), pp. 95–105, 1997.

12. I. A. Lubashevsky, A. V. Priezzhev, and V. V. Gafiychuk. "Free boundary model for local thermal coagulation. Growth of a spherical and cylindrical necrosis domain", in: *Laser–Tissue Interaction VIII*, S. L. Jacques, Editor, Proc. SPIE **2975**, pp. 43–53, 1997.

13. I. A. Lubashevsky, A. V. Priezzhev, V. V. Gafiychuk, and M. G. Cadjan. "Dynamic free boundary model for laser thermal tissue coagulation", in:*Laser-Tissue Interaction and Tissue Optics II*, H. J. Albrecht, G. Delacrétaz, T. H. Meier, R. W. Steiner, and L. O. Svaasand, Editors, Proc. SPIE **2923** pp. 48–57, 1996.

14. I. A. Lubashevsky, A. V. Priezzhev, V. V. Gafiychuk. "Effective interface dynamics of laser-induced heat diffusion-limited thermal coagulation", *J. Biomed. Opt.*, **3**(1), 1998.

15. J. Grezee. *Experimental Varification of Thermal Models* (Utrecht University, Utrecht, 1993).

Correlation of thermal and mechanical effects of the holmium laser for various clinical applications

Matthijs CM Grimbergen, Rudolf M Verdaasdonk and Christiaan FP van Swol

Department Of Clinical Physics and Biomedical Engineering [#]
University Hospital Utrecht, The Netherlands

ABSTRACT

The Holmium laser has become established in orthopedic surgery and urology due to its unique combination of mechanical and thermal properties induced by explosive vapor bubbles. In a specialized setup, real-time high-speed and thermal images of dynamic vapor bubbles and thermal relaxation at a water tissue interface were obtained simultaneously. The thermal effects in the tissue model were correlated to the characteristics of the bubbles dependent on pulse energy (0.2-4 J), pulse repetition frequency (5-40 Hz), distance and angle of fiber delivery system (diameter 365 μm) to the tissue surface. Up to a fiber-to-tissue distance of 50% of the radius of the bubble, only a superficial tissue layer was heated. During bubble implosion, the tissue surface was attracted to the fiber, ripping of irregularities, and was effectively cooled by turbulence. In case of hard tissues, the bubble detached from the fiber imploding towards the hard surface. At closer distances (<50% of bubble radius), the tissue itself was vaporized resulting in mechanical damage and thermal relaxation into the tissue, especially above repetition rates of 5 Hz.

There is a strong correlation between the path length of the free beam within the bubble and the degree of mechanical and thermal damage in the tissue directly irradiated by this beam.

During clinical applications the surgeon should be aware of the size of the vapor bubble in relation to the distance and angle with the tissue for safe and optimal use of the mechanical and thermal properties of the Holmium laser

Keywords: holmium, laser-tissue interaction, bubbles, thermal effects, clinical applications.

1. INTRODUCTION

Since the introduction of the holmium laser in the medical field, the number of applications has grown rapidly. This is mostly attributed to its unique combination of cutting and hemostatic capabilities [1]. The use of the Holmium laser for lithotripsy in urology [2] and for cartilage defects in orthopedic surgery [3] is commonly accepted. Applications like prostatectomy, and discectomy in neurosurgery [4] are evolving. Other fields of surgery e.g. dacryorhinocystotomy (DCR) in ophthalmology [5] are currently under investigation. Above mentioned procedures comprise as well hard as soft tissue applications. Depending on the tissue properties the surgeon needs a controlled extent of either thermal or mechanical tissue effects. However, the surgeon has a large range of laser settings and methods of energy delivery at his disposal.

Therefore, the aim of the study was to investigate the correlation between mechanical and thermal effects of the Holmium laser in relation to pulse energy, the pulse repetition rate and the angle of irradiation frequency to provide a 'rule of thumb' for the surgeon for a safe and optimized treatment strategy

---

[#] Further author information: RMV. (correspondence): email R.M.Verdaasdonk@id.azu.nl, website http://www.urolog.nl/lasercenter, tel: 31-30-2507302, fax: 31-30-2542002

2. HOLMIUM LASER TISSUE INTERACTION

The Holmium laser light is usually delivered to the tissue through fiber delivery systems under endoscopic guidance. Therefore, the fiber tip will be submerged is a liquid medium like water or saline. The 2.1 μm mid-infrared wavelength of the holmium laser light is absorbed in the first 500 μm layer of (tissue)water in front of the laser beam.

At the start of the typically 300 μs laser pulse, the water is instantly vaporized forming a rapidly expanding vapor bubble. The initial bubble creates an 'opening' through the liquid in front of the fiber. While the laser pulse continues, The beam vaporizes the front-end or 'top' of the bubble increasing the size and changing its shape to a 'pear'. This process is usually referred to as the 'Moses effect' [6]. This process is depicted in the sequence of still-frames in Figure 1.

At the end of the laser pulse the mechanical expansion still continues due to mass inertia until the underpressure will finally cause implosion of the vapor bubble. During implosion, the momentum of the liquid mass is focussed towards the center in implosion. The accelerated liquid forms jets and potentially shock waves capable of tearing soft and breaking hard tissues [7].

Although the penetration of the laser beam at the start of the laser pulse is only 500 μm, the beam can penetrate up to 15 mm into the (tissue)water at 4 J. Up to this distance tissue within the range of the bubble can be effected [8]. A distinction can be made between direct interaction with the tissue due to direct exposure to the laser beam and indirect interaction due to the bubble.

During bubble implosion the heat of condensation is dissipated in the surrounding liquid resulting in thermal effects in the liquid or tissue. In the liquid and at tissue surfaces, the thermal energy is effectively dissipated due to turbulence induced by the bubble implosion. In tissue, however, the temperature increase can be substantially. Depending on the temperature level, the tissue can be coagulated or thermally remodeled [9].

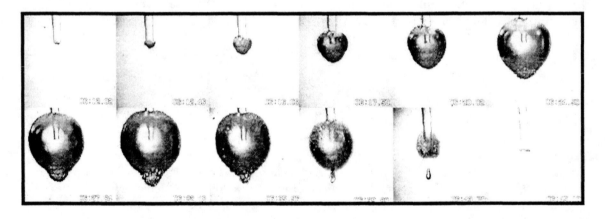

Figure 1. Holmium laser light induced expanding and collapsing vapor bubble.
Time frame of the sequence is about 1ms

3. MATERIAL & METHODS

To unravel the relation between the thermal and mechanical effects after holmium irradiation, the bubble dynamics, resulting in accumulation of thermal energy and destructive mechanical effects, were visualized simultaneously. Fast photography and Color-Schlieren techniques [10] were combined to obtain real-time mechanical and thermal action of the laser pulse near and within the tissue.

3.1 Fast photography

Time delayed high-speed photography with a temporal resolution of 1µs was used to capture the development of the bubble during the vaporization process and the implosion. A 'start of pulse' signal from the laser was time-delayed with a preset time to trigger an arc flash lamp illuminating the vaporization process at the fiber tip Figure 2. It is assumed that the vapor bubble formation is reproducible, so the sequential images of the ablation process were obtained from different individual bubbles at time-delays from 0 - 1000 µs.

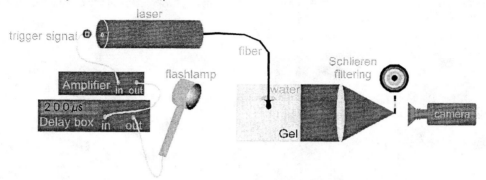

Figure 2. Experimental setup combining Schlieren optics and fast photography

3.2 Color Schlieren imaging

The thermal effects were visualized by means of Color Schlieren techniques based on an optical processor. Using this method, very small changes in optical density, induced by flow, pressure or temperature gradients inside an optically transparent medium, can be color-coded resulting in color images. These images are obtained with resolutions in the millisecond region and are comparable with thermal-images produced by a thermo-camera. The feasibility of this technique was shown in previous studies of thermal effects of cw and pulsed lasers [10].

3.3 Artificial tissue, PAA gel

For the setups used in this study, the ablation effects of the irradiated tissue can only be visualized in transparent media. Therefore, a polyacrylamide gel (PAA) was used which resembles tissue such that it consists of merely water in a matrix of organic molecules and consequently thermal characteristics are comparable to biological tissue. For the highly absorbed wavelength of the Holmium laser, it was assumed that beam scattering could be neglected so the optical properties are also similar. The use of polyacrylamide gel ensures reproducibility of the samples and enables molding of the material in the required geometry for a Schlieren setup.

3.4 Laser and experimental settings

An 80W Holmium laser (Coherent Versa Pulse, Palo Alto, Ca) was used; the maximum pulse energy was 4J at a repetition frequency of 20 Hz and maximally 40 Hz with 2 J pulses. The experiments were performed under conditions and settings, simulating the clinical situation as observed during orthopedic surgery and urologic treatments. In a water environment, the distance and angle of a 365 µm bare fiber tip was varied in relation to the surface of the tissue model, which was exposed to series of laser pulses. Table 1 gives an overview of the parameters varied during the experiments. During laser exposure real-time images were recorded on video. From the videotape, hard copies of still-frames were obtained for measurements.

Table 1. Overview experimental settings

	Energy	Angle	Distance	Rep. Rate
range	0.2 - 4 J	0 – 90°	1 - 5 mm	5 - 40 Hz

4. RESULTS

4.1 Basic laser-tissue interaction: bubble size and thermal zone

Because of the thermal as well as mechanical action mechanism, the experiments were aimed at determination of the relation of both effects. The size of bubble was directly related to the energy content of the laser pulse as shown in Figure 3.

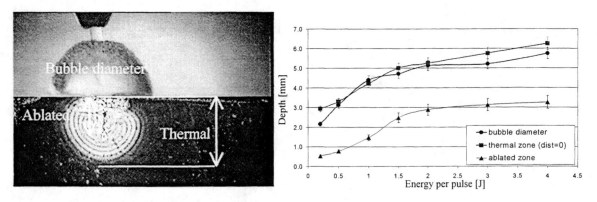

Figure 3. Measured values of the bubble and its tissue effects.

The left image shows a composition of a fast photography and a thermal image from the same `bubble formation'. The dark area represents the artificial tissue with water on top. Arrows refer to the dimensions obtained for bubble size, extent of the thermal and ablated zone. The right graph shows bubble diameter, the extent of the thermal as well as the ablated zone as function of the energy per pulse. The thermal zone was determined after 5 pulses and shows a good correlation with the bubble diameter.

The ablated zone was defined as the area where cracks could be observed in the model. These cracks can be attributed to vapor formed in the polyacrylamide gel structure itself by absorption of the laser beam as illustrated in the top row images of Figure 6. The curve of the ablated zone in Figure 3 correlates to about half the bubble diameter. The originally pear shaped vapor bubble is deformed by the tissue surface since the vapor can expand less freely like in an all liquid environment due to mechanical properties of the artificial tissue.

4.2 Accumulation of thermal energy

Figure 4 shows the accumulation of thermal energy after consecutive pulses of 0.5 J at 5 Hz, irradiated under a 45° angle. At this distance, the bubble partly overlaps the tissue. The thermal area grows especially during the first 5 pulses. Between 5 to 10 pulses, this area expands slowly to thermal equilibrium. The images after 5 and 10 pulses also show the ablated area clearly. This tissue area is located in the path of the beam and is vaporized by direct irradiation.

At the surface of the tissue, the presence of 'thermal flares' suggests turbulence induced by the imploding bubbles contributing to effective heat dissipation in the water. The combined effect of heat conduction into the tissue and effective surface cooling due to turbulence, might explain the onset of a thermal equilibrium already after 5-10 pulses.

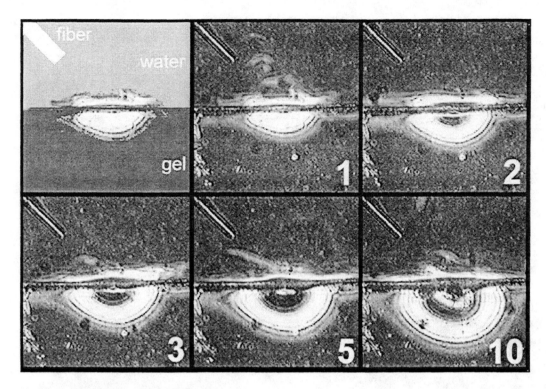

Figure 4. Accumulation of thermal energy.

4.3 Thermal effects in relation to irradiation angle

The tissue surface was irradiated at particular angles and distances. Figure 5 shows the extent of the thermal area for various angles of irradiation while the distance from the fiber tip to the tissue along the axis of the fiber (path of the laser beam) is constant at 2 mm. The images were captured after 5 pulses of 2 J at 5 Hz. The thermal effect is most pronounced at perpendicular irradiation and when the fiber is in contact with the tissue (0 degrees).

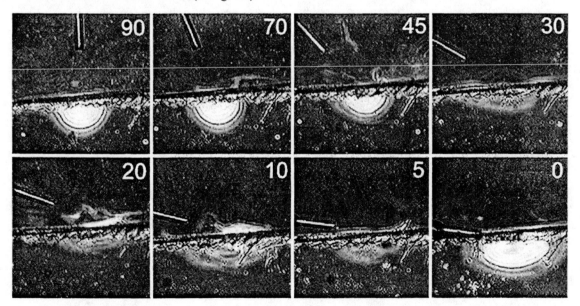

Figure 5. Thermal effect in tissue in relation to the irradiation angle at constant
(2 mm) distance of beam to tissue.

When the distance to the tissue was minimized to a few tenths of a millimeter the thermal effect was substantial for all angles and also shows a good correlation with the dimensions of the bubble as illustrated before in Figure 3. The composition in Figure 6 shows the bubble shape and the resulting thermal effect in the tissue at 90, 45 and 10-degree angles after 5 pulses of 0.5 J at 5 Hz. The bubble is clearly deformed by the presence of the tissue while the tissue surface itself is pushed down. Also the formation of the cracks in the tissue within the path of the laser beam emitted through the vapor bubble is evidently visible.

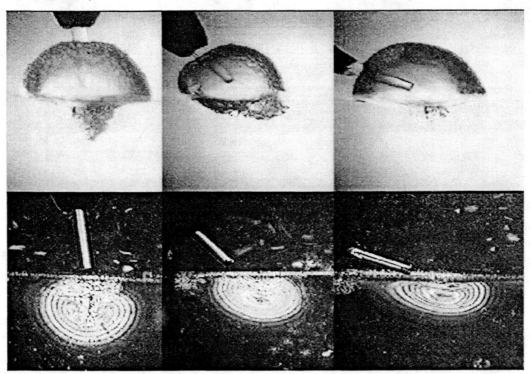

Figure 6. Bubble shape (top row) and thermal effect (bottom row) at close distance to tissue at 90 (left), 45 (middle) and 15 (right) irradiation angles after 5 pulses of 0.5 J at 5 Hz.

From the captured still-frames for the various angles at close distance to the tissue, the dimensions of the thermal zone were determined as illustrated in Figure 7 (left). The thermal area was characterized by the extent of thermal effect into the depth and in the direction of the fiber (or path of the beam). The results in relation to the angle of irradiation are presented in Figure 7 (right). The asymmetry of the thermal area in the tissue is closely related to the path of the beam irradiating the tissue and is especially pronounced at shallow irradiation angles.

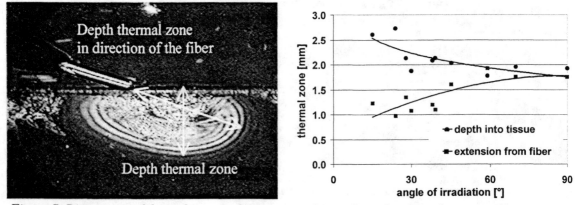

Figure 7. Dimensions of thermal zone in the tissue in relation to angle of irradiation at close distance to the tissue.

4.4 Bubble implosion

Depending on the pulse energy, the bubble implodes between 500 to 1000 µs after the start of the laser pulse. During bubble implosion, a distinctive difference was observed between the mechanical effects near hard and soft tissue surfaces. In case of soft tissue, the tissue surface was attracted towards the fiber tip (Figure 8, left) while in case of hard tissue the bubble detached from the fiber tip and the implosion was concentrated at the hard tissue surface (Figure 8 right). During bubble implosion fluid is sucked into the cavity of condensing vapor. Soft tissue easily deforms under these pressures and will give in towards the implosion center. If the elastic properties are high enough the tissue will bounce back into its original shape after the implosion. However, soft tissues with a weaker structure will fractured into small pieces and detach from the underlying structure.

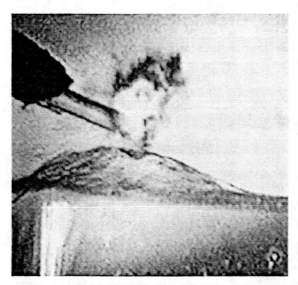 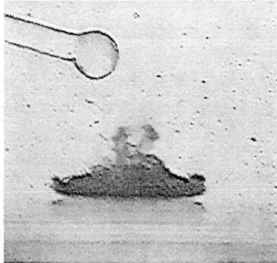

Figure 8. Mechanical tissue effects during a bubble implosion near a soft (left) and hard (right) tissue surface.

5. DISCUSSION

The Holmium laser is becoming more accepted for various clinical application since surgeons begin to appreciate this unique combination of mechanical and thermal properties. However, this versatility of the laser makes a controlled medical application difficult especially for novices. There are many parameters that contribute to the resulting thermal and mechanical effects in the biological tissue and that can be both beneficial and adverse at the same time. In this study a correlation was determined between mechanical effects induced by bubbles and the thermal effects in tissue depending on angle of irradiation, distance to the tissue and pulse energy.

5.1 Rule of thumb for Mechanical and Thermal effects

To provide the surgeon with a rule of thumb what tissue effects to expect for the parameter mentioned, the results of this study are summarized in the simple graphical representation of the bubble in Figure 9. The tissue effects are divided in mechanical and thermal.

Mechanical Effect   **Thermal Effect**

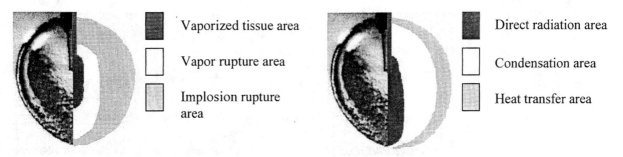

Mechanical Effect
- Vaporized tissue area
- Vapor rupture area
- Implosion rupture area

Thermal Effect
- Direct radiation area
- Condensation area
- Heat transfer area

Figure 9. Thermal and mechanical effective areas in relation to the original bubble shape.

Thermal tissue effects (fig.9, right)

Direct irradation area

The central area within the bubble represents the laser beam emitted from the fiber. Liquid or tissue that comes within this area will be directly exposed to the laser beam. Although, the first 500 μm layer will be vaporized at first instance, the vapor will create an opening to more distal layers as long as the laser pulse continues.

Condensation area

During and after implosion of the bubble, condensation heat will be dissipated into the liquid or tissue layer that was in direct contact will the bubble surface. This layer will at first be near 100 °C with a steep temperature gradient and consequently, due to thermal conduction to surrounding layers, cool rapidly to ambient temperatures effecting tissue up to a few millimeters.

Heat transfer area

If multiple pulses are given at a particular repetition rate, the temperature gradient in the condensation zone is sustained and heat is conducted to deeper layer surrounding this area. An equilibrium is reached after a series of pulses depending on the repetition rate and pulse energy. For 5 Hz, dimensions of this area are comparable with the original bubble size.

This description of the thermal areas can be interpreted independent from the angle of irradiation by projecting the boundaries of the areas over the tissue surface at a particular distance and angle and discern the overlap with the specific areas.

Mechanical effects (fig.9, left)

Vaporized tissue area

The central area within the bubble represents the laser beam emitted from the fiber. Most of the tissue within the beam starting from the laser tip is ablated leaving hole in the tissue. Due to the explosive mechanism of ablation the walls of these cavities are fractures. Due to mechanical resistance of the tissue the beam does not reach as far as the expanding bubble in a liquid. Therefore the mechanical effect extends to about half the bubble diameter as shown in Figure 3.

Vapor rupture area

Alongside and in front of the vaporized tissue area, tissue is ruptured due to the explosive expansion of the vapor. Depending on the mechanical properties of the tissue, the vapor will find its way of lowest resistance like weak spots in the tissue or along anatomical structures. Typically, this area might reach about two times the dimensions of the vaporized tissue area.

Implosion ruptured area

As illustrated in Figure 8, the vapor bubble will effect the tissue depending on the mechanical structure.

Soft tissue at the boundary of the bubble will be sucked toward the fiber tip during implosion and parts will detach from the underlying structure.

During implosion near a hard surface, there is no inflow of liquid from the hard surface. Due to the influx of fluid from the other side of the bubble, the implosion is directed towards the hard surface. This fluid dynamical process can result in forceful water jets projected towards the surface. The impact of the momentum of these water jets at collision might break the hard surface to pieces. This could be one of the mechanisms of lithotripsy [11].

Elastic tissue will deform during implosion but will resist the forces associated with the implosion and rebound to this original shape without noticeable mechanical damage at macroscopic level. However, there might be damage at cellular level and indirect thermal damage as described in the thermal section.

This description of the mechanical areas can be interpreted independent from the angle of irradiation by projecting the boundaries of the areas over the tissue surface at a particular distance and angle and discern the overlap with the specific areas. However, it can be expected that the magnitude of the mechanical effect will depend on the distance to the tissue.

5.2 Clinical implications

Orthopedic surgery

The treatment goal in arthroscopic procedures concerns cartilage defects by shaving off affected filaments and 'sealing' the surface to prevent the creation of new anomalies [12]. The firmaments consist of soft tissue fragments attached to the underlying stiff cartilage structure. To remove or shave off these irregularities, the cartilage should be irradiated at shallow angles (5-10°) and relatively low power settings (0.5-0.8 J, 5-10 Hz). Taking Figure 9 in consideration, the firmaments will be within the vapor implosion area and thermal condensation area. During implosion, the fragments will detach from the underlying cartilage that will be heated superficially and remodeled to a smooth surface. In order to control the thermal energy deposited in the cartilage, the fiber should be moved over the surface during irradiation at repetition rates not exceeding 10 Hz.

Urology

Lithotripsy in urology is a typical hard tissue application, where the objective is the breaking of the stone [13]. These stones are typically located in the bladder and the ureter. The stone should be located within the range of the vaporized tissue area while the walls of either the bladder or ureter are outside this range. The surface of the stone itself will be ablated together with the surrounding liquid. The implosion of the vapor bubble toward the stone surface will contribute to the breaking of the stone. The recommended pulse energies would be 0.5 - 1 J. At higher energies the expanding bubble (diameter over 4 mm) would for instance dilate the ureter resulting in adverse mechanical effects. The pulse should be applied in short bursts of a few pulses to prevent accumulation of heat in the ureter wall [14]. The situation in the bladder is less critical.

6. CONCLUSION

There is a strong correlation between the path length of the free beam within the bubble and the degree of mechanical and thermal damage in the tissue directly irradiated by this beam

Knowing the dimensions of the vapor bubble, the surgeon is able to control the mechanical and thermal effects in tissue in relation to the distance and angle of the fiber with the tissue for safe and optimal application of the Holmium laser

The versatility of the Holmium laser

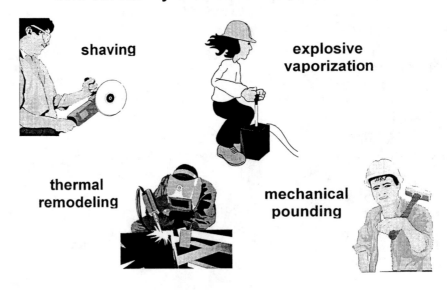

shaving

explosive vaporization

thermal remodeling

mechanical pounding

7. REFERENCES

1. Holmium:YAG surgical lasers. *Health Devices.* 1995;24:92-122

2. Johnson DE, Cromeens DM, Price RE: Use of the holmium:YAG laser in urology. *Lasers Surg.Med.* 1992;12:353-363

3. Smith CF: Lasers in orthopedic surgery [editorial]. *Orthopedics.* 1993;16:531-534.

4. Casper GD, Hartman VL, Mullins LL: Results of a clinical trial of the holmium:YAG laser in disc decompression utilizing a side-firing fiber: a two-year follow-up. *Lasers.Surg.Med.* 1996;19:90-96.

5. Silkiss RZ: THC:YAG nasolacrimal duct recanalization. *Ophthalmic Surg* 1993;24:772-774.

6. Leeuwen AGJM v, Veen MJ vd, Verdaasdonk RM, Borst C: Non-contact tissue ablation by holmium:YSGG laser pulses in blood. *Lasers Surg Med* 1991;11:26-34.

7. Jansen ED, Asshauer T, Frenz M, Motamedi M, Delacretaz G, Welch AJ: Effect of pulse duration on bubble formation and laser-induced pressure waves during holmium laser ablation. *Lasers.Surg.Med* 1996;18:278-293.

8. Leeuwen AGJM van, Veen MJ vd, Verdaasdonk RM, Borst C: Tissue ablation by holmium:YSGG laser pulses through saline and blood, in Jacques SL (ed): *Laser-tissue interaction II.* Bellingham, SPIE Vol 1427, 1991, pp 214-219

9. Vangsness CT, Jr., Watson T, Saadatmanesh V, Moran K: Pulsed Ho:YAG laser meniscectomy: effect of pulsewidth on tissue penetration rate and lateral thermal damage. *Lasers.Surg.Med* 1995;16:61-65.

10. Verdaasdonk RM: Imaging laser induced thermal fields and effects, in Jacques SL (ed): *Laser-Tissue interaction VI.* Bellingham, SPIE Vol 2391, 1995, pp 165-175.

11. Zeman RK, Davros WJ, Garra BS, Goldberg JA, Horii SC, Silverman PM, Cattau EL J, Hayes, WS, Cooper CJ: Relationship between stone motion, targeting, and fragmentation during experimental biliary lithotripsy. *Radiology.* 1990;176:125-128.

12. Vangsness CT, Jr., Ghaderi B: A literature review of lasers and articular cartilage. *Orthopedics.* 1993;16:593-598.

13. Yiu MK, Liu PL , Yiu TF, Chan AY: Clinical experience with holmium:YAG laser lithotripsy of ureteral calculi. *Lasers.Surg.Med* 1996;19:103-106.

14. Swol CFP v, Verdaasdonk RM, Zeijlemaker B, Boon TA: Optimalization of the dosimetry and safety using the Holmium laser for urology. In Watson GM (ed): *Lasers in Urology* Bellingham, SPIE Vol 3245, 1998.

Accidental Bilateral Q-Switched Neodymium Laser Exposure: Treatment and Recovery of Visual Function

Harry Zwick[a], Bruce E. Stuck[a], Weldon Dunlap[c], David K. Scales[b],
David J. Lund[a] and James W. Ness[a]

[a]US Army Medical Research Detachment, Walter Reed Army Institute of Research, 7914 A Drive,
Brooks AFB, TX 78235
[b]Retina and Uveitis Consultants of Texas, P.A., San Antonio, TX 78299
[c]Department of Ophthalmology, Brooke Army Medical Center, Fort Sam Houston, TX 78234

ABSTRACT

A 21 year old female was accidentally exposed in both eyes when she looked into the 10 cm exit aperture of a military laser designator emitting 1064 nm q-switched (30 ns) pulses at a 10 pulse per second rate. Steroid therapy (methylprednisolone sodium succinate) was initiated within 6 hours post exposure. Initial ophthalmoscopic observation revealed small contained macular hemorrhages in each eye. Fluorescein angiography (FA) showed minimal leakage. Visual acuity was 20/100 and 20/60 in OD and OS respectively. Contrast sensitivity in both eyes was depressed across all spatial frequencies by more than 1.5 log units. At four weeks post exposure, no significant macular scarring was apparent and visual acuity returned to 20/25 in both eyes. Contrast sensitivity had improved to normal levels with a peak at 3 cycles/degree. At one year post exposure, visual acuity was 20/13 in both eyes and measures of contrast sensitivity were within normal limits. During the course of recovery, the patient's fixation shifted from a slightly superior temporal site back to the central foveal region. The foveal lesion sites were still evident by ophthalmoscopy and Amsler grid measurements but were deemed functional when the patient placed small targets generated by the scanning laser ophthalmoscope in the lesion site for discrimination. This outcome indicates remarkable recovery of visual function and suggests that early administration of steroids may assist in preserving the natural neural recovery process of the photoreceptor matrix by minimizing intraretinal scar formation.

Keywords: lasers, laser eye injury, visual acuity, contrast sensitivity, visual impairment, treatment, recovery, mechanisms, preferred retinal location, confocal scanning laser ophthalmoscopy, optical coherence tomography

1. INTRODUCTION

The degree of visual impairment caused by laser exposure of the retina depends not only on the amount of energy absorbed within the eye and the location of the lesion(s) within the retinal field but also on the subsequent biological response and adaptation to the injury. In published laser eye accident cases,[1-16] there is significant recovery in some cases[1,2,8,9,10,13,15] whereas in others, there is permanent loss of visual function.[1-14,16] Injury to the central retina (foveal region) is often considered the most debilitating due to high spatial and chromatic vision inherent to the fovea. Appropriate and efficacious treatment for laser-induced retinal injury remains an open issue. Longitudinal evaluations of the time course of laser accident cases[1-16] contribute to the understanding of injury and recovery mechanisms. Effects secondary to the acute laser-tissue interaction such as intraretinal scar, epiretinal membrane formation, retinal traction and nerve fiber layer loss contribute to the long-term effects on visual function. Adaptations to the injury such as the development of altered visual strategies[17] concomitant with the neural plasticity inherent in the visual system contribute to the recovery of function. An assessment of human accident cases permits evaluations of these responses which implicate medical treatment targets or strategies.

This paper describes a recovery of visual function after bilateral foveal exposure from a q-switched laser. In this case, recovery of visual acuity and contrast sensitivity functions over a fourteen month period is based on the return of foveal functionality rather than the development of a pseudofovea. This case history is compared with a previously reported laser exposure incident where recovery of visual function results by the establishment of a pseudofovea located superior and temporal to the anatomical fovea.

2. METHODS

Laser Exposure Incident: A 21 year old female technician accidentally exposed both eyes when she looked into the 10 cm exit aperture of a military laser designator emitting 10 pulses per second at 1064 nm. The exit aperture of the neodymium YAG laser was supposed to be covered for this procedure and was mistaken for the eyepiece. No corrective or protective eyewear was worn. The incident occurred in an indoor test facility under typical fluorescent light ambient illumination. The post hoc measured total emission energy per pulse from the laser was 75 mJ with an irregular beam intensity distribution at the approximate eye position a few centimeters in front of the exit aperture. The average radiant exposure was approximately 1 mJ/cm^2 and the peak radiant exposure (based upon beam profile measurements) was 2.5 mJ/cm^2. The measured emission duration was 30 nanoseconds (full width half maximum). The pupil diameter was estimated to be 4 mm for the indoor test environment. The Total Intraocular Energy (TIE) through a 4 mm pupillary aperture was 315 µJ or less depending on where the eye intercepted the beam. The exit beam diameter was large enough (larger than the interpupillary distance - 6.2 cm) to permit a simultaneous bilateral exposure. The exposure dose or TIE for each eye may have been different due to the irregular beam intensity distribution and the relative position of each eye during the brief exposure incident. The 30 ns pulse TIE for induction of a minimal ophthalmoscopically visible lesion (MVL) at 1064 nm is 100 µJ in a non-human primate eye[18]. The threshold TIE for a vitreous hemorrhage is about 1 mJ[19]. This exposure is just above the MVL threshold and resulted in a small confined hemorrhage in the fovea.

With the laser operating at a pulse repetition frequency near 10 pulses per second, three pulses could have been incident on the eye in approximately 200 ms. The patient reported "seeing two or three yellowish flashes" and immediately sought medical assistance. This incident will be designated Case 1 for this report

A previously described[1,3,4,5,6] accidental exposure (Case 2) from a hand-held laser rangefinder at close range (arms length) is compared with Case 1. A 21 year old male received bilateral macular injury from separate exposure(s) to each eye from the q-switched neodymium YAG laser operating at 1064 nm in a bright ambient noontime outdoor environment. The estimated TIE for this exposure was 1 mJ or less depending on the exact geometry[1]. This patient perceived a "bright flash, white in color" which "washed over" his eyes. He delayed a few hours before seeking medical assistance. Although he sustained bilateral injury, only the assessment of the effects and recovery of the left eye (OS) are compared with Case 1 in this report. These left eye assessments are designated Case 2.

Treatment: In Case 1, a steroid treatment regimen was initiated six hours after the exposure. An initial dose of 80 mg methylprednisolone sodium succinate (Solu-Medrol$_{TM}$) was administered intravenously (IV) over a 30 minute period. This was followed by 250 mg every 6 hours (Q6) for the next 72 hours. The dose was tapered over the next two weeks from 80 mg (Q6) to 40 mg (Q6).

There was no pharmacological treatment initiated in Case 2[1,4].

Ophthalmoscopic and Visual Function Assessments: A series of standard and nonstandard imaging and visual function assessments were made over a period of 14 months (Case 1) to 3 years (Case 2). Patients were evaluated by direct and indirect ophthalmoscopy, fluorescein angiography, biomicroscopy, confocal scanning laser ophthalmoscopy (CSLO, Rodenstock Inc.) and optical coherence tomography (OCT, Humphrey's Inc). High contrast Snellen visual acuity was measured throughout the evaluation period. Visual field defects were measured with the Amsler grid and the Humphrey's 10-2 regimen. Large field (6°) sinewave contrast sensitivity was measured under normal room illumination (100 nits) with the Neuroscientific CS-2000. Focal contrast sensitivity was measured with the CSLO which allows focal test stimuli (Landolt rings and "gapless" rings) to be written to the raster pattern which is projected onto the retina under operator control. The CSLO system contrast was calibrated with a CCD camera and was linear with system settings[7]. The contrast maximum was 0.64 for all scanning laser power settings[7]. This test allowed simultaneous measurement of focal contrast sensitivity and direct visual inspection of target placement on the retina (Figure 1), thus permitting observation of the preferred retinal location (PRL) during discrimination. Focal electrophysiological measurements of macular dysfunction were obtained with a Doran maculoscope incorporating a 3 degree Maxwellian view retinal spot. Both the electroretinogram (ERG) and the visual evoked potential (VEP) were recorded for macula stimulation. Color vision was assessed

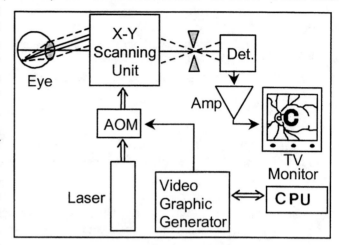

Figure 1. Schematic of the confocal scanning laser ophthalmoscope with an acousto-optic modulator (AOM) and video graphic generator which facilitates "writing" Landolt rings or other test targets directly on the retina. The retina and the test target are simultaneously viewed on the monitor.

using the Farnsworth-Munsel 100 Hue and a Rayleigh-Moreland anomaloscope (Interzeag, AG, CVM 712).

In both cases, no pre-exposure baseline data were available. Data are compared with average data from an age-matched control group. Medical histories of both individuals indicated excellent health with no visual problems prior to the accident. Neither patient wore corrective lenses. Neither was wearing protective eyewear at the time of exposure.

3. RESULTS

When evaluated approximately 30 minutes after the exposure, the Case 1 patient described small dark (nearly absolute) central scotomas in both eyes. Ophthalmoscopy augmented with CSLO images with the argon laser operating at 514 nm revealed a small confined retinal hemorrhage in both eyes, perhaps slightly larger in the right eye and centered on the fovea. There was no vitreous hemorrhage. In Case 2, a small vitreous hemorrhage was observed and the retinal injury site was located on the fovea. Visual function loss and recovery were measured at various intervals over 14 months (Case 1) and 3 years (Case 2) after exposure. In Case 1, high contrast Snellen visual acuity (VA) decreased from 20/50 (OD) measured within a few hours after the exposure to 20/200 at the 2 day observation (Figure 2). In both cases, high contrast Snellen VA recovered to 20/15 or better. In Case 1, VA recovers to 20/20 in both OD and OS by 55 days post exposure and was better than 20/15 at the 317 day measurement and at 14 months. The more significant early loss in visual acuity in OD versus OS is not apparent in acuity measurements made at and beyond 32 days post exposure. In Case 2, recovery of VA (OS) required almost 3 times the amount of time to recover to a VA of 20/15 and remained stable at 20/15 when last measured at 3 years post exposure. Color vision measurements showed minimal disturbances and were generally within normal limits.

The visual field decrement and recovery was evaluated with the Amsler grid and Humphrey's visual field. In Case 1, a dense circular scotoma approximately 4 degrees in diameter was described two days after exposure for OD, whereas only a relative scotoma (i.e. Amsler grid lines were lighter in the central area but could be read) of about the same size was described for OS. At one month, wavy lines in the central 2 degrees

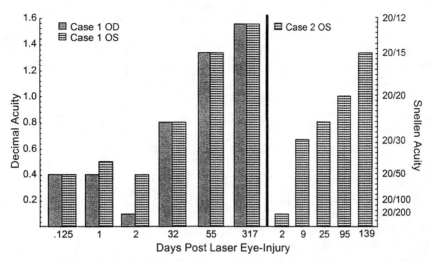

Figure 2. Recovery of high contrast Snellen visual acuity after laser-induced foveal injury is shown for Case 1 (OS and OD) and Case 2 (OS). The difference in absolute recovery between the patients may reflect the eventual recovery of the anatomical fovea for Case 1 versus the use of a superior temporal preferred retinal location (pseudofovea) for Case 2.

with possibly a line missing were described in the OD Amsler grid. The OS Amsler grid was normal with no abnormalities noted. These results are consistent with the absorption of the blood, reduction in edema and suggested reorganization of the fovea based on ophthalmoscopic observations. At fourteen months, a small disturbance in the central Amsler grid lines was still apparent in OD and the OS Amsler grid was unremarkable. The Humphrey 10-2 (ten degree field) test demonstrated the central field loss in OD at the 2 day measurement. Subsequent Humphrey fields were within normal limits. In Case 2, a dense 3 degree scotoma immediately temporal to fixation was apparent on the Amsler grid and in the Humphrey 10-2 measurements six days after the exposure. At six months, the Humphrey 10-2 was normal, however, a "small disturbance" temporal to the fixation point was still apparent on the Amsler grid[4]. These visual field tests require foveal fixation which may be altered when foveal function is compromised.

Large field (6 degree) contrast sensitivity (CS) for sinewave gratings (Figure 3) shows a similar recovery time course for Case 1 similar to that of the high contrast Snellen visual acuity. At 2 days post exposure, contrast sensitivity for Case 1 is uniformly suppressed across all spatial frequencies with a shallow peak at 1 cycle/degree. At 32 days post exposure, CS falls within the normal range for age matched subjects.

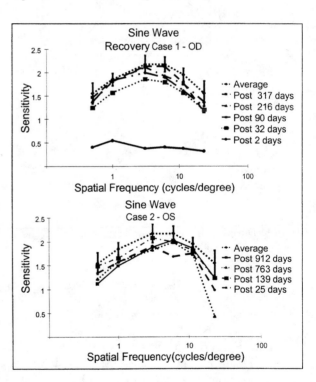

Figure 3. Large field sinewave contrast sensitivity (CS). In Case 1 (upper), the CS returned to normal limits at 90 days after exposure. In Case 2 (lower), CS also returned to normal, however, more variability was exhibited for high spatial frequency sensitivities. Vertical bars on the average CS function indicate ± 1 standard deviation.

Case 2 requires more time to recover maximal contrast sensitivity, similar to that observed in Figure 1 for recovery of high contrast Snellen visual acuity. Recovery for high spatial frequencies is also delayed in Case 2. The first measurement of contrast sensitivity was made 24 days after the exposure. Both cases show normal peak sensitivities between 3 and 6 cycles per degree.

Focal CSLO contrast sensitivity (Figure 4) reveals an initial peak at 0.5 cycles per degree that shifts to a peak at about 3 cycles per degree at 216 days post exposure in Case 1. Case 2 shows a similar peak at 0.5 cycles per degree but does not develop a secondary peak at 3 cycles per degree.

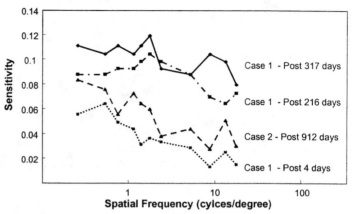

The preferred retinal location (PRL) was determined with the CSLO during small target discrimination by observing the patient's placement of the "gap" of the Landolt ring on the retina (Figure 5). In Case 1 at one year (Figure 5, left), the PRL as determined by the location of the "gap" in the Landolt ring is located in the lesioned fovea indicating foveal function. In early (4 days) PRL determinations in Case 1, the PRL was located in the superior temporal retina region outside the foveal lesion. In Case 2 (Figure 5, right), the PRL selected for small target discrimination was a retinal site superior and temporal to the fovea. This PRL changed very little over the 3 year observation period. When the test target was placed within the Case 2 lesion site, the patient could not discriminate a 20/40 target at the maximum contrast.

Comparison of CSLO fluorescein angiograms (FA) at two days (Figure 6, upper left) and at one month (Figure 6, upper right) shows a reduction in the area of blockage in the foveal region with peripheral white punctate

Figure 4. Focal contrast sensitivity (FCS) measured with the CSLO. Case 1 shows a shift in peak FCS from less than 1 cycle/degree (4 days) to 3 cycles/degree (216 days). This change is consistent with the shift in her preferred retinal location (PRL) from superior temporal retina to the fovea. In Case 2, the peak of the FCS function remains at less than 1 cycle/degree with a PRL superior temporal to the fovea.

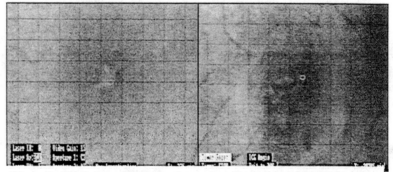

Figure 5. CSLO images showing the preferred retinal location (PRL) (i.e. location of "gap" of the Landolt ring with respect to the anatomical fovea) during discrimination. In Case 1 (left), the PRL at one year after the injury) is in the anatomical fovea. In Case 2, the PRL at 216 days after the injury is superior temporal to the fovea.

reflective areas. Corresponding optical coherence tomography (OCT) scan[20] through the fovea shows a disrupted retinal pigmented epithelial (RPE) at two days after exposure (Figure 6, lower left). A comparable OCT scan at one month shows an intact foveal RPE. A CSLO FA (Figure 7) of Case 1 (OD) at 12 months after the exposure indicates minimal blockage with a white, highly reflective, somewhat punctate region in the central retina, suggesting development of new retinal morphology not apparent at 1 month post exposure.

Consistent with functional recovery and morphological reorganization, Case 1 showed a significant increase in both focal ERG and VEP measured in the macula region (Figure 8).

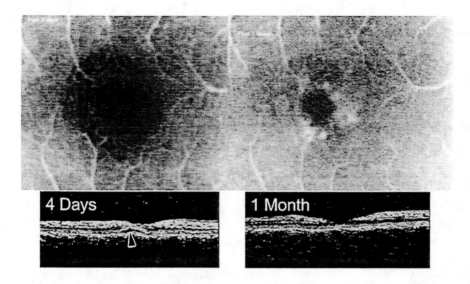

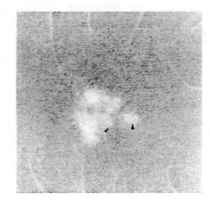

Figure 6. Comparison of the CSLO fluorescein angiogram (FA) and optical coherence tomography (OCT) of the fovea of Case 1 (OD) at 2-4 days and at 1 month post exposure. The CSLO FA at 2 days (upper left) and an OCT image at 4 days (lower left) post exposure shows a region of vascular blockage in the macular region (FA) which corresponds with a disruption or discontinuity in the macular retinal pigment epithelium (OCT – arrow). At one month, the FA (upper right) shows a 50% decrease in vascular blockage and development of punctate, white-reflecting regions in the macula. The OCT image at one month (lower right) shows nearly complete resolution of the discontinuity in the retinal pigment epithelium.

Figure 7. CSLO fluorescein angiogram of Case 1 (OD) at 12 months shows minimal blockage of fluorescein and enhanced evidence of a highly reflective concentric retinal structure around the lesion site (two black arrows).

4. DISCUSSION

Recovery of critical visual function was demonstrated in two cases of human foveal injury induced by exposure to military laser systems. Both Case 1 and Case 2 show recovery in high contrast Snellen visual acuity to 20/15 or better as well as full recovery for large field sinewave contrast sensitivity. In addition, Case 1 presents evidence of a return in foveal functionality not evident in Case 2. CSLO measures of contrast sensitivity show a shift in contrast sensitivity from < 1 cycle per degree to about 3 cycles per degree over the fourteen month period of post exposure measurements. Consistent with this shift in focal CSLO contrast sensitivity is an increase in utilizing the lesioned foveal region for placement of all CSLO target sizes. This observation suggests

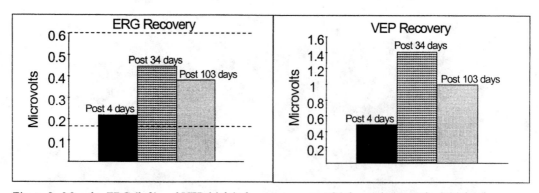

Figure 8. Macular ERG (left) and VEP (right) shows recovery at 34 days relative to the initial 4 day measurement. This recovery appears stable as shown by the measurements at 103 days after the exposure. (Dashed lines in the ERG graph indicate the normal ERG range)

that the fovea in this patient is at least capable of resolving targets of 20/40. Case 2 is capable of resolving such targets only with a retinal area outside the fovea (i.e. in an area superior and temporal to the fovea measured over a post exposure period of 3 years).

The ability of the fovea to recover some of its post exposure functionality may involve several factors. The injury in Case 1 reflects a less severe retinal impact in that damage involved a somewhat smaller and confined retinal hemorrhage. Resolution of the size of the injury site was indicated by a significant reduction in the size of vascular blockage measured by CSLO fluorescein angiography and evidence of a return of RPE continuity at 1 month post exposure (Figure 6, OCT images). At one month post exposure, however, the PRL was not foveal and CSLO contrast sensitivity peaked in the low spatial frequency region (<1cycle per degree). We suggest that the later CSLO images reflecting little or no vascular blockage may reflect a possible cellular reorganization at the posterior retina involving RPE cells and possibly photoreceptor cells from regions adjacent to the damage fovea[21,-24,26-28]. Other mechanisms recently described in artificial occlusion experiments may function to change the photoreceptor alignment allowing maximal photoreceptor sensitivity in the foveal region[24,26-29]. The increase in macular retinal electrical activity (ERG) and the increase in the cortical representation of macula activity (VER) may reflect this recovery of neural processes.

The specific mechanisms for cellular reorganization at the level of the retina are largely unknown and generally assumed to be passive. Photoreceptors from adjacent areas move into the damaged foveal region and repopulate the fovea restoring the photoreceptor density required for high contrast visual acuity[23]. Similarly, receptor orientation must also be maintained for optimal photoreceptor quantum efficiency[24]. While this process may occur passively, the presence of a complex network of striated rootlets at the level of the photoreceptor extending the length of the inner segment[27] and a parallel system within the retinal pigmented epithelium may well serve to neurally control the recovery process[28]. When the fovea is nonfunctional (Case 2), these same mechanisms may facilitate establishment of a new PRL to optimize high contrast acuity and photoreceptor quantal efficiency.

While the efficacy of the treatment of laser-induced retinal injury remains unknown, the observed recovery in Case 1 with minimal retinal traction or scar formation may, in part, be attributable to the early application of the steroidal therapy. Early introduction of the steroid may have limited retinal inflammatory processes and the subsequent scar formation[25] and thus permitted passive and active processes attributed to photoreceptor movement and orientation to facilitate functional recovery.

Finally, the potential to inflict bilateral retinal injury at close range from a laser system with a large exit beam diameter has received minimal discussion. In typical laboratory and industrial laser configurations or the laser rangefinder accident described in Case 2[1], accessible beam diameters are 1 cm or less. For small beam diameters there is a low probability of monocular exposure (i.e. low probability of a small beam intercepting the small pupillary aperture) and simultaneous bilateral exposure is not possible if the beam diameter is smaller than the interpupillary distance. For lasers with large exit beam diameters, there is potential for binocular exposure and injury at close range (e.g. Case 1). In addition, the probability of monocular exposure increases due to the larger beam size. Laser eye protection and control procedures must be emphasized.

5. SUMMARY AND CONCLUSIONS

We have reported the return of foveal function in a case of bilateral foveal damage induced by accidental exposure to a repetitively pulsed neodymium laser. Steroid treatment was administered six hours after the exposure and tapered over a two week period. Visual function recovered to 20/25 within 1 month post exposure and ultimately recovered to 20/13 within 12 months postexposure. Sinewave contrast sensitivity reflective of foveal function showed a similar recovery over this same period being well within normal limits at the end of 12 months postexposure. Unlike Case 2 where functional recovery was mediated by the development of a new preferred retinal location (PRL) located external to the non-functional fovea, Case 1 foveal function recovered and the PRL returned to the fovea. We conclude that foveal repair is possible even under conditions of confined macular hemorrhage. When treatment is early, the maintenance of posterior retinal cells in a marginal condition is possible thus allowing natural retinal repair mechanisms to be invoked. The potential for simultaneous bilateral ocular exposure at close distances must be considered in hazard assessments for lasers with large exit beam diameters.

6. ACKNOWLEDGMENTS

The authors gratefully acknowledge the assistance of Dr. Mark S. Foster at the Darnal Army Hospital, Fort Hood, Texas for his initial ophthalmological assessment and rapid referral. P. Edsall and C.W. Van Sice provided valuable measurement and calibration support. The assistance of S. Ruiz and J. Loveday in the collection and management of visual function measurements is gratefully appreciated. A. Akers is gratefully acknowledged for ophthalmic imaging, image processing and figure preparation assistance. R. Elliot assisted in the CSLO evaluations. B. Gomez assisted with the Optical Coherence Tomography imaging.

7. DISCLAIMER

The opinions or assertions contained herein are the private views of the authors and are not to be construed as official or as reflecting the views of the Department of the Army or the Department of Defense. Citation of trade names in this report does not constitute an official endorsement or approval of the use of such items. Human Volunteers participated in these studies after giving their free and informed voluntary consent. Investigators adhered to AR 70-25 and USAMRMC Regulation 50-25 on the use of volunteers in research.

8. REFERENCES

1. B.E. Stuck, H. Zwick, J.W. Molchany, D.J. Lund, D.A. Gagliano, "Accidental human laser retinal injuries from military laser systems," *SPIE Proc. of Laser-inflicted Eye Injuries: Epidemiology, Prevention and Treatment*, Vol. 2674, pp 7-20, 1996.
2. H. Zwick, B.E. Stuck, D. Gagliano, V.C. Parmley, D.J. Lund, J. Molchany, J.J. Kearney and M.Belkin. "Two informative cases of q-switched laser eye injury," Presidio of San Francisco, CA. Letterman Army Institute of Research, Institute Report No. 463, 1991.
3. H. Zwick, J.W. Ness, J.W. Molchany, B.E. Stuck, "Comparison of artificial and accidental laser-induced macular scotomas on human contrast sensitivity," *SPIE Proc. of Laser-inflicted Eye Injuries: Epidemiology, Prevention and Treatment*, Vol. 2674, pp 136-143,1996.

4. P.H. Custis, D.A. Gagliano, H. Zwick, S.T. Schuschereba, , C.D. Regillo "Macular hole surgery following accidental laser injury with a military rangefinder," *SPIE Proc. of Laser-inflicted Eye Injuries: Epidemiology, Prevention and Treatment*, Vol. 2674, pp 166-174,1996.

5. H. Zwick, D.A. Gagliano, S. Ruiz, and B.E. Stuck. "Utilization of scanning laser ophthalmoscopy in laser induced human retinal nerve fiber layer damage," *SPIE Proc. of the Ophthalmic Technologies V*, Vol. 2393, pp. 189-193, 1995.

6. B.E. Stuck, H. Zwick, J.W. Molchany, D.A. Gagliano, M. Belkin. "Accidental human laser retinal injuries from a hand held military rangefinder." (Abstract) Investigative Ophthalmology and Visual Sciences, Vol. 36, pp 354, 1995.

7. H. Zwick, D.J. Lund, D.A. Gagliano, B.E. Stuck, "Functional and ophthalmoscopic observations in human laser accident cases using scanning laser ophthalmoscopy," *SPIE* Vol. 2126, pp. 144-153, 1994.

8. J.A. Wolfe. "Laser retinal injury," Military Medicine. 150:170-185; 1984.

9. E.E. Boldrey, H.L. Little, M. Flocks, A.Vassiliadis. "Retinal eye injury due to industrial laser burns," Ophthalmology 88:101-107; 1981.

10. J.R. Manning, F.H. Davidorf, R.H. Keates, A.E. Strange. "Neodymium:YAG Laser Lesions in the Human Retina: Accidental/Experimental," Contemporary Ophthalmic Forum. Vol. 4. No. 3:86-91; 1986.

11. G.K. Lang, G. Lang, G.O.H. Naumann. "Akzidentelle bilaterale asymmetrische rubin-laser-makulo-pathie," Klin. Mbl. Augenheilk. 186:366-370; 1985.

12. J.J. Kearney, H.B. Cohen, B.E. Stuck, G.P. Rudd; D.E. Beresky, F.D. Wertz. "Laser injury to multiple retinal foci," Lasers in Surgery and Medicine. 7:499-502; 1987.

13. V.P Gabel, R. Birngruber, B. Lorenz. "Clinical observations of six cases of laser injury to the eye," Health Physics 56: No. 5, 705-710, 1989.

14. A.B. Thach, P.F. Lopez, L.C. Snady-McCoy, B.M. Golub, D.A. Fraumbach. "Accidental Nd:YAG laser injuries to the macula," Amer. J. of Ophthalmol. 119: No. 6, 767-773, 1995.

15. D.R. Hirsch, D.G. Booth, S. Schocket, D.H. Sliney. "Recovery from pulsed-dye laser retinal injury," Arch of Ophthalmol. 110: 1688-1689; 1992.

16. A. Alhalel, Y. Glovinsky, G. Treister,E. Bartov, M. Blumenthal, M. Belkin, "Long-term follow up of accidental parafoveal laser burns," Retina, Vol. 13, pp. 152-154, 1993.

17. J. Guez, J. Le Gargasson, F. Rigaudierre, K.O'Regan. "Is there a systematic location for the pseudo-fovea in patients with central scotoma?," Vision Research, Vol. 33, pp. 1271-1279, 1993.

18. D.J. Lund, E.S. Beatrice, "Near infrared laser ocular bioeffects," Health Physics Vol. 56, No. 5, pp 631-636, 1989.

19. W.D. Gibbons, R.G. Allen, "Retinal thresholds from suprathreshold q-switched laser exposure," Health Physics, Vol. 35, 1978.

20. C.A. Puliafito, M.R. Hee, J.S. Schuman, J.G. Fujimoto, *Optical Coherence Tomography of Ocular Diseases*, Chapts 2 and 11, SLACK Inc., Thorofare, NJ, 1996.

21. H. Zwick, "Visual function changes associated with low-level light effects," Health Physics, Vol 56, pp. 657-663, 1989.

22. H. Zwick, R.B. Bedell, K.R. Bloom, "Spectral and visual deficits associated with laser irradiation," Modern Prob. Ophthal. Vol. 13, pp 299-308, 1974.

23. M.O.M. Tso, "Photic maculopathy in rhesus monkey, a light and electron microscope study," *Invest. Ophthal. and Vis. Sci.*, Vol. 12, pp. 17-34, 1972.

24. J.M. Enoch, D.G. Birch, E.E. Birch, "Monocular light exclusion for a period of days reduces directional sensitivity of the human retina," Science, Vol. 206, pp. 705-707, 1979.

25. N. Naveh, C. Weissman, "Prolonged corticosteroid treatment exerts transient inhibitory effect on prostaglandin E_2 release in rabbits' eyes," Prostaglandins Leukotrienes and Essential Fatty Acids, pp. 101-105, 1990.

26. H. Zwick, S.T. Schuschereba, E. Manougian, D.J. Lund, B.E. Stuck, "Low-level light effects on vision: Laser versus non-coherent light," *SPIE Proceedings of Low-Energy Laser Effects on Biological Systems*, Vol. 1883, pp14-20, 1993.

27. S.T. Schuschereba, H. Zwick, "Ciliary rootlets in primate rods and cones," Letterman Army Institute of Research Technical Note No. 82-34TN, pp. 1-15, 1982.

28. S.T. Schuschereba, H. Zwick, B.E. Stuck, E.S. Beatrice, "Basal body and striated rootlet changes in primate macular retinal pigmented epithelium after low level diffuse argon laser radiation," Letterman Army Institute of Research Technical Note No. 82-35TN, pp. 1-17, 1982.

29. H. Zwick, J.W. Ness, J. Loveday, J.Molchany, B.E. Stuck, "Optimization of neural retinal visual acuity following acute laser induced macula injury," *Proc. SPIE Laser and Noncoherent Ocular Effects: Epidemiology Prvention and Treatment,* Vol. 2974, pp. 75-81, 1997.

SESSION 4

Photoacoustic Mechanisms

Effects of Stress Waves on Cells

Heather L. Campbell, Steven R. Visuri, Luiz B. Da Silva

Lawrence Livermore National Laboratories

Livermore, CA 94551

1. ABSTRACT

Laser induced stress waves are being used in a variety of medical applications, including drug delivery and targeted tissue disruption. Stress waves can also be an undesirable side effect in laser procedures such as ophthalmology and angioplasty. Thus, a study of the effects of stress waves on a cellular level is useful. Thermoelastic stress waves were produced using a Q-switched frequency-doubled Nd:YAG laser (λ=532 nm) with a pulse duration of 4 ns. The laser radiation was delivered to an absorbing media. A thermoelastic stress wave was produced in the absorbing media and propagated into plated cells. The energy per pulse delivered to a sample and the spot size were varied. Stress waves were quantified. We assayed for cell viability and damage using two methods. The threshold laser parameters for cell damage were defined for three cell lines.

Key Words: stress wave, cell damage, photoacoustic

2. INTRODUCTION

Short pulse lasers are used in a number of clinical procedures, including lithotripsy, ophthalmology and drug delivery. Pressure transients produced by these short pulse lasers may produce damage to surrounding cells and tissues. Stress waves are produced when optical energy is absorbed into an appropriate medium. If the deposition of this energy is less than the stress confinement time, an acoustic pressure wave is produced.

There has been some research done in this field previously, most notably at Wellman Laboratories of Photomedicine. They have used excimer lasers, with rise times from 10-25 ns in their experiments on stress waves and cell death. They have reported effects of stresses up to kbars, though they have mainly published results on the compressive component of the waves. Fluences ranged from 90-560 mJ/cm^2. Their results were cell-type dependent.[1]

3. MATERIALS AND METHODS

Figure 1 shows the experimental arrangement. A glass slide coverslip coated with black enamel paint on the underside was placed onto a second coverslip. Water-based gel placed between the paint and second coverslip assured good acoustic coupling. This second coverslip had cells plated on the underside. Stress waves were produced by the deposition of optical energy into the black paint, which is in turn vaporized, propagating a stress wave. The approximate distance between the absorption of the laser and the target cells was 450 µm. This experimental arrangement prevented any measurable temperature rise or optical energy from reaching the cells.

The laser source was a Q-switched, frequency-doubled Nd:YAG laser (Spectra Physics, Mountain View, CA). The wavelength was 532 nm and the spatial beam profile was approximately Gaussian. Pulse duration was approximately 4 ns. Energy per pulse was varied from 2.13 mJ to 217 mJ, using neutral density filters. Spot size was varied by focusing the beam and moving the target to discrete distances. Spot sizes obtained varied from 960 µm to 2400 µm, as measured by photo-sensitive paper. Consequently, the fluence range was 226 mJ/cm^2 to 2590 mJ/ cm^2.

SPIE Vol. 3254 • 0277-786X/98/$10.00

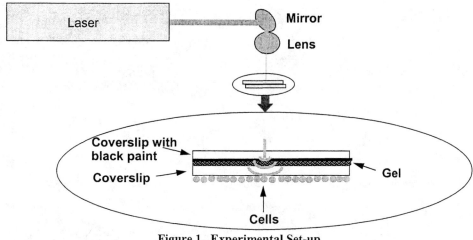

Figure 1. Experimental Set-up

We estimated the stress confinement time of our experimental arrangement to be approximately 7 ns ($\tau_s=d/c_s$). This was calculated using a penetration depth, d, of 10 µm and 1500 m/s as the speed of sound, c_s, in our medium. Since the laser pulse duration was 4 ns, the energy deposition was stress-confined.

The pressure magnitude in the stress waves was measured using a PVDF (polyvinylidene fluoride) hydrophone (NTR Systems, Seattle WA). The hydrophone is calibrated between from 1-20 MHz where it has a relatively flat frequency response and the sensing area is 0.6 mm in diameter. Figure 2 shows a typical pressure profile obtained with the hydrophone. The hydrophone was placed at varying distances from the target and a plot of distance vs. pressure was obtained. To prevent damage to the hydrophone, the proximity to the target was limited to 1 mm. Pressures were then extrapolated back to the location of the cells.

Three different cell lines (ATCC, Rockville, MD) were used as targets: 769P (human renal adenocarcinoma), NCTC (mouse fibroblasts from connective tissue), and MES-SA (human uterine sarcoma). All cells were grown under standard cell culture techniques, in a 37°C, 5% CO_2 incubator. Cells were passed and plated onto slide coverslips that were coated with poly-L-lysine to promote adhesion. Cells were then placed back in the incubator, allowed to reach near-confluency, and later used as targets in the laser experiments.

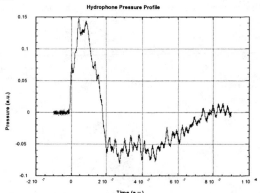

Figure 2. Pressure profile measured by hydrophone.

After completion of the experiments, cells were returned to the incubator for 12 hours and then were assayed for cell death using two methods: fluorescence microscopy and Trypan Blue. The fluorescence microscopy assay involved the use of the LIVE/DEAD Viability/Cytotoxicity kit (Molecular Probes, Eugene, OR), which is comprised of calcein-AM and ethidium homodimer-1, both of which weakly fluoresce in the media. Figure 3 shows the mechanism of the assay. The AM portion of the calcein-AM molecule facilitates transport across the plasma membrane. Once inside a live cell, the AM is cleaved by intracellular esterases and calcein becomes highly fluorescent (green). Ethidium homodimer-1 cannot enter cells through intact membranes. However, in a dead cell with a compromised membrane, ethidium homodimer-1 enters the cell, binds to the DNA and increases its red fluorescence intensity 40-fold. Calcein-AM also enters the dead cell but the AM is not cleaved and it remains virtually non-fluorescent. A solution of 150 µl of 4 µM calcein-AM and 4 µM ethidium homodimer-1 was added to the coverslips and allowed to incubate at room temperature for 30 minutes. Coverslips were mounted on slides and observed under a fluorescent microscope (Zeiss). Trypan Blue staining was performed in the usual manner. Trypan Blue enters cells with compromised membranes and is unable to enter those with intact membranes. Both methods produced similar results.

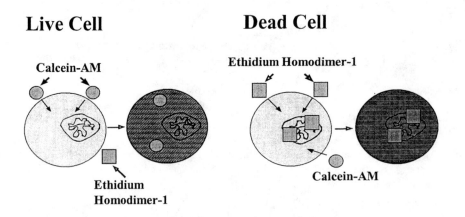

Figure 3. Fluorescence Microscopy Assay

4. RESULTS

The stress waves produced had both a positive (compression) and negative (tension) component. The tension results from reflection off of the glass-air interface. The magnitude of the tensile portion of the wave was approximately half the magnitude of the compression portion of the wave. Figure 4 shows the percent of samples demonstrating some degree of death as a function of the fluence produced, for the NCTC target cells. The laser-treated samples are grouped according to average spot size. A positive correlation was observed between the fluence produced and the percent of samples that were damaged. For the large spot size (2000 µm), there was no damage observed at the lowest fluences (226 and 483 mJ/cm^2). Damaged samples were observed at the higher fluences (701, 913, and 1200 mJ/cm^2). For the small spot size (960 µm), no damage was observed at the lowest fluence (424 mJ/cm2), but damage was noted at 829, 1180, and 2590 mJ/cm^2. Figure 5 shows the correlation between fluence and the calculated pressure differential seen by the cells. Damaged samples were observed at the two spot sizes between a pressure differential of 200 bar (+133, -66 bar) and 400 bar (see Figure 2 for a representative trace of ΔP. At approximately 400 bar, 100 percent of the samples were damaged. The 2000 µm spot size had resulting pressures up to 554 bar, though damage peaked at 400 bar. The 960 µm spot size had resulting pressures up to 432 bar.

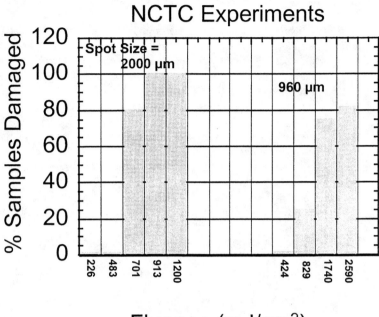

Figure 4. Fluence vs. % Samples Damaged

At times, we observed a hole in the cell layer, visible to the naked eye, immediately after laser treatment. In other instances, a hole was not observed immediately following treatment, but was observed during the cell death assays. A combination of two events may be happening. The cells may be removed from the coverslip by the pressure of the stress waves. Alternatively, cells may be dying during the 12 hour incubation and floating off of the coverslip, resulting in a hole during the assay. Dead cells typically lose their adhesion to their substrate. The three cell lines used as targets had similar thresholds for damage.

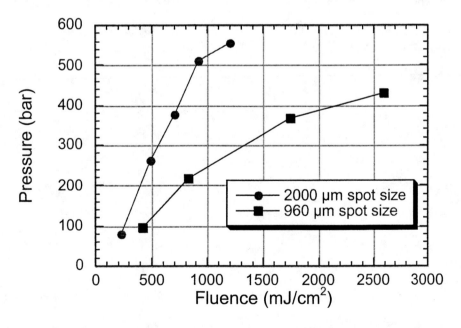

Figure 5. Fluence vs. Pressure at Cells

5. DISCUSSION

We believe that spot size effects were responsible for the differences in damage that we observed. With a small spot size, the stress wave produced propagates in a spherical manner almost from the outset. The peak pressure in a spherical wave falls off in a 1/r manner. However, a larger spot size will initially produce a planar wave, in which the peak pressure falls off more slowly, in a linear fashion. This planar wave eventually evolves into a spherical wave, due to defraction, and the pressure begins to fall off at a rate of 1/r. This phenomenon may account for the higher number of samples damaged with the larger spot size, and lower fluences, and the decreased damage observed at the smaller spot size.

The cell damage threshold for tensile waves is believed to be significantly lower than that for solely compressive waves.[2] Our findings are relevant to fiber-delivered laser applications, in which the resulting stress waves have both a compressive and tensile component. Cavitation probably occurred in our experimental set-up. Water fails at approximately -10 to -100 bar, which was sometimes exceeded in our experiments.

We intend to further quantify the cell death and damage observed, using assays that detect earlier stages of cell death than membrane integrity assays. In addition, temporal effects on cell damage, obtained by varying the incubation time post-treatment, will be explored. Obtaining data on the damage caused by the different components of the wave is also of interest. Spot size effects, multiple pulses, and pulse duration differences will be investigated.

6. REFERENCES

[1] Doukas, A.G., McAuliffe, D.J., Flotte, T.J., "Biological effects of laser-induced shock waves: structural and functional cell damage *in vitro*". Ultrasound in Medicine and Biology, 19(2): p. 137-146, 1993.

[2] Niemz, M.H., Lin, C.P., Pitsillides, C., Cui, J., Doukas, A.G., Deutsch, T.F., "Laser-induced generation of pure tensile stresses". Applied Physics, 70(20): p. 2676-2678, 1997.

7. ACKNOWLEDGMENTS

The authors wish to thank Jim Tucker and Marilyn Ramsey of the Biology and Biotechnology Research Program at LLNL for their assistance with fluorescence microscopy.

This work was performed under the auspices of the U.S Department of Energy by Lawrence Livermore National Laboratory under Contract W-7405-Eng-48.

Interferometric Technique to Measure Shock-Induced Surface Velocities in Tissues for the Determination of Dynamic Mechanical Properties

Ujwal S. Sathyam   Peter M. Celliers   Luiz B. Da Silva

Lawrence Livermore National Laboratory

ABSTRACT

We present an interferometric technique to measure free surface velocities of a tissue phantom when subjected to a high power laser pulse. Such information is useful for the determination of the dynamic mechanical properties of tissues and tissue phantoms. We deliver a 4-nanosecond doubled Nd:YAG laser pulse to a tamped surface of a slab sample and probe the opposite free surface with a HeNe laser beam. The stress-wave induced motion of the rear-surface imparts a Doppler shift to the reflected HeNe probe. We monitor the Doppler shift with a velocity interferometer sensitive to velocities as low as 1-2 m/s.

Keywords: stress wave, velocity interferometry, spallation, VISAR

1. INTRODUCTION

The generation and control of laser-induced stress waves in tissues is becoming increasingly important in laser surgery and localized drug delivery applications. In order to understand and precisely control these stresses, one requires knowledge of the dynamic mechanical properties of the tissue. This data is also required as input to numerical and theoretical models that seek to optimize laser parameters for various surgical and drug delivery techniques. However, these properties are generally not known for most biological materials.

Research into the dynamic mechanical properties of non-biological materials such as metals, ceramics, and optical materials is a mature field.[1,2] One important method involves monitoring free surface motion as a stress wave interacts with the surface. This method is often used to measure wave profiles,[3] and to detect spallation. The advantages of an interferometric detection scheme over a traditional pressure transducer measurement are:

- it is a non-contact measurement and thus does not disturb the sample,

- wide band frequency response (depending on the detection technology employed in the experiment, bandwidths up to several GHz are possible in principle),

- high spatial resolution operating either as a single point measurement or in an imaging mode

In this paper, we apply an interferometric method to measure free-surface velocities generated in a tissue model by the deposition of a high power laser pulse. To the best of the authors' knowledge, such velocity measurements have not been performed in the regimes relevant to stress wave generation in biological media. Previous studies involving velocity measurements in biomedical research have focussed on measuring blood flow in arteries using Doppler velocimetry.[4] These techniques generally use a standard Michelson interferometer that can measure low velocities of the order of 1 cm/s. However, such an arrangement is not suitable for measuring high free-surface velocities of the order of 10 m/s expected from an interaction with a high power laser pulse.[5] In this study, we use an approach developed by Barker and Hollenbach to make velocity measurements in a back-spallation geometry (1) to observe stress-induced failure of the free surface.[6] The results of this study should provide valuable insight to the response of tissues and tissue phantoms to laser-induced stresses.

Correspondence: U. S. S.: Email: ujwal@llnl.gov

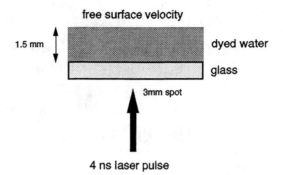

Figure 1. The back-plane spallation experiment: A Q-switched laser pulse is deposited into absorbing water and a stress wave is generated. The evolution of the stress wave can be monitored by measuring the free surface velocity as a function of time. When a strong enough stress wave is generated, the free surface will break away from the rest of the medium. Quantifying the surface velocity at failure, and hence the stress, is useful in the determination of the dynamic mechanical properties of the medium.

2. THEORY

2.1. VELOCITY INTERFEROMETRY

All velocity interferometers operate by measuring a Doppler shift imparted to light reflected off the moving target. The Doppler shift is given by:

$$|\frac{\partial \nu(t)}{\nu}| = |\frac{2u(t)}{c}| \tag{1}$$

where u is the velocity of the target, c is the speed of light, and ν the frequency of the light. In its basic configuration, the velocity interferometer consists of a Michelson interferometer with two arms unbalanced by a length of L, and with laser light reflected off the target as the source (figure 2). The total path length difference between the light returning from the two arms is thus $2L$, and the time difference is $\tau = \frac{2L}{c}$. The total phase difference between the two paths is:

$$\phi = 2\pi\nu\tau = 2\pi\nu\frac{2L}{c}. \tag{2}$$

Any motion of the target will impart a Doppler shift to the frequency of the light entering the interferometer. The frequency manifests itself as a change in phase at the detector, as seen by taking the derivative of equation 2,

$$|\partial\phi(t)| = 2\pi|\partial\nu(t)|\frac{2L}{c} \tag{3}$$

which can be related to the velocity of the moving target by equation (1):

$$|\partial\phi(t)| = |2\pi\frac{2u(t)}{\lambda}\frac{2L}{c}| = |2\pi F(t)| \tag{4}$$

where $F(t)$ is the fringe count. Depending on noise levels fringe shifts of around $F(t) = 0.1$ are relatively easy to detect, while detection limits as low as 0.01 F are possible. The phase is encoded in an interferogram at the output of the interferometer, so that the output signal $S(t)$ is sinusoidally modulated depending on the phase,

$$S(t) = \frac{1}{2}A\cos(\Phi_0 + \partial\phi(t)) \tag{5}$$

where A is the fringe peak-to-peak signal and Φ_0 is the initial phase difference before the target begins to move.

The interferometer system shown in figure (2) requires the light at the detector to be spatially and temporally coherent to produce fringes. This imposes two restrictions on the system:

- The light source has to temporally coherent at least over the path length difference of $2L$.

- The target surface has to have a near mirror-like finish so as to not destroy the spatial coherence of the laser light upon reflection. This restricts the type of specimen that can be studied, and particularly biological samples generally do not have such surfaces.

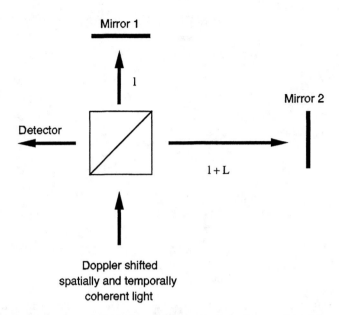

Mirror 1

Detector

Mirror 2

1

1 + L

Doppler shifted
spatially and temporally
coherent light

Figure 2. The principle of velocity interferometry: When light is reflected off a moving object, a Doppler shift is imparted to the frequency that is proportional to the velocity of the object. This Doppler shifted light is sent into a Michelson interferometer with unbalanced arms. The mismatch between the arms causes a slight change in the incident light to cause a large change in phase at the detector. However, since this is a long path length difference interferometer, the light incident on it has to be both spatially and temporally coherent to produce fringes at the detector. This need for spatial coherence imposes the requirement of an almost mirror-like finish of the target's surface, and therefore limits the applicability of this system.

2.2. VISAR

Barker and Hollenbach solved the spatial coherence problem by using an etalon to create the delay and adjusting the position of the mirror in that arm such that the image of the mirror in the delay arm is superimposed with the mirror on the opposite arm of the interferometer (figure 3). This removes the requirement of high spatial coherence of the light entering the interferometer, and very good fringe contrast can be obtained with light reflected from diffuse surfaces such as biological samples. This system still requires a source with high temporal coherence (over a distance of $2L$). Barker and Hollenbach called this arrangement "Velocity interferometer system for any reflecting surface" (VISAR), and it has become a standard tool in high pressure shock research and ballistics research.[7]

2.3. QUADRATURE

The sinusoidal equation (5) contains an ambiguity because it cannot discriminate between increasing and decreasing velocities. Depending on the material response the free surface can undergo both accelerations and decelerations (1), hence this ambiguity must be eliminated. The problem can be resolved by employing quadrature detection, whereby two fringe signals that are 90° out of phase are simultaneously monitored:

$$S_1(t) = \frac{1}{2} A \cos(\Phi_0 + \partial\phi(t))$$
$$S_2(t) = \frac{1}{2} A \sin(\Phi_0 + \partial\phi(t))$$

(6)

Quadrature detection also improves measurement resolution. The velocity sensitivity at fringe maxima and minima is always poor because $dS/dF \approx 0$. Having two fringe records in quadrature solves this problem because one or the other of the signals will always be in a region of good sensitivity.

We implement quadrature detection through polarization manipulations. Assuming that the interferometer is illuminated with linearly polarized light we place in one arm of the interferometer a $\lambda/8$ wave such that the light returning from the arm is circularly polarized, and in the other a $\lambda/4$ plate such that the light returning is polarized at 45° to the vertical. After exiting the interferometer, the quadrature signals are extracted with a polarizing beamsplitter and sent to their individual detectors.

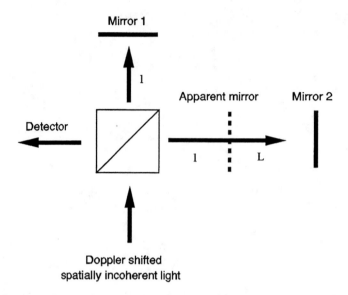

Figure 3. The VISAR modification: The requirement of spatial coherence in the velocity interferometer can be overcome by using imaging optics to create a virtual mirror in the long arm at the same position as the mirror in the short arm. Therefore, objects with diffusing surfaces such as biological media can be studied. However, temporal coherence of the light is still required since the light still has to travel the extra distance in the long arm.

3. EXPERIMENT

Figure (4) shows the experimental setup used in this study. The sample was a simple tissue model made of water containing an absorbing dye. Since most biological media have a high water content, this model is a reasonable first approximation. Further experiments will use more realistic tissue models made of gel (to impart some mechanical strengths) and real tissue. The laser used to generate the stress waves was a Q-switched double Nd:YAG laser (532 nm, 4 ns). The dye in the water provided an absorption depth of $100\,\mu$m at wavelength of the laser, also commonly encountered in laser-tissue interactions. The sample was placed in an open holder with a glass bottom. The laser pulse was delivered to the bottom of the sample through the glass plate, and generated a purely compressive stress at this interface. The sample was 1.5 mm thick and the laser spot size was 3 mm in diameter, and thus an approximately planar stress wave was generated that travelled towards the top free surface. The radiant exposure was varied between 1.5–3.5 J/cm^2 and covered a range spanning mechanical failure threshold at the free surface.

A HeNe laser (632.8 nm), used as the light source, was focused onto the rear surface to a spot of approximately $100\,\mu$m diameter. We imaged the reflected light into a VISAR system with a 4 meter long delay, which produced a velocity sensitivity of 15 m/s per fringe calculated from equation (4). A combination of a field lens ($f = 1\,m$) and two spherical mirrors ($f = 0.5\,m$) was used to create a virtual mirror surface at the position of the field lens. This arrangement was positioned such that the virtual mirror in the long arm and the real mirror in the short arm were equidistant from the beamsplitter NBS. Quadrature signals were separated by the polarizing beamsplitter PBS1 and sent to photomultiplier tubes $D1$ and $D2$. A third photomultiplier tube M monitored the total reflected light.

4. RESULTS AND CONCLUSIONS

Figure (5a) shows the quadrature fringe signals obtained from the quadrature detectors and the monitor at a laser pulse radiant exposure of 1.7 J/cm^2. Time $t = 0$ represents the arrival time of Nd:YAG laser pulse. The monitor signal remained unchanged during the entire acquisition period indicating that the reflectivity of the free surface has not changed. No fringes were observed on the quadrature detectors until about 1 μs after the laser pulse, consistent with the acoustic transit time. At this time motion of the free surface is evident through changes in the fringe phase. Following this initial surface acceleration we observed further accelerations at intervals of twice the acoustic transit time, indicating a reverberation of the initial stress pulse back an forth through the sample. The presence of these rebounds clearly indicates that the free surface did not fail in this particular experiment when the first stress wave arrived.

We can extract the surface velocity from the quadrature signals through a simple procedure: division of the two signals $\cos[\Phi_0 + \partial\phi(t)]$ and $\sin[\Phi_0 + \partial\phi(t)]$ produces $\tan[\Phi_0 + \partial\phi(t)]$. However, the arctangent does not give the true value of

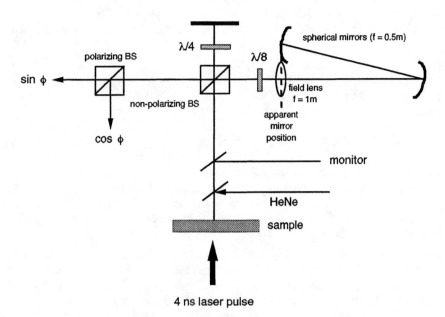

Figure 4. Experimental setup: A 4 ns laser pulse from a doubled Nd:YAG laser was delivered over a 3 mm spot to the tissue model consisting of water containing an absorbing dye with an absorption depth of $100\,\mu$m. The evolution of the stress wave is monitored by measuring the free surface velocity as a function of time with the VISAR. The probe source was a HeNe laser at 632.8 nm with a coherence length greater than 4 m path length difference. Quadrature fringe patterns are obtained by using wave plates to get linearly polarized at 45° and circularly polarized light returning from the arms.

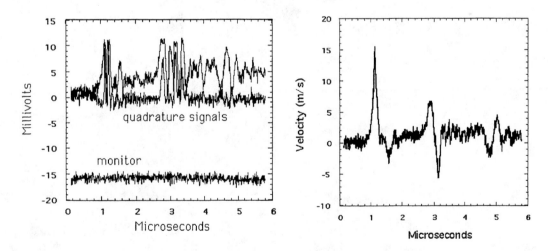

Figure 5. (a) Velocity fringes at a radiant exposure of 1.7 J/cm^2. The laser pulse arrived at time $t = 0$. The stress wave generated takes about 1 μs to travel through the water to reach the free surface at the speed of sound. The free surface did not fail in this experiment as is indicated by the first and second rebounds. (b) Calculated velocities: Peak velocities of 15 m/s are reached. The first stress wave is largely unipolar and compressive. The rebounds are more bipolar with compressive and tensile components.

$[\Phi_0 + \partial\phi(t)]$, but instead computes its principal value between $-\pi/2$ and $\pi/2$. The true value of $[\Phi_0 + \partial\phi(t)]$ can be obtained by phase unwrapping.[8,9] In this study, we used the method described by Takeda *et al.* to calculate the true value of $[\Phi_0 + \partial\phi(t)]$.[8] The initial phase Φ_0 is generally random and must be subtracted by setting $\partial\phi(0) = 0$. Conversion of phase to velocity $u(t)$ uses equation (3).

Figure (5b) shows the velocity calculated from the data in figure (5a). Peak velocities of 15 m/s were reached on the first arrival of the stress wave, with each successive echo diminishing. The rise time of the velocity profile is indicative of the energy deposition profile. An interesting feature is that the velocity profile of the first arriving stress wave is largely unipolar, while it becomes more bipolar for the subsequent rebounds. The unipolar nature of the first wave was expected since upon deposition of the laser energy, a compressive stress is built up in the deposition region. In a strictly one-dimensional situation the echoes should remain unipolar, either positive or negative.[5] However the finite spot size (3 mm) and relatively thick sample (1.5 mm) allow lateral rarefactions to transform the evolving stress wave into a diverging profile after the first pulse. This probably accounts for the development of the bipolar structure in the following echoes. The slight tensile component in the initial compressive wave could be due some degree of vaporization of the the water in the laser deposition region. The radiant exposure of 1.7 J/cm^2 in this case is not enough to heat the irradiated surface to 100°C, and vaporization is therefore not expected. However, the spatial profile of the laser was not uniform, and hot spots may have induced localized vaporization. Future experiments will use cleaner laser spots, and attempt to maintain one-dimensional motion.

Figure (6a) shows velocity fringes just above failure of the free surface at a radiant exposure of 2.9 J/cm^2. No rebounds of the stress wave are present in the signal, indicating that the reflecting surface is disconnected from the main sample volume after the initial release. Failure of the free surface was also confirmed by visual observation. Peak velocities of 25 m/s were reached. This is in good agreement with theoretical prediction by Glinsky *et al.* who calculated free surface velocities of 20 m/s at failure.[5] Figure (7) shows the case where the radiant exposure was 3.3 J/cm^2, which was well above the threshold for failure of the free surface. Higher velocities of 35 m/s were recorded.

In summary, an experimental technique to measure particle velocities during stress wave generation in regimes relevant to laser-tissue interactions was demonstrated. The information provided by this system can be used to study the evolution of stress waves in biological media, and ultimately play an important role in dosimetry calculations for laser surgery and drug delivery applications. The system is based on an interferometric detection scheme and has several advantages over traditional pressure transducer measurements in terms of speed, sensitivity, and the non-contact mode of operation.

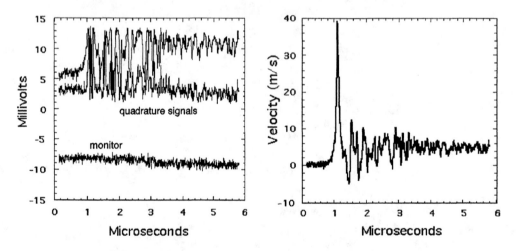

Figure 6. Fringe signals and calculated velocities at a radiant exposure of 2.9 J/cm^2, just above the threshold for spallation of the free surface. No rebounds are observed, and peak velocities of 35 m/s were reached. Glinsky *et al.* theoretically predicted a free surface velocity of 20–25 m/s at spallation threshold.[5]

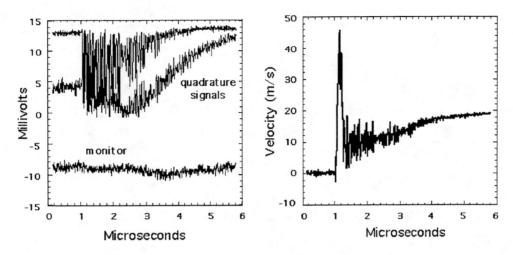

Figure 7. Radiant exposure of 3.3 J/cm^2: The surface spalls away from the rest of the material at speeds of 45 m/s.

ACKNOWLEDGMENTS

The authors would like to thank Dr. Richard London and Dr. Michael Glinsky of Lawrence Livermore National Laboratory for their helpful comments.

REFERENCES

1. L. M. Barker and R. E. Hollenbach, "Shock-wave studies of pmma, fulsed silica, and sapphire," *J. Appl. Phys.* **41**, pp. 4208–4226, 1970.
2. L. M. Barker and R. E. Hollenbach, "Shock wave study of the $\alpha \rightleftharpoons \epsilon$ phase transition in iron," *J. Appl. Phys.* **45**, pp. 4872–4887, 1974.
3. L. M. Barker and R. E. Hollenbach, "Interferometer technique for measuring the dynamic mechanical properties of materials," *Rev. Sci. Instrum.* **36**, pp. 1617–1620, 1965.
4. Z. Chen, T. E. Milner, S. Srinivas, X. Wang, A. Malekafzali, M. J. C. vanGemert, and J. S. Nelson, "Noninvasive imaging of in vivo blood flow velocity using optical doppler tomography," *Opt. Lett.* **22**(14), pp. 1119–21, 1997.
5. M. E. Glinsky, D. S. Bailey, and R. A. London, "LATIS modeling of laser induced midplane and backplane spallation," in *Proceedings of Laser-Tissue Interaction VIII*, S. L. Jacques, ed., vol. 2975, pp. 374–387, (San Jose, CA), 1997.
6. L. M. Barker and R. E. Hollenbach, "Laser interferometer for measuring high velocities of any reflecting surface," *J. Appl. Phys.* **43**, pp. 4669–4675, 1972.
7. S. Wang, C. Cao, and J. Sun, "A VISAR with multireflection étalon and its application in interior ballistics research," *Rev. Sci. Instrum.* **62**, pp. 2944–2945, 1991.
8. M. Takeda, H. Ina, and S. Kobayashi, "Fourier-transform method of fringe-pattern analysis for computer-based topography and interferometry," *J. Opt. Soc. Am.* **72**, pp. 156–160, 1982.
9. D. C. Ghiglia, G. A. Mastin, and L. A. Romero, "Cellular-automata method for phase unwrapping," *J. Opt. Soc. Am. A* **4**, pp. 267–280, 1987.

Generating subsurface acoustic waves in indocyanine green stained elastin biomaterial using a Q-switched laser

John A. Viator, Steve L. Jacques, Scott A. Prahl

Oregon Graduate Institute, Portland, OR 97291
Oregon Medical Laser Center, Portland, OR 97225

ABSTRACT

A Q-switched frequency-doubled Nd-YAG laser coupled to an optical parametric oscillator generated 4.75 ns 800 nm laser pulses to create a subsurface acoustic wave in planar indocyanine green gel samples and flat segments of elastin biomaterial stained with indocyanine green. The acoustic waves traveled through the target and were detected by a piezoelectric transducer. The waveforms were converted to measurements of pressure (and temperature) as a function of depth in the material. An algorithm was developed and applied to the acoustic signals to extract information about the the absorption coefficient as a function of depth in the samples.

Keywords: photoacoustic imaging, photothermal imaging, depth profiling, absorption coefficient

1. INTRODUCTION AND BACKGROUND

Laser tissue welding is a thermal process in which two tissues are fused together using laser energy. Laser welding is proposed as an alternative to suture techniques, since it is potentially faster and less traumatic.[1] Numerous investigations on tissue welding have been undertaken, including those using indocyanine green (ICG) as a chromophore to localize laser energy deposition at the welding site. Since the welding process depends on temperature, accurate measurement of the thermal profile at the welding site is critical for understanding the mechanism of laser welding. Furthermore, the initial distribution of ICG at the welding site is a crucial parameter in the welding process. In this paper we use a photoacoustic technique[2] to obtain thermal profiles as a function of depth in tissues stained with ICG. We also develop and apply a simple algorithm for extracting information about the absorption coefficient (or ICG concentration) as a function of depth from the acoustic signals.

An acoustically-confined[3] laser pulse will create a pressure wave in an absorbing sample (biomaterial or gelatin, Figure 1). This pressure wave will propagate in both directions along the laser beam axis, each with half of the original amplitude.[2] The acoustic signal, detected at a short distance from the site of the initial pressure wave, contains information about the initial temperature and pressure and consequently about the distribution of dye in the material.

2. MATERIALS AND METHODS

An ICG-dyed gel and ICG-stained elastin biomaterial are used as targets from which acoustic waves are generated and detected. The gel, being homogeneous, has uniform absorption while the elastin biomaterial is expected to have a dye layer that drops in concentration with depth.

2.1. Q-switched Laser

The laser used for these experiments was a Q-switched frequency doubled Nd-YAG laser (Quantel Brilliant) operating at 532 nm coupled to an optical parametric oscillator (OPOTEK) tuned to 800 nm. All laser pulses for these experiments were performed as single shots of 40 mJ. The pulse duration (FWHM) was 4.75 ns. The laser spot was elliptical, with major and minor diameters of 3 and 2 mm, respectively.

2.2. Indocyanine Green Gel

The absorbing gel was prepared as 3.5% gelatin (175 Bloom) in 15 ml of water with 0.0171 g of indocyanine green dye. This corresponds to a 2 mM concentration, similar to that used in many tissue welding experiments. The absorption coefficient at 800 nm was 190 cm^{-1}. The gel was formed directly on glass slides and allowed to cool so that the glass-gel interface would be free of air bubbles. The glass slide provided support for the thin gelatin sample during irradiation. The thickness of the gel was measured with a micrometer and was approximately 750 μm.

SPIE Vol. 3254 • 0277-786X/98/$10.00

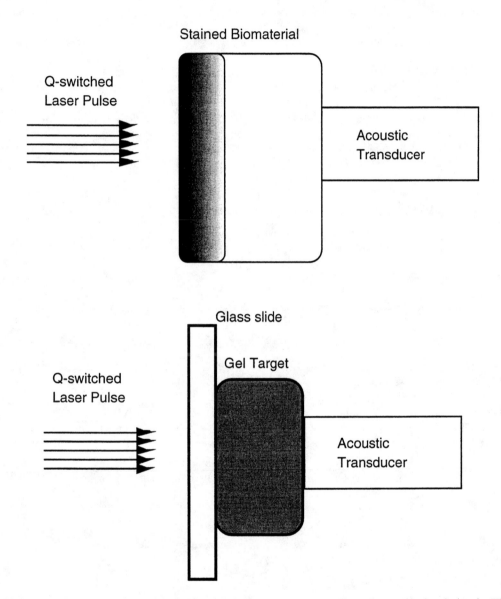

Figure 1. ICG stained elastin biomaterial. The dye layer concentration decreases with depth (top). The ICG dyed gelatin target. The dye concentration is uniform throughout. The gel was set on a glass slide (bottom).

2.3. Elastin Biomaterial

Elastin biomaterial is formed from the elastin constituent of an aorta. In these experiments the elastin biomaterial was derived from porcine aorta harvested from domestic swine. The aorta was cleaned and placed in a 0.5 M sodium hydroxide at 65°C. The vessels were sonicated for 60 minutes. The vessels were then rinsed in deionized water. This process resulted in the removal of all constituents of the artery except for the elastin layer. The thickness of the tissue was measured with a micrometer and was approximately 1 mm. The biomaterial was cut open so that a flat, rectangular piece could be positioned in the path of the laser beam. The intimal surface was stained by brushing a 2 mM ICG dye solution onto the biomaterial. The opposite surface contacted a piezoelectric transducer.

2.4. Piezoelectric Transducer

The piezoelectric transducer (Science Brothers, WAT-12) is a LiNbO crystal used for detecting acoustic pulses of nanosecond duration. The sensing element is protected by a germanium window that is opaque to the 800 nm laser light. The delay in the transducer is 700 ns, determined by placing the stained biomaterial surface directly onto the germanium window, with no intervening stained tissue. The signal was detected after 700 ns, the delay being attributed to the time for the acoustic signal to travel from the site of laser deposition through the germanium window and onto the sensing element.

3. RESULTS

3.1. Gel Response

The signal detected by the acoustic transducer for the absorption in the gel is shown in the top graph of Figure 2. Equivalent temperatures are shown on the right vertical axis. The relation

$$T = \frac{P}{\rho c \Gamma} \tag{1}$$

is used, where P is pressure [J/cm^3], ρ is the density [g/cm^3], c is the specific heat [J/g°C], and Γ is the unitless Grüneisen coefficient. The value $\Gamma = 0.12$ was used in this paper.[2] The relation

$$10 \, \text{bar} = 1 \, \text{J/cm}^3 \tag{2}$$

should be used to convert pressures in bars to energy density. The total delay after the trigger pulse is shown on the horizontal axis. The less smooth negative pressure (tensile wave) that follows is probably caused by an acoustic diffractive effect of the beam boundaries. The tensile wave is not a reflection at a free surface, since the gel to glass coupling was free from air bubbles. The total delay of the initial stress wave is 1100 ns, so subtracting the transducer delay of 700 ns, gives a propagation time through the gel of 400 ns, indicating a gel thickness of 600 μm. This result assumes a sound propagation speed c_s of 1.5 mm/μs. This is less than the measured thickness of 750 μm, but the transducer placed against the gel surface may have caused some compression, thus reducing the gel thickness.

The bottom graph of Figure 2 is the initial acoustic wave generated in the ICG gel, where the times t from the top graph have been converted to depths z within the gelatin using $z = (1.1 \mu s - t)c_s$. The solid line is an exponential curve fit, given by

$$P(z) = 4.21 \exp(-178 \text{cm}^{-1} z) \qquad \text{(bar)} \tag{3}$$

The fit is close for most of the curve, but shows significant disagreement at the surface ($z = 0$). This may be due to diffraction or complications from the glass-gel boundary.

3.2. Elastin Biomaterial Response

The acoustic signal detected from the stained elastin biomaterial is shown in the top graph of Figure 3. In this case, the front of the tissue is bounded by air, thus creating a free surface, which results in a following tensile wave described earlier. This feature is shown here, although the tensile wave is attenuated. The total delay for the initial stress wave after the trigger, 1400 ns, is indicated on the horizontal axis. Since the detector delay is 700 ns, the propagation time through the tissue is 700 ns. This gives a tissue thickness of 1050 μm, which agrees with the measured thickness of 1000 μm.

The bottom graph of Figure 3 shows the initial acoustic wave generated in the stained biomaterial. In this case, the times t from the top graph have been converted to depths z within the biomaterial using $z = (1.42 \mu s - t)c_s$. The right vertical axis directly gives the temperature rise in the elastin biomaterial as a function of depth.

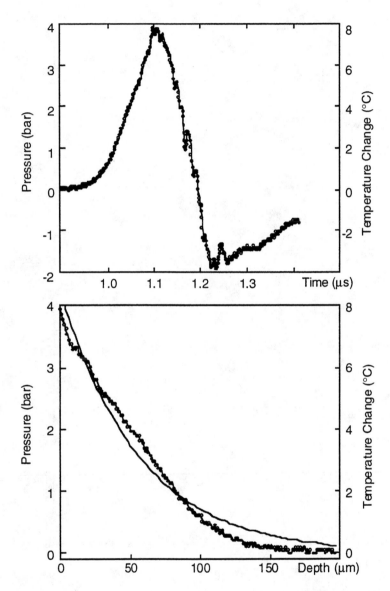

Figure 2. (Top) The acoustic wave from the ICG gel. The time scale is set to zero at the beginning of the Q-switched pulse. (Bottom) The initial acoustic wave generated in the ICG gel, showing pressure as a function of depth. The solid line is an exponential curve fit.

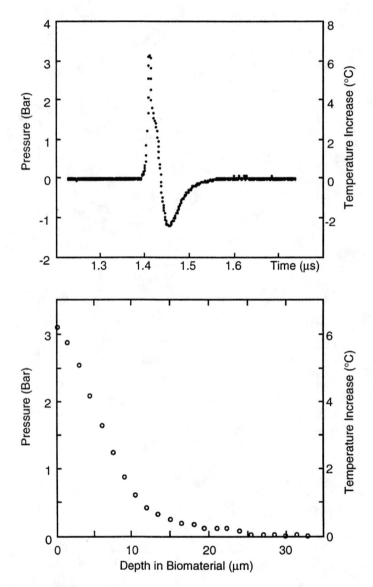

Figure 3. (Top) The acoustic signal from the stained biomaterial. The time scale is set to zero at the beginning of the Q-switched pulse. (Bottom) The initial positive pressure wave as a function of depth derived from the signal at the top. No exponential curve fit was made because the dye concentration is not expected to be uniform.

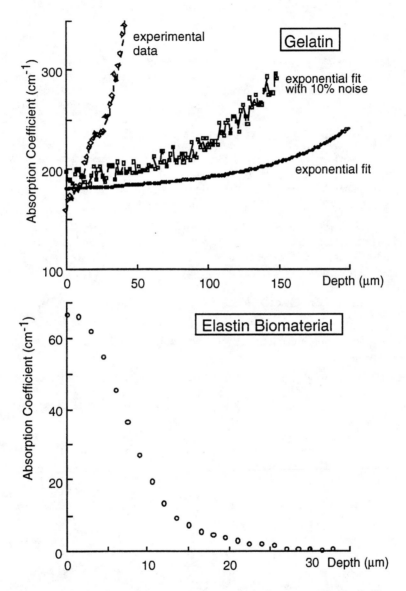

Figure 4. The absorption coefficient calculated using equation (8). The top graph shows the results for data obtained using the exponential fit of equation (3), the exponential fit (3) with 10% noise, and for the experimental data in Figure (2). The bottom graph shows the results for the stained biomaterial.

4. DISCUSSION

4.1. Absorption Coefficient of ICG Gel

The absorption coefficient of the ICG gel was selected as $190\,\mathrm{cm}^{-1}$ to be comparable to the absorption of a lightly stained ICG biomaterial.[4] This corresponds to an absorption depth of about $50\,\mu\mathrm{m}$. The elastin biomaterial waveform shows the initial stress which indicates a dye deposition depth of $30\,\mu\mathrm{m}$ (Figure 6).

4.2. Diffraction Effects

The analysis of the stress wave assumes a planar wave front. Diffractive effects become important when the size of the initial stress field is comparable to the distance that the pressure waves must propagate to the acoustic detector. The gelatin stress waves propagated $750\,\mu\mathrm{m}$ and the biomaterial stress waves propagated about $950\,\mu\mathrm{m}$. Since the initial stress field was only $2000\,\mu\mathrm{m}$ across, diffractive effects will affect the detected signal.

4.3. Frequency Response of the Piezoelectric Transducer

The sensitivity of the piezoelectric transducer is dependent on the frequency of the detected signal. The manufacturer's supplied sensitivity calibration was used to convert the signal amplitude in millivolts to a pressure in bars. In the case of the gel and elastin biomaterial, $20\,\mathrm{MHz}$ and $50\,\mathrm{MHz}$ were used as signal frequencies, respectively. The calibration curve gave a value of $20\,\mathrm{mV/bar}$ and $40\,\mathrm{mV/bar}$, respectively.

Fourier analysis was performed on the signal generated from the gel sample and on the predicted signal pressures from the gel to determine the frequency response of the transducer. Since the gel absorption coefficient was known to be $190\,\mathrm{cm}^{-1}$ and assuming a homogeneous distribution of ICG in the gel, the transducer sensitivity as a function of frequency was calculated. The sensitivity was flat except for a decrease by a factor of two at the higher frequencies.

4.4. Derivation of Absorption Coefficient

The pressure and temperature rise following the laser pulse is explicit in Figures 2 and 3, but the variation in ICG concentration is implicit. To calculate the intrinsic absorption as a function of depth, we developed a simple model based on an absorbing-only medium.

For a uniformly absorbing medium exposed to a laser pulse with a radiant exposure of H_0, the energy A_1 absorbed per unit area in a layer with thickness Δx_1 is

$$A_1 = H_0\big(1 - \exp(-\mu_a \Delta x_1)\big) \tag{4}$$

For a two layer medium, the energy absorbed per unit area in the second layer is reduced by the amount lost in passing through the first layer with thickness Δx_1,

$$A_2 = H_0\big(1 - \exp(-\mu_{a2}\Delta x_2)\big)\exp(-\mu_{a1}\Delta x_1) \tag{5}$$

Extending this to a multi-layer case, the energy per unit area absorbed in the nth layer is

$$A_n = H_0\big(1 - \exp(-\mu_{an}\Delta x)\big)\exp\left(-\sum_{i=1}^{n-1}\mu_{ai}\Delta x\right) \tag{6}$$

Since equation (6) is expressed in terms of energy per unit area, the relationship $P_n = \Gamma A_n/\Delta x$ may be used to obtain the pressures that propagate in each direction,

$$P_n = \frac{\Gamma H_0}{2\Delta x}\big(1 - \exp(-\mu_{an}\Delta x)\big)\exp\left(-\sum_{i=1}^{n-1}\mu_{ai}\Delta x\right) \tag{7}$$

(The factor of two arises because half the energy propagates in each direction along the axis of the laser beam.) Note, that if the radiant exposure is given in $\mathrm{J/cm^2}$ and the layer thickness is in cm, then equation (7) will generate pressures with units of $\mathrm{J/cm^3}$. To obtain pressures in bars, then equation (2) should be used.

An equation for the absorption coefficient of each layer can be derived from equation (7).

$$\mu_{an} = -\frac{1}{\Delta x} \ln \left(1 - \frac{2\Delta x P_n}{\Gamma H_0} \exp \left(\sum_{i=1}^{n-1} \mu_{ai}\Delta x \right) \right) \tag{8}$$

Again, the pressure P should be in J/cm^3, the layer thickness Δx should be in cm, and the radiant exposure H_0 should be in J/cm^2. If the target material is divided into layers corresponding to the resolution of the waveform on the digitizing signal analyzer, the absorption coefficient can be derived for each of these layers using the algorithm described above. The absorption coefficients are obtained with increasing depths, starting with the first layer and propagating downwards into the sample.

To illustrate the stability of the algorithm, noiseless data was generated using equation (3) and processed using equation (8). This is shown in the top graph of Figure 4 for the data labeled "exponential fit." To show the sensitivity of the algorithm to noise, 10% noise was added to the exponential data and the results are also shown in the top graph of Figure 4. Finally, the actual data shown in Figure 2 is processed using equation (8) and shown in the same graph. The absorption coefficients increase with depth, contrary to the known uniform absorption coefficient of the gel.

The algorithm is unstable for the experimental data. While the initial absorption coefficient of $180\,\mathrm{cm}^{-1}$ is reasonable, the values diverge almost immediately. The curve fit result, showing an absorption coefficient of about $180\,\mathrm{cm}^{-1}$ for the first $150\,\mu\mathrm{m}$, is much better behaved. Even with the noise added, the curve fit result shows an calculated absorption coefficient of 180–$200\,\mathrm{cm}^{-1}$ for the first $100\,\mu\mathrm{m}$. The algorithm is very sensitive to artifacts in the experimental data, while the curve fits are generally faithful to the known absorption. As noted before, the data at the surface of the gel departs from the exponential fit. This may cause an early error in the algorithm computation, though the result would probably only manifest itself as an magnitude, not the extreme divergence shown here. Interestingly, all three curves show an increasing absorption with depth. This indicates a bias in the algorithm to process error in one direction, regardless of the nature of the perturbation in the data.

The bottom graph in Figure 4 shows the calculated absorption coefficient of the ICG stained elastin biomaterial. The exponential decay of the absorption is expected for the staining. The divergence shown in the gel calculations is not evident here, perhaps due to the fact that the staining depth is less than $30\,\mu\mathrm{m}$, so the algorithm may not have manifested its latent instability.

5. ACKNOWLEDGEMENTS

We would like to acknowledge the help of Gary Gofstein for assistance in the acoustic wave detection experiment. We also acknowledge the help of Dr. Alexander Oraevsky of Rice University for his help on the acoustic transducers. This work was supported by the Department of the Army Combat Casualty Care Division, US AMRMC contract 95221N–02, and by the Department of Energy, DE–FG03–97–ER62346.

REFERENCES

1. L. S. Bass and M. R. Treat, "Laser tissue welding: A comprehensive review of current future clinical applications," *Lasers Surg. Med.* **17**, pp. 315–349, 1996.
2. A. A. Oraevsky, S. L. Jacques, and F. K. Tittel, "Mechanism of laser ablation for aqueous media irradiated under stress confined conditions," *J. Appl. Phys.* **78**, pp. 1281–1289, 1995.
3. S. L. Jacques, "Laser-tissue interactions. Photochemical, photothermal and photomechanical," *Lasers General Surg.* **72**, pp. 531–557, 1992.
4. K. S. Kumar, "Spectroscopy of indocyanine green photodegradation," Master's thesis, Oregon Graduate Institute of Science and Technology, 1996.

Internal photomechanical fracture of spatially limited absorbers irradiated by short laser pulses

Guenther Paltauf and Heinz Schmidt-Kloiber

Institut für Experimentalphysik, Karl-Franzens-Universität Graz
Universitätsplatz 5, 8010 Graz, Austria

ABSTRACT

A photomechanical damage mechanism in absorbing regions or particles surrounded by a non-absorbing medium after irradiation with a short laser pulse is investigated experimentally and theoretically. In tissue, such absorbers are for example melanosomes, blood vessels or tattoo pigments. It follows from theoretical considerations that the photoacoustic wave caused by irradiation of a spatially limited volume contains both compressive and tensile stress. Experiments were performed to test whether these tensile stresses cause cavitation in absorbers of spherical or cylindrical shape. High-speed video images of liquid spheres or gelatin cylinders (diameters 200 to 300 μm) suspended in oil showed that cavitation occurs at the center of the spheres or on the cylinder axis, respectively, shortly after irradiation with a light pulse (6 ns duration) from an optical parametric oscillator. The cavitation effect was observed at maximum temperatures below and above the boiling point and at ratios of the absorber size on the absorption length larger and smaller than one. The experimental findings are supported by theoretical calculations, from which strong tensile stresses are predicted in the interior of the absorbers, even if the values of acoustic impedance inside and outside the absorbing volume are equal.

The reported effect is believed to cause damage to absorbers if the pulse duration is short enough to provide stress confinement, that is if the time an acoustic wave needs to cross the absorbing region is longer than the pulse duration. For small absorbers such as melanosomes with a size of about 1 μm this requires a laser pulse duration in the picosecond regime.

Key words: Cavitation, thermoelastic stress, stress confinement.

1. INTRODUCTION

In several kinds of laser therapies the photomechanical interaction between short laser pulses and small pigmented areas embedded in the tissue play an important role. Examples of such areas are tattoo pigments, melanosomes in the retinal pigmented epithelium (RPE) of the eye or small blood vessels. Photomechanical damage to melanosomes in the RPE has been related to bubble formation and shockwave emission following absorption of sub-nanosecond laser pulses [1,2]. Although the most plausible explanation for this effect seems to be the explosive vaporization of the absorber, there has been also the hypothesis that the strong thermoelastic stress that can be created by short laser pulses at average temperatures below the boiling point may also cause photomechanical damage [3].

High thermoelastic pressure is achieved in an absorbing volume if it is exposed to a laser pulse that satisfies the condition of stress confinement,

$$t_p < \frac{a}{c} \tag{1}$$

where t_p is the laser pulse duration, a the size of the absorbing region and c the speed of sound. The thermoelastic pressure causes damage in a material if negative stresses exceeding the tensile strength appear. Tensile stress can be generated by negative reflection of a compressive stress wave at a boundary to a medium with lower acoustic impedance. The photoacoustic fracture and ejection („photospallation") of a material after generation of such a negative thermoelastic stress has been recognized as an important mechanism of tissue ablation by short laser pulses [4-6]. A second mechanism of tensile stress generation inside and outside the source of a thermoelastic wave is related to the source geometry. It follows from principles of sound generation and propagation that a source of finite size always emits a wave that contains positive and negative stress. For certain source geometries (for example a flat disc as it is produced by irradiation of a strongly absorbing medium with a laser pulse) the generation of tensile stress has been described as an acoustic diffraction effect [7]. An example of photoacoustic damage induced by acoustic diffraction is the cavitation that occurs near an optical fiber tip in an absorbing liquid after transmission of a short laser pulse [8]. In the case of an optical fiber, the absorbing volume is limited by the fiber diameter and the optical penetration depth. Tensile stress-induced cavitation is also expected if the absorber itself has finite size and is irradiated by a laser beam with a larger diameter. In the following, theoretical and experimental evidence is presented that such tensile stresses are generated and that they are capable of causing fracture in the interior of the absorber.

2. GENERATION OF PHOTOACOUSTIC WAVES

If thermal conduction from the irradiated volume can be neglected, a laser pulse generates a photoacoustic wave that is described by the following wave equation [9],

$$\nabla^2 \psi - \frac{1}{c^2} \frac{\partial^2 \psi}{\partial t^2} = \frac{\beta}{\rho C_p} S \tag{2}$$

where ψ is the velocity potential, β the thermal expansion coefficient, ρ the density, C_p the specific heat capacity at constant pressure and S the heat generated per unit volume and time. The pressure p and the velocity of a volume element $\vec{u}$ can be derived from ψ using the relations

$$p = -\rho \frac{\partial \psi}{\partial t} \qquad and \qquad \vec{u} = grad\, \psi \tag{3}$$

For irradiation with a very short laser pulse, the heat source term S can be expressed as the product of the volumetric energy density W and the Dirac delta function $\delta(t)$:

$$S(\vec{r},t) = W(\vec{r})\delta(t) \tag{4}$$

Instantaneous heat deposition at time zero gives rise to a time-dependent photoacoustic velocity potential at an arbitrary point $\vec{r}$ that is given by

$$\psi(\vec{r},t) = -\frac{t}{4\pi\rho} \frac{\beta c^2}{C_p} \iint_{|\vec{r}-\vec{r}'|=ct} W(\vec{r}')\,ds \tag{5}$$

where $\vec{r}\,'$ is a point in the source volume, ds is the surface element on a unit sphere and the integration has to be carried out on the surface of a sphere with radius ct around the observation point $\vec{r}$. The photoacoustic pressure can be derived from (5) using the first relation in (3). If the source volume, where a certain energy density is generated by absorption of a laser pulse, has a finite size, the integral on the right-hand side of (5) will yield a nonzero value only if a sphere with radius ct drawn around the observed point intersects the heated volume, that is if $t_3 < t < t_4$ (Fig.1).

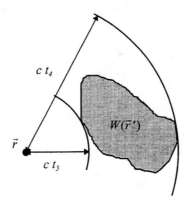

Fig.1 For an observer located at point $\vec{r}$, the photoacoustic wave emitted from a distribution of absorbed energy density $W(\vec{r}')$ starts at $t = t_3$ and ends at $t = t_4$. For times smaller than t_3 or larger than t_4 both velocity potential and pressure must vanish.

113

Integration of the photoacoustic pressure over a time ranging from t_1 to t_2, where $t_1 < t_3$ and $t_2 > t_4$, gives zero:

$$\int_{t_1}^{t_2} p\, dt = \rho\left[\psi(t_1) - \psi(t_2)\right] = 0 \tag{6}$$

Therefore a wave generated in a finite volume must contain both positive and negative stress. The same argument can be used for a point inside the source, provided that the integration starts at a time before the laser pulse is absorbed. In contrast, a plane layer of infinite size produces a purely compressive stress wave, because $\psi(t_2)$ never vanishes.

The calculated results shown below are derived from equations (3) and (5), using either an absorbing sphere or a cylinder of finite length as sources. The absorbers are irradiated from one side, resulting in an energy distribution as it is shown in a cross section in Fig. 2. In the calculation it is assumed that both the optical refractive index and the acoustic impedance are equal inside and outside the absorber. The ratio of the radius a on the absorption length $1/\mu_a$ (where μ_a is the absorption coefficient) is varied, including the two extreme cases where either a thin shell is heated or the laser energy is homogeneously distributed over the whole absorber volume. To obtain a solution of the thermoelastic wave equation for a finite pulse duration, the delta-pulse solution is convoluted with a Gaussian function that describes the temporal intensity profile of the laser pulse:

$$p(t) = \frac{\displaystyle\int_{-\infty}^{+\infty} e^{-(2t'/t_p)^2}\, p_\delta(t-t')\, dt'}{\displaystyle\int_{-\infty}^{+\infty} e^{-(2t'/t_p)^2}\, dt'} \tag{7}$$

where p_δ is the solution obtained for instantaneous energy deposition. For better comparability, the calculated pressure signals are normalized by setting the maximum of the initial thermoelastic pressure equal to one. The absolute pressure values can be obtained by multiplication with the pressure amplitude $\hat{p}_0$,

$$\hat{p}_0 = \frac{\beta c^2}{C_p}\mu_a H_0 = \Gamma \mu_a H_0 \tag{8}$$

where H_0 is the incident radiant exposure and Γ is the Grüneisen parameter.

Laser pulse

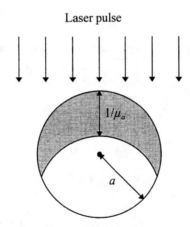

Fig.2 Cross-sectional drawing of a sphere or a cylinder with radius a irradiated from one side with a laser beam. The shaded area represents the heated volume.

3. EXPERIMENT

For the experiments we used two kinds of samples, either water droplets ($\rho = 1$ g/cm^3, $c = 1500$ m/s) suspended in silicone oil ($\rho = 0.96$ g/cm^3, $c = 1000$ m/s) or gelatin filaments ($\rho = 1.08$ g/cm^3, $c = 1600$ m/s) in castor oil ($\rho = 0.96$ g/cm^3, $c = 1540$ m/s). The samples were colored with Orange G (10g/l) and their diameter ranged from approximately 200 to 300 µm. The gelatin was prepared with 75 weight percent dye solution and 25% dry gelatin. The samples were irradiated by 6 ns long pulses from an optical parametric oscillator (OPO) that was pumped with the third harmonic of a Q-switched Nd:YAG laser. A 600 µm core diameter optical fiber was used to transmit the pulses from the OPO close to the samples. Wavelength tuning of the OPO allowed to change the absorption coefficient of the samples in a range from approximately 20 to 1000 cm^{-1}. At variable delay times after the laser pulse the samples were imaged with a time-gated video camera using exposure times between 10 and 20 ns. The experimental setup is shown in Fig.3. Back-illumination with a xenon flash lamp resulted in shadowgraphs in which not only cavitation inside the absorbers, but also stress waves around the absorbers are visible.

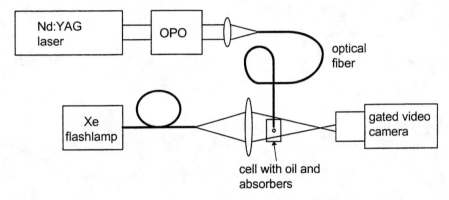

Fig.3 Experimental setup for time-resolved imaging of spherical or cylindrical absorbers suspended in oil.

4. RESULTS

The first series of images in Fig. 4 shows liquid spheres after irradiation with pulses from the OPO. By tuning the wavelength between 500 and 540 nm three cases could be distinguished where the ratio of the sphere radius on the absorption length was either smaller, equal or larger than one: $a\,\mu_a = 0.22$ ($a = 110$ µm, $\mu_a = 20$ cm^{-1}), $a\,\mu_a = 1.2$ ($a = 110$ µm, $\mu_a = 109$ cm^{-1}) and $a\,\mu_a = 14.8$ ($a = 150$ µm, $\mu_a = 985$ cm^{-1}). In all cases, cavitation is seen around the center of the spheres shortly after incidence of the laser pulse. The cavitation bubbles disappear after a few microseconds. At $a\,\mu_a = 0.22$, an incident radiant exposure $H_0 = 0.71$ J/cm^2 led to an average temperature rise of $\Delta T = 3.4°$C. The temperature rise is given by the relation

$$\Delta T = \frac{\mu_a\,H_0}{\rho\,C_p} \tag{9}$$

In the sample with $a\,\mu_a = 1.20$, the temperature rise was 16.5°C ($H_0 = 0.64$ J/cm^2). Only at the highest absorption, where $\Delta T = 99°$C ($H_0 = 0.42$ J/cm^2), the temperature exceeded the boiling point. Due to vaporization of water, the upper half of the sphere turned dark (image after 15 µs).

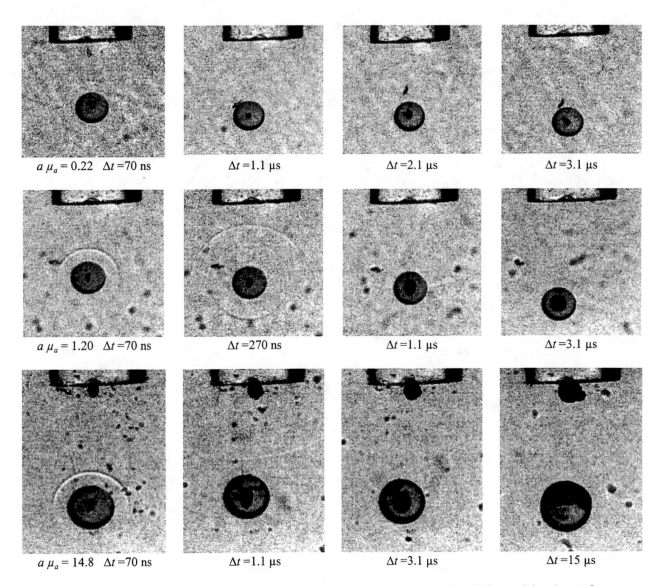

$a\,\mu_a = 0.22$ $\Delta t = 70$ ns $\Delta t = 1.1$ µs $\Delta t = 2.1$ µs $\Delta t = 3.1$ µs

$a\,\mu_a = 1.20$ $\Delta t = 70$ ns $\Delta t = 270$ ns $\Delta t = 1.1$ µs $\Delta t = 3.1$ µs

$a\,\mu_a = 14.8$ $\Delta t = 70$ ns $\Delta t = 1.1$ µs $\Delta t = 3.1$ µs $\Delta t = 15$ µs

Fig.4 Video images showing absorbing water spheres suspended in silicon oil at different delay times after irradiation with 6 ns long pulses from an OPO. The OPO wavelength was changed in order to vary the ratio of sphere radius on the absorption length, $a\,\mu_a$. Images taken at the same value of $a\,\mu_a$ are arranged in the same row. The fiber tip in the upper part of each image has a diameter of 600 µm.

A similar series of images was made with gelatin filaments in castor oil (Fig.5). The use of castor oil provided a closer acoustic impedance match at the gelatin-oil boundary as it was achieved by the combination of water and silicon oil. Images of water droplets in castor oil could not be made because the large difference in refractive indices (1.33 in water and 1.47 in castor oil) made an observation of the interior of the sphere impossible. In this series the ratio of cylinder radius on absorption length was varied from $a\,\mu_a = 0.18$ ($a = 100$ µm, $\mu_a = 18$ cm^{-1}) to $a\,\mu_a = 1.09$ ($a = 90$ µm, $\mu_a = 121$ cm^{-1}) and to $a\,\mu_a = 10.4$ ($a = 100$ µm, $\mu_a = 1040$ cm^{-1}).

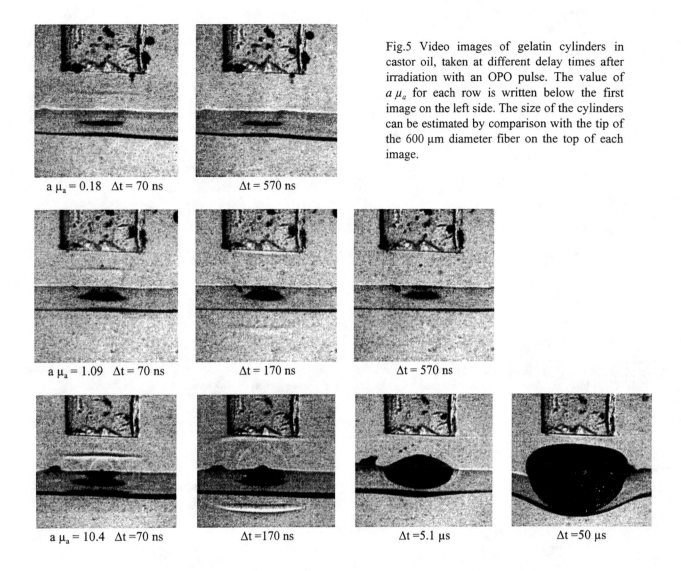

Fig.5 Video images of gelatin cylinders in castor oil, taken at different delay times after irradiation with an OPO pulse. The value of $a \mu_a$ for each row is written below the first image on the left side. The size of the cylinders can be estimated by comparison with the tip of the 600 μm diameter fiber on the top of each image.

$a \mu_a = 0.18$ $\Delta t = 70$ ns $\Delta t = 570$ ns

$a \mu_a = 1.09$ $\Delta t = 70$ ns $\Delta t = 170$ ns $\Delta t = 570$ ns

$a \mu_a = 10.4$ $\Delta t = 70$ ns $\Delta t = 170$ ns $\Delta t = 5.1$ μs $\Delta t = 50$ μs

In all images, cavitation can be seen as a dark shadow along the cylinder axis. At the two lower values of $a \mu_a$, the maximum average temperature stays below the boiling point, $\Delta T = 8°C$ at $a \mu_a = 0.18$ and $\Delta T = 32°C$ at $a \mu_a = 1.09$. At the highest absorption, a theoretical temperature rise of 310°C (assuming a constant heat capacity of 3.5 J g^{-1} K^{-1} and no phase change) created a large vapor bubble (images at 5.1 and 50 μs) that deformed the gelatin filament and lasted for more than 100 μs.

The calculated normalized thermoelastic pressure as a function of time at the center of a sphere is shown in Fig.6. For comparison with the experiments, $a \mu_a$ values of 0.2, 1 and 10 were assumed in the calculations. All curves are bipolar, with a tensile stress amplitude exceeding the maximum compressive stress. The curve at $a \mu_a = 0.2$ is characterized by a plateau phase with $p(t) = 1$, followed by a sharp negative peak after a delay that corresponds to the collapse time of a spherical wave with an initial radius a. At the highest absorption, positive and negative phases of the signal are nearly symmetric. The positive amplitude exceeds the maximum thermoelastic pressure initially created at the surface of the sphere by nearly a factor of two, which is due to a focusing effect.

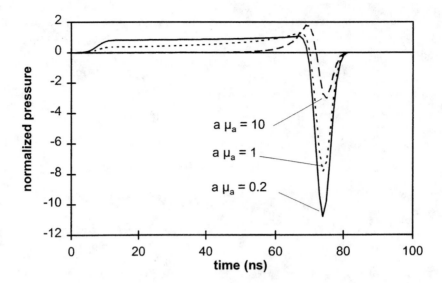

Fig.6 Calculated thermoelastic pressure at the center of an absorbing sphere with radius $a = 100\ \mu m$, created by absorption of a 6 ns long laser pulse.

Curves that were calculated for a point on the axis of a 1 mm long cylinder are displayed in Fig.7. The pressure signals are again bipolar. Compared to the spherical waves, the signals have generally lower amplitudes, because of the smaller focusing effect of the cylinder.

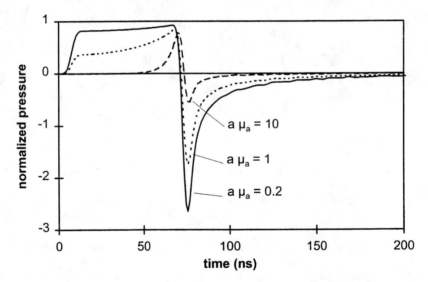

Fig.7 Calculated thermoelastic pressure signals at the axis of an absorbing cylinder with radius $a = 100\ \mu m$. The observed point lies in the middle of a 1 mm long cylinder segment.

5. DISCUSSION

This study has shown that tensile stress-induced cavitation occurs in volumes of finite size in which thermoelastic stress is created by absorption of a short laser pulse. The generation of tensile stress is due to a general property of pulsed photoacoustic sound generated in a spatially limited region, namely that the time integral over the pressure must be zero at any point inside or outside the source volume, provided the integration is performed over a sufficiently long interval. As it was shown above, the tensile stress amplitude depends on the shape of the absorber and is higher in a sphere than in a cylinder. The maximum tensile stress is always located around a symmetry center of the absorber, where the rarefaction waves arriving from the absorber surface interfere constructively. The focusing effect is shown in Fig.8, where positive and negative pressure amplitudes as a function of the position in a sphere are displayed.

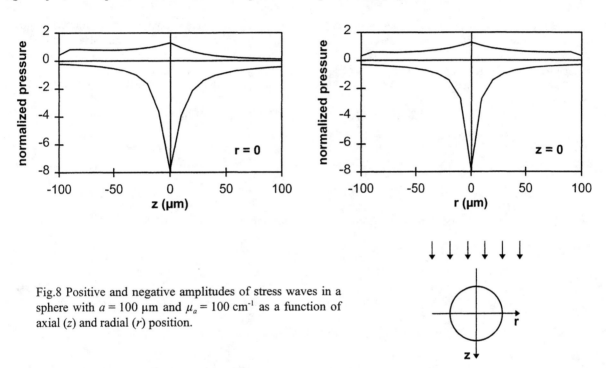

Fig.8 Positive and negative amplitudes of stress waves in a sphere with $a = 100$ μm and $\mu_a = 100$ cm^{-1} as a function of axial (z) and radial (r) position.

It is evident that the focusing effect is strongest in a sphere, because it has the highest symmetry. In order to be able to extend the estimations made in this study to absorbers with a lower degree of symmetry, experiments and calculations in cylinders were included in this study. From these results, the behavior of melanosomes, which have either spherical or ellipsoidal shape, or of blood vessels can be estimated. In addition to the lower pressure amplitudes, pressure waveforms in cylinders show a longer tensile phase as in spheres.

The influence of an acoustic impedance mismatch at the surface of the absorber could not be investigated in this study. In order to be able to compare measured and theoretical results, it has been tried to obtain as close as possible an impedance match between the absorber and the surrounding medium. This was not exactly possible, since two immiscible media had to be found with similar density, speed of sound and optical refractive index. The main result of our investigations, which is also strongly supported by the theoretical findings, is that tensile stresses arise from the limited size of the source and are not subject to an impedance mismatch. In contrast, a plane thermoelastic wave only becomes negative upon reflection at a boundary to a medium with lower acoustic impedance.

Estimations can be made about the tensile stress amplitude that can be expected inside absorbing tissue regions. Assuming the Grüneisen coefficient of water at room temperature, $\Gamma = 0.11$, a volumetric energy density of $W_0 = \mu_a H_0 = 4.2$ J/cm^3 that heats water by 1°C leads to a thermoelastic pressure of $\hat{p}_0 = 4.6$ bar. Since the Grüneisen parameter shows an approximately linear rise with temperature from 0.11 at 20°C to 0.42 at 100°C [6], a thermoelastic stress as high as 900 bar is expected at the boiling point. Taking into account the focusing effect, tensile amplitudes in the kbar region can be expected for absorbers of high symmetry.

The absorbers investigated in this study are about 100 µm in size. An important question is, whether these results can be scaled, for example to smaller absorbers. It is not sufficient to just keep the product $a\,\mu_a$ constant to get comparable results in absorbers of different size. At the same time, also the laser pulse duration has to be changed in a way that the condition of stress confinement (1) is still fulfilled. For a melanosome with a characteristic size of 1 µm this would require a pulse duration shorter than 700 ps.

6. CONCLUSION

Pigmented tissue regions can be damaged by thermoelastic stress that is generated during absorption of a laser pulse under conditions of stress confinement. The damage mechanism is characterized by:

- The formation of tensile stress inside the absorber. The negative stress amplitude depends strongly on the shape of the absorber and shows a strong local variation. Tensile stress generation is a result of the finite size of the absorbing region.
- The generation of cavitation preferably at locations where the tensile stress is highest. Cavitation is observed at temperatures below the boiling point. At temperatures exceeding the boiling point, tensile stress-induced cavitation is generated in addition to a vapor bubble.

The photomechanical damage mechanism described in this study is believed to play an important role in several applications of pulsed laser radiation, both as a therapeutic tool (e.g. for the destruction of tattoo pigments) and as an effect determining safety considerations (e.g. as a possible damage mechanism for melanosomes in the RPE).

ACKNOWLEDGMENT

This work has been supported by the Austrian Science Foundation (FWF), Project Number P10769 Med.

REFERENCES

1. M.W. Kelly and C.P. Lin, "Microcavitation and cell injury in RPE cells following short-pulsed laser irradiation," in *Laser-Tissue Interaction VIII*, edited by S.L. Jacques, Proc. SPIE 2975, pp. 174-179, SPIE, Bellingham, 1997.
2. M. Strauss, P.A. Amendt, R.A. London, D.J. Meitland, M.E. Glinsky, C.P. Lin, and M.W. Kelly, "Computational modeling of stress transient and bubble evolution in short-pulse laser irradiated melanosome particles," in *Laser-Tissue Interaction VIII*, edited by S.L. Jacques, Proc. SPIE 2975, pp. 261-270, SPIE, Bellingham, 1997.
3. S.L. Jacques, A.A. Oraevsky, R. Thompson, and B.S. Gerstman, "A working theory and experiments on photomechanical disruption of melanosomes to explain the threshold for minimal visible retinal lesions for sub-ns laser pulses," in *Laser-Tissue Interaction V*, edited by S.L. Jacques, Proc. SPIE 2134A, pp. 54-65, SPIE, Bellingham, 1994.
4. R.S. Dingus and R.J. Scammon, "Gruneisen-stress-induced ablation of biological tissue," in *Laser-Tissue Interaction II*, edited by S.L. Jacques and A. Katzir, Proc. SPIE 1427, pp. 45-54, SPIE, Bellingham, 1991.
5. A.A. Oraevsky, S.L. Jacques, and F.K. Tittel, "Mechanism of laser ablation for aqueous media irradiated under confined-stress conditions," J. Appl. Phys. 78, pp. 1281-1290, 1995.
6. G. Paltauf and H. Schmidt-Kloiber, "Model study to investigate the contribution of spallation to pulsed laser ablation of tissue," Lasers Surg. Med. 16, pp. 277-287, 1995.
7. M.W. Sigrist, "Laser generation of acoustic waves in liquids and gases," J. Appl. Phys. 60, pp. R83-R121, 1986.
8. M. Frenz, G. Paltauf, and H. Schmidt-Kloiber, "Laser generated cavitation in absorbing liquid induced by acoustic diffraction," Phys. Rev. Lett 76, pp. 3546-3549, 1996.
9. G.J. Diebold and T. Sun, "Properties of photoacoustic waves in one, two, and three dimensions," Acustica 80, pp. 339-351, 1994.

SESSION 5

Ocular I: Pulsed Laser Effects on Tissues

Windows of Opportunity:
Applying Ultrashort Laser Pulses for Selective Tissue Effects

Cynthia A. Toth[a], Eric K. Chiu[a], Katrina P. Winter[a], Clarence P. Cain[b], Gary D. Noojin[b], W.P. Roach[c], Benjamin A. Rockwell[d]

[a]Duke University Eye Center, Box 3802, Durham, NC 27710
[b]TASC Inc., San Antonio, TX 78212
[c]Air Force Office of Scientific Research, Bolling AFB, D.C.
[d]Air Force Research Laboratory, Brooks AFB, Texas

ABSTRACT

Ultrashort pulsed laser retinal effects vary widely depending on the configuration of the laser energy as it reaches the retina and surrounding structures. Tissue response is determined by: wavelength, pulsewidth, energy per pulse, peak irradiance, linear optics of the beam path, and non linear optics of the ultrashort beam. In vivo, we have reported a range of lesions from visible and from near infrared ultrashort laser pulses. New data from additional infrared studies in vivo is combined with our previous data to present an overview of retinal effects and how these might be selected for retinal surgical use.

Keywords: Ultrashort Laser Pulses, Laser-tissue interaction, Ophthalmic surgery, Retinal laser, wound healing,

1. INTRODUCTION

Ultrashort pulsed laser retinal effects vary widely depending on the laser energy as it reaches the retina and surrounding structures[1-5]. The wavelength, pulsewidth, peak irradiance and energy per pulse determine the tissue response. The expected effects have been calculated and actual laser effects have been demonstrated in laboratory models. In vivo, we have reported a range of lesions from visible and from near infrared ultrashort laser pulses. New data from additional infrared studies in vivo is combined with our previous data to present an overview of retinal effects and how these might be selected for retinal surgical use.

2. PREVIOUS STUDIES

Lasers were first used in ophthalmology as a replacement for the xenon arc photocoagulation of the retina. The absorption of the laser energy over 100 to 500 msec by melanosomes of the RPE and by hemoglobin within blood vessels created a thermal lesion. Advances since the first argon laser application have involved the use of different laser wavelengths for selective thermal absorption in tissues containing different chromophores, or use of the compact, air-cooled diode laser for portability. Surgeons continue to study laser activation of chemicals within ocular tissue as a future clinical treatment. The use of laser induced breakdown from q switched Nd:YAG laser has been extremely useful to rupture nonpigmented membranes in clear ocular media an the anterior portions of the eye. This can cause retinal injury[6,7] when used deep within the vitreous adjacent to the retina. Many other lasers have been evaluated for use in cutting vitreous and preretinal membranes. To date, the erbium laser has been the most widely used clinically for retinal membrane incision.

3. ULTRASHORT LASER PULSE EFFECTS

Precise selective delivery of the laser energy to tissues of interest might improve the clinical outcome and diminish the loss of vision from ocular laser treatments[8]. External delivery of ultrashort laser pulses into the eye may be an improved way to induce more precise focal injury at selective sites. The selection of the ultrashort pulsewidth, the wavelength and the optics of delivery path may be used to select the window of preferred effect, such as, the creation of microbubbles in cells or laser induced breakdown within retinal tisssue or at preretinal sites. There are two general sites of particular interest for this treatrment: 1. focal laser effect on the retinal pigment epithelium without damage to underlying choroidal blood vessels and 2. cutting or removal of preretinal membranes without injury to the underlying retina.

4. METHODS
Animals involved in this study were procured, maintained, and used in accordance with The Federal Animal Welfare Act, Public Law 89-544, 1966, as amended and the "Guide for the Care and Use of Laboratory Animals", NIH No. 86-23, Washington, D.C., 1986.

We performed histopathologic study of retinal lesions from visible, and near infrared laser and compared the morphology to that of control lesions from an argon laser. A portion of this data was reported previously[9-11], but in this report, new data from infrared laser lesions is added to create a summary of retinal effects.

5. RESULTS
To summarize our retinal data, there are two major issues in laser tissue effect, location of effect and type of effect. Table number 1 summarizes the location of injury by pulsewidth, wavelength and relative energy delivered to the eye.

Table 1. Distribution of Retinal Pathology by Laser Parameters

Pulsewidth	30×10^{-3} ms		$4\text{-}7 \times 10^{-12}$ ns				80×10^{-12} ps		60×10^{-12} ps		3×10^{-12} ps		150×10^{-15} fs		90×10^{-15} fs	
λ (nm)	511		1064		532		1064		532		580		1064		580	
relative energy	↓	↑	↓	↑	↓	↑	↓	↑	↓	↑	↓	↑	↓	↑	↓	↑
nerve fiber layer	-	♦	-	*	-	♦	-	-	-	-	-	*	-	♦	*	♦
inner retinal layers	-	■	-	♦	-	♦	-	·	-	*	-	♦	-	♦	*	♦
photo-receptors	■	■	♦	■	■	■	*	*	*	■	♦	■	♦	■	♦	•
RPE	■	■	■	■	■	■	■	■	♦	■	♦	•	♦	■	♦	•
chorio-capillaris	■	■	♦	■	■	■	-	*	-	-	-	-	-	*	-	-
choroid	*	■	-	■	♦	■	-	-	-	-	-	-	-	-	-	-
hemorrhage	-	C	-	C	-	C	-	-	-	R	-	R	-	C-R	R	R

↓ = energy to create a minimal visible lesion (MVL) up to 2 times MVL
↑ = energy of ~ 5 times MVL
- = no effect   C = hemorrhage from choroidal vessels
* = infrequent or minimal effect   R = hemorrhage from retinal vessels
♦ = focal moderate effect   RPE = retinal pigment epithelium
■ = broad pronounced effect

The above table references our data on retinal lesions from ultrashort laser pulses delivered to the cornea, and relates these to longer pulsewidths and cw laser retinal effects delivered to the corneal surface by similar optics. This tabulation of the vertical location of injury within retinal layers, provides information beyond that of the "yes" or "no" grading of the ocurrence of a retinal lesion. By necessity, however, there are numerous pathologic findings that are hidden by the broad overview of such a table. Summarizing the pathology by anatomic layer--applies only to laser delivery along an optical path similar to that in this study. Specifically this applies for a minimally diverging laser beam directed to the surface of the cornea and thus focussed at the retina in the emmetropic rhesus monkey eye. This table of findings would not apply, for example to 580 nm 90 fs pulses delivered through a focusing lens so that the beam narrows to a 10 micron diameter in the mid vitreous cavity. In that specific example, with adequate energy in the pulse, a plasma may form in the mid vitreous cavity and no retinal effect may be seen. Diverging the beam to broaden the spot size at the retina will also affect the pattern of injury.

From the table of location of pathology we see the following patterns:

1. At low levels of laser energy, 80 ps and shorter visible laser pulses do not cause damage that extends into the choriocapillaris.

2. At high energy with 511-580 nm laser, the longer pulses cause pronounced damage to the choroidal vessels adjacent to the RPE, while shorter pulses cause no choroidal effect.

3. The 1064 nm laser pulses, cause broader and more pronounced RPE effect than the visible laser at threshold, although this required greater energy per pulse for minimal visible lesion

4. The energy difference from MVL to columnar damage was greater as pulsewidth increased for visible ultrashort laser pulses, and was greater for 1060 nm, 150 fs than for 580 nm,90 fs pulses.

5. The location of the vessels which bled in these laser lesions depended on the laser pulsewidth. For nanosecond or 100 ms laser delivery, higher energy caused bleeding from choroidal vessels into the choroid, subretinal space, retina and sometimes into the vitreous cavity. For 80 ps or shorter pulses, higher energy caused bleeding from retinal vessels into the retina and sometimes into the vitreous cavity or subretinal space. Theese was no bleeding into the choroid.

6. DISCUSSION

These findings demonstrate how ultrashort laser pulsewidths could be selected to avoid injury (or inadvertent treatment) to choroidal vessels, while producing a damaging effect at the retinal pigment epithelium. This might eventually be applied as an alternative to traditional delivery of laser energy to affect the retinal pigment epithelium. This may possibly be used to induce injury of the retinal pigment epithelium in eyes with age-related macular degeneration. The injury of the retinal pigment epithelium, may cause the resolution of pathologic drusen found beneath the retinal pigment epithelium in this disease.

These findings also demonstrate how narrow columns of damage can be created with pico and femtosecond laser pulses. By focussing the laser beam at the surface of the retina, this focal effect may be useful for cutting of preretinal membranes using an external laser beam rather than an intraocular surgical instrument. The incision, created by laser induced breakdown, should have a precise limit to the posterior extent, as seen in the focal retinal columns of damage from laser induced breakdown in the retina from 90 fs pulses.

The second aspect of the pathology of laser effect is the tissue effect of the laser energy. That is, in both the argon laser retinal lesion and the 90 fs 580 nm laser lesion, the RPE is injured. The injury pattern of the 90 fs lesion, with vacuolization within the RPE cell, rupture and striation of melanosomes, preservation of the tight junctions between RPE cells, and abrupt drop-off in pathology is in striking contrast to the argon laser 100 ms lesion, where the damage extends from the RPE into the choriocapillaris. The low energy damage to the retinal pigment epithelium from the ultrashort pulses, is thought to be due to the acute heating of the melanosomes over the short duration of the laser pulse. This results in cavitation bubble formation around the melanosome and often to rupture or striation of the melanosome[12].

Future studies may demonstrate a different pattern of adjacent cell death and wound healing than is seen after classic photocoagulation injury. If the wound healing response is different from lesions created by ultrashort laser pulses, a future surgeon may select a laser depending on the desired type of cellular response wanted for treatment of the disease process.

Acknowledgements: This work was supported by USAF Armstrong Laboratory, the Air Force Office of Scientific Research, Air Force Systems Command, USAF, under grant number 2312AA-92AL014 and F49620-95-1-0226 and Contract F33615-92-C-0017.

REFERENCES

1. Goldman AJ, Ham WT, Mueller HA. Ocular damage thresholds and mechanisms for ultrashort pulses of both visible and infrared laser radiation in the rhesus monkey. *Exp Eye Res*; 1977; 24:45-56.

2. Bruckner AP, Schurr JM, Chang EL. Biological damage threshold induced by ultrashort 2nd and 4th harmonic light pulses from a mode-locked Nd:glass laser. USAF SAM-TR-80-47; 1980.

3. Goldman AJ, Ham WT, Mueller HA. Mechanisms of retinal damage resulting from the exposure of rhesus monkeys to ultrashort laser pulses. *Exp Eye Res*. 1975; 21: 457-469.

4. Ham, Jr WT, Mueller HA, Goldman AJ, Newman BE, Holland LM, Kuwabara T. Ocular hazard from picosecond pulses of Nd:YAG laser radiation. *Science*. 1974; 185: 362-363.

5. Taboada & Gibbons WD. Retinal tissue damage induced by single ultrashort 1060 nm laser light pulses. *Appl Opt.* 1978; 17: 2871-2873.

6. Schuschereba ST, Lund DJ, Stuck BE. Picosecond Nd:YAG (1064 & 532) Laser effects on Monkey Retinal Morphology, Lasers in Surgery & Medicine, Supp.7, 1995 abs (15th annual meeting) April, 1995.

7. Lund DJ and Beatrice ES. Near infrared laser ocular bioeffects. *Health Phys.* 1989; 56(5): 631-636.

8. ANSI Standard Z136.1. American national standard for the safe use of lasers. American National Standards Institute, Inc., New York, 1993.

9. Cain CP, Toth CA, DiCarlo CD, Stein CD, Noojin GD, Stolarski DJ, Roach WP. Visible retinal lesions from ultrashort laser pulses in the primate eye. *Invest Ophthalmol Vis Sci.* 1995; 36(5):879-888.

10. Zuclich JA, Elliott WR, Cain CP, Noojin GD, Roach WP, Rockwell BA, Toth CA. Ocular damage induced by ultrashort laser pulses. 1993; USAF AL/OE-TR-93-0099.

11. Cain CP, Noojin GD, Stolarski DJ, Toth CA, DiCarlo CD, Stein CD, Roach WP. Ultrashort Pulse Laser Effects in the Primate Eye. 1994; USAF AL/OE-TR-1994-0141.

12. Toth CA, Chiu EK, Jumper JM, Rockwell BA. Damage mechanisms of pico- and femtosecond laser retinal lesions as viewed by electron microscopy. SPIE 1998; 3254, in press.

Visible Lesion Threshold Dependency on Retinal Spot Size for Ultrashort Laser Pulses in the Near Infrared

Clarence P. Cain,[*] Cynthia A. Toth,[†] Gary D. Noojin,[*] David J. Stolarski,[*]
Dale J. Payne,[‡] Benjamin A. Rockwell[‡]

* TASC, San Antonio, TX 78228
† Duke University Eye Center, Durham, NC 27710
‡ Air Force Research Laboratory, Optical Radiation Division
Brooks, AFB, TX 78235

ABSTRACT

Single pulses in the near-infrared (1060 nanometers) were used to measure retinal spot size dependence of minimum visible lesion (MVL) thresholds in rhesus monkey eyes at a pulsewidth of 150 femtoseconds. We report the MVL thresholds determined at 1 hour and 24 hours post exposure which were obtained with 2 different lenses placed in front of the eye to vary the retinal spot size. Also we report the flourescein angiography thresholds (FAVL) for the above measurements. These new data points will be added to the databank for Retinal Maximum Permissible Exposure (MPE) as a function of spot size for this pulsewidth and a comparison will be made with previous spot size dependency studies. Our measurements show that the retinal ED_{50} threshold fluence decreases for increasing retinal spot sizes. The fluence at the MVL threshold decreased by a factor of 3 for an increase in retinal image diameter by a factor of 4.5 times from the smallest to largest spot size.

1. INTRODUCTION

Retinal effects of ultrashort pulse laser pulses may vary significantly depending on the pulse energy, wavelength, and laser spot size at the retina. Pulsewidth effects have been reported for visible wavelengths at pulsewidths from nanosecond down to 100 femtoseconds.[1] For the near infrared, pulsewidth dependency has been measured for pulsewidths down to 150 fs. With high energy, femtosecond visible pulses, the likelihood increases for peak irradiances to exceed the threshold required for laser induced breakdown within the eye. We have reported[2] the thresholds for 100 fs, 580 nm laser pulses to create bubbles within the vitreous of live eyes as being very near or at the thresholds for creating a minimum visible lesion for the same pulses. The retinal image size of the laser beam was estimated to be minimal (~ 10 μm) which creates very high irradiances and can exceed the threshold for LIB. As the wavelength increases to the near infrared, the ability of the eye to focus the laser beam to a minimal spot size on the retina decreases and hence the likelihood for laser induced breakdown decreases. Likewise if the retinal image size is artificially increased to larger spot sizes, the pulse energy as well as peak power in the pulse required for LIB increases.

A decrease in threshold radiant exposure (J/cm^2) has been shown by Sliney and Wolbarsht[3] to be a function of the pulse duration "t" raised to the ¾ power for exposure durations ranging from 20 μs to 10 s. Another scaling relation derived from published data for the retinal injury threshold for all exposure durations has been shown[4,5] to vary approximately as the reciprocal of the image diameter for image sizes of 20 um to at least 1 mm for pulse durations from 30 ps to 10 s. Herein we are reporting data for visible lesion thresholds at a pulsewidth of 150 femtoseconds and a wavelength of 1060 nm.

2. EXPERIMENTAL METHODS

2.1 Experimental Systems

The Laser System operated with a mode-locked Ti:Sapphire oscillator operating at 76 Mhz, 1060 nm, and a pulsewidth of 150 fs. These pulses were amplified by a doubled Nd:YAG pumped Ti:Sapphire Regenerative Amplifier and provided single pulses at 150 fs with energies up to 3 mJ. Pulsewidths were always measured with a slow scan autocorrelator

SPIE Vol. 3254 • 0277-786X/98/$10.00

after tuning the compressor for minimum pulsewidth. Marker lesions were accomplished with a shuttered cw, 3 watts before the beam splitter, Krypton laser beam for 3 ms.

For this system, the cornea was positioned approximately 1 cm from the beamsplitter so that the reflected portion of the beam entered the eye. The retina was in the focal plane of the fundus camera and the transmitted portion of the beam was directed to an energy meter so that the energy of each pulse could be recorded. The ratio of the reflected and transmitted portions of the beam were measured for each experiment and recorded. This was accomplished in order that the actual energy delivered to cornea could be calculated for each pulse. These energies and ratios were measured with a Molectron JD2000 joulemeter/ratiometer with J4-09 or J3-09 detectors. Throughout this paper, "laser energy delivered" is the energy delivered to the corneal surface without any contact lens or other device to control the image size on the retina.

2.2 *In Vivo* Model

Mature macacca mulatta primates from 2.2 to 6.9 kilograms (kg) were maintained under standard laboratory conditions (12 hours light, 12 hours dark). All primates were screened pre-exposure to ensure that no eye was more than one-half diopter from being emmetropic. All procedures were performed during the light cycle. Animals involved in this study were procured, maintained, and used in accordance with The Federal Animal Welfare Act, Public Law 89-544, 1966, as amended and the "Guide for the Care and Use of Laboratory Animals", 7th Edition, 1996.

2.3 *In Vivo* Preparation

All animals were chemically restrained using 10 milligrams (mg)/kg ketamine hydrochloride (HCl) intramuscularly. Once restrained, 0.25 mg atropine sulfate was administered subcutaneously. Two drops of proparacaine HCl 0.5%, phenylephrine HCl 2.5%, and tropicamide 1% were each administered to both eyes. Under ketamine restraint, the primate had intravenous catheters placed for administration of warmed lactated Ringers solution (10 milliliters (ml)/kg/hour (hr) flow rate) and for administration of propofol. An initial induction dose of propofol (5 mg/kg) was administered to effect. The state of anesthesia was maintained in the monkey using 0.2 - 0.5 mg/kg/min of propofol via syringe pump. The animal was intubated with a cuffed endotracheal tube. A peribulbar injection of 2% lidocaine was administered to reduce extraocular muscular movement. The monkey was securely restrained in a prone position on an adjustable stage for the fundus photography, laser exposure, and FA. Prior to FA, 0.6 ml of Fluorescite 10% (Alcon Laboratories) was administered intravenously. The subject's blood pressure, temperature, and pulse were continuously monitored throughout the experimental protocol. Normal body temperature was maintained by the use of circulating hot water blankets.

Fundus photography (including fluorescein angiography) and observations of lesion formation by the researchers were performed by monocular viewing through a Topcon fundus camera's optical system. Photographs of the fundus were taken immediately before the dye injection during fluorescein angiography and continued at intervals of a few seconds until 5 minutes had elapsed, thus providing a sequence of photographs for the development of fluorescein leakage. After fluorescein injection and angiography the lesions were also assessed for fluorescence by viewing through the camera system with excitation and barrier filter in place. However, fluorescein leakage for the smaller lesions could not be identified by this method and it was not used for this paper.

Baseline fundus photographs in color were taken prior to laser exposures. The eyelids were held open with a wire lid speculum, and the cornea was moistened throughout the procedures with 0.9% saline solution. A minimum of two examiners evaluated all eyes at 1-hr and 24-hr postexposure. Visible lesions at a given exposure site were reported as a yes only if the two examiners identified a lesion. Color fundus photographs were taken at 1-hr and 24-hr postexposure along with black and white photographs of the fluorescein angiography.

2.4 Statistical Analysis

The Probit Procedure[6] was used to estimate the ED_{50} dose for creating an MVL in the retina for all retinal image sizes and to estimate the 95% confidence intervals for the ED_{50}s. Enough data was taken to ensure that the fiducial limits were reasonable and within the following limits at the 24-hr post-exposure reading for visible lesions only. The upper fiducial limit could be no larger than 50% greater than the ED_{50} dosage and the lower fiducial limit could be no less than 50% of the ED_{50} dosage.

3. RESULTS

Measurements were made to determine the effects of varying retinal spot sizes on the MVL thresholds by placing positive and negative lens in front of the eye to change the divergence of the laser beam. One positive and one negative lens were used to change the calculated spot size from 48 μm in diameter to 224 μm diameter for an image area increase of 22 times. Spot sizes were calculated using the gaussian beam propagation formula[7] and multiple lens formulas[8] to determine the focal point behind the retina and the image radius projected onto the retina. The fluence or radiant exposure in J/cm^2 was calculated for each image size. Table 1 lists the lens power, distance to focal point behind retina, image size at retina, area, MVL- ED_{50} thresholds at 24 hours post exposure and the Fluence or Radiant Exposure in joules/centimeter[2]. The one hour MVL thresholds were larger than the 24 hr reading in all cases and the slopes of all probit curves were all larger than 2. Fluorescein angiography did not give a lower threshold in any measurement.

As shown in the table, the threshold energy did not change when a +0.75 diopter lens was placed in front of the cornea even though the image area was reduced by almost one-half. For a negative lens, the threshold energy did not increase proportionally with the image areas and for a 10 fold increase in area, the ED_{50} increased by only a factor of 7 times. Thus the fluence at the ED_{50} threshold for the -5 D lens was only 2/3 of the value for no lens.

Table 1. Minimum Visible Lesion Thresholds for 150 fs, 1.06 μm, for Different Retinal Image Sizes and Calculated Retinal Fluence using Retinal Image Areas are listed

Lens used	Focus behind Retina in mm	Image diam. at retina in μm	Image area at Retina in μm^2	ED_{50} for MVL in μJ	Radiant Expos. J/cm^2
+0.75 Diopter	0.32	48	1.79E-05	1.0 (0.6 - 1.8)	0.056
None	0.44	70	3.93E-05	1.0 (0.8 - 1.2)	0.026
–5 Diopter	0.99	224	39.5E-05	7.2 (5.2 - 9.0)	0.018

Lens were placed 9.5 cm in front of the eye, fs=femtoseconds, μm=micrometers
Fiducial limits are shown in parenthesis, mm=millimeters

4. DISCUSSION

It has been almost universally accepted that while the energy necessary to create a lesion goes up as the spot size increases, the fluence in J/cm^2 decreases as the spot size increases. All measurements previous to ours were for pulsewidths of 30 ps and longer and as Sliney[4] reported in 1984, this dependence of retinal radiant exposure on approximately $1/d_r$ was surprising for the 15 ns and 30 ps pulses. Thus, our findings for the spot size measurements were not surprising in that the radiant exposure at the MVL thresholds decreased as the retinal spot size increased while the threshold energy increased. However our results did not confirm the reciprocal diameter relationship that other have found since we tripled the image diameter and the fluence decreased by only one-third. There was a concern that laser induced breakdown may be influencing the MVL thresholds at these short pulsewidths but the irradiance at the smallest spot size was almost an order in magnitude smaller than necessary to cause LIB. Thus there may be other nonlinear effects which account for our differences from the inverse diameter relationship but we do not know what they may be at this time.

5. ACKNOWLEDGMENTS

This research reported here was supported by AFOSR (2312A101), U.S. Air Force Research Laboratory, and Contract F33615-92-0017).

6. REFERENCES

1. C.P. Cain, C.A.Toth, C.D. DiCarlo, C.D.Stein, G.D.Noojin, D.J. Stolaraski, & W.P. Roach, "Visible Retinal Lesions from Ultrashort Laser Pulses in the Primate Eye", *Investigative Ophthalmology & Visual Sciences,* **36(5)**, pp. 879-888, 1995.

2. C.P. Cain, C.D. DiCarlo, B.A. Rockwell, P.K. Kennedy, G.D. Noojin, D.J. Stolarski, D.X. Hammer, C.D. Toth, & W.P. Roach, "Retinal Damage and Laser-Induced Breakdown Produced by Ultrashort-Pulse Lasers", *Graefe's Archive for clin. & experi. Ophthalmol.,* **234:Suppl.1**, pp. S28-37, 1996.

3. D.H. Sliney and M.L.Wolbarsht, *Safety with Lasers and Other Optical Sources*, Plenum Publishing Corp., New York, 1980.

4. D.H. Sliney, Laser-induced Damage in Optical Materials, NBS Publ. SP 669, Jan. 1984, 355-367

5. D.H. Sliney, Editor, Selected Papers on Laser Safety, SPIE Vol. MS117 SPIE Opt. Eng. Press, pp. 363-374, 1995.

6. SAS Institute, SAS probit procedure, Cary, NC, 1996.

7. C.P. Cain, G.D. Noojin, D.X. Hammer, R.J. Thomas, & B.A. Rockwell, "Artificial Eye for *In-Vitro* Experiments of Laser Light Interaction with Aqueous Media, *J. Biomed. Optics*, **2:1**, pp. 88-94, 1997.

8. W.J. Smith, *Modern Optical Engineering*, 2nd Edition, pp. 45, McGraw-Hill, New York, 1990.

Threshold energies in the artificial retina

Dale J. Payne, Richard A. Hopkins, Jr., Brent Eilert, Gary D. Noojin[†], Benjamin A. Rockwell

Air Force Research Laboratory, Human Effectiveness Directorate, Directed Energy Bioeffects Division,
Optical Radiation Branch, 8111 18th Street, Brooks AFB, TX, 78235-5215
[†]TASC, 4241 Woodcock Drive, Suite B-100, San Antonio, TX, 78228-1330

ABSTRACT

Laser threshold energies for artificial retinal damage from ultrashort (i.e. ≤ 1 ns) laser pulses are investigated as a function of both pulse width and spot size. A piece of film acts as the absorbing layer and is positioned at the focus of the Cain artificial eye[1] (17 mm in water). We performed experiments at the focal point, and at two and ten Rayleigh ranges in front of the focus with the damage endpoint being the presence of a bubble coming off the film. Thresholds were determined for wavelengths of 1064 nm, 580 nm, and 532 nm with pulse durations ranging from the nanosecond (ns) to the femtosecond (fs) regimes. For the at-focus data in the visible regime, the threshold dropped from 0.25 µJ for a 5 ns pulse at 532 nm to 0.11 µJ for a 100 fs, 580 nm pulse. Similarly, for the near infrared (NIR) the threshold changed from 5.5 µJ for a 5 ns pulse to 0.9 µJ for a 130 fs pulse. These results are discussed in the context of applicable nonlinear optical phenomena.

Keywords: laser, ultrashort, threshold, retina, damage

1. INTRODUCTION

Damage induced by ultrashort laser pulses incident on the eye has been of great concern in recent years due to the commercial availability of such laser systems. In particular, damage at or near the retina is of primary interest since this region is responsible for vision. However, threshold trends may be difficult to ascertain since numerous biological processes are occurring in the eye, and these processes may either hinder or encourage damage[2-4]. In order to understand the interaction between the laser pulse and the retina, but without the complications of a biological system, we measured thresholds on an artificial retina for a variety of wavelengths and pulse widths. In our experiment we used a piece of exposed camera film as the artificial retina since both the real retina and regular film can be treated as absorbing layers. Understanding the origins of retinal damage from ultrashort laser pulses is essential for developing an accurate model for the mechanisms involved.

2. EXPERIMENT

Our experimental setup is shown in Fig. 1. A frequency doubled Nd:YAG laser is used to pump a dye laser and produce a 580 nm beam. This beam is then passed through a dye amplifier. Upon exiting the amplifier the laser light is directed through a spatial filter so that a purely Gaussian beam profile is achieved. A polarizing cube and a half-wave plate are utilized to adjust the beam energy entering the spatial filter. Part of the beam is picked off by a beam splitter and directed into an Inrad autocorrelator for measuring the pulse width, while the remainder of the light is focused onto the piece of film by means of the Cain artificial eye[1]. The type of film used in this experiment was Kodak black-and-white TMAX 100™. The silver halide granules had an average circular diameter of 1 µm and an average thickness of 0.16 µm. The cuvette used in this experiment simulates the focusing characteristics of the human eye, and was designed and constructed in-house. The lens, which has a 17 mm focal length, is embedded into the front face of the cuvette and was designed such that the lens-water interface enables the laser beam to focus into the water. The spot size (radius) of the lens measured in water at the beam waist is 2.5 µm for the visible wavelengths, and the cone angle is calculated to be 8°.

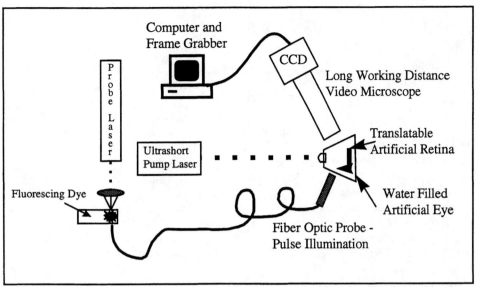

Figure 1. Experimental setup for observing bubble formation from irradiated absorbing layer.

Damage was determined by employing the pump-probe technique for observing bubbles coming off the film. Observation of the threshold event was accomplished by utilizing a Titan imaging microscope, which has a long working-distance objective, attached to a Sony CCD camera. The resolution of the system is 4 μm. The probe pulse is produced by a separate DCR Nd:YAG laser which is frequency doubled by a crystal to provide a 532 nm laser beam. This beam in turn excites a rhodamine 620 dye cell whose fluorescence is focused onto and delivered by a fiber optic cable to the sample site. The DCR laser was triggered from the lamp sync of the ultrashort pulse laser via a time delay generator. Since the delay is controlled electronically, the event can be strobed at any later time. For this investigation we observed the event 500 ns after the pump pulse.

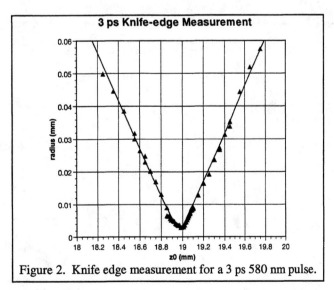

Figure 2. Knife edge measurement for a 3 ps 580 nm pulse.

A Unidex 11 stage controller was used to translate the film along the optical, scan, and vertical axes within the artificial eye. Knife-edge measurements were taken for each pulse duration, and yield a beam diameter of 5 μm. Figure 2 shows the result of a typical knife-edge measurement. The triangles are the actual data and the solid line is the theoretical fit to the data using the equation

$$r(z) = M^2 r_0 \left\{ 1 + \left[\frac{\lambda_n (z - z_0)}{\pi M^2 r_0^2} \right]^2 \right\}^{1/2} \tag{1}$$

where M^2 describes the deviation from a perfect Gaussian diffraction limit, r_0 is the diffraction-limited spot size, and z is the position from the minimum radius position z_0[1].

3. RESULTS

We observed that as the laser pulse width decreases the threshold energy decreases, too. For the at-focus data in the visible regime, the threshold dropped from 0.25 µJ for a 5 ns pulse at 532 nm to 0.11 µJ for a 100 fs, 580 nm pulse. Similarly, for the NIR (1064 nm) the threshold changed from 5.5 µJ for a 5 ns pulse to 0.9 µJ for a 130 fs pulse. Previous experiments for determining minimum visible lesion (MVL) thresholds over the same spectral range and pulse duration have demonstrated a similar trend; that is, less energy is required for retinal damage as the pulse width becomes shorter[5]. Figure 3 illustrates that as the spot size increases, threshold behavior remains unaffected. Figure 4 shows the at-focus trend for the artificial retina threshold for visible and near infrared wavelengths. The error bars represent the upper and lower fiducial limits for the ED_{50} values as calculated by SAS[6]. Because an infrared pulse entering the eye will focus 400 µm behind the retina[7], the energy values for the two Rayleigh ranges NIR data are shown on the graph along with the at-focus visible data in order to account for this difference.

What is important to note about Fig. 4 is how closely the artificial retina data, which lacks any biological components, mimics the data taken using a biological system. This indicates that the underlying physics responsible for damage to an absorbing layer within the artificial eye is the same as that responsible for damage to the retina in a normal eye. Previous studies have suggested that for pulses with nanosecond to microsecond durations the primary damage mechanism is thermal in nature[8,9]. This is because the absorbing material has insufficient time to conduct heat away from itself while the energy from the laser pulse is being deposited. Furthermore, the high extent of agreement between the two separate systems indicates that the artificial retina model is a good emulator of the interaction between ultrashort laser pulses and the biological retina. An advantage here is that it may now be possible to construct theories that explain the damage mechanism(s), but do not necessarily rely on biological contributions.

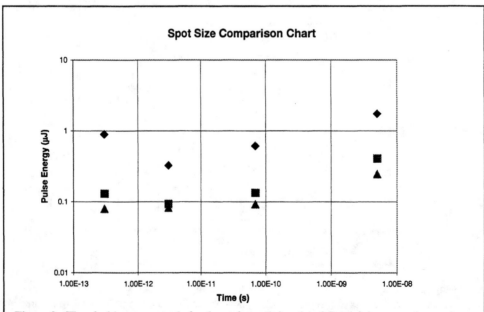

Figure 3. Threshold energy trends for the at-focus (triangle), 2 Rayleigh ranges (square), and 10 Rayleigh ranges (diamond) data. Note: Only visible wavelengths are shown in this graph.

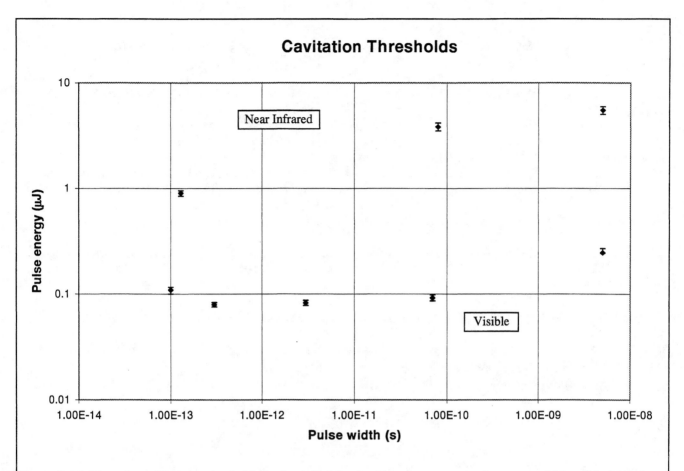

Figure 4. Visible and near IR energy thresholds for the artificial retina. Error bars represent the upper and lower fiducial limits.

4. CONCLUSIONS

We have measured the energy thresholds necessary for bubble formation on an artificial retina. For the at-focus data in the visible regime, the threshold dropped from 0.25 μJ for a 5 ns pulse at 532 nm to 0.11 μJ for a 100 fs, 580 nm pulse. Similarly, for the near IR (1064 nm) the threshold changed from 5.5 μJ for a 5 ns pulse to 0.9 μJ for a 130 fs pulse. The trends observed in our model are similar to trends reported by Cain *et al.* for experiments performed on biological systems. This indicates that the artificial retina system approximates well the physical response of a biological retina when irradiated by laser pulses spanning the nanosecond to femtosecond durations. Previous investigations have explained the drop in threshold within the context of a pulse width dependent thermal damage mechanism. At this writing, studies are continuing with the artificial retina in order to determine the contribution of non-linear effects to the damage process.

5. ACKNOWLEDGEMENTS

This research was supported by the Air Force Office of Scientific Research (2312A103) and Armstrong Laboratory. This research was conducted while Dale Payne held an NRC-Armstrong Laboratory Postdoctoral Research Associateship.

6. REFERENCES

1. C. Cain, G.D. Noojin, D.X. Hammer, R.J. Thomas, and B.A. Rockwell, "Artificial eye for in-vitro experiments of laser light interaction with aqueous media," *J. Biomed. Optics*, **2**, 88 (1997).

2. R.D. Glickman and K-W Lam, "Melanin may promote photooxidation of linoleic acid," *SPIE Laser-Tissue Interactions VI*, **2391**, 254 (1995).

3. T. Sarna, "Properties and function of the ocular melanin - A photobiophysical view," *J. Photochem. Photobiol. B*, **12**, 215 (1992).

4. H.C. Longuet-Higgins, "On the origin of the free radical property of melanins," *Arch. Biochem. Biophys.*, **86**, 231 (1960).

5. C.P. Cain, C.A. Toth, G.D. Noojin, D.J. Stolarski, B.A. Rockwell, "Femtosecond Laser Pulses in the Near-Infrared Produces Visible Lesions in the Primate Eye," to appear in the proceedings of BiOS Europe V conference.

6. SAS Institute, 1996, SAS probit procedure, Cary, NC.

7. B.A. Rockwell, D.X. Hammer, P.K. Kennedy, R. Amnotte, B. Eilert, J.J. Drussel, D.J. Payne, S. Phillips, D.J. Stolarski, G.D. Noojin, R.J. Thomas, and C.P. Cain, "Retinal Spot Size with Wavelength," *SPIE Laser-Tissue Interactions VIII*, **2975**, 148 (1997).

8. D. Sliney and M. Wolbarsht, Safety with Lasers and Other Optical Sources, Ch.4, Plenum Press, New York, NY, 1985.

9. B.A. Rockwell, W.P. Roach, and M.E. Rogers, "Determination of self-focusing effects for light propagaing in the eye," *SPIE Laser-Tissue Interactions V*, **2134**, 2 (1994).

Microscopic simulation of short pulse laser damage of melanin particles

Leonid V. Zhigilei and Barbara J. Garrison

Department of Chemistry, 152 Davey Laboratory, Penn State University, University Park, PA 16802

Abstract

Microscopic mechanisms of short pulse laser damage to melanin granules, the strongest absorbing chromophores of visible and near - IR light in the retina and skin, are studied using the molecular dynamics simulations. The pulse width dependence of the fracture/cavitation and vaporization processes within the small particles, their coupling to the surrounding medium and the resulting tissue injury are discussed based on the simulation results. The effect of laser irradiation on an isolated submicron particle at different laser fluences and pulse durations is first analyzed. The mechanical disruption of the particle due to the laser induced pressure is found to define the character of damage for short pulse widths (tens of picoseconds) at laser fluences that are significantly lower than those required for boiling. Thermal relaxation and explosive disintegration of the overheated particle at higher laser fluencies are the processes that dominate at longer laser pulses (hundreds of picoseconds). Damage of an absorbing particle embedded into a transparent medium with different mechanical characteristics is then simulated. Coupling of the acoustic and thermal pulses generated within absorbing particles to the surrounding medium is studied and the possible cumulative effects from an ensemble of absorbing particles are discussed. The simulation results provide the basis for future work in which the microscopic and continuum descriptions are combined for multiscale modeling of laser tissue interaction.

Keywords: computer simulation, melanin, pressure waves, photomechanical damage

1. Introduction

Computer simulations have been shown to enhance our understanding of the elementary processes occuring in a wide range of physical phenomena. The simulations are especially beneficial in the cases when important processes occurs at the time or length-scales inaccessible for direct experimental investigation. This is the case for the short pulse laser injury to epithelial (pigmented) tissues of the eye and skin where the laser energy is absorbed within micrometer-sized melanosomes composed of strongly absorbing granules of the biological pigment melanin with dimension of order 10-15 nm. The processes within the absorbing granules and their coupling to the surrounding transparent medium should be understood in order to predict the cumulative effect from all granules in the melanosome and the character of the resulting laser damage of the tissue.

The effects of the thermal and stress confinement within melanin granules or the whole melanosome have been discussed theoretically,[1,2] investigated experimentally,[3,4] and simulated using a continuum hydrodynamic model.[5] For sub-nanosecond pulses, the spatially non-uniform absorption and hot spot formation within the melanosome are the factors that are presumably responsible for the substantially lower threshold for minimal visible tissue damage then with longer laser pulses. It has been proposed that relation between the size of the melanin granules and the laser pulse duration is the critical factor that defines the mechanism of short pulse laser injury.[1] When laser pulse duration τ_p becomes shorter than the time for cooling of the absorbing granule by thermal conduction, the hot spots are formed at and around the absorber. Explosive vaporization of the overheated granule and/or the surrounding medium can lead to the vapor bubble formation and generation of a pressure wave.[3,4,5] Moreover, when τ_p is shorter than the time of mechanical relaxation of the stresses generated due to the fast heating of the granule, a high pressure can build up within the absorbing structure at low laser fluences when the deposited energy is below the threshold for explosive vaporization.[1] The emission of strong shock waves from melanosomes isolated in water and irradiated with 40 and 100 ps laser pulses have been observed experimentally[3,4] and reproduced in computer simulations.[5] These observations suggest the importance of photomechanical effects in the short pulse laser damage to pigmented tissues. What is lacking, however, is the information on microscopic mechanisms and nature of the laser induced damage at submicron scale. The complexity and diversity of the processes that define the tissue damage, namely, formation and development of laser induced pressure within and outside the absorbing granules, nucleation, growth, and interaction of microcracks and cavities, explosive vaporization, spinodal decomposition and cooling of the overheated material, hinder the analytical description of the phenomenon.

An alternative method of microscopic analysis of laser induced processes is the molecular dynamics (MD) computer simulation technique.[6] The advantage of this approach is that only details of the microscopic interactions need to be specified, and no assumptions are made about the character of the processes under study. Rather the physical phenomena arise naturally out of the simulations. Moreover, the MD method is capable of providing a complete microscopic description of the dynamic processes induced by the laser pulse as well as the final results of the laser irradiation. Recent development of a breathing sphere model for MD simulations of laser ablation[7] have significantly expanded the time and length scales of the model and have laid the foundation for bridging the gap between the microscopic and mesoscopic aspects of laser ablation and damage of organic solids. Application of the model to the analysis of the ablation of molecular films and matrix-assisted laser desorption demonstrate the ability of the method to provide insight into the microscopic mechanisms of laser ablation.[7,8,9]

In this work, we use the MD method and the breathing sphere model to investigate the basic processes and mechanisms that define a strong dependence on pulse duration of the threshold energy for producing a minimal visible damage to pigmented tissues. Irradiation of individual submicron particles and absorbing particles embedded into a transparent medium is simulated at laser fluences close to the threshold for damage. Apparent qualitative differences in the damage mechanisms for shorter, tens of picoseconds, and longer, hundreds of picoseconds, laser pulses are delinated and related to the experimental observations for pigmented tissues.

2. Computational Method

The molecular dynamics computer simulation technique is used in this work to investigate microscopic mechanisms of short pulse laser damage to absorbing particles embedded in a transparent medium. We study the effects of laser irradiation at submicron resolution that is inaccessible for neither the traditional atomic level MD nor continuum simulations.[5,10] Two innovations are used to expand the time of the MD simulation and the size of the simulated system. These are the breathing sphere model for molecular dynamics simulations of laser ablation and damage in organic materials and non-reflecting boundary conditions that allows us to simulate the propagation of the laser induced stress waves out from the MD computational cell.

The breathing sphere model. The model and the results relevant to the application of the laser ablation phenomena in mass spectrometry are described in detail elsewhere.[7,8,9] Briefly, the model assumes that each molecule (or appropriate group of atoms) can be represented by a single particle that has the true translational degrees of freedom but an approximate internal degree of freedom. This internal (breathing) mode allows us to reproduce a realistic rate of the conversion of internal energy of the molecules excited by the laser to the translational motion of the other molecules. Because we are following molecules and not atoms, our system size can be significantly larger. Moreover, because we are not following explicit atomic vibrations our timestep in the numerical integration is longer. Molecular level resolution of the material description provides an easy means for simulation of complex inhomogeneous organic materials. The strength of the material, the bonding interactions, as well as the wavelength dependent absorptivity of the different tissue components can be easily included. The rate of energy transfer within an individual tissue component as well as between components can be precisely controlled.[7]

Non-reflecting boundary conditions. The generation of stress waves is a natural result of the fast energy deposition in the case of short pulse laser irradiation and inhomogeneous absorption.[1,3,4,5,7,8,10,11] Simulation of the propagation of the stress waves requires the size of the MD computational cell to be increased linearly with the time of the simulation. For times longer than ~100 ps the size of the model required to follow the wave propagation becomes computationally prohibitive. On the other hand, since displacements of the molecules in a region outside the immediate vicinity of the absorbing granule are small, the propagation of the laser induced stress waves can be readily described at the continuum level and do not require a molecular level analysis. In this work the non-reflecting propagation of the stress wave out from the MD computational cell is simulated using recently developed boundary conditions where the traveling wave equation is used to obtain the forces acting at the molecules in the boundary region.[12] The formation and propagation of the pressure wave within the MD computational cell as well as out from the MD region through the non-reflecting boundary is illustrated in Figure 1 for the simulation set up used in Ref. 7-9. In this case the high pressure builds up during the 15 ps laser pulse within the penetration depth of the irradiated sample. The high pressure causes ablation of a part of the irradiated volume and drives a strong compression wave into the bulk of the sample. The non-reflecting boundary conditions set at the

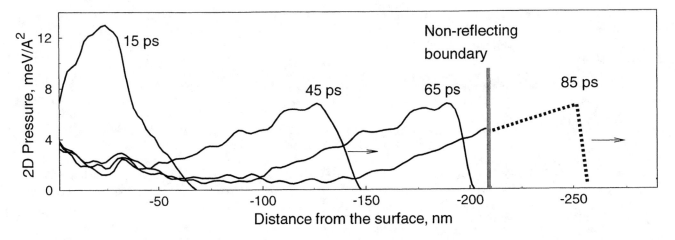

Figure 1. The time development of the high pressure within the penetration depth, 32 nm, of the irradiated sample and propagation of the pressure wave into the bulk of the sample. Non-reflecting boundary conditions set at the depth of 210 nm are used to mimic the propagation of the wave through the boundary of the MD computational cell as schematically shown by dashed line.

depth of 210 nm allow us to avoid an unphysical reflection of the pressure wave from the boundary of the MD computational cell and to monitor the amount of energy carried away by the wave.[12]

Simulation setup. An accurate molecular level simulation of the laser induced damage in a cell requires the knowledge of structural, mechanical, optical, and thermodynamic properties of subcellular structures. As of now, these properties cannot be reliably ascertained from the available experimental data. For example, particles described by a water equation of state and solid protein granules were both considered as possible alternative representations of melanin granules in recent simulations of Strauss et al.[5] Due to uncertainty in sizes, structures and mechanical properties of the submicron compounds we choose to use the present simulations to address general mechanisms and dynamics of short pulse laser damage from inhomogeneous absorption in tissue. As a first step we perform simulations for an isolated melanin granule and study the effect of the mechanical characteristics of the surrounding medium on the laser induced processes.

Simulations are performed both on a two-dimensional (2D) and a three-dimensional (3D) versions of the breathing sphere model. The 2D simulation offers a clear visual picture of the damage process whereas 3D model has a potential for a quantitative comparison between the computed and experimental results. The parameters of the model used to represent an organic solid are given elsewhere.[7] Two-dimensional simulations have been performed for an absorbing particle with radius of 55 nm consisting of 33,799 molecules. We perform simulations both for isolated particles and particles embedded into a transparent medium. The computational setup for the latter case is shown in Figure 2. In this setup the MD computational cell has an outer radius of 140 nm and consists of 220,525 molecules. Non-reflecting boundary conditions are applied at the border of the computational cell in order to mimic the propagation of the laser induced pressure waves through the border. To study the role of the acoustic impedance mismatch at the interface between the absorbing granule and the surrounding medium, simulations are performed with two sets of parameters for intermolecular interactions in the surrounding medium. With one set the granule and the surrounding medium have identical

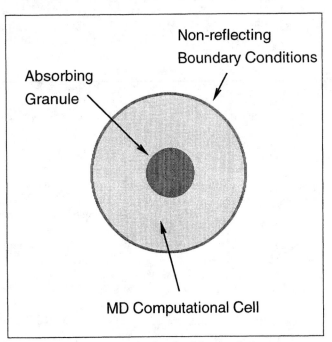

Figure 2. Schematic sketch of the simulation setup.

mechanical properties, with another set intermolecular interactions in the surrounding medium are half as much leading to ~30% mismatch in the acoustic impedance at the interface between the particle and surrounding medium. For the 3D simulations we use an amorphous molecular cluster with the radius of 10 nm consisting of 28,955 molecules. Parameters of the 3D model are chosen to reproduce the density, ρ, of 1.2 g/cm^3 and sound velocity, c_s, of 1650 m/s in the granule.

The laser irradiation is simulated by vibrational excitation of molecules that are randomly chosen during the laser pulse duration. In this case an implicit assumption is that the particle absorbs homogeneously and the effect of laser beam attenuation within the particle can be neglected. The vibrational excitations are performed by depositing a quantum of energy equal to the photon energy into the kinetic energy of internal vibration of the molecule to be excited.[7] Laser pulses of 10 ps and 100 ps in duration at a wavelength of 337 nm are used in the 3D simulations. In 2D simulations pulses of 15 ps and 300 ps are used and the photon energy is scaled down by factor of two in order to account for the lower cohesive energies in the 2D system as compared to the 3D case. A series of simulations at different laser fluences is performed for each pulse duration, starting from a fluence that does not cause any visible damage to the absorbing particle up to fluences that lead to significant visible damage to the particle.

Analysis of simulation results. The MD simulation technique allows one to perform a detailed analysis of the laser induced processes. In particular, visual observations can be correlated with data on microscopic dynamics at the molecular level. The positions, velocities, and energies of molecules are obtained directly from the MD algorithm. The concept of local atomic stresses[13] is used in calculations of the local hydrodynamic pressure that is defined as a first invariant of the stress tensor. The coordination numbers of molecules defined through the Dirichlet construction are used to characterize the defect structure and describe the structural changes and phase transitions occurring in the 2D model.[7,14]

3. Results

In this section we start from the simulation results for isolated absorbing particles. The damage mechanism and the laser fluence threshold values for producing minimal damage within a particle are compared for irradiation with laser pulses of different durations. The physical processes and mechanisms leading to the apparent pulse duration dependence of particle damage are analyzed. Coupling of the acoustic and thermal pulses generated within absorbing particles to the surrounding medium is then studied and the role of the acoustic impedance mismatch between the absorbing granule and the surrounding medium is discussed.

3.1 Isolated particles. Mechanical disruption vs thermal disintegration.

Snapshots from the 2D simulations given in Figure 3 clearly indicate that the laser fluence threshold values for producing minimal damage or cavitation within an isolated particle are essentially different for irradiation with 300 ps and 15 ps pulses. For the 15 ps laser pulse, the threshold laser fluence for producing a minimal visible damage to the irradiated particle is found to correspond to ~0.12 eV per molecule within the particle, Figure 3a. The damage at the threshold has a pronounced character of mechanical disruption of a relatively cold particle. We find that at about 50 ps (or 35 ps after the end of the pulse) a cluster of microcracks is generated. All the microcracks originate in the central part of the particle and radiate outward from the center. Within the succeeding 500 ps the microcracks develop into a cluster of micropores that have lower potential energy due to the reduced area of internal free surfaces. With increasing energy deposited by the laser pulse, more substantial damage is produced. Microcracks crop out to the surface of the particle, Figure 3b, and, at energies deposited higher than ~0.14 eV per molecule, split the particle apart.[14]

In order to reveal the physical processes responsible for the laser damage to the particle we correlate the visual pictures shown in Figure 3 with the spatial and time development of the local hydrostatic pressure in the irradiated particles presented in Figure 4 in the form of contour plots. For the 15 ps laser pulse, a high compressive pressure (positive pressure in Figure 4) builds up in the central part of the particle during the laser pulse. This pressure is the result of inertial stress confinement, when the laser heating of the irradiated particle occurs faster then the mechanical relaxation of the thermoelastic stresses.[1,5,7,8] The minimum characteristic time of mechanical response to the heating can be estimated as the ratio of the size of the heating volume to the speed of acoustic wave propagation. For particles with a radius of ~55 nm and with a speed of sound in the 2D model of 2760 m/s, the time of mechanical relaxation is ~20 ps. Thus, the conditions for inertial confinement exist for 15 ps laser pulses and lead to the high pressure build up in the central part of the particle, Figure 4a. As a consequence of the laser induced compressive pressure an unloading wave propagates from the surface of the particle. Focusing of the unloading wave leads to the concentration of the tensile stresses in the center of the particle at ~50 ps, Figure 4a. The generation of the microcracks, Figure 3a, coincides temporally and spatially with the maximum tensile stresses, indicating that it is the tensile stresses that cause the damage of the particle.

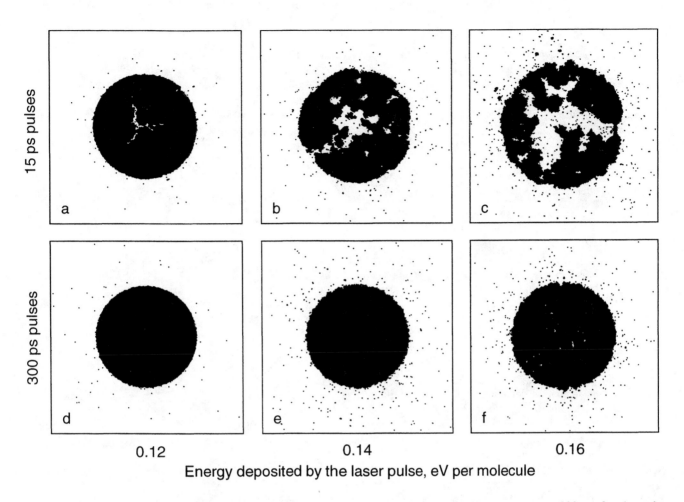

Figure 3. Snapshots from the MD simulations of isolated particles vs. deposited laser energy. Results at 200 ps after the end of the laser pulses are shown for 15 ps (a-c) and 300 ps (d-f) pulse durations.

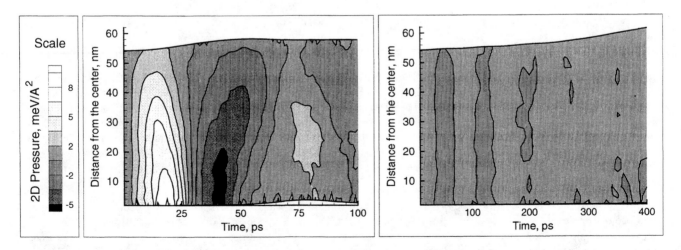

Figure 4. Spatial and time distribution of the local hydrostatic 2D pressure within the particles irradiated with (a) 15 ps and (b) 300 ps laser pulses. Energies deposited by the laser pulses are (a) 0.12 and (b) 0.16 eV per molecule. The contour plots are drawn through the points corresponding to the average of the local pressure for molecules in 20 ring-shaped zones within the particle. The data points are calculated at 1 ps intervals during the MD trajectories starting from the beginning of the laser pulse.

For the longer laser pulse, significantly higher laser fluences are required to cause a visible damage to the particle, Figure 3d-e. The pressure contour in Figure 4b shows that there is scarcely any pressure buildup induced by the 300 ps laser pulse even for the highest laser fluence shown in Figure 3. A 300 ps laser pulse is significantly longer then the time of mechanical relaxation of the particle and thermal expansion occurs during the energy deposition. Thus, the mechanical mechanism of particle damage and ablation that is crucial for 15 ps pulse irradiation does not play any role in the case of 300 ps pulses. For energy of 0.16 eV per molecule deposited, the onset of homogeneous melting and formation of small cavities at the end of the laser pulse is observed. An additional increase of the deposited energy leads to the overheating of the particle up to the limit of its thermodynamic stability,[15] when the particle spontaneously decomposes into a mixture of gas phase molecules and molecular clusters.[14]

This thermal decomposition or explosion leads to the transfer of a significant part of the deposited laser energy to the radial expansion of the disintegrated particle. This can be seen from the time dependence of the average kinetic energy of molecular motion in the radial and tangential directions shown for 3D simulations in Figure 5. The tangential component does not contain a contribution from the radial expansion of the overheated particle and can be associated with the thermal motion whereas the difference between radial and tangential parts of the kinetic energy corresponds to the energy of the radial flow apart. At high laser fluences, when an explosive disintegration of the overheated particles occurs, a splitting of the radial and tangential components of the kinetic energy is observed for both shorter and longer laser pulses as shown in Figure 5. Several points can be made regarding the figure. First, the phase explosion provides fast cooling of the particle and short time of the thermal spike. A big part of the thermal energy is transferred in this case into potential energy of particle decomposition and kinetic energy of the radial flow apart. Second, for the same laser energies deposited, the energy of radial expansion is significantly higher for the shorter laser pulses, when the inertially confined thermoelastic pressure adds to the pressure of the thermal explosion. Third, the transfer of the laser energy to the energy of radial expansion is much faster for the 10 pulse then for the 100 ps pulse. As shown in the next subsection, a stronger pressure wave with a steeper front is emitted into the surrounding medium as a result of the faster and stronger radial expansion of the absorbing particle for shorter pulses.

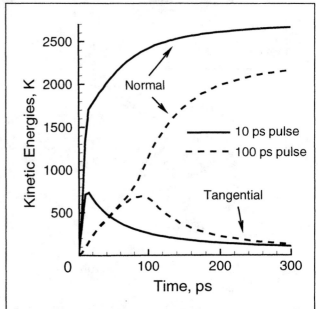

Figure 5. Normal and tangential kinetic energies of particles irradiated with 10 and 100 ps laser pulses from 3D simulations. Energy deposited by laser pulse is 0.5 eV per molecule.

3.2 Coupling of the acoustic and thermal pulses to the surrounding medium.

To study the coupling of the processes within the absorbing particles to the surrounding medium, 2D simulations are performed for different laser fluences, pulse durations and properties of the surrounding medium. The pressure and defect contour plots for three simulations with the same deposited energy of 0.2 eV per molecule are shown in Figure 6. The plots in Figure 6a are for the 300 ps laser pulse and the same intermolecular interaction within and outside the absorbing particle. A 300 ps laser pulse is longer than the time needed for thermal expansion to occur, and only a moderate pressure builds up in the hot particle by the end of the pulse. The slow thermal expansion does not cause any noticeable pressure wave in the surrounding medium and only a transitory appearance of a small number of defects is observed in the central part of the absorbing particle.

As discussed above for isolated particles, irradiation with the 15 ps laser pulse leads to a high compressive pressure build up during the pulse, Figure 6b. Relaxation of the compressive pressure leads to the emission of a strong pressure wave into the surrounding medium and propagation of an unloading wave from the border of the particle toward the center. The pressure wave in the medium carries a significant part of the absorbed laser energy away from the absorption site. This is illustrated in Figure 7 where the time development of the energy in the absorbing particle, within a 90 nm zone around the particle, and outside this zone is plotted. More than 30% of the absorbed laser energy is transferred from the absorbing particle to the surrounding medium during the first 100 ps after the laser pulse. Consequently less energy is left to induce mechanical or thermal damage within the particle. Although the energy deposited in this simulation is higher than for the

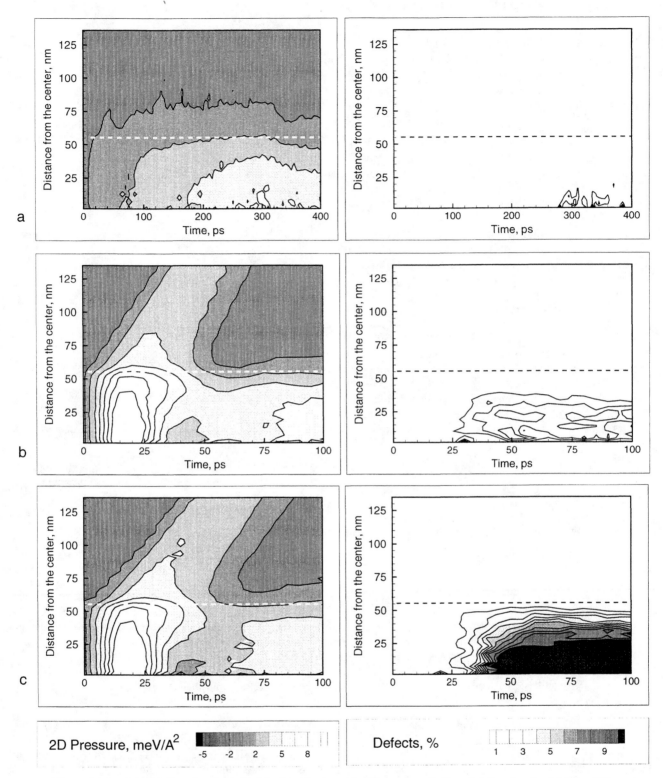

Figure 6. Spatial and time distribution of the local hydrostatic 2D pressure (left) and defect density (right) within and outside the absorbing particles embedded into a transparent medium. The contour plots are for the energy of 0.2 eV per molecule deposited by 300 ps (a) and 15 ps (b,c) laser pulses. Simulations are performed for the particles and surrounding medium with identical mechanical properties (a, b) and for the surrounding medium with intermolecular interactions twice as strong as within the absorbing particle (c). Dashed lines mark the boundary of the absorbing particle.

simulations shown in Figure 3, the defect density in Figure 6 is lower than the ones for isolated particles. Melting and formation of numerous small cavities rather than fracturing in the central part of the particle is responsible for the rise of the defect density in Figure 6b.

Simulations with two sets of parameters for intermolecular interactions in the surrounding medium are performed to investigate the role of the acoustic impedance mismatch at the interface between the absorbing granule and the surrounding medium. In the simulations when the granule and the surrounding medium have identical mechanical properties the most efficient transfer of the expansion energy into producing the pressure wave is observed, Figure 7. When the surrounding medium is weaker/softer than the absorbing particle, less energy goes out from the particle, Figure 7, and a higher defect density within the particle is observed, Figure 6c. Unloading wave that propagates from the border of the irradiated particle and focuses in the central region is stronger in the case of the softer surrounding medium and leads to the more significant pressure lowering. The reduced pressure facilitates cavitation within the overheated particle that is reflected in higher defect density in Figure 6c as compared to Figure 6b. The difference in mechanical properties of the absorbing particle and surrounding medium thus appears to define the role of the intragranular fracturing/cavitation in short pulse laser damage. The greater is the difference, the bigger part of the compressive pressure experience reflection at the interface and is transferred into the expansion wave that focuses in the center of the particle and cause cavitation or fracturing. The results for isolated particles with free boundary conditions, Figures 3 and 4, can be viewed as an extreme case of the maximum impedance mismatch at the particle/surround interface and the maximum photomechanical damage to the particles.

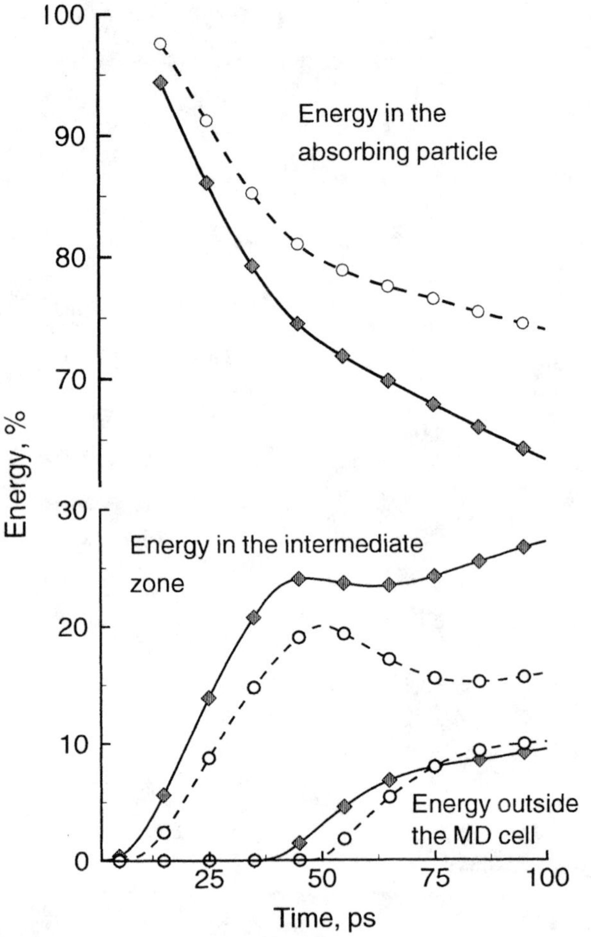

4. Summary

The basic processes and mechanisms that define a low energy threshold for visible damage to pigmented tissues are studied using the MD method and the breathing sphere model. Different threshold energies and qualitative differences in the damage mechanisms for shorter, tens of

Figure 7. The time development of the energy in the absorbing particle, within a 90 nm zone around the particle, and outside this zone for particles irradiated with 15 ps laser pulses. Solid lines are for the simulations when the granule and the surrounding medium have identical mechanical properties, dashed lines are for the half as strong intermolecular interaction in the surrounding medium as compared to the granule. Energy deposited by laser pulse is 0.2 eV per molecule.

picoseconds, and longer, hundreds of picoseconds, laser pulses are observed for both isolated particles and absorbing granules embedded in a transparent medium.

For the shorter pulses a high compressive pressure builds up in the irradiated particles under conditions of inertially confined photothermal expansion. Relaxation of the compressive pressure leads to the formation of a strong pressure wave that carries a significant part of the absorbed laser energy away from the absorption site. Upon interaction with intracellular structures the pressure wave has the potential to develop a tensile component and cause a photomechanical damage in the areas distant from the absorbing compounds. Within the absorbing granule, an unloading wave propagates from the boundary of the absorbing granule and focuses in the centre. The focusing leads to the expansion in the central part of the granule and causes fracturing or cavitation. This effect of intragranular mechanical damage becomes more pronounced with increasing acoustic impedance mismatch between granule and surrounding medium. Photomechanical damage due to the pressure wave emission from the absorbing granule and intragranular fracturing/cavitation can occur at the deposited energies significantly lower than the ones required for explosive vaporization of the absorption site and is likely to be responsible for the energetically efficient regime of the short pulse laser ablation of the tissue.

For the longer, hundreds of picoseconds, laser pulses thermal expansion occurs during the laser energy deposition and no high pressure build up and photomechanical effects are observed in the simulated energy range. Overheating of the absorbing granule up to the level for explosive vaporization is required to cause a visible damage.

The results from the simulation demonstrate the ability of the MD method and the breathing sphere model to provide insight into the basic microscopic mechanisms of short pulse laser damage at the absorption site and coupling of the processes within the absorbing granule to the surrounding medium. Experimental data on the molecular structure and properties of the intracellular components are needed for more detailed quantitative analysis of the threshold values and damage mechanisms. Combination of the present molecular level model with a continuum description can open the way for multiscale modeling of laser-tissue interactions.

Acknowledgments

We gratefully acknowledge financial support from the Chemistry Division of the National Science Foundation. The computational support for this work was provided by the IBM-SUR Program and the Center for Academic Computing at Penn State University.

References

1. S. L. Jacques, A. A. Oraevsky, R. Thompson, and B. S. Gerstman, "A working theory and experiments on photomechanical disruption of melanosomes to explain the threshold for minimal visible retinal lesions for sub-ns laser pulses," *Laser-Tissue Interaction V,* S. L. Jacques, Editor, Proc. SPIE **2134A**, pp. 54-65, 1994.
2. C. R. Thompson, B. S. Gerstman, S. L. Jacques, and M. E. Rogers, "Melanin granule model for laser induced thermal damage to the retina," *Bulletin Mathematical Biology* **58**, pp. 513-553, 1996.
3. C. P. Lin and M. W. Kelly, "Ultrafast time-resolved imaging of stress transient and cavitation from short pulsed laser irradiated melanin particles," *Laser-Tissue Interaction VI,* S. L. Jacques, Editor, Proc. SPIE **2391**, pp. 294-299, 1995.
4. M. W. Kelly and C. P. Lin, "Microcavitation and cell injury in RPE cells following short-pulsed laser irradiation," *Laser-Tissue Interaction VIII,* S. L. Jacques, Editor, Proc. SPIE **2975**, pp. 174-179, 1997.
5. M. Strauss, P. A. Amendt, R. A. London, D. J. Maitland, M. E. Glinsky, C. P. Lin, and M. W. Kelly, "Computational modeling of stress transient and bubble evolution in short-pulse laser irradiated melanosome particles," *Laser-Tissue Interaction VIII,* S. L. Jacques, Editor, Proc. SPIE **2975**, pp. 261-270, 1997.
6. D. W. Heermann, *Computer Simulation Methods in Theoretical Physics,* Berlin: Springer-Verlag, 1990.
7. L. V. Zhigilei, P. B. S. Kodali, and B. J. Garrison, "Molecular dynamics model for laser ablation of organic solids," *J. Phys. Chem. B* **101**, pp. 2028-2037, 1997.
8. L. V. Zhigilei, P. B. S. Kodali, and B. J. Garrison, "On the threshold behavior in the laser ablation of organic solids," *Chem. Phys. Lett.* **276**, pp. 269-273, 1997.
9. L. V. Zhigilei and B. J. Garrison, "Velocity distributions of molecules ejected in laser ablation," *Appl. Phys. Lett.* **71**, pp. 551-553, 1997.
10. M. E. Glinsky, D. S. Bailay, and R. A. London, "LATIS modeling of laser induced midplane and backplane spallation," *Laser-Tissue Interaction VIII,* S. L. Jacques, Editor, Proc. SPIE **2975**, pp. 374-387, 1997.
11. R. S. Dingus, D. R. Curran, A. A. Oraevsky, and S. L. Jacques, "Microscopic spallation process and its potential role in laser-tissue ablation," *Laser-Tissue Interaction V,* S. L. Jacques, Editor, Proc. SPIE **2134A**, pp. 434-445, 1994.
12. L. V. Zhigilei and B. J. Garrison, "Simple non-reflecting boundary conditions for elastic waves in molecular dynamics simulations," in preparation.
13. S.-P. Chen, T. Egami, and V. Vitek, "Local fluctuations and ordering in liquid and amorphous metals," *Phys. Rev. B* **37**, pp. 2440-2449, 1988.
14. L. V. Zhigilei and B. J. Garrison, "Computer simulation study of damage and ablation of submicron particles from short pulse laser irradiation," *Applied Surface Science* **125**, March issue, pp. xxxx, 1998.
15. R. Kelly and A. Miotello, "Comments on explosive mechanisms of laser sputtering," *Applied Surface Science* **96-98**, pp. 205-215, 1996.

SESSION 6

Ocular II: Mechanisms of Laser Effects

Parameter sensitivity of the Thompson granular retinal damage model

Paul K. Kennedy[1], Jeffrey J. Druessel[1], James M. Cupello[1], Stephen Till[2], Bernard S. Gerstman[3], Charles R. Thompson[4], and Benjamin A. Rockwell[1]

[1]Optical Radiation Branch, U.S. Air Force Research Laboratory, Brooks AFB, TX 78235
[2]Defense Evaluation and Research Agency, Malvern, Worcs WR14 3PS, England, UK
[3]Physics Dept., Florida International Univ., Miami, FL 33199
[4]Lockheed-Martin, Litchfield Park, AZ 85340

ABSTRACT

As part of a research program to understand and model eye damage produced by exposure to cw and pulsed lasers, the U. S. Air Force has created a granular model of laser retinal damage. The Thompson granular model simulates absorption of light by melanosomes distributed in the retinal pigmented epithelium, melanosome heating, and subsequent photothermal damage from bulk tissue heating. Various biological input parameters required for the model, such as the density, size, spatial distribution, and absorption coefficient of melanosomes, are not well known, creating uncertainty in the results. This problem is being addressed both experimentally, through measurements of biological parameters for various species, and theoretically, through analysis of parameter sensitivity in the model. In the current study, the parameter sensitivity was analyzed using a technique known as "design of experiments," which allows statistical estimation of the relative importance of independent experimental variables. A matrix of 20 cases has been analyzed, using 7 input parameters as independent variables. Cases have been confined to the long pulse regime (≥ 10 μs), where photothermal damage is dominant. Results were assessed using both temperature rise and Arrhenius damage integral values. Corneal fluence was found to be the most important physical parameter and melanosome absorption the most important biological parameter.

Keywords: Lasers, retinal damage, photothermal damage, granular model, parameter sensitivity, design of experiments.

2. INTRODUCTION

Since the advent of the laser in 1960, laser technology has made almost continual progress in two areas: i) an increase in the average power obtainable from large, cw laser systems and ii) an increase in the peak power and a decrease in the pulsewidths produced by small, pulsed laser systems. These advances have led to a steady increase in civilian and military laser applications[1-3]; but have also produced a greater risk of accidental or deliberate eye damage.[4-6]

Over the past two decades the U.S. Department of Defense has funded a large amount of research into laser safety, laser eye protection, and laser bioeffects, with the goal of protecting pilots and other military personnel from laser-induced eye damage. As part of a research program to understand and model eye damage produced by exposure to cw and pulsed lasers, the U. S. Air Force has created a granular model of laser-induced damage to the retina. The Thompson granular model[7,8] simulates absorption of light by melanosomes distributed in the retinal pigmented epithelium (RPE), melanosome heating, diffusion of heat into the surrounding tissue, and subsequent photothermal damage from protein denaturization.

Melanin in the melanosomes is the primary absorber of visible and near-infrared light in the transparent tissues of the retina.[5] The Thompson model therefore assumes that retinal absorption of laser energy takes place only within melanin granules. Melanosomes in the RPE are modeled as identical absorbing spheres surrounded by cellular material which is assumed to have the thermal properties of water. Melanosomes are

SPIE Vol. 3254 • 0277-786X/98/$10.00

also assumed to have the thermal properties of water for heat transfer calculations. These assumptions are similar to those used by Hayes and Wolbarsht.[9] They allow an analytical solution to the heat transfer equation[7,8] and a calculation of the time-temperature history at any spatial point using linear superposition of the thermal effects of multiple granules. Photothermal damage is calculated from the time-temperature data using an Arrhenius integral approach.[7,10,11]

The Thompson retinal damage model was created primarily as an alternative to previous homogeneous layer models.[10,11] The granular nature of the simulation allows modification of the model to include phase transitions and photomechanical effects around individual melanosomes. A strictly photothermal damage model is only valid for cw and long pulse ($\tau_p \geq 10$ μs) exposures and for moderate fluences; where thermal relaxation can occur during the pulse interaction time and where cellular temperatures remain below the boiling point of water. At shorter pulsewidths or very high fluences, photothermal damage may be compounded by photomechanical damage from bubble formation about heated melanosomes and/or from shock wave emission. Research is currently underway to develop a theoretical model of retinal bubble formation, which can be incorporated into the Thompson granular model.[12,13] This will extend the range of validity into the nanosecond regime, where photomechanical effects are believed to dominate.

Even for calculation of long pulse photothermal damage, anchoring of the model to experimental measurements of biological damage is difficult. Various biological input parameters required for the model, such as the density, size, spatial distribution, and absorption coefficient of melanosomes, are not well known or show biological variation, creating uncertainty in the results. The difficulty is compounded by the fact that biological damage data is available for a number of animal models[14,15] and both the biological parameters and the damage thresholds vary from species to species. Knowledge of physical (laser) parameters is better, but still imperfect; with spot size on the retina being the most difficult either to measure *in vivo* [16,17] or to calculate.[18]

The validation and anchoring problem is currently being addressed both experimentally, through measurements of biological parameters for various species, and theoretically, through analysis of parameter sensitivity in the model. Two sets of experimental studies are now in progress. The first, by Dr. Cynthia Toth of the Duke University Eye Center, will use histopathology, combined with optical and electron microscopy, to determine melanosome number, size, and spatial distribution in rhesus, rabbit, pig, and human RPE cells. The second, by Dr. Charles Lin of MIT-Wellman Labs, will attempt to measure the absorption coefficient of melanosomes for visible and near-infrared wavelengths. This paper documents the results of the theoretical analysis, which has been performed in parallel with the experimental studies. The goal of the theoretical study was to determine the most important physical and biological parameters in the model, both to aid in understanding and interpreting code results and to guide experimental research.

The parameter sensitivity of the model was analyzed using a technique known as "design of experiments".[19,20] This technique, developed by Sir Ronald Fischer during the early decades of this century, involves the use of "factorial designs" in which all independent variables of interest are varied simultaneously. This method is very efficient with regard to sample size and allows for the estimation of interactions among the main variables. The design used involved 16 primary runs (cases) and 4 center point runs. Seven input parameters were chosen as independent variables. Cases have been confined to the long pulse regime (≥ 10 μs), where photothermal damage is dominant. Results were assessed using both the peak temperature rise in the center of the beam and the size of the retinal damage spot as output parameters.

The size of the damage spot, i.e., the diameter of the region over which the Arrhenius integral value is greater than or equal to 1, was not particularly useful as an output parameter. In 7 of the 16 primary runs, the diameter of the damage spot was calculated to be zero and this high frequency of null responses resulted in poor statistical results. Variations in peak temperature indicated that corneal fluence was the most important physical parameter and melanosome absorption the most important biological parameter. A more detailed description of our statistical study of parameter sensitivity is provided in the next section. The results are discussed in Section 4 and conclusions are given in Section 5.

3. DESCRIPTION OF ANALYSIS

The goal of our theoretical study was to identify which model input parameters have the greatest impact on 1) temperature rise in the irradiated tissue and 2) induced tissue damage. This is determined by varying input parameter values over specified ranges and analyzing the subsequent variation in the output parameters. The typical approach to such an analysis involves varying one factor while holding all others fixed. A second factor is then varied in the same way, followed by a third, a fourth, etc. Design of experiments (DOE) is an alternative approach involving the use of "orthogonal designs." In an orthogonal design all factors are varied simultaneously, in such a way that each independent variable can be estimated independently of all the others; hence the use of the term "orthogonal." One additional benefit of this DOE approach is the ability to detect the presence of interactions among independent variables.

We selected seven input parameters to vary in the study. Three were physical parameters: corneal fluence, retinal spot size (diameter), and pulse duration. Four were biological parameters: melanosome density, melanosome radius, melanosome absorption coefficient, and the thickness of the layer containing melanosomes in each RPE cell. The two output parameters used to assess results were peak temperature rise in the center of the beam (on-axis) and the diameter of the retinal damage spot.

The goal of identifying the most important input parameters involved the use of a DOE "screening" design. The screening design used in this study was a Resolution IV, Taguchi L-16 orthogonal array.[19] It is also known as a 16-run fractional factorial design. Resolution IV means that the direct effects of the seven main parameters are aliased (or confounded) with 3-factor interactions and that 2-factor interactions are aliased with other 2-factor interactions. Our design is a two-level design, which involves choosing a high and a low value (two levels) for each input parameter. Since there are two possible values for each of seven input parameters, a total of 2^7 combinations can be constructed. The fractional factorial design chooses 16 of these 128 possible cases (a one-eighth fraction of a full factorial) for analysis. The DOE method yields a large amount of useful statistical information from this limited number of cases.

Since only maximum and minimum parameter values are used in the 16 runs of the fractional factorial design, these essentially sample the edges (extremes) of the parameter space. Four additional runs were performed in the center of the parameter space, in order to detect the possible existence of quadratic (non-linear) effects. Inputs for these runs consisted of minor perturbations ($\pm 5\%$) about the mid-point values of each parameter range.

The parameter ranges specify the subset of the total parameter space explored, and the conclusions of the statistical analysis are only valid in this region. The input values chosen should therefore apply to a region of high interest and should give significant (i.e., non-zero) output values for most, if not all, cases. If the parameter ranges are set too high or too low, then the results generated by the Thompson model may not be useful for statistical analysis. For example, if the melanosome absorption coefficient is set too low, then the absorbed energy will be too small to produce a significant temperature rise. All cases will then give a null response, and the runs will be useless for analysis. Parameter ranges which give a large response in all cases are also undesirable. An ideal subset of the total parameter space will give non-zero results for most cases, as well as a significant variation between maximum and minimum output values.

The values chosen for the biological parameters corresponded to a reasonable guess for the range of values in humans[5,7] or in the rhesus monkey, which is the primary animal model used for threshold damage studies.[14] The laser parameters corresponded to values at or near the *in-vivo* retinal damage threshold in rhesus,[7] for exposure to visible laser pulses ($\lambda \approx 500$ nm). The initial ranges chosen for the laser parameters were too broad and produced too many cases in which there was no significant heating or temperature rise, violating the range selection criteria given above. The ranges were therefore narrowed somewhat in the final study, in order to produce non-zero temperature increases in all cases. The final parameter ranges used in this study were: corneal fluence [10^{-4} - 10^{-3} J/cm^2], retinal spot size [20-50 μm], pulse duration [10^{-5} - 10^{-3} sec], melanosome density [20-100 granules/cell], melanosome radius [0.5-1.0 μm], melanosome absorption coefficient [500-5000 cm^{-1}], and melanosome layer thickness [7-15 μm].

After the input parameters had been specified for all 20 cases, the Thompson model was used to obtain the corresponding peak temperatures and damage spot sizes. The results were then analyzed statistically, with the aid of the Design Expert (DX-5) software package.[21] The first step in the data reduction was to apply a base-10 logarithmic transform to the calculated temperatures and damage diameters. The need for such a transformation is indicated by the large variation in the response values (greater than 3 orders of magnitude for the temperature data). The log transform helps to produce homogeneity of variance across the the design space, a key assumption in the DOE analysis of variance.[20] It also ensures that the linear model constructed during DOE analysis (see below) predicts only positive temperature changes and damage diameters as a result of laser irradiation.

Next, the maximum and minimum values for each input parameter are coded as having values of – 1(min) and +1(max). The coded input parameters and the log transformed responses are then used to develop a linear model of the response. The linear model is a sum of 16 terms. The first term is the grand mean of the response values. Each of the other 15 terms is the product of a coefficient (weighting factor) with one of the seven input parameters or with one of their multi-parameter interactions. The input and output parameters for the 16 primary cases are placed in this linear model to produce 16 equations in 16 unknowns (the grand mean + 15 coefficients). The unknowns are then solved for by matrix manipulation. One of the strengths of the DOE technique is that, because of the parameter coding, the magnitudes of the coefficients are directly proportional to the effects of the corresponding terms in the linear model on the response variable. The results of this analysis are discussed below.

4. DISCUSSION OF RESULTS

Input and output parameter values for the 20 cases used in this study are shown in Table 1. The input parameter ranges chosen gave a peak on-axis temperature rise of at least 1 °C in all cases, with a variation of 3 orders of magnitude between minimum (1.3 °C) and maximum (4,660 °C) values. The temperature data thus satisfies the range selection criteria mentioned above and appears to give meaningful statistical results when analyzed. We should note in passing that peak temperatures above 100 °C were calculated in a number of cases. This is clearly a nonphysical result and indicates the importance of adding models for phase transition and bubble formation to the calculation, even for interactions with moderately long pulses (≥ 10 µs), where photothermal damage is dominant. For the purposes of this parameter sensitivity study, however, we have ignored phase transitions and photomechanical damage and simply performed the statistical analysis using the high peak temperatures calculated by the model.

The calculated size of the damage spot for the 20 cases varied from 0 to 69 µm in diameter. As mentioned previously, damage spot size was not particularly useful as an output parameter for statistical analysis. Nearly half of the cases gave no calculated damage, and this many zeros in the data set produced unreliable statistical results. The null results were due in large part to the fact that the parameter ranges were selected to ensure a good range of responses for the temperature data only. The statistical results that follow refer only to analysis of the temperature data, using construction of a linear model as described in Section 3.

The easiest method for comparison of the DOE linear model coefficients is through the use of a Pareto diagram, which depicts one-half the absolute value of the coefficients, arranged in descending order of importance. The Pareto diagram for the temperature response data is shown in Figure 1. The seven main input parameters have been labeled as factors A through G in Figure 1, in order to simply identification of the multi-parameter interaction terms (AC, BC, ABC, etc.). To save space, the word melanin has been substituted for melanosome when identifying the biological parameters, both in Fig. 1 and in Table 1.

The diagram indicates that the six terms in the linear model which have the largest effect on the temperature response are those representing six of the main input parameters being studied. In descending order of importance these are: corneal fluence, melanosome (or melanin) absorption coefficient, melanin radius, retinal spot size, pulse duration, and melanin density. The thickness of the melanin layer was found to be much less important in determining response than the other seven input parameters. All the 2, 3, and 4-factor interactions (products of the main parameters) also had smaller coefficients than the six key parameters.

A more detailed depiction of the results of the analysis can be found by using a normal probability plot of the results. A normal probability plot is a statistical analysis tool to quickly determine how data compares to a normal (gaussian) distribution. Analogous to a logarithmic plot, the normal probability plot has the vertical axis scaled such that data that falls on a normal distribution will form a straight line when plotted. Figure 2 is a graph showing the relative effects (coefficients) of the various terms plotted on a normal probability scale. Coefficients for terms that are insignificant will fall on a straight line centered around zero. Coefficients that depart significantly from a straight line on the plot represent terms that are statistically significant in the model.

Nineteen points are plotted in Fig. 2, representing 19 effects, which are described below. The normal probability values are calculated by assigning each effect a ranking (a number from 1 to 19, representing lowest to highest) and then calculating a percentile, p, for that effect using:

$$p = 100[Rank - 0.5]/19. \qquad (1)$$

The circle in the figure represents the origin. The three triangles near the origin are error estimates generated from statistical analysis of the four center point runs (usually termed replications in DOE analysis). This analysis will be discussed in more detail later. The six dark squares labeled A through F represent coefficients for the six main parameters identified as the most significant terms from the Pareto analysis. (The label key for these factors is the same as in Fig.1.) Note that these coefficients appear well off the line in the figure, indicating that they are probably significant. The nine light squares are the coefficients corresponding to melanin thickness and to the multi-factor interactions. The fact that the error estimates (triangles) and smaller coefficients (light squares) all fall near the line indicates that they fit a normal distribution centered about zero and that their contribution to the linear model is equivalent to that of noise.

Figure 2 also shows the signs of the coefficients representing the six significant factors. The coefficients corresponding to pulse duration and retinal spot size were both negative, indicating that a decease in these parameters, while holding all others fixed, will produce an increase in the peak on-axis temperature. This agrees with physical intuition. For a fixed corneal fluence (constant intraocular energy), a decrease in pulse duration corresponds to an increase in temperature rise. The shorter pulse duration allows less time for heat to flow out of the interaction volume, while absorption is taking place. Similarly, a constant intraocular energy and a smaller retinal spot will produce higher retinal fluence and thus, higher temperatures. In contrast, the other four parameters have positive coefficients, which again agrees with our expectations based on our understanding of the biophysical model. Increases in corneal fluence, melanin absorption, melanin radius, or melanin density all correspond to increases in the total energy absorbed and logically should produce an increase in temperature.

Another significant finding of this study arose from inclusion of the 4 center point runs in the analysis. As mentioned previously, each of these cases had slightly different perturbations from the mid-point values of the input parameters. The center point runs serve two purposes. First, they provide an estimate of the potential importance of quadratic effects to the linear DOE model. Second, as indicated above, they provide an estimate of the variance (error) associated with the linear model, for comparison with the model coefficients.

In this case, analysis of the center point data indicated that quadratic terms are required to properly model the temperature response over the parameter range examined. The quadratic terms are identified and their coefficients estimated by the inclusion of additional runs, which explore the design space beyond the − 1 and +1 ranges already studied. Inclusion of these additional cases may shift the ordering and relative importance of the significant factors identified in this screening experiment. Unfortunately, we did not have time to perform the additional analysis prior to the BiOS conference. This is planned as future work.

The issue of estimating variance in the Thompson model is also complicated. Most applications of the DOE technique in the literature deal with measurements on physical systems (hardware). Thus, most of the methods for estimating variance are based on replications of experimental measurements, where each measurement yields a different value due to experimental error. Here we are applying the technique to a deterministic computer code and there is no obvious opportunity for replication to provide this information. We attempted to address this issue in the center point runs by artificially inducing variation on the input parameters; i.e., by adding normally distributed noise to the mid-point value for each parameter. However, this method of inducing variance does not tell us the <u>true</u> uncertainty in the input parameters to the Thompson model. Hopefully the experimental parameter measurements mentioned in Section 2 will soon provide this information.

5. CONCLUSIONS

Statistical analysis of variations in peak temperature, using the design of experiments technique, indicates that the melanosome absorption coefficient, the melanosome radius, and the melanosome density in the RPE cell, are all important biological parameters in the Thompson thermal model. Not suprisingly, corneal fluence (equivalent to total intraocular energy) was found to be the most important physical parameter and melanosome absorption the most important biological parameter. As a caveat, we should note that the ranking of parameters in terms of relative importance is still somewhat uncertain due to the presence of quadratic effects in our results. A more advanced (3-level) analysis, including quadratic effects, is planned for the future. In summary, the DOE technique provides a rigorous and highly efficient method for planning and executing exploration of a design (parameter) space. Future work will include both a 3-level design analysis and use of experimentally determined parameter values and variances in the code. The latter will hopefully allow anchoring of the damage model to biological damage data for a number of species.

6. ACKNOWLEDGMENTS

This work was supported by the U.S. Air Force Research Laboratory and by the Air Force Office of Scientific Research (AFOSR) through grant No. 2312AA-92AL014.

7. REFERENCES

1. S. J. Gitomer and R. D. Jones, "Laser-produced plasmas in medicine," IEEE Trans. on Plasma Science, vol. 19, pp. 1209-1219, 1991.

2. D. A. Cremers, L. J. Radziemski, and T. R. Loree, "Spectrochemical analysis of liquids using the laser spark," Appl. Spectroscopy, vol. 38, pp. 721-729, 1984.

3. P. K. Kennedy, D. X. Hammer, and B. A. Rockwell, "Laser-induced breakdown in aqueous media," Prog. Quantum Electron., vol. 21, pp. 155-248, 1997.

4. <u>ANSI Standard Z136.1-1993: American National Standard for Safe Use of Lasers</u>, (American National Standards Institute, New York, 1993).

5. D. Sliney and M. Wolbarsht, <u>Safety with Lasers and Other Optical Sources</u>, (Plenum Press, New York, 1980), p. 126.

6. D. H. Sliney, "Ocular injuries from laser accidents," in <u>Laser-Inflicted Eye Injuries: Epidemiology, Prevention, and Treatment</u>, B. E. Stuck and M. Belkin, Eds., Proc. SPIE, vol. 2674A, pp. 25-33, 1996.

7. C. R. Thompson, B. S. Gerstman, S. L. Jacques, and M. E. Rogers, "Melanin granule model for laser-induced thermal damage in the retina," Bull. Math. Biol., vol. 58, no. 3, pp. 513-553, 1996.

8. C. R. Thompson, "Melanin granule model for heating of tissue by laser," in <u>Laser-Tissue Interaction V</u>, S. L. Jacques, Ed., Proc. SPIE, vol. 2134A, pp. 66-77, 1994.

9. J. R. Hayes and M. L. Wolbarsht, "Thermal modeling for retinal damage induced by pulsed lasers," Aerospace Med., vol. 39, no. 5, pp. 474-480, 1968.

10. R. Birngruber, F. Hillenkamp, and V. P. Gabel, "Theoretical investigations of laser thermal retinal injury," Health Physics, vol. 48, pp. 781-796, 1985.

11. A. J. Welch, "The thermal response of laser irradiated tissue," IEEE J. Quantum Electron., vol. QE-20, pp. 1471-1481, 1984.

12. B. S. Gerstman, C. R. Thompson, S. L. Jacques, and M. E. Rogers, "Laser induced bubble formation in the retina," Las. Surg. Med., vol. 18, pp. 10-21, 1996.

13. C. R. Thompson and B. S. Gerstman, "Gruneisen equation of state for melanosomes irradiated by sub-nanosecond laser pulses," in <u>Laser-Tissue Interaction VII</u>, S. L. Jacques, Ed., Proc. SPIE, vol. 2681A, pp. 449-459, 1996.

14. C. P. Cain, C. A. Toth, C. D. DiCarlo, C. D. Stein, G. D. Noojin, D. J. Stolarski, and W. P. Roach, "Visible retinal lesions from ultrashort laser pulses in the primate eye," Invest. Ophthalmol. Vis. Sci., vol. 36, pp. 879-888, 1995.

15. C. A. Toth, C. P. Cain, C. D. Stein, G. D. Noojin, D. J. Stolarski, J. A. Zuclich, and W. P. Roach, "Retinal effects of ultrashort laser pulses in the rabbit eye," Invest. Ophthalmol. Vis. Sci., vol. 36, pp. 1910-1917, 1995.

16. L. D. Forster, "Light intensity measurements with a fiber optic microprobe in the laser irradiated rhesus monkey eye," Dissertation, The Univer. of Texas at Austin, 1978.

17. G. D. Polhamus, D. K. Cohoon, and R. G. Allen, "Measurement of the point spread function in the rhesus eye," Technical Paper, USAF School of Aerospace Medicine, 1979.

18. B. A. Rockwell, W. P. Roach, and M. E. Rogers, "Determination of self-focusing effects for light propagating in the eye," in <u>Laser-Tissue Interaction V</u>, Steven L. Jacques, Ed., Proc. SPIE, vol. 2134A, pp. 2-9, 1994.

19. S. R. Schmidt and R. G. Launsby, <u>Understanding Industrial Designed Experiments</u>, 4th ed.(Air Academy Press, Colorado Springs, CO, 1997).

20. G. E. P. Box, W. G. Hunter, and J. S. Hunter, <u>Statistics for Experimenters</u>, (Wiley & Sons, Inc., New York, 1978).

21. Design Expert is a commercial product of the Stat-Ease Corp., 2021 East Hennepin Ave., Suite 191, Minneapolis, MN 55413.

Case #	Corneal Fluence (J/cm^2)	Retinal Spot Size (µm)	Pulse Duration (sec)	Melanin Density (number/cell)	Melanin Radius (µm)	Melanin Thickness (µm)	Melanin Absorption (cm^{-1})	Peak Temp (C)	Damage Spot Size (µm)
1	1.00E-04	20.00	1.00E-05	20.00	0.50	7.00	500.00	13.08	0
2	1.00E-04	20.00	1.00E-05	100.00	0.50	15.00	5000.00	131.8	19
3	1.00E-04	20.00	1.00E-03	20.00	1.00	7.00	5000.00	63.16	10
4	1.00E-04	20.00	1.00E-03	100.00	1.00	15.00	500.00	23.87	0
5	1.00E-04	50.00	1.00E-05	20.00	1.00	15.00	500.00	2.822	0
6	1.00E-04	50.00	1.00E-05	100.00	1.00	7.00	5000.00	339.9	55
7	1.00E-04	50.00	1.00E-03	20.00	0.50	15.00	5000.00	1.528	0
8	1.00E-04	50.00	1.00E-03	100.00	0.50	7.00	500.00	1.293	0
9	1.00E-03	20.00	1.00E-05	20.00	1.00	15.00	5000.00	4660	39
10	1.00E-03	20.00	1.00E-05	100.00	1.00	7.00	500.00	2474	37
11	1.00E-03	20.00	1.00E-03	20.00	1.00	15.00	500.00	8.968	0
12	1.00E-03	20.00	1.00E-03	100.00	0.50	7.00	5000.00	317.5	37
13	1.00E-03	50.00	1.00E-05	20.00	0.50	7.00	5000.00	55.73	41
14	1.00E-03	50.00	1.00E-05	100.00	0.50	15.00	500.00	53.11	6
15	1.00E-03	50.00	1.00E-03	20.00	1.00	7.00	500.00	14.74	0
16	1.00E-03	50.00	1.00E-03	100.00	1.00	15.00	5000.00	673.3	69
17	5.50E-04	35.00	5.05E-04	60.00	0.75	11.00	2750.00	136.8	38
18	5.50E-04	34.81	5.05E-04	58.05	0.77	11.00	2668.37	135.1	38
19	5.50E-04	35.75	5.05E-04	59.77	0.76	11.00	2720.55	136.8	39
20	5.50E-04	34.55	5.05E-04	60.33	0.78	11.00	2702.53	147.1	39

Table 1-- Input parameters and output (response) values for the 20 cases used in the study. Temperature and damage values were calculated using the Thompson model.

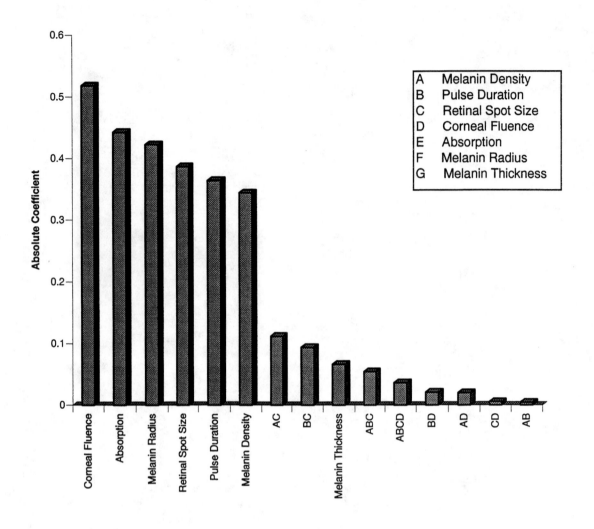

Figure 1 -- Pareto diagram showing the relative order of importance of the seven input parameters, and of multi-parameter interaction terms, to the temperature response.

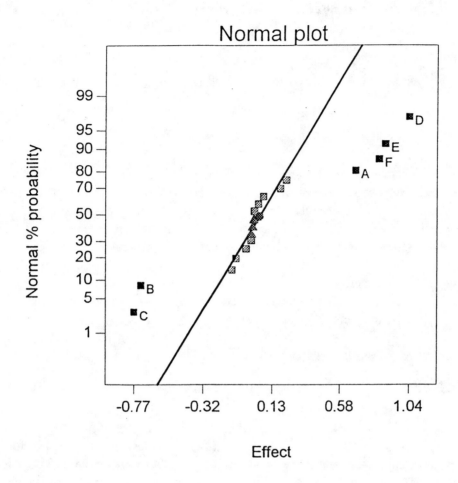

Figure 2 -- Normal probability plot of the coefficients (effects), which represent terms of the DOE linear model of temperature response.

Pressure Generation in Melanosomes by Sub-Nanosecond Laser Pulses

Jinming Sun and Bernard S. Gerstman

Department of Physics, Florida International University, Miami, FL 33199

ABSTRACT

We have computationally modeled the generation of high pressures in melanosomes resulting from the absorption of sub-nanosecond laser pulses. The melanosome is treated as a solid sphere characterized by a bulk modulus, specific heat, coefficient of thermal expansion, and a uniform absorption coefficient. Using a series of partial differential equations to represent how the absorbed laser energy is converted to thermal and mechanical energy, we can calculate expected pressures resulting from laser pulses of any duration or fluence. We find that for the same fluence, the maximum pressure generated increases as the pulse duration decreases. For sub-nanosecond pulses, kilobar pressures can be generated inside the melanosome. We examine how the pressures that are generated depend on pulse characteristics and melanosome properties.

Key Words: laser, retina, pressure, melanosome

1. INTRODUCTION

The high intensities available from lasers make their interactions with the eye an important field of research.[1,2] From the standpoint of safety and health issues, threshold levels for causing damage are especially important. The determination and prediction of threshold levels is greatly facilitated by an understanding on a fundamental level of the physical mechanisms by which damage is created and how the laser energy is transmuted in the biological material. In this paper, we report on our investigations of how sub-nanosecond pulses can lead to extremely high pressures within retinal pigment epithelial (RPE) cells[3] and be the likely physical mechanism for damage at threshold levels. The limited number of experimental measurements of damage thresholds for ultrashort pulses seem to show a decrease in required fluence as the pulse duration is shortened below a nanosecond.[4] An understanding of the underlying physics of how the energy of the laser pulse couples to the biological media will help in determining if the drop in threshold fluence level is real and to explain the physical mechanisms that are responsible. This will then help in predicting damage thresholds for other pulse durations and wavelengths, as well as explaining and predicting the effects of suprathreshold pulses.

Laser energy absorbed in the retina can affect and damage the biological media via three types of physical mechanisms: temperature increases,[2] vaporization,[1] and mechanical waves.[5] Nanosecond time scales have an especial significance for laser pulses in the eye. The dominant absorbers in the eye are melanosomes in the RPE that are approximately one micron (10^{-6} meters) in size. The speed of sound in these material is on the order of 10^3 m/s and therefore it takes mechanical waves approximately a nanosecond to travel across the absorbing melanosomes. The energy of an ultrashort laser pulse is deposited in a time shorter than this and pressures generated by the early part of the absorbed laser energy cannot be dissipated while the latter portion of the laser pulse is absorbed. This stress confinement during the duration of the laser pulse can lead to the buildup of pressures that are much higher than would be generated if the same amount of absorbed energy was deposited over longer times. Therefore, ultrashort laser pulses introduce the possibility of a new physical mechanism dominating the damage process and we report results from our calculations of high pressures expected to be generated by ultrashort pulses.

In order to get a detailed understanding of the effects of ultrashort pulses, we have approached the generation of pressure waves and elevated temperatures using a series of models. The first model we used was artificial (a "toy" model) in order to obtain detailed physical understanding about the type of behavior that could be expected. Once we developed and learned from this toy model we then changed the assumptions of the model in a systematic fashion in order to make the model more physically realistic. The detailed mathematical solutions to the more realistic models are complicated and therefore the toy model is extremely valuable for interpreting the more complicated solutions in terms of meaningful physical results that could cause biological damage to the retina.

2. Homogeneous Model

2.1 Description of Model

This toy model is unphysical but allows intuitive understanding of the physical interactions between the laser properties of pulse duration and fluence, the melanin properties such as absorption coefficient, bulk modulus, density, specific heat, etc., and the resulting pressure and temperature that is generated. The distinguishing, and unrealistic assumptions of this model are
1) pressure and temperature rise homogeneously throughout the melanosome (with uniform pressure throughout the melanosome, this model precludes pressure waves inside the melanosome)
2) the fluid (water) outside the melanosome is incompressible (which causes any pressure changes at the surface of the melanosome to propagate through the external liquid instantaneously to infinity)

Physical thermodynamics can be employed with these approximations to obtain P and T increases as a function of laser pulse characteristics. Energy conservation can be expressed in a standard fashion

$$dE_e = dE_i + dE_k + dE_w$$
$$\text{absorbed} \quad \text{internal} \quad \text{kinetic} \quad \text{work} \tag{1}$$

where the absorbed energy is the laser energy absorbed by the melanosome, the internal and kinetic energies pertain to the melanosome, and the work is performed by the melanosome on the surrounding environment. This expression can be rewritten in terms of thermodynamic variables

$$dE_e = c_v dT + T\frac{\gamma}{V}c_v dV + dE_k \tag{2}$$

where γ is the Grueneisen parameter for the melanosome, $\gamma = V(\partial P/\partial E)_v$ and c_v is the heat capacity for the entire melanosome (a sphere of radius a=1 μm with a specific heat of 2.51 J/g-K and ρ_{mel}=1.35 g/cm^3 has c_v=1.42x10^{11} J/K) The first two terms on the right represent the change in entropy of the process. The dynamic behavior of the system can be followed by examining the time rate of change of the variables

$$\dot{E}_e = c_v \dot{T} + 4\pi T c_v \frac{\gamma}{V} R^2 \dot{R} + \frac{4\pi}{5} \rho_m a^3 \dot{R} \ddot{R} \qquad (3)$$

Equation (3) is only valid for the case of a homogeneous sphere in which changes in the pressure and temperature occur uniformly throughout the melanosome.

In addition to conservation of energy, the thermodynamic variables also obey the equation of state

$$dV = \left(\frac{\partial V}{\partial P}\right)_T dP + \left(\frac{\partial V}{\partial T}\right)_P dT \qquad (4)$$

Under the conditions of a homogeneous spherical melanosome, the equation of state can be rewritten as

$$\dot{R} = \frac{R}{3}\alpha_v \dot{T} - \frac{R}{3B}\dot{P} \qquad (5)$$

where α_v is the bulk coefficient of thermal expansion and is three times the linear coefficient of thermal expansion for isotropic materials and B is the bulk modulus. With α_v and B constrained to remain constant ("acoustic approximation") and not vary with temperature or pressure, there can be no non-linearities in the dynamics of the system and hence no shock waves.[6]

Finally, there is the equation of motion of the system which, at the surface, reduces to

$$\frac{P - P_o}{\rho_L} = \frac{3}{2}\dot{R}^2 + R\ddot{R} \qquad (6)$$

where ρ_L is the density of the surrounding liquid. Equation (6) results from the assumption of incompressibility of the surrounding liquid.[7] The pressure at the surface of the melanosome acts as the driving force that accelerates the liquid.

2.2 Results

Equations (3), (5), and (6) can be used to determine the pressure, temperature, and volume of a melanosome that absorbs energy at the rate of $\dot{E}$ (J/sec) using a numerical finite difference iterative approach. The power absorbed is related to the laser fluence I_o, duration τ_o and the melanosome absorption coefficient α_m and radius 'a' through

$$\dot{E} = \frac{I_o}{\tau_o}\pi a^2 \left[1 - \frac{1}{2\alpha_m^2 a^2}(1 - e^{-2\alpha_m a}(1 + 2\alpha_m a)) \right] \qquad (7)$$

which is derived in Ref. (1). In Figs. (1a-d) we plot the pressure predicted by this model in a melanosome of radius a=1μm and absorption coefficient of α_m=1000 cm^{-1} for a retinal laser fluence of I_o=1J/cm^2 and for pulse lengths τ_o ranging from 10 nanoseconds down to 10 picoseconds. Thus, the same total energy is absorbed by the melanosome in all the figures, the important difference being the time during which the absorption occurs. The time axis is given in units of pulse duration and therefore has a different absolute scale for each pulse.

The oscillations, which are most obvious in the 10 ns and 1 ns figures, give important insight into the underlying physics of the system's response to the absorption of laser energy. As the melanosome absorbs energy and heats up, the increase in energy on an atomic scale leads to a separation of atoms. This is the cause of thermal expansion, but this random thermal process requires a finite time to propagate throughout the melanosome to cause an overall expansion. During the time required for full expansion, determined by the speed of sound and the diameter of the melanosome, the increased random thermal motion of the atoms causes an increase in the pressure that depends on the bulk modulus. As the melanosome expands, the internal pressure is relieved. The dynamical behavior of the melanosome is similar to a spring in which the spring force is analogous to the difference between the melanosome's internal pressure compared to the one atmosphere of constant pressure of the surrounding water. This is exhibited explicitly in Eq. (6). Ultimately, the inertial motion of the outwardly expanding surrounding liquid causes the melanosome to expand such that its pressure drops below the ambient pressure, at which time there is a net force of compression due to the pressure difference. Thus the dynamics of the radius of the melanosome are a combination of two influences: the increasing temperature causing a steadily increasing radius (as long as the laser is on, until t=1), and the oscillatory behavior due to the interaction with the surrounding liquid. Once the laser pulse turns off at t=1, there is no longer any driving force for a net increase in radius and only the oscillating behavior continues. Since this model does not include heat loss by thermal conduction, the temperature of the melanosome never decreases and therefore the average radius during the oscillations after the laser pulse has ended remains that which it is at the end of the pulse. It should be noted that thermal conduction has been left out because it occurs on microsecond time scales and therefore would have negligible effect during the nanosecond time scales that we are investigating, even if it were included in this model.

The maximum temperature generated in the melanosome is virtually the same for all pulse lengths. This is because less than 1% of the pulse energy is used in generating kinetic energy or high pressures. This channeling of more than 99% of the absorbed energy into heating may be due to the high bulk modulus (assumed to be 39.4x10^9 Pa, similar to graphite) and the assumption of incompressibility of the surrounding liquid, both of which tend to reduce melanosome expansion. Further work will vary the melanosome bulk modulus and also allow the surrounding liquid to be compressible in order to determine if this changes the fraction of energy channeled into heating versus mechanical effects. Even the small fraction of energy that goes into pressure elevation is enough to allow pressure waves to cause damage since the melanosome is an intense absorber and per molecule absorbs a large amount of energy.

The pressure calculations show that as the pulse length is reduced below 10 ns, higher pressures are generated for the same fluence. A rise in temperature induces an expansion of the melanosome. If this thermal expansion occurs on time scales slower than the rate at which the temperature rises, an increase in pressure occurs. The thermal expansion time scale is approximately the time for sound waves to travel across the melanosome. For a 1 μm particle with a speed of sound of approximately 1500 m/s, the stress confinement time is approximately 1 ns. A laser pulse duration significantly longer than this will cause little buildup in pressure because thermal expansion will keep pace with the temperature rise so that the pressure remains in equilibrium with the surroundings. For pulses around a nanosecond in duration, the pressure buildup should depend inversely on the pulse duration because a shorter pulse gives less time for thermal expansion. Our calculations show a progressively smaller increase in the radius of the melanosome during the pulse as the pulse duration is shortened from 10 nanoseconds to 0.1 nanoseconds and a corresponding increase in the maximum pressure generated. For pulse lengths significantly shorter than the stress confinement time, the increase in radius during the pulse is negligible compared to the ultimate increase induced by the temperature rise, and the maximum pressure generated, which occurs at the end of the pulse, will once again become independent of the pulse duration. This is exhibited in Figs. (1c,d) for pulse durations of 0.1 nanosecond and 10 picoseconds. This simple model predicts that a retinal fluence of 1 J/cm^2 will generate pressures on the order of 3×10^8 Pa (3000 bar) for sub-nanosecond pulses.

2.3 Linearization of the Model: Analytical Solution and Energy Channeling

The large bulk modulus of the melanosome allows the equations in the model to be well approximated in a way that leads to a linearized system. This linearization has two valuable consequences: an analytical solution for the pressure oscillations can be derived which explicitly shows how the amplitude and frequency depend on various parameters, and the fraction of absorbed energy that goes into mechanical effects versus heating can be calculated directly.

The linearization of the equations is carried out as follows. The high bulk modulus of the melanosome limits size changes to a small fraction (< 0.1%) of the original radius. Therefore, in Eqs. (3), and (6), terms that depend on $\dot{R} = \Delta R / \Delta t$ can be neglected. Eq. (5) must retain the $\dot{R}$ term in order to be of any value as an equation of state that relates P, V, and T. The small variations in R allow us to assume constant R=a. It must be noted that we cannot set $\ddot{R} = 0$ because

$$\ddot{R} \sim \frac{\Delta R}{\Delta t} \frac{1}{\Delta t} \tag{8}$$

and the second Δt in the denominator can produce large $\ddot{R}$ during numerical stepping that cannot be neglected. The linearized versions of Eqs. (3), (5), and (6) are

$$\dot{E}_e = c_v \dot{T} \tag{9a}$$

which physically reflects the fact that the mechanical energy is relatively tiny and virtually all of the laser energy goes into heating,

$$\dot{R} = \frac{a}{3} \alpha_v \dot{T} - \frac{a}{3} \frac{1}{B} \dot{P} \tag{9b}$$

which shows that the increase in radius is so small that the Equation of State can be evaluated, to first order, at the initial volume, i.e. changes in volume $\dot{R}$ can be determined based upon the initial volume, and finally

$$\frac{P - P_o}{\rho_L} = a \ddot{R} \tag{9c}$$

for the linearized equation of motion.

The linearized Eqs. (9a-c) can be solved to give analytical expressions for the time dependence of all the variables. The solution of Eq. (9a) for the decoupled temperature is a temperature that increases linearly with time as long as the laser is on ($\dot{E}_o \neq 0$) and then remains constant at the elevated value after the pulse ends. Equations (9b) and (9c) show that the pressure and radius of the melanosome remain coupled and undergo harmonic oscillations like a spring, along with a constant driving force $\dot{T}$ causing an increase in P and R that is present as long as the laser is on. The analytical solutions for the linearized equations while the laser is on ($0<t<\tau_o$) are

$$T(t) = 310K + \frac{E_e \, t}{c_v \, \tau_o} \tag{10a}$$

$$R(t) = a + \frac{E_e \alpha_v a}{3 c_v \tau_o}\left[t - a\sqrt{\frac{\rho_L}{3B}}\sin\left(\frac{1}{a}\sqrt{\frac{3B}{\rho_L}}t\right)\right] \tag{10b}$$

$$\dot{R} = \frac{a\alpha_v E_e}{3 c_v \tau_o}\left(1 - \cos\frac{1}{a}\sqrt{\frac{3B}{\rho_L}}t\right) \tag{10c}$$

$$P(t) = \frac{a E_e \alpha_v}{\tau_o c_v}\sqrt{\frac{B\rho_L}{3}}\,\sin\left(\frac{1}{a}\sqrt{\frac{3B}{\rho_L}}t\right) \tag{10d}$$

These expressions shows how the oscillation frequency depends on characteristics of the melanosome's driving force (B) and the inertia of the surrounding water (ρ_L)

$$\omega = \frac{1}{a}\sqrt{\frac{3B}{\rho_L}} \tag{11}$$

Additionally, the increase in the amplitude of the pressure oscillations as the pulse length is decreased is manifested by the term E_e/τ_o in the prefactor of Eq. (10d). When the pulse length is significantly shorter than the period of the oscillations, $\tau_o \ll 2\pi/\omega$, the first term in the expansion of the sine function leads to a maximum pressure, which occurs at the end of the pulse, that is independent of τ_o

$$P(t) \simeq \frac{\alpha_v B E_e}{c_v} \tag{12}$$

This shows that for pulse durations in the stress confinement regime for which negligible expansion of the melanosome can occur during the duration of the pulse, the maximum pressure created is the same as if the melanosome was slowly heated to the final temperature E_e/c_v, allowed to undergo full thermal expansion as determined by α_v, and *then* compressed back to its original radius by a pressure determined by B. In contrast, for longer pulses the pressure does not build up to as high a level because some thermal expansion of the melanosome occurs during the pulse.

The linearized model also allows a determination of the factors that control how much laser energy is channeled into mechanical and pressure effects versus heating. Equation (3) shows how the absorbed laser energy is channeled into temperature increases versus mechanical energy such as pressure increases or kinetic energy of expansion of the melanosome. In the absence of any mechanical effects, so that R would remain constant and $\dot{R}=0$, Eq. (3) reduces to Eq. (9a) and the final temperature increase would be given by $\Delta T = E_e/c_v$. For a laser fluence of $I_o=1$ J/cm^2, a melanosome radius a=1 μm, and an absorption coefficient $\alpha_m=1000$ cm^{-1}, Eq. (7), when multiplied by the length of the pulse τ_o, gives a total absorbed energy $E_e=3.89\times10^{-9}$ J. With $c_v=1.42\times10^{-11}$ J/K, this results in $\Delta T=274$ K and $T_{max}=310K+\Delta T=584$ K.

The actual amount of energy that does go into mechanical effects can be determined by the linearized equations. The last two terms in Eq. (3) quantitatively exhibit the rate at which energy is channeling into mechanical effects

$$\dot{E}_m = 4\pi T c_v \frac{\gamma}{V} R^2 \dot{R} + \frac{4\pi}{5}\rho a^3 \dot{R}\ddot{R} \tag{13}$$

We can determine the fraction of energy that will go into mechanical effects, E_m, through the following analysis. We will use the fact that in the linearized case $R\approx a$, $V\approx V_o$, and $E_e\approx c_v T$, which together allow us to write, for constant laser fluence

$$\frac{E_m}{E_e} = \frac{\dot{E}_m}{\dot{E}_e} = \frac{4\pi T c_v \frac{\gamma}{V_o} a^2 \dot{R} + \frac{4\pi}{5}\rho_m a^3 \dot{R}\ddot{R}}{c_v \dot{T}} \tag{14}$$

The Equation of State, Eq. (5), expresses $\dot{R}$ as a function of $\dot{T}$ and $\dot{P}$ and in the linearized model R can be replaced by 'a' giving

$$\dot{R} = \frac{a}{3}\alpha\dot{T} - \frac{a}{3B}\dot{P} \tag{15}$$

We can use Eq. (15) to substitute into Eq. (14) for $\dot{R}$ and $\ddot{R}$ in terms of $\dot{P}$, $\ddot{P}$ and $\dot{T}$ ($\ddot{T}=0$ if the laser fluence is constant). We can then substitute from Eq. (9a) $\dot{T}=\Delta T/\tau_o = E_e/c_v\tau_o$ and for $\dot{P}$ and $\ddot{P}$ from Eq. (10). This leads to a final expression

162

$$\frac{E_m}{E_e} = \frac{4\pi a^3}{3} \frac{\bar{T}\alpha_v^2}{c_v} B(1-\cos\omega t) + \frac{4\pi a^3}{3} \frac{a\alpha_v^2 \rho_m \sqrt{B}}{5\sqrt{3}\sqrt{\rho_L}c_v^2} \frac{E_e}{\tau_o}(1-\cos\omega t)(\sin\omega t)$$

$$= c_1(1-\cos\omega t) + c_2(1-\cos\omega t)\sin\omega t \tag{16}$$

Using a=10^{-6}m, α_v=29.8x10^{-6}/K, B=39.4x10^9 Pa, ρ_m=1.35 g/cm^3, c_v=$\rho_m cV_o$=1.42x10^{-11}J/K (with c=2.51 J/g-K), ρ_L=1.0 g/cm^3, α_m=1000 cm^{-1}, and laser pulse characteristics τ_o=10^{-8}seconds and I_o=1 J/cm^2, we get a total absorbed energy of E_e=3.89x10^{-9} J. In addition, $\bar{T}$ represents the temperature the melanosome would have at the end of the pulse if all the absorbed laser energy went into raising the melanosome's temperature. For the parameters listed above, $\bar{T}$=584 K. The coefficients in Eq. (16) give the fraction of absorbed laser energy that goes into mechanical effects and using the listed values of the melanosome and laser parameters, these coefficients are

$$c_1 = 6.03 \times 10^{-3} \qquad c_2 = 7.03 \times 10^{-6}$$

The small value of these coefficients justifies the use of the approximation $E_e \approx c_v T$ in Eq. (9a).

3. Inhomogeneous Model

The homogeneous model described above has the advantages of producing results that are physically intuitively easy to understand and can be solved analytically for a sphere composed of high bulk modulus material such as a melanosome. We now describe a physically more realistic model in which the pressure and temperature inside the melanosome is not constrained to rise and fall homogeneously but can vary as a function of radial position. This inhomogeneous model continues to assume that the surrounding water is incompressible.

3.1 Description of Model

In this model the pressure, temperature, displacement, and velocity of the melanosome sphere can be different at different radial positions. We use a Lagrangian representation in which the dynamics are described by the non-fixed coordinates u_i whose significance are defined by their initial position $u_i(t=0)=r_i$. In the differential equations used to describe the system, we follow the particle that was originally at r by calculating its corresponding u(t).

The first equation is the equation of mass continuity

$$\rho_m r^2 = u^2 \rho \frac{\partial u}{\partial r} \tag{17}$$

This equation will not be used in the numerical finite difference calculations to determine P, T, u but is used to replace the time and position varying ρ in terms of the initial melanosome density ρ_m, u, r. The equation of motion inside the melanosome is

$$\rho_m r^2 \ddot{u} = -u^2 \frac{\partial P}{\partial r} \tag{18}$$

The conservation of energy must now be expressed in local terms

$$\dot{I}_e = \rho c_v \dot{T} + 3\rho \alpha B T \dot{V} \tag{19}$$

where $\dot{I}_e$ is the energy absorbed per unit volume per second, V is the specific volume (m³/kg) and varies with r and t, V=V(r,t),

$$\dot{V} = \left[\frac{2}{\rho_m r^2} u \dot{u} \left(\frac{\partial u}{\partial r} \right) + \frac{u^2}{\rho_m r^2} \left(\frac{\partial \dot{u}}{\partial r} \right) \right] \tag{20}$$

and $\rho = 1/V$. The Equation of State, Eq. (4), which was expressed as Eq. (5) for the homogeneous model, now is expressed as

$$\frac{2\dot{u}}{u} + \frac{\left(\dfrac{\partial \dot{u}}{\partial r} \right)}{\left(\dfrac{\partial u}{\partial r} \right)} = -\frac{1}{B} \dot{P} + 3\alpha \dot{T} \tag{21}$$

where the left side is the time rate of change of the volume. Finally, the equation of motion at the boundary for u=u(r=a,t) combines Newton's Second Law and the approximation of incompressibility of the surrounding liquid and supplies a boundary condition for the system of partial differential equations.

$$\frac{P - P_o}{\rho_L} = \frac{3}{2} \dot{u}^2 + u \ddot{u} \tag{22}$$

3.2 Results

Results from this model are presented in Figs. (2a-d). As with the homogeneous model, for the same fluence the amplitude of the pressure oscillations increases as the laser pulse decreases. The amplitude of the pressure oscillations is highest at the center and lowest at the surface. The temporal oscillations of the pressure are still present. For the simpler model with homogeneous pressure changes throughout the melanosome and thus no internal waves, the oscillation frequency depended only on ρ_L. In this model which permits the pressure to vary inhomogeneously at different radial locations inside the melanosome, the oscillation frequency depends both on ρ_L and ρ_m. This is most apparent in Fig. (2b) in which the pressure is clearly not sinusoidal.

Our calculations also show that that the temperature rise predicted by this model is indistinguishable for the different radial positions in the melanosome and indistinguishable from the temperature rises for any of the pulse durations of Fig. (1). This is a reflection of the fact that even with the allowance of pressure waves inside the melanosome, mechanical effects still utilize less than 1% of the absorbed laser energy. Furthermore, because of the high bulk modulus of the melanosome, the changes in radius of the melanosome are also less than 1%.

4. Summary

The work presented gives a detailed, quantitative understanding of how the pressure and temperature of a melanosome are affected by laser pulses of various fluences and pulse lengths. In addition, the importance of the properties of the melanosome and the surrounding liquid are exhibited explicitly in Eqs. (9-22). We have shown explicitly that the pressures generated for the same fluence increases as the pulse length is decreased with a leveling off at approximately $\tau_o = 0.1 \times 10^{-9}$ seconds. Thus, for sub-nanosecond pulses the pressures generated are 100 times the pressures generated for a 10 nanosecond pulse. The next step is to determine how these pressures are transmitted into the surrounding cellular medium where the large pressures can cause biological damage.

Funded by AFOSR Grant F49620-96-1-0438

REFERENCES

1. B. S. Gerstman, C. R. Thompson, et. al., "Laser Induced Bubble Formation in the Retina", *Lasers in Surgery and Medicine,* **18**:10-21, 1996.

2. C. R. Thompson, B. S. Gerstman, et. al., "Melanin Granule Model for Laser Induced Thermal Damage to the Retina", *Bulletin of Mathematical Biology*, **58(3)**: 513-553, 1996.

3. E. A. Boettner and J. R. Wolter, "Transmission of the Ocular Media", United States Air Force Technical Documentary Report MRL-TDR-62-34.

4. C.P. Cain, C. A. Toth, et. al., "Visible Retinal Lesions from Ultrashort Laser Pulses in the Primate Eye", *Invest. Opthalmol. Vis. Sci.*, **36**, 879-888, 1995.

5. A. Vogel, S. Busch and U. Parlitz, "Shock Wave Emission and Cavitation Bubble Generation by Picosecond and Nanosecond Optical Breakdown in Water", *J. Acoust. Soc. Am.*, **100**, 148, 1996.

6. R. Courant and K. Friedrichs, *Supersonic Flow and Shock Waves*, Springer-Verlag, New York, chapter 3, 1948.

7. L. D. Landau and E. M. Lifshitz, *Fluid Mechanics*, Pergamon Press, Oxford, pp. 27-29, 1959.

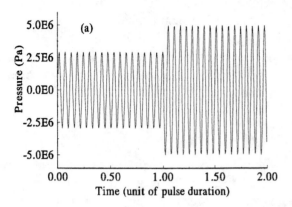 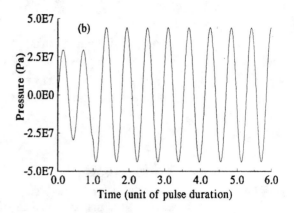

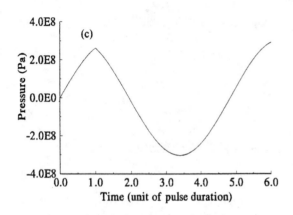 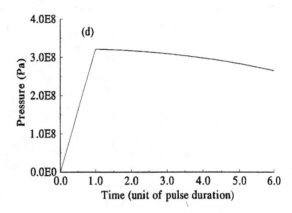

Figure 1. Pressure increase in a melanosome using a simplified model in which the pressure changes homogeneously and uniformly throughout the melanosome. Parameter values are melanosome radius a=1 μm, specific heat=2.51 J/g·K, ρ=1.35 g/cm^3, α$_v$=29.8x10^{-6}/K, B=39.4x10^9 Pa, α$_m$=1000 cm^{-1}, and laser fluence I$_o$=1 J/cm^2. The pulse duration is different for each figure: (a) 10 nanoseconds, (b) 1 nanosecond, (c) 0.1 nanosecond, (d) 10 picoseconds.

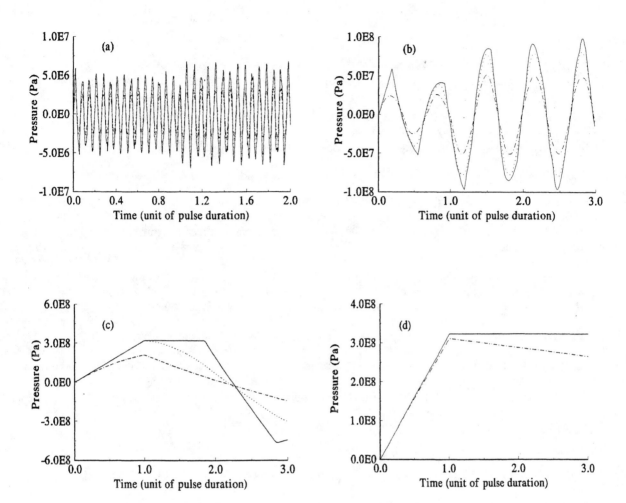

Figure 2. Pressure increase in a melanosome using the inhomogeneous model of section 3. Parameter values are the same as in Figure 1 with the melansome radius a=1 μm, specific heat=2.51 J/g·K, ρ=1.35 g/cm^3, α$_v$=29.8x10^{-6}/K, B=39.4x10^9 Pa, α$_m$=1000 cm^{-1}, and laser fluence I$_o$=1 J/cm^2. In this model the pressure varies differently at different locations within the melanosome: ——— r(t=0)=0.0a, ······ r(t=0)=0.5a, -----· r(t=0)=1.0a. The pulse duration is different for each figure: (a) 10 nanoseconds, (b) 1 nanosecond, (c) 0.1 nanosecond, (d) 10 picoseconds.

Energy balance of optical breakdown in water

Alfred Vogel[1], Joachim Noack[1], Kester Nahen[1], Dirk Theisen[1], Stefan Busch[1], Ulrich Parlitz[2], Daniel X. Hammer[3], Gary D. Noojin[3], Benjamin A. Rockwell[3], and Reginald Birngruber[1]

1) Medizinisches Laserzentrum Lübeck, D-23562 Lübeck, Germany
2) Drittes Physikalisches Institut, University of Göttingen, D-37073, Germany
3) Optical Radiation Division, Armstrong Laboratory, Brooks AFB, TX 78235, USA

ABSTRACT

During optical breakdown, the energy delivered to the sample is either transmitted, reflected, scattered, or absorbed. The absorbed energy can be further divided into the energy required to evaporate the focal volume, the energy radiated by the luminescent plasma, and the energy contributing to the mechanical effects such as shock wave emission and cavitation. The partition of the pulse energy between these channels was investigated for 4 selected laser parameters (6 ns pulses of 1 and 10 mJ, 30 ps pulses of 50 μJ and 1 mJ, all at 1064 nm). The results indicated that the scattering and reflection by the plasma is small compared to plasma transmission. The plasma absorption can therefore be approximated by $A \approx (1-T)$. The ratio of the shock wave energy and cavitation bubble energy was found to be approximately constant (between 1.5:1 and 2:1). For a more comprehensive study of the influence of pulse duration and focusing angle on the energy partition, we therefore restricted our measurements to the plasma transmission and the cavitation bubble energy. The bubble energy was used as an indicator for the total amount of mechanical energy produced. We found that the plasma absorption first decreases strongly with decreasing pulse duration, but increases again for pulses shorter than 3 ps. The conversion of the absorbed energy into mechanical energy is $\approx$ 90% with ns-pulses at large focusing angles. It decreases both with decreasing focusing angle and pulse duration (to $\leq$ 15% for fs-pulses). The disruptive character of plasma-mediated laser surgery is therefore reduced with ultrashort laser pulses.

Keywords: laser-induced breakdown, plasma, shock wave, cavitation, energy balance, ultrashort laser pulses, plasma-mediated laser surgery.

1. INTRODUCTION

Optical breakdown enables localized energy deposition even into media which are transparent at low light intensities[1]. This feature has been used for intraocular microsurgery avoiding the need to open the eye[2,3], and it has also been applied for the ablation and micromachining of various other biological and nonbiological materials[4-7]. The advent of compact and reliable ultrashort pulse lasers has made it possible to achieve very fine laser effects, because the threshold for optical breakdown decreases with a reduction of pulse duration[8,9]. Besides on the breakdown threshold, the laser effects also depend on the partition of the incident energy in various pathways. Only the absorbed energy is effective; light transmission through the plasma as well as scattering and reflection by the plasma reduce the efficacy of the plasma-mediated process. Absorbed energy going into evaporation contributes to the tissue cutting or material ablation, whereas the energy going into the mechanical pathways of shock wave generation and cavitation contributes to the disruptive character of the breakdown process. The latter may be advantageous in some cases (e.g. in posterior capsulotomy and lithotripsy), but it is mostly the source of unwanted side effects. Knowledge of the energy partition during optical breakdown is thus a prerequisite for an optimal parameter choice for each particular application.

Correspondence: Alfred Vogel, PhD, Medical Laser Center Lübeck, Peter-Monnik-Weg 4, D-23562 Lübeck, Germany. FAX: xx49-505 486; e-mail: vogel@mll.mu-luebeck.de

In this paper, we establish a complete energy balance of optical breakdown in water for a few selected laser parameters, and we present the dependence of energy partition on the focusing angle θ and on laser pulse duration τ_L for a large parameter range ($4° < \theta < 32°$, 100 fs $< \tau_L < 76$ ns).

2. METHODS

2.1 Optical system for plasma generation

The plasmas were generated by focusing laser pulses with various durations between 76 ns and 100 fs into a cuvette containing distilled water (Fig. 1). The optical delivery system allowed for the realization of different focusing angles and was designed to minimize spherical aberrations. For that purpose, an ophthalmic contact lens was built into the cuvette wall. A detailed description of the optical system for plasma generation and of the methods used for the measurement of the focusing angle, the spot size, and the optical breakdown threshold has been given previously[8,10,11]. The laser parameters used and the corresponding spot sizes and breakdown thresholds are summarized in Table 1.

pulse duration	wavelength [nm]	focusing angle [°]	measured spot diameter [µm]	I_{th} [10^{11} Wcm^{-2}]	F_{th} [Jcm^{-2}]
76ns	750	19	20	0.23	1750
6 ns	1064	32	5.5	0.66	398
6 ns	1064	22	7.6	0.47	284
6 ns	1064	8	11.5	0.79	472
6 ns	1064	5.4	14.6	1.1	648
30 ps	1064	28	4.6	4.6	13.8
30 ps	1064	22	4.7	4.5	13.6
30 ps	1064	14	5.8	3.0	9.0
30 ps	1064	8.5	9.6	4.5	13.6
30 ps	1064	4	19.5	3.7	11.1
60ps	532	13	5.6	2.8	16.8
3ps	580	16	5.0	8.5	2.6
300 fs	580	16	5.0	47.6	1.4
100 fs	580	16	4.4	111.0	1.1

Table 1: Laser parameters investigated in the present study, and corresponding spot sizes and breakdown thresholds. A complete energy balance was obtained for 6-ns pulses at 22° and 30-ps pulses at 14°. The dependence of energy partition on focusing angle was investigated for 6-ns and 30-ps pulses. The dependence on pulse duration was investigated for 76-ns pulses, 6-ns pulses at 22°, 60 ps, 3 ps, 300 fs, and 100 fs.

2.2 Plasma transmission, scattering and reflection

The plasma transmission was measured with the setup depicted in Figure 1a[12]. For each focusing angle θ of the incident light, only light transmitted within that angle was collected; scattered light was rejected by an iris diaphragm. To account for light losses by reflections at optical surfaces and water absorption, detector 2 was calibrated against detector 1 assuming that at pulse energies far below breakdown threshold 100% of the incident energy is transmitted through the laser focus.

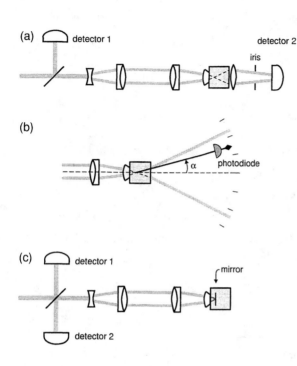

The amount of light scattered out of the cone angle of the laser beam was determined through goniometric measurements performed for $\alpha \leq 45°$[12] (Fig. 1b). To assess the amount of forward scattering by the plasma, we compared the angular energy distribution at a given superthreshold energy $\beta = E / E_{th}$ to the distribution it has below threshold. The measurement technique is described in detail in a previous paper[12].

The amount of light reflected by the plasma back into the cone angle of the focused laser beam was measured using the setup in Figure 1c. First, an aluminium mirror was placed into the focus and a measurement was performed at an energy where no plasma formation on the mirror occurred. In this way the calibration factor between the two detectors was determined for a case with a known reflection of 80 %. The mirror was then removed and the plasma reflection measured at higher pulse energies.

Figure 1: Setup for the measurement of plasma transmission (a), forward scattering (b), and back reflection into the focusing optics (c).

Direct investigation of the energy absorbed in the breakdown volume would require measurements with a water-filled integrating sphere. At a wavelength of 1064 nm where the absorption coefficient of water is 0.13 cm^{-1}, such measurements are, however, difficult, because no equilibrium light distribution can be achieved within the sphere. We therefore deduce the absorption A from the measurements of transmission T, scattering S and reflection R: $A = (1-T-S-R)$.

2.3 Evaporation energy

To assess the evaporation energy, we assume that all water within the plasma volume is evaporated, neglecting heat conduction into the surrounding liquid. The time available for heat conduction is very short because i) the laser pulse duration is extremely short, and ii) the content of the cavitation bubble cools down to room temperature within a few microseconds[13]. The plasma volume was determined from photographs of the plasma radiation[8]. The heat of evaporation is given by

$$E_v = \rho V \left[c(T_2 - T_1) + r \right] , \qquad (1)$$

with ρ = 998 kg m^{-3}, c = 4.18 kJ (kg K)$^{-1}$, T_2 = 100°C, T_1 = 20°C, and r = 2256 kJ kg^{-1}. We use the isobaric evaporation enthalpy and specific heat, because the initially high bubble pressure decays to hydrostatic pressure (or even lower pressure values) already after a small fraction of the bubble lifetime.

2.4 Cavitation bubble energy

The energy of a spherical cavitation bubble is $\quad E_B = \frac{4\pi}{3}(p_0 - p_v) R_{max}^3$, $\qquad\qquad\qquad$ (2)

where R_{max} is the radius at the time of maximum bubble expansion, p_0 is the hydrostatic pressure, and p_v the vapor pressure inside the bubble (2330 Pa at 20°C). The bubble size is related to its oscillation period T_B by the Rayleigh

equation $\qquad\qquad\qquad\qquad R_{max} = \dfrac{T_B}{2 \times 0.915\sqrt{\dfrac{\rho_0}{p_\infty - p_v}}}$. $\qquad\qquad\qquad$ (3)

The oscillation period was determined through a hydrophone measurement of the acoustic transients emitted upon optical breakdown and bubble collapse[14]. It was confirmed in preliminary measurements that Eq. (3), which was derived for spherical bubbles, gives good results also for elongated bubbles arising after fs-breakdown[15]. In that case, R_{max} corresponds to the radius of a sphere having the same volume as the elongated bubble.

2.5 Acoustic energy

The shock wave energy is given by[16] $\qquad\qquad E_s = \frac{4\pi\, r_m^2}{\rho_0\, c_0}\int p_s^2\, dt$ $\qquad\qquad\qquad$ (4)

where r_m denotes the distance from the emission center at which the pressure p_s is measured. Use of Eq. (4) for a determination of the total acoustic energy requires knowledge of the shock wave profile $p(t)$ in the immediate vicinity of the laser plasma, because further away a large part of the shock wave energy is already dissipated[10,17]. The shock wave profile close to the plasma is difficult to measure and was therefore obtained through numerical calculations based on the Gilmore model of cavitation bubble evolution[10,17]. Experimental parameters entering the calculations are the photographically determined plasma volume, the maximum radius R_{max} of the cavitation bubble, and the laser pulse duration. The shock wave energy obtained by this method is denoted $E_s^{Gilmore}$.

We also used a second approach based on an evaluation of the energy dissipated at the shock front[17]. The Rankine-Hugoniot equation relates the increase of internal energy per unit mass at a shock front to the change of pressure ($p_0 \rightarrow p_s$) and density ($\rho_0 \rightarrow \rho_s$) at the shock front[2]:

$$\Delta\varepsilon(r) = \frac{1}{2}\left(\frac{1}{\rho_0} - \frac{1}{\rho_s(r)}\right)\left(p_s(r) + p_0\right) \approx \frac{1}{2}\left(\frac{1}{\rho_0} - \frac{1}{\rho_s(r)}\right)p_s(r).$$ $\qquad\qquad$ (5)

The pressure p_s and density ρ_s behind the shock front were determined indirectly through a measurement of the shock front velocity u_s[10]. The pressure is related to u_s by[10]

$$p_s = c_1\rho_0 u_s\left(10^{(u_s - c_0)/c_2} - 1\right) + p_0 \quad ,$$ $\qquad\qquad\qquad$ (6)

where c_0 denotes the sound velocity in water, c_1 = 5190 m/s, and c_2 = 25306 m/s.

The density is linked with u_s by[17]

$$\rho_s = \frac{\rho_0}{1 - \dfrac{p_s}{u_s^2 \rho_0}} \,. \tag{7}$$

Integration of Eq. (5) yields the total change of internal energy during propagation of a spherical shock front from r_0 to r_1

$$E_{Diss} = \int_{r_0}^{r_1} 4\pi r^2 \rho_s(r)\, \Delta\varepsilon(r)\, dr \,. \tag{8}$$

The total amount of acoustic energy was estimated by adding the dissipated energy E_{Diss} in the near field (r ≤ 300 μm) and the energy $E_{S/10mm}$ remaining at 10 mm distance from the source which was obtained from hydrophone measurements using Eq. (4). The resulting value is a lower estimate, because the dissipation in the range 0.3 mm $< r <$ 10 mm is not considered. This error is, however, small because most of the dissipation takes place very close to the plasma[17]. Furthermore, it is probably compensated by the fact that our calculations of E_{Diss} do not consider that a part of the acoustic energy deposited as internal energy behind the shock front flows back into the shock wave at its trailing edge[16].

2.6 Energy of plasma radiation

Barnes and Rieckhoff[18] and Stolarski et al.[19], who measured the spectral energy density of the plasma radiation in the wavelength range 300 nm $< \lambda <$ 900 nm found that it closely resembles the spectral distribution of a blackbody radiator. The radiant energy emitted by the blackbody depends on its temperature T, the surface area A and the duration τ_{rad} of the radiation[20]:

$$E_{rad} = \sigma A\, \tau_{rad}\, T^4 \tag{9}$$

with the Stefan Boltzmann constant $\sigma = 5.670\ 10^{-8}$ W m^{-2}K^{-4}. The temperature T of the blackbody can be determined from the maximum of the spectral distribution $\rho(\nu)$ using Wien's displacement law

$$T = 1.70 \times 10^{-9}\ \nu_m \,. \tag{10}$$

Equation (9) yields an upper estimate of the energy E_{rad} of the plasma radiation for a given temperature, because it assumes a perfect blackbody radiator. More refined models considering the emissivity $\varepsilon(\nu)$ of the plasma ($0 \le \varepsilon \le 1$) as a function of pressure and temperature of the plasma constituents and of the plasma size have been developed by Weyl and Tucker[21], and by Roberts et al.[22]. However, the simpler approach of Eq. (9) suffices already to show that the plasma radiation plays only a minor role in the energy balance of optical breakdown (see below). Data for the plasma temperature were taken from the literature[19], the plasma surface area was determined from plasma photographs, and the duration of the plasma radiation was determined with a fast photodiode.

3. RESULTS AND DISCUSSION

3.1 Complete energy balance for selected parameters

Figure 2 shows the complete energy balance for 6-ns pulses with 1 mJ and 10 mJ energy, and for 30-ps pulses with 50 μJ and 1 mJ pulse energy.

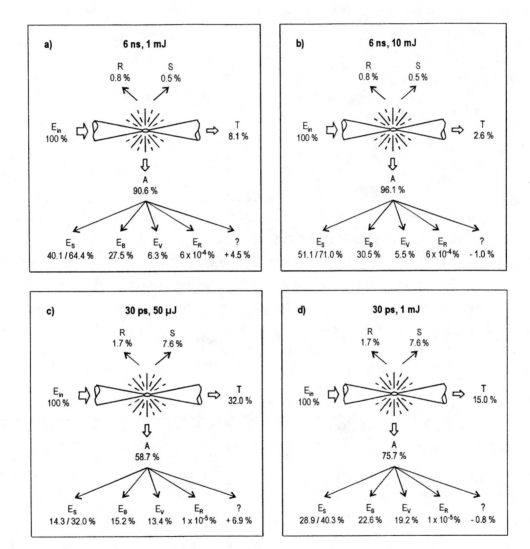

Figure 2: Energy balance for selected laser parameters. For the shock wave energy two values $E_s^{Gilmore}$ and $(E_{Diss} + E_{S/10mm})$ obtained by different methods (see text) are given for each laser parameter. The difference of the complete energy balance to 100 % is denoted by "?". It was calculated using the average of the two energy values quoted for the shock wave energy.

Near threshold, considerably more light is transmitted through the plasma than reflected or scattered. Well above threshold the relative importance of transmission decreases. For all laser parameters, considerably less light is reflected or scattered by the plasma than absorbed. The absorption is thus approximately given by A ≈ (1-T). This differs from plasma formation at solid surfaces, where reflection plays a large role[23]. In liquids, the electron density is limited by the fact that the breakdown front moves within the medium during the laser pulse. The plasma frequency remains therefore smaller than the frequency of the laser light, and the laser-plasma-coupling is not impaired.

The energy of the plasma radiation was calculated using the data reported by Stolarski et al. [19] for the temperatures of plasmas produced with Nd:YAG laser pulses at 1064 nm wavelength (9860 K at 5 ns pulse duration and 4 mJ pulse energy; 6230 K at 80 ps pulse duration and 1 mJ pulse energy). The duration of the plasma radiation was measured to be 10 ns after a 5 mJ/6 ns pulse, and 0.5 ns after a 2 mJ/30 ps pulse (In the latter case, the photodiode signal was deconvoluted with the impulse response of the photodiode/oscilloscope system. Streak photographic measurements by other authors yielded similar results of 0.24 ns[24] and 0.5 ns[25]). The results of our calculations (Fig. 2) demonstrate that the energy loss through plasma radiation is negligible for all laser parameters investigated. The situation is slightly different for plasmas produced with microsecond laser pulses used in laser lithotripsy[1]. Here the energy carried away by plasma radiation may reach up to 1% of the incident laser light energy because of the longer duration of the plasma emission[21].

The relevant pathways for the absorbed laser energy are evaporation, shock wave generation and cavitation. For all laser parameters, a considerably larger part of the incident light energy is transformed into mechanical energy than into evaporation energy. This feature is particularly pronounced with the 6-ns-pulses where the mechanical energy is 12-16 times larger than the evaporation energy (with the 30-ps pulses it is 3 times as large). The high conversion efficiency of light energy into mechanical energy is the cause for the disruptive character of plasma-mediated laser surgery. The mechanical energy divides itself into shock wave energy and bubble energy with a ratio of ≈ 1.5:1 for ps-pulses and ≈ 2:1 for ns-pulses (for calculation of these ratios we used the average of the shock wave energies obtained through the two different methods described in section 2).

The difference of the complete energy balance to 100 % is less than 7 % for all laser parameters. Considering the measurement uncertainties of the individual parts of the energy balance which is particularly large for the shock wave energy, this result is very satisfactory.

3.2 Parameter dependence of energy deposition

The parameter dependence of the energy deposition at the optical breakdown site can be deduced from the parameter dependence of plasma transmission, because the complete energy balance for selected parameters showed that $A ≈ (1-T)$. Figure 3 presents transmission data $T(E / E_{th})$ for different focusing angles at 30 ps pulse duration, and Figure 4 shows the transmission as a function of laser pulse duration for two different values of the dimensionless pulse energy $\beta = E / E_{th}$.

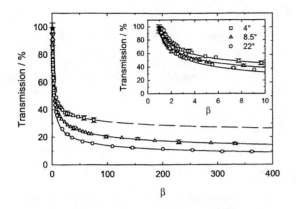

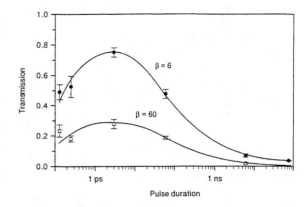

Figure 3: Plasma transmission at various focusing angles, plotted as a function of the normalized laser pulse energy $\beta = E / E_{th}$. Pulse duration 30 ps, wavelength 1064 nm.

Figure 4: Plasma transmission as a function of laser pulse duration for $\beta = 6$ and $\beta = 60$. The measured data points[15] are connected with lines to facilitate orientation.

Figure 3 demonstrates that the plasma transmission increases with decreasing focusing angle, i.e. the energy deposition decreases. This finding is quite surprising at first sight, because a decreasing focusing angle goes along with an approximately quadratic increase of the plasma length when β is kept constant[8]. The results can only be understood, if the increased plasma length is compensated for by a decrease of the absorption coefficient in the plasma. This is indeed the case, because the energy density of the plasma decreases with decreasing focusing angle: at a certain energy, the plasma can grow into the cone of the laser beam until it reaches the cross section for which $I = I_{th}$. This cross section is the same regardless of the focusing angle, but the distance between laser focus and the cross section is larger for smaller angles. Therefore, the volume of the cone is larger and the energy density less for smaller angles. This results in a smaller absorption coefficient for inverse bremsstrahlung absorption, because this mechanism depends on the free electron concentration and on the collision frequency between electrons and heavy particles which, in turn, are both positively correlated with the energy density within the plasma volume[12,26]

Figure 4 shows that the transmission strongly depends on the laser pulse duration τ. It is small in the nanosecond range, but considerably larger for ps-pulses. When the pulse duration is further reduced into the femtosecond range, the transmission decreases again. We identified two factors contributing to the observed $T(\tau)$-dependence. i) Ns-plasmas are, at equal β and equal focusing angle, considerably longer than ps and fs plasmas[8,15]. Therefore, they absorb more light even at equal absorption coefficient. ii) The time evolution of the free electron concentration during the laser pulse changes with pulse duration[27,28]: With ns-pulses the electron concentration reaches high values already early in the pulse (which leads to a large value of the average absorption coefficient), with ps-pulses the maximum is achieved much later, and with fs-pulses a high electron density is again reached earlier due to the increasing role of multiphoton ionization. The latter explains the increase of absorption (decrease of transmission) for fs-pulses.

3.3 Energy partition into evaporation energy and mechanical energy

The cavitation bubble energy is used as marker for the total mechanical energy to elucidate the parameter dependence of the conversion of light energy into mechanical energy. This simplification is justified by the fact that the division of mechanical energy into bubble energy and shock wave energy was in section 3.1 found to be similar for different energies and pulse durations.

Figure 5 shows that the conversion efficiency of light energy into cavitation bubble energy decreases with decreasing focusing angle. The conversion efficiency depends on the focusing angle, because the energy density in the plasma volume decreases with smaller focusing angles, as explained already in section 3.2. With a smaller energy density, a larger percentage of the laser energy is required for the evaporation of the liquid in the plasma volume, and a smaller fraction is available for the generation of mechanical effects.

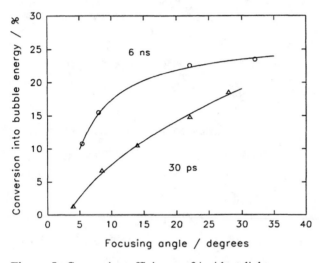

Figure 5: Conversion efficiency of incident light energy into cavitation bubble energy as a function of focusing angle, for energies well above the breakdown threshold.

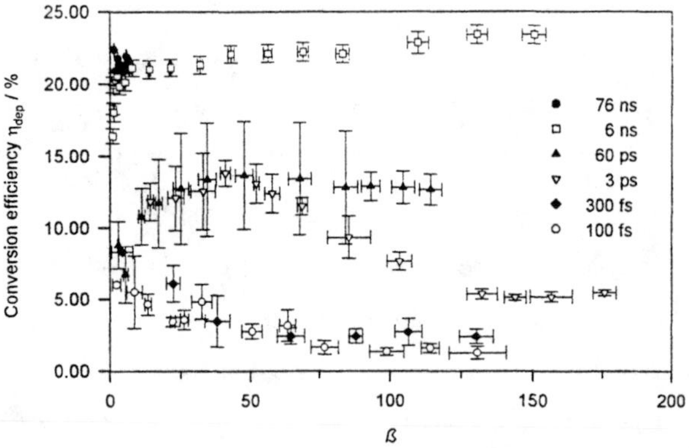

Figure 6: Conversion efficiency of absorbed light energy into cavitation bubble energy as a function of the normalized laser pulse energy $\beta = E / E_{th}$ for various laser pulse durations.

The conversion efficiency into bubble energy is, at all focusing angles, larger for 6-ns pulses than for 30-ps pulses. Figure 6 shows that the conversion efficiency decreases even further in the fs-range. This trend is caused by the fact that the radiant energy required to produce breakdown decreases with decreasing pulse duration which goes along with a decrease of the average energy density in the breakdown region: We determined the energy density to be 30-40 kJ/cm^3 for ns-pulses[10] and less than 1 kJ/cm^3 for 100 fs-pulses[11].

Several factors may contribute to that trend:

i) The energy density in the plasma volume will decrease with pulse duration, if the maximum concentration of free electrons reached during the laser pulse is smaller for shorter pulse durations. This possibility has been suggested by Kennedy[29], but it has not yet been investigated to date; a measurement of free electron concentration after optical breakdown in water has only been performed for ns-plasmas[18].

ii) Even if the maximum concentration of free electrons does not depend on pulse durations, the energy density in the plasma volume does. With long pulses, a temperature equilibrium between electrons and heavy particles is achieved during the pulse through recombination processes, and therefore the energy density is high[28]. With ultrashort pulses, however, very little energy has at the end of the laser pulse been transferred to the heavy particles. An equilibrium temperature develops only after the laser pulse. The equilibrium temperature will thus be much lower than in the case of the ns-pulses, particularly because the specific heat of the electrons is much smaller than that of the ions and other heavy particles[6].

iii) After fs-breakdown, heating of the liquid has been observed in front of the actual breakdown zone where a bubble is produced[15,28]. Similar observations have not been made for ns- or ps-pulses. This means that in fs-breakdown a larger part of the absorbed energy cannot be converted into bubble energy than with the longer pulse durations[15,28].

For pulse durations ≤ 3 ps, the conversion efficiency of absorbed light energy into bubble energy reaches a maximum at small β-values and decreases again at energies well above threshold. A similar energy dependence has been observed for 30-ps pulses at 1064 nm (not shown)[30]. It reflects a decrease of the energy density in the breakdown volume with increasing β which can be understood as follows: For ps- and fs-pulses, the plasma length varies approximately proportional to[8,15] $(\beta-1)^{1/2}$, and the plasma volume is, hence, proportional to $(\beta-1)^{3/2}$. The energy density in the plasma can therefore be written as

$$W = \frac{A E_{in}}{V} \propto \frac{A \beta E_{th}}{(\beta-1)^{3/2}} \approx \frac{A E_{th}}{\sqrt{\beta}} \quad \text{for } \beta \gg 1 \tag{11}$$

At large β-values, the coupling coefficient $A \approx (1-T)$ of laser energy into the plasma is approximately constant, because the transmision changes only very slowly (Fig. 3). It can be concluded from Eq. (14) that under these circumstances the average energy density decreases with increasing β. For fs-pulses, another factor might also contribute to the energy dependence of the conversion efficiency into bubble energy. We observed that the relative size of the zone in front of the breakdown region where the liquid is heated but no bubble is formed, increases with increasing β. Therefore, a smaller fraction of absorbed energy is available for bubble formation.

In all applications aiming at tissue cutting or ablation with little mechanical side effects, the ratio of mechanical energy E_{mech} to evaporation energy E_v should be as small as possible. The above results show that (E_{mech}/E_v) is small for short laser pulse durations, small focusing angles, and large values of the normalized pulse energy β. Only the first aspect, however, is of real advantage for achieving very precise and fine laser effects. A smaller focusing angle leads to a higher energy threshold for breakdown and a larger volume of the breakdown region which contradicts the aim of increased precision. If we assume that the shock wave energy is always 1.5 to 2 times larger than the bubble energy, we find that the ratio (E_{mech}/E_v) is about 12.5:1 for 6-ns pulses and 0.25:1 to 1:1 for 100-fs pulses. Besides the reduction of the energy threshold with decreasing pulse duration, this change of energy partition contributes largely to the less disruptive character of fs-breakdown.

3.4 Conclusions

The conversion efficiency of light energy into mechanical energy during optical breakdown is larger (up to 90%) than with any other laser-tissue interaction[31-33]. This is the cause for the disruptive character of plasma-mediated laser surgery in a liquid environment. At large focusing angles, short and highly absorbing plasmas are achieved which allow a well localized energy deposition. However, this goes along with a particularly large conversion efficiency into mechanical energy, and therefore with a large potential for mechanically induced side effects. The mechanical effects can be dramatically reduced by shortening the laser pulse duration, but this is possible only at the expense of a decreased efficacy of energy deposition.

4. ACKNOWLEDGEMENTS

This work was supported by the German Science Foundation (#Bi321/2-4), The United States Air Force Office of Scientific Research (#2312AAAL014), and TASC (#J06829S95135).

5. REFERENCES

1. A. Vogel, "Nonlinear absorption: intraocular microsurgery and laser lithotripsy", *Phys. Med. Biol.* **42**, pp. 895-912, 1997.
2. R. F. Steinert and C. A. Puliafito, "*The Nd:YAG Laser in Ophthalmology*", Saunders, Philadelphia, PA, 1985.
3. A. Vogel, P. Schweiger, A. Frieser, M. N. Asiyo, R. Birngruber, "Intraocular Nd:YAG laser surgery: Light-tissue interaction, damage range, and reduction of collateral effects", *IEEE J. Quantum Electron.* **26**, pp. 2240-2260, 1990.
4. J. Neev, L.B Da Silva, M. D. Feit, M. D. Perry, A. M. Rubenchik, and B. C. Stuart, "Ultrashort pulse lasers for hard tissue ablation", *IEEE J. Selected Topics Quantum Electron.* **2**(4), pp. 790-800, 1996.
5. A. A. Oraevsky, L. B. DaSilva, A. M. Rubenchik, M. D. Feit, M. E. Glinsky, M. D. Perry, B. M. Mammini, W. Small IV, and B. C. Stuart, "Plasma-mediated ablation of biological tissues with nanosecond-to-femtosecond laser pulses: Relative role of linear and nonlinear absorption", *IEEE J. Selected Topics Quantum Electron.* **2**(4), pp. 801-809, 1996.
6. B. N. Chichkov, C. Momma, S. Nolte, F. von Alvensleben, and A. Tünnermann, "Femtosecond, picosecond and nanosecond ablation of solids", *Appl. Phys. A* **63**, pp. 109-115, 1996.
7. X. Liu, D. Du, and G. Mourou, " Laser ablation and micromachining with ultrashort laser pulses", *IEEE J. Quantum Electron.* **33**, pp. 1706-1716, 1997.
8. A. Vogel, K. Nahen, D. Theisen, J. Noack, "Plasma formation in water by picosecond and nanosecond Nd:YAG laser pulses- part I: optical breakdown at threshold and superthreshold irradiance", *IEEE J. Selected Topics Quantum Electron.* **2**(4), pp. 847-860, 1996
9. P. K. Kennedy, S. A. Boppart, D. X. Hammer, B. A. Rockwell, G. D. Noojin, W. P. Roach, "A first order model of laser-induced breakdown thresholds in ocular and aqueous media: Part II- comparison to experiments", *IEEE J. Quantum Electron.* **31**, pp.2250-2257, 1995.
10. A. Vogel, S. Busch, U. Parlitz, "Shock wave emission and cavitation bubble generation by picosecond and nanosecond optical breakdown in water", *J. Acoust. Soc. Am.* **100**, pp. 148-165, 1996.
11. J. Noack, D. X. Hammer, G. D. Noojin, B. A. Rockwell, A. Vogel, "Influence of pulse duration on mechanical effects after laser-induced breakdown in water", *submitted to J. Appl. Phys.* 1997.
12. K. Nahen and A. Vogel, "Plasma formation in water by picosecond and nanosecond Nd:YAG laser pulses - Part II: Plasma transmission, scattering and reflection", *IEEE J. Selected Topics Quantum Electron.* **2**(4), pp. 861-871, 1996.
13. S. Fujikawa and T. Akamatsu, "Effects of the non-equilibrium condensation of vapour on the pressure wave produced by the collapse of a bubble in a liquid", *J. Fluid Mech.* **97**, pp. 481-512, 1980.
14. A. Vogel, W. Hentschel, J. Holzfuss, W. Lauterborn, "Cavitation bubble dynamics and acoustic transient generation in ocular surgery with pulsed neodymium YAG lasers", *Ophthalmology* **93**, pp. 1259-1269, 1986.
15. J. Noack, "Optical breakdown in water with laser pulses between 100 ns and 100 fs", *PhD Dissertation*, Medical University of Lübeck, Lübeck, Germany 1998 (in German).

16. R. H. Cole, "*Underwater Explosions*", Princeton University Press, Princeton, NJ, 1948.

17. A. Vogel and J. Noack, "Shock wave energy and acoustic energy dissipation after laser-induced breakdown", *SPIE Proc.* **3254A** (this issue), 1998.

18. P. A. Barnes and K. E. Rieckhoff, "Laser induced underwater sparks", *Appl. Phys. Lett.* **13**, pp. 282-284.

19. D. J. Stolarski, J. Hardman, C. G. Bramlette, G. D. Noojin, R. J. Thomas, B. A. Rockwell, W. P. Roach, "Integrated light spectroscopy of laser-induced breakdown in aqueous media", *SPIE Proc.* **2391**, pp. 100-109, 1995.

20. D. Sliney and M. Wolbarsht, "*Safety with Lasers and Other Optical Sources*", Plenum Press, New York, 1980.

21. G. Weyl and T. Tucker, "Penetration of plasma radiation in tissue", *Lasers Life Sci.* **3**, pp. 125-138, 1989

22. R. M. Roberts, J. A. Cook, R. L. Rogers, A. M. Gleeson, T. A. Griffy, "The energy partition of underwater sparks", *J. Acoust. Soc. Am.* **99**, pp. 3465-3475, 1996.

23. R. P. Godwin, C. G. M. van Kessel, J. N. Olsen, P. Sachsenmaier, R. Sigel, "Reflection losses from laser-produced plasmas", *Z. Naturforsch.* **32a**, pp. 1100-1107, 1977

24. F. Dochio, "Lifetimes of plasmas induced in liquids and ocular media by single Nd:YAG pulses of different duration", *Europhys. Lett.* **6**, pp. 407-412.

25. R. J. Thomas, D. X. Hammer, G. D. Noojin, D. J. Stolarski, B. A. Rockwell, W. P. Roach, "Time-resolved spectroscopy of laser-induced breakdown in water", *SPIE Proc.* **2681**, pp. 402-410, 1996.

26. Y. R. Shen, "*The Principles of Nonlinear Optics*", Wiley, New York, 1984.

27. J. Noack, A. Vogel, D. X. Hammer, G. D. Noojin, B. A. Rockwell, "Thresholds and transmission of laser-induced breakdown in water for pulse durations between 100 fs and 100 ns", *submitted to Opt. Lett.* 1997.

28. A. Vogel, J. Noack, K. Nahen, D. Theisen, R. Birngruber, D. X. Hammer, G. D. Noojin, B. A. Rockwell, "Laser-induced breakdown in the eye at pulse durations from 80 ns to 100 fs", *SPIE Proc.* **3255**, 1998 (in print)

29. P. K. Kennedy, " A first-order model for computation of laser-induced breakdown thresholds in ocular and aqueous media: Part I-Theory", *IEEE J. Quantum Electron.* **31**, pp. 2241-2249, 1995.

30. D. Theisen, "Experimental investigations of plasma formation in water with ps-and ns-Nd:YAG laser pulses", *Diploma thesis*, Polytechnical of Lübeck, Lübeck 1994 (in German).

31. V. S. Teslenko, "Investigation of photoacoustic and photohydrodynamic parameters of laser breakdown in liquids", *Sov. J. Quant. Electron.* **7**, pp. 981-984, 1977.

32. L. M. Lyamshev, "Optoacoustic sources of sound", *Sov. Phys. Usp.* **24**, pp. 977-995, 1981.

33. E. J. Chapyak, R. P. Godwin, A. Vogel, "A comparison of numerical simulations and laboratory studies of shock waves and cavitation bubble growth produced by optical breakdown in water", *SPIE Proc.* **2975**, pp. 335-342, 1997.

Shock wave energy and acoustic energy dissipation
after laser-induced breakdown

Alfred Vogel and Joachim Noack

Medical Laser Center Lübeck, D-23562 Lübeck, Germany

ABSTRACT

We investigated the spatial distribution of energy dissipation during propagation of the shock front arising from optical breakdown in water, because it is related to the stress-induced cellular changes in plasma-mediated laser surgery. The dissipation can be calculated from the shock wave velocity u_s by a relation derived from the Rankine-Hugoniot equation. u_s was measured as a function of time and space for various laser parameters. With a 1 mJ/ 6-ns pulse, 64 % of the absorbed light energy are converted into acoustic energy, but the largest part of this energy are converted into heat already within the first 200 μm of shock front propagation. Afterwards, the dissipation occurs at a much slower rate. Only ≈ 10% of the acoustic energy reaches a distance of 10 mm. Far-field measurements can thus be very misleading for an energy balance. The energy dissipation at the shock front leads to a temperature rise of the medium. At 10 mJ pulse energy, the temperature close to the plasma exceeds the critical point of water. This means that the shock wave passage goes along with an enlargement of the cavitation bubble. High-pressure-induced bubble formation can also occur at locations further away from the laser plasma where shock waves from adjacent plasmas interfere. We have thus demonstrated a mechanism of stress wave induced cavitation which does not rely on tensile stress, but on very high overpressures. Since most of the dissipation takes place within the first 200 μm, the shock wave effects are mostly covered by the effects of the cavitation bubble which reaches a radius of 800 μm in water at the same laser parameters. Acoustic tissue effects are, nevertheless, important, because the bubble is smaller in tissue than in water, the weakening of the tissue structure by the shock wave passage probably contributes to the cavitation-induced damage, and the range for acoustic damage is larger in nonspherical geometries.

Keywords: Laser-induced breakdown, shock wave, energy dissipation, energy balance, cell damage, cavitation

1. INTRODUCTION

Shock waves, unlike acoustic waves, feature a strong dissipation of energy during propagation[1-4]. The dissipated energy changes the state of the matter behind the shock front, and is thus related to stress-induced tissue changes arising in plasma-mediated laser surgery and short-pulsed laser ablation. In this paper, we investigate the spatial distribution of the acoustic energy dissipation after optical breakdown in water, and we look at the interplay between acoustic energy dissipation and cavitation bubble formation. We show that most of the energy is dissipated already in the immediate vicinity of the laser-generated plasma. The total shock wave energy can therefore be estimated by integration over the dissipated energy near the source.

Figure 1 illustrates the energy dissipation at a shock front. The shock front is a pressure discontinuity which propagates with velocity u_s into a medium with a particle velocity u_0. If the medium is at rest, the particle velocity u_0 in front of the shock is zero in a laboratory coordinate system (Fig. 1a). The particle velocity behind the shock front is u_p.

Correspondence: Alfred Vogel, PhD, Medical Laser Center Lübeck, Peter-Monnik-Weg 4, D-23562 Lübeck, Germany.
FAX: xx49-505-486; e-mail: vogel@mll.mu-luebeck.de

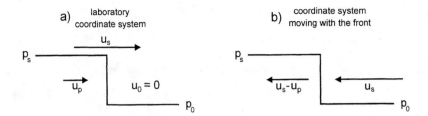

a) laboratory coordinate system

u_s

p_s

u_p $u_0 = 0$

p_0

b) coordinate system moving with the front

p_s

$u_s - u_p$ u_s

p_0

Figure 1: Shock wave and particle velocities in different coordinate systems

It is several hundred m/s at shock pressures of a few hundred MPa (for example 430 m/s at 1000 MPa[1]). The dissipation process is easily understood in a coordinate system moving with the shock front (Fig. 1b). The medium now "flows" into the shock front with velocity u_s and leaves the front with $u_s - u_p$. This obviously goes along with a massive loss of kinetic energy which is converted into heat. On a molecular level it means that ordered translational motion is converted into random motion. This change of molecular velocity is of viscous nature[5]. Heat conduction also plays a role in the dissipation process, but only in the redistribution of dissipated energy[5].

The above picture is completely true only for a pressure step, i. e. for a shock "wave" of infinite duration. In a real shock wave, part of the energy deposited in the liquid behind the shock front will flow back into the shock wave at its trailing edge[1]. The energy flow becomes less important when the ratio (shock wave duration/rise time of the shock wave) increases. Because shock waves generated during optical breakdown in water have a duration of 20 - 60 ns[3] and a rise time of ≈ 20 ps[3,6], this ratio has a value of more than 1000. In the present paper, we therefore neglect that energy flow in a first order approximation.

When the shock wave profile $p(t)$ is known, the shock wave energy can be determined through[1]

$$E_s = \frac{4 \pi r_m^2}{\rho_0 c_0} \int p_s^2 \, dt \qquad (1)$$

where r_m denotes the distance from the emission center at which the pressure p_s is measured. Equation (1) is well suited for a determination of the shock wave energy far away from the source where the pressure profile $p(t)$ can be readily measured using a hydrophone. In the far field, however, a large part of the shock wave energy is already dissipated[1,3], and therefore that measurement does not yield the total acoustic energy generated during optical breakdown. In immediate vicinity of the plasma, $p(t)$ is difficult to measure and has to date only been determined through numerical calculations[3].

In the following we present a different approach to determine the shock wave energy near the source from experimental data. This approach is based on the Rankine-Hugoniot equation which relates the increase of internal energy per unit mass at a shock front to the change of pressure ($p_0 \rightarrow p_s$) and density ($\rho_0 \rightarrow \rho_s$) at the shock front[2]:

$$\Delta \varepsilon(r) = \frac{1}{2} \left(\frac{1}{\rho_0} - \frac{1}{\rho_s(r)} \right) \left(p_s(r) + p_0 \right) \approx \frac{1}{2} \left(\frac{1}{\rho_0} - \frac{1}{\rho_s(r)} \right) p_s(r). \qquad (2)$$

The pressure p_s and density ρ_s behind the shock front can be obtained through a measurement of the shock front velocity u_s. The pressure is given by

$$p_s = c_1 \rho_0 u_s \left(10^{(u_s - c_0)/c_2} - 1\right) + p_0 \; ,$$ (3)

where c_0 denotes the normal sound velocity in water, $c_1 = 5190$ m/s, and $c_2 = 25306$ m/s. Equation (3) is based on the Hugoniot data of Rice and Walsh[7] and on the conservation of momentum at the shock front. The density is through conservation of mass[2]

$$u_s \rho_0 = (u_s - u_p)\rho_s,$$ (4)

and momentum[2]

$$p_s - p_0 = u_s u_p \rho_0,$$ (5)

also linked with u_s:

$$\rho_s = \frac{\rho_0}{1 - \dfrac{p_s}{u_s^2 \rho_0}}.$$ (6)

The total change of internal energy during propagation of a spherical shock front from r_0 to r_1 can be obtained by integration of Eq. (2):

$$E = \int_{r_0}^{r_1} 4 \pi r^2 \rho_s(r) \, \Delta\varepsilon(r) \, dr.$$ (7)

Since the largest part of the shock wave energy is already dissipated near the laser plasma[3], equation (7) can be used for a lower estimate of the shock wave energy, if measurement data for u_s are available up to a distance which is at least 10 - 20 times larger than the plasma radius.

The data obtained with Eq. (2) for the increase of the internal energy per unit mass can be used to calculate the temperature increase behind the shock front.

2. EXPERIMENTS

The experimental arrangement for the investigation of shock wave emission is depicted in Figure 2. It was described in detail elsewhere[3] and is therefore only briefly summarized here. All experiments were performed with Nd:YAG laser pulses of 30 ps or 6 ns duration and at a wavelength of 1064 nm. The laser beam was first expanded and then focused into a cuvette filled with distilled, filtered water using a laser achromat. An ophthalmic contact lens (Rodenstock RYM) was built into the cuvette wall in order to minimize aberrations. The convergence angle in water was 14° for the ps-pulses and 22° for the ns-pulses, and the focus diameters ($1/e^2$ value of intensity) were measured to be 5.8 and 7.6 µm respectively. The energy threshold for plasma formation (50% breakdown probability) was 7 µJ for the ps-pulses and 150 µJ for the ns-pulses.

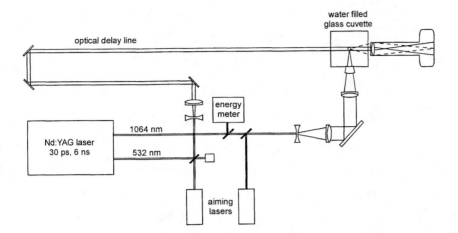

Figure 2: Experimental arrangement for the investigation of shock wave emission.

The shock wave velocity was determined by taking series of photographs with an increasing time interval between the optical breakdown and the exposure of the photograph. For illumination of the photographs we used a frequency doubled part of the Nd:YAG laser pulse that was optically delayed by 2 - 136 ns with respect to the pulse at 1064 nm producing the optical breakdown. We investigated the shock wave emission after 30-ps pulses with 50 µJ and 1 mJ pulse energy, and after 6-ns pulses with 1 and 10 mJ energy.

Pressure amplitudes and shock wave profiles at 10 mm distance from the laser plasma were measured using a PVDF hydrophone (Ceram) with an active area of 1 mm^2, a rise time of 12 ns, and a sensitivity of 280 mV/MPa.

3. RESULTS AND DISCUSSION

3.1 Shock wave energy and its dissipation

The measured data for $u_S(r)$ have been reported earlier in Ref. [3]. They were used to determine the shock peak pressure at the plasma rim (Eq. 3), and to calculate the energy dissipated at the shock front during shock wave propagation. (Eq. 7). Figure 3 shows the accumulated energy loss as a function of propagation distance.

With most laser parameters, the loss rate has decreased considerably at the end of the measurement range. The accumulated energy loss E_{Diss} at maximum propagation distance can therefore be regarded a lower estimate of the energy content of the shock wave (Table 1). Only for the 1 mJ/ 30 ps pulse where the plasma is more cylindrical and the geometrical decay of the shock wave pressure is slower than in the other cases[3], the dissipation rate continues to be relatively high.

The shock wave energy at 10 mm distance from the plasma was determined from the measured hydrophone signals using Eq. (1). The values for the peak pressure and shock wave duration (FWHM) at 10 mm distance and the corresponding values of the shock wave energy $E_{S/10mm}$ are listed in Table 1.

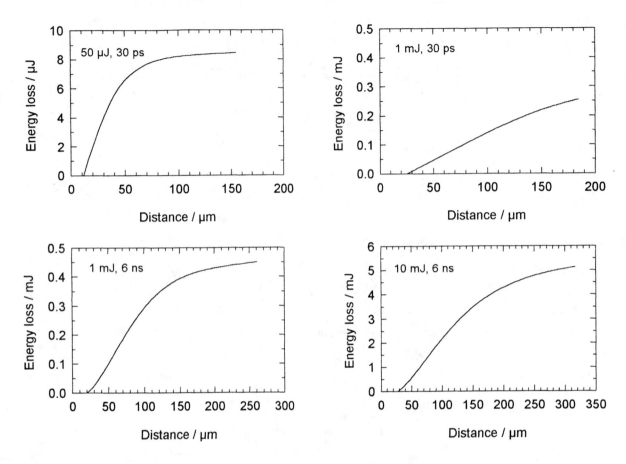

Figure 3: Accumulated energy loss E_{Diss} at the shock front vs propagation distance r for various laser parameters.

The total amount of acoustic energy can be estimated by adding the dissipated energy E_{Diss} in the near field and the energy $E_{S/10mm}$ remaining in the far-field. It is still a lower estimate, because the dissipation in the range 0.3 mm $< r < 10$ mm is not considered. This error is, however, probably compensated by the fact that our calculations of E_{Diss} do not consider that a part of the acoustic energy deposited as internal energy behind the shock front flows back into the shock wave at its trailing edge.

The conversion efficiency of absorbed light energy E_L into shock wave energy ($E_{Diss}+E_{S/10mm}$) ranges from 32 % for 30 ps pulses of 50 μJ pulse energy to 71% for 6-ns pulses of 10 mJ pulse energy (Table 1). The conversion efficiency is higher for ns-pulses than for ps-pulses, because they produce more compact plasmas with a higher energy density and peak pressure[3,8]. It is also higher at pulse energies far above the breakdown threshold, probably also as a result of higher a energy density in the plasma.

For comparison to the earlier results[3], Table 1 contains also values for the shock wave energy E_S which were obtained from calculated pressure profiles by means of Eq. (1). The calculations were performed for a distance r_m from the emission center at which $r_m/R_0 = 6$ (R_0 denotes the plasma radius). At this distance, the shock wave has already acquired an approximately exponential form with a steep shock front, and r_m is large compared to the shock wave width[3]. The

	30 ps		6 ns	
	50 μJ (31 μJ)	1 mJ (0,74 mJ)	1 mJ (0,77 mJ)	10 mJ (8,2 mJ)
Near-field data				
Pressure p_s at plasma rim [MPa]	1300	1700	2400	7150
Dissipated energy E_{Diss} [μJ]	8.4	250	450	5200
Shock wave parameters at r = 10 mm				
Pressure p_s [MPa]	0.24	1.06	0.99	2.62
Duration τ_s [ns]	43	70	77	148
Energy $E_{S/10mm}$ [μJ]	1.5	48	46.2	622
Total shock wave energy				
$E_{Diss} + E_{S/10mm}$ [μJ]	9.9	298	496	5822
Conversion of light energy into shock wave energy $(E_{Diss} + E_{S/10mm})/E_L$ [%]	32.0	40.3	64.4	71.0
Calculated shock wave parameters at $r_m/R_0 = 6$				
Width a_S [μm]	32	93	54	114
a_S/R_0	3.8	3.6	3.0	3.1
Energy E_S [μJ]	4.44	214	309	4190

Table 1: Shock wave parameters close to the plasma and at 10 mm distance from the source. The data given for the laser pulse energy are the energy in front of the cuvette and the absorbed energy (in brackets) which was taken from Ref. [9]. The conversion efficiency $(E_{Diss}+E_{S/10mm})/E_L$ refers to the absorbed energy. The data in the last three lines are quoted from Ref. [3].

agreement between the results of both methods is generally quite good. It is remarkable, however, that the calculations of Ref. [3] yielded always smaller values for the shock wave energy than the integration of dissipated energy performed in this paper. One reason for this discrepancy might be, that part of the shock wave energy is already dissipated until it reaches the location $r_m/R_0 = 6$ where the pressure profile was calculated.

The energy dissipation during the first 10 mm of shock wave propagation amounts to 85% - 89% of the total acoustic energy. The percentage of dissipated energy is larger when the initial pressure is high and the normalized shock wave width a_S/R_0 is small (in this case the energy reservoir behind the shock front is small and more rapidly exhausted). It is obvious from Figure 3 that a major part of the shock wave energy is dissipated already within the first 200-300 μm from the source. This means that the shock wave energy is strongly underestimated if it is determined only through far-field measurements as done in earlier studies[10,11].

3.2 Temperature rise and bubble formation by dissipation of shock wave energy

Passage of a shock front leads to a temperature and entropy rise in the medium because of viscous damping[5]. Justus et al.[12] measured a temperature increase of 33°C after a shock of 840 MPa, Duvall and Fowles[2] quote a temperature rise of 257°C and 690°C for water subjected to a shock pressure of 5500 MPa and 12000 MPa, respectively, and Holmes et al.[13] found temperature jumps of 347 °C at 7500 MPa and 547°C at 11700 MPa.

According to the above data, the critical point of water (374.2°C) is exceeded when the shock pressure is higher than ≈ 7500 MPa. Shock wave propagation after optical breakdown may thus lead to evaporation of surrounding water. The evaporated material becomes part of the cavitation bubble which was originally created by the evaporation of the liquid within the plasma volume (At first the fluid in the plasma volume and the fluid subjected to shock wave heating are supercritical water, but they become vapor as soon as the pressure has dropped below the critical value of 22 MPa). Since the temperature reached during shock-wave-induced evaporation is not as high as the plasma temperature, this process leads to a reduction of the average temperature and pressure within the bubble[14].

Pressure amplitudes higher than 7500 MPa are reached during nanosecond optical breakdown at pulse energies above ≈ 10 mJ (Table 1). Figure 4 shows that in the case of a 20 mJ pulse the bubble dynamics in the initial phase after breakdown shows some characteristic features indicative for shock-wave-induced evaporation. During the laser pulse, the "bubble wall" corresponds to the boundary between plasma (defined by a high concentration of free electrons) and liquid

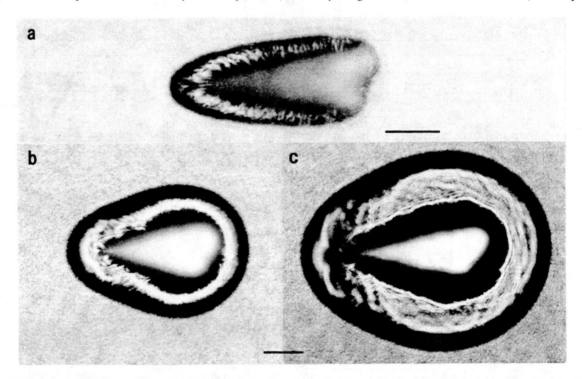

Figure 4: Shock wave and cavitation bubble 12 ns (a), 48 ns (b), and 92 ns (c) after optical breakdown produced with a 20 mJ 6 ns pulse. The laser light was incident from the right. Focusing angle: 22°, length of scales: 100 μm.

under normal conditions. This boundary is very sharp due to the nonlinearities of the breakdown process. It is visible on the photographs due to refractive index changes caused by the free electrons and the heating of the liquid. A little later, when a the free electrons have largely disappeared through recombination processes, the "bubble wall" corresponds to the boundary between supercritical water and surrounding liquid, and when temperature and pressure drop below the critical point, a real phase transition between water vapour and liquid water is formed. At small pulse energies, the bubble wall is smooth[8], because the plasma rim is smooth. At a pulse energy of 20 mJ, however, the boundary between supercritical water and surrounding liquid is modified by the shock-wave-induced heating, and acquires a frayed structure (Fig. 4a). Only after ≈ 90 ns, the bubble wall has become smooth (Figs. 4b and c).

The initial irregularity of the bubble wall is probably a consequence of local variations of the energy density within the plasma leading to irregularities in the pressure distribution. This is illustrated in Figure 5 showing many "elementary" pressure or shock waves emitted from "hot spots" within the plasma. The interference of these elementary waves has produced a smooth shock front, but the pressure distribution *behind* this front is still very irregular even outside the plasma. The situation is probably similar in Figure 4, but with a much smaller distance between the hot spots.

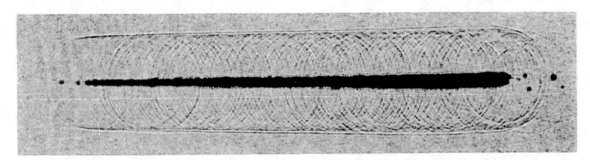

Figure 5: Shock wave emission after a 1 mJ 30 ps pulse focused into the water with a convergence angle of 5°. Inhomogeneities in the laser-produced plasma lead to many "elementary" pressure waves. Their interference results in an irregular pressure distribution behind the main shock front , although that front is smooth. Length of scale: 200 μm.

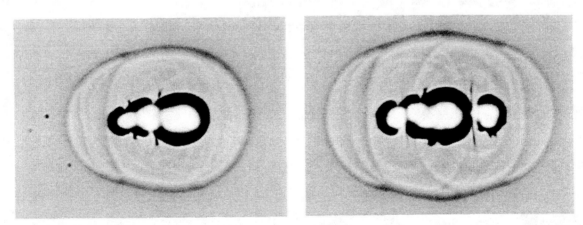

Figure 6: Shock wave emission and cavitation bubble formation after breakdown produced by 5 mJ, 12 ns pulses with irregular intensity distribution in the cross section of the laser beam. Due to the poor beam quality, several individual plasmas were formed, each emitting a shock wave. Dark stationary structures appear at locations where these shock waves interfered. They are most likely bubbles formed because the critical temperature and pressure of water were exceeded.

If the amplitude of individual shock waves is sufficiently high, the critical point is exceeded when they interfere, and the liquid evaporates. This effect is obvious in Figure 6, because it occurs at a certain distance from the main cavitation bubble, and it is most likely also the reason for the frayed shape of the bubble wall in Figure 4a.

It is not yet fully understood through which mechanism the bubble wall smoothens within 90 ns after breakdown. During this time the temperature has probably already dropped below the critical temperature of 374.2°C, but the pressure at the bubble wall remains higher than 22 MPa [3]. This would imply that no clear phase transition has formed yet, and the bubble wall has smoothened without the influence of surface tension. It is possible that heat convection due to the particle velocity in the elementary shock waves behind the main shock front contributes to the smoothening (heat conduction is probably too slow to play a significant role).

Shock wave induced tissue effects

Since most of the acoustic energy dissipation takes place within the first 100-300 μm (depending on pulse energy), the shock-wave-induced tissue effects are mostly obscured by the effects of the cavitation bubble expansion. In the case of a 1 mJ/ 6 ns Nd:YAG laser pulse, for example, the major part of the shock wave energy is dissipated within a radius of ≈ 200 μm (Fig. 3c), but the bubble reaches a radius of 800 μm in water[3]. Acoustic tissue effects are, nevertheless, important, because 1. The bubble is smaller in tissue than in water. 2. The weakening of the tissue structure by the shock wave passage probably contributes to the cavitation-induced damage, and 3. The range for acoustic damage is larger in nonspherical geometries, as found in short-pulsed laser ablation, where the geometrical decay of the pressure amplitude is slower.

It is of interest to compare the present results obtained through an analysis of acoustic dissipation with the thresholds for functional cell damage caused by monopolar stress waves. Doukas and co-workers[15,16] detected cellular damage at peak pressures above 50-100 MPa and pressure gradients steeper than 2 MPa/μm. After optical breakdown with a 1 mJ/ 6 ns pulse, a pressure of 50 MPa is exceeded only within a radius of 250 μm. This zone approximately coincides with the volume in which the acoustic energy dissipation is most pronounced. It should be emphasized, however, that close to the threshold for cellular damage, the temperature rise through acoustic energy dissipation is too small (≈ 3° C) to cause any damage. The damage is rather related to the acceleration at the shock front (∝ pressure gradient and peak pressure), and to the shear and tensile stresses arising at acoustic inhomogeneities.

4. ACKNOWLEDGEMENTS

We thank Dr. Apostulos Doukas for fruitful discussions. The work was supported by the German Science Foundation, grant Bi-312/2-4.

5. REFERENCES

1. R. H. Cole, *"Underwater Explosions"*, Princeton University Press, Princeton, NJ, 1948.
2. G. E. Duvall and G. R. Fowles, "Shock waves", in R. S. Bradley (Ed) *"High Pressure Physics and Chemistry"*, pp. 209-291, New York, Academic Press, 1963.
3. A. Vogel, S. Busch, U. Parlitz, "Shock wave emission and cavitation bubble generation by picosecond and nanosecond optical breakdown in water", *J. Acoust. Soc. Am.* **100**, pp. 148-165, 1996.
4. A. Doukas, A. D. Zweig, J. K. Frisoli, R. Birngruber, T. Deutsch, "Non-invasive determination of shock wave pressure generated by optical breakdown", *Appl. Phys. B* **53 pp.** 237-245, 1991.
5. Y. B. Zel'dovich and Y. P. Raizer, *"Physics of Shock Wavew and High Temperature Hydrodynamic Phenomena"*, Academic Press, New York and London, 1966.
6. P. Harris and H. N. Presles, "Reflectivity of a 5.8 kbar shock front in water", *J. Chem. Phys.* **77**, pp. 5157-5164, 1982.
7. M. H. Rice and J. M. Walsh, "Equation of state of water to 250 kilobars", *J. Chem. Phys.* **26**, pp. 824-830, 1957.
8. A. Vogel, K. Nahen, D. Theisen, J. Noack, "Plasma formation in water by picosecond and nanosecond Nd:YAG laser pulses- part I: optical breakdown at threshold and superthreshold irradiance", *IEEE J. Selected Topics Quantum Electron.* **2**(4), pp. 847-860.
9. K. Nahen and A. Vogel, "Plasma formation in water by picosecond and nanosecond Nd:YAG laser pulses - Part II: Plasma transmission, scattering and reflection", *IEEE J. Selected Topics Quantum Electron.* **2**(4), pp. 861-871, 1997.
10. V. S. Teslenko, "Investigation of photoacoustic and photohydrodynamic parameters of laser breakdown in liquids", *Sov. J. Quant. Electron.* **7**, pp. 981-984, 1977.
11. A. Vogel and W. Lauterborn, "Acoustic transient generation by laser-produced cavitation bubbles near solid boundaries", *J. Acoust. Soc. Am.* **84**, pp. 719-731, 1988.
12. B. L. Justus, A. L. Huston, A. J. Campillo, "Fluorescence thermometry of shocked water", *Appl. Phys. Lett.* **47**, pp. 1159-1161, 1985.
13. N. C. Holmes, W. J. Nellis, W. B. Graham, G. E. Walrafen, "Raman spectroscopy of shocked water", in: Y. M. Gupta (Ed) *"Shock Waves in Condensed Matter"*, pp. 191-200 (Plenum Press, New York and London, 1986.
14. R. M. Roberts, J. A. Cook, R. L. Rogers, A. M. Gleeson, T. A. Griffy, "The energy partition of underwater sparks", *J. Acoust. Soc. Am.* **99**, pp. 3465-3475, 1996.
15. A. Doukas, D. J. Mc Aucliff, T. J. Flotte, "Biological effects of laser-induced shock waves: Structural and functional cell damage in vitro", *Ultrasound Med. Biol.* **19**, pp. 137-146, 1993.
16. A. Doukas, D. J. McAucliffe, S. Lee, V. Venugopalan, T. J. Flotte, "Physical factors involved in stress-wave-induced cell injury: the effect of the stress gradient", *Ultrasound Med Biol* **21**, pp. 961-967, 1995

SESSION 7

Ablation I

Pulsed Holmium:YAG-Induced Thermal Damage in Albumen

T. Joshua Pfefer[1*], Kin Foong Chan[2], Daniel X. Hammer[2] and A. J. Welch[1]

[1] Biomedical Engineering Program
[2] Department of Electrical and Computer Engineering
The University of Texas at Austin, Austin, TX 78712

ABSTRACT

The development of thermal damage during pulsed Holmium:YAG ($\lambda = 2.12$ μm, $\tau_p = 250$ μs) irradiation of albumen was analyzed experimentally and numerically with the intent of validating the Arrhenius integral and investigating the influence of beam profile and dynamic changes in absorption. Fast flash videography was performed to document the transient development of coagulation during and after the laser pulse. A two-dimensional dynamic optical-thermal model was developed.

The optical component involved a discretized Beer's law method in which absorption is a function of temperature. The thermal component was comprised of 1) a cylindrical coordinate (r,z) finite difference formulation of the heat conduction equation in which the output from the optical model was used as the source term and 2) a routine for calculating thermal damage using the Arrhenius relation. At the end of each time step, the temperature distribution was used to recalculate the absorption coefficient array, which in turn is used in the optical component.

The model showed good agreement with experimental data and the literature. The Arrhenius integral was shown to be valid for the sub-vaporization pulsed laser regime. Experimental and numerical results indicated that spatial beam profile has a significant impact on thermal damage. Simulations predicted that at higher radiant exposures dynamic changes in absorption become more significant, accounting for a 10% increase in coagulation depth.

Keywords: thermal damage, albumen, pulsed holmium laser, laser-tissue interaction, high speed imaging, heat transfer, dynamic optical properties, numerical modeling, finite difference, Arrhenius integral

1. INTRODUCTION

The generation of highly localized regions of thermal damage is essential to pulsed laser surgery techniques such as Port Wine Stain treatment[1], corneal photocoagulation[2], and tissue welding[3]. Although good experimental results have been achieved, a true understanding of the mechanisms that influence the thermal damage process has not been reached. Using numerical models in conjunction with experiments employing tissue phantoms, knowledge can be gained which will be useful in optimization of laser parameters.

The process by which heat destroys biological tissue has long been accurately predicted using the Arrhenius integral - a chemical rate process relation that describes the concentration of altered tissue as a linear function of time and an exponential function of temperature[4,5]. Although this relation has had extensive successful use in regards to continuous wave laser irradiation procedures, its relevance to the pulsed laser regime has not been thoroughly investigated.

In a study of continuous wave laser irradiation, Halldorsson et al.[6] initiated the use of fast flash photography to investigate the development of thermal damage in albumen (egg white). Recently, Asshauer et al.[7] documented the thermal damage distribution in albumen 40 ms after irradiation with 0.13 and 1.0 ms-long Ho:YAG laser pulses

---
[*] Author contact information:
TJP: (pfefer@piglet.cc.utexas.edu), AJW: (welch@mail.utexas.edu)
Biomedical Engineering Program; University of Texas at Austin, ENS 610; Austin, TX USA 78712

using a similar technique. The depth of coagulation was found to be a nearly linear function of irradiance for both pulse durations. Time-resolved imaging using similar laser parameters[8] demonstrated that the onset of coagulation can occur after the end of the laser pulse, indicating a rate process damage mechanisms.

Possibly the most promising technique for noninvasive assessment of thermal damage in scattering tissue involves monitoring changes in tissue birefringence. Sankaran et al.[9] used real-time measurement of changes in birefringence to measure development of thermal damage during Ho:YAG irradiation of rat tail tendon (collagen) and found that thermal damage began within 200 µs of the beginning of the 250 µs pulse and that the Arrhenius relation agreed well with experimental results for energy levels below the vaporization threshold. Additionally, a technique for two-dimensional imaging of birefringence using optical coherence tomography has recently been developed[10].

Research into numerical modeling of pulsed laser tissue interaction has been limited. Brinkmann et al.[11,12] simulated Erbium and Holmium pulsed laser irradiation of corneal tissue using an optical-thermal numerical model that did not incorporate the Arrhenius relation, but assumed a coagulation threshold temperature of 100 °C. This model used a novel technique in which ray tracing was performed to account for spatial beam profile changes. Other pulsed laser models have been used to investigate temperature dependent changes in optical properties. These have been one dimensional models that did not account for thermal diffusion or tissue damage. [13,14].

In this study, the time dependence of the development of thermal damage in albumen was documented. This data and corresponding simulated data was used to evaluate:
- the validity of the Arrhenius relation for pulsed lasers (sub-vaporization threshold)
- the ability of numerical modeling to predict the transient development of coagulation
- the effect of spatial beam profile on thermal damage
- the significance of dynamic, temperature-dependent changes in absorption

2. METHODS

2.1 Experimental methods
Investigation of the development of thermal damage was performed using a Holmium:YAG laser (Schwartz SEO 1-2-3; λ = 2.12 µm) in the free-running mode with a pulse duration (τ_p) of 250 µs (full width half maximum). The light was coupled into a low OH optical fiber with a core diameter of 0.5 mm diameter (core + cladding = 0.55 mm) and delivered below the surface of the tissue sample. Fresh chicken albumen was obtained from a local source.

The fast flash videography experimental setup developed for this study (Figure 1) used a PC with LabVIEW to program and trigger a pulse generator (Stanford Research Systems DG-535). The pulse generator, in turn, controlled the Ho:YAG laser and a nitrogen dye laser (Laser Photonics LN 102; λ = 540 nm; τ_p = 600 ps) which was used as the flash source. A CCD camera was used to record a single image at a specified point in time during or after a single Ho:YAG pulse. The nitrogen laser light was delivered with a fiber in an orientation such that reflective illumination of the highly scattering coagulated region was produced. The relative timing of the laser pulses was verified using photodiodes connected to an oscilloscope.

By changing the delay between the two lasers, individual images were taken at various times during and after single laser pulses. Numerous images were taken at each time delay for the same laser energy so as to establish a "typical" laser event and thus accurately document the development of thermal damage.

2.2 Numerical methods
A dynamic optical-thermal numerical model was developed to simulate the mechanisms leading to thermal damage. Assuming that the beam profile of the Ho:YAG laser is Gaussian or flat top and the albumen is homogeneous, the resulting temperature and damage distributions will be axially symmetric about the center of the laser beam. Thus, the optical and thermal routines were formulated using a two dimensional (r,z) cylindrical coordinate grid system (Figure 2).

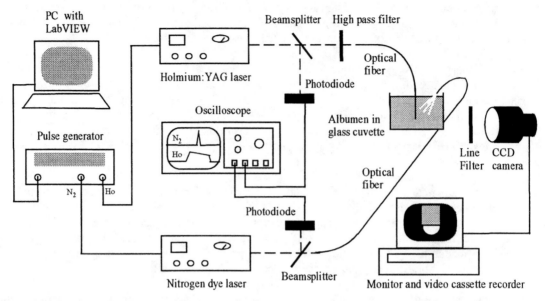

Figure 1: Fast flash videography setup for imaging the transient development of coagulation in albumen.

A simplified flow chart of the algorithm used in the model is seen in Figure 3. Beginning with a set of pre-determined parameters and material constants, the optical component calculates the fluence rate (ϕ ; W/cm^2) distribution in the tissue. This is performed using a discretized form of Beer's law:

$$\phi(r, z + \Delta z, t) = \phi(r, z, t)e^{-\mu_a(r, z+\Delta z/2, t)\Delta z} \tag{1}$$

where μ_a (1/mm) is the absorption coefficient. The volumetric energy absorption is computed by dividing the change in fluence rate over the depth of an element by the axial thickness (Δz) of the element. This approach provides the ability to calculate the rate of energy absorption in each grid element based on the local absorption coefficient[13,14]. The optical model is used to compute the source term, S(r,z,t), for the thermal component.

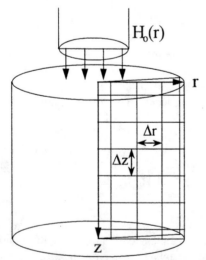

Figure 2: Schematic of thin wedge-shaped region represented by the two-dimensional cylindrical coordinate grid system used. A 2 mm x 2mm grid region was simulated ($\Delta r = \Delta z = 0.02$ mm).

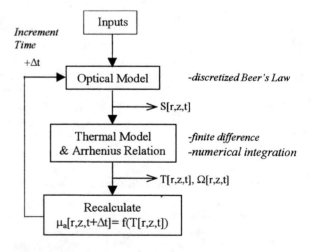

Figure 3: Overview of dynamic μ_a optical-thermal numerical model.

Temperature rise is calculated based on the two dimensional axisymmetric form of the Fourier heat conduction equation:

$$\frac{\partial^2 T}{\partial r^2} + \frac{1}{r}\frac{\partial T}{\partial r} + \frac{\partial^2 T}{\partial z^2} + \frac{S}{k} = \frac{1}{\alpha}\frac{\partial T}{\partial t} \qquad (2)$$

where T is temperature ($^\circ$C), t is time (s) , k is thermal conductivity (W/m/$^\circ$C), and α (= k/ρc) is thermal diffusivity (m^2/s)[15]. This equation is solved numerically using an explicit (forward difference) finite difference scheme which incorporates adiabatic boundary conditions on all sides.

The second part of the thermal component involves the calculation of accumulation of thermal damage over the previous time step. The Arrhenius relation is integrated numerically to quantify the extent of denaturation[4, 16]:

$$\Omega(t) = A\int_0^t \exp\left[\frac{-E_a}{RT(\tau)}\right]d\tau \qquad (3)$$

where A is the frequency factor (1/s), E_a is the activation energy (J/mole), and R is the universal gas constant (8.321 J/mole/$^\circ$K). Note that for the Arrhenius relation, the units of T are $^\circ$K.

After the thermal component has computed the new temperature and damage distributions, the new distribution of absorption coefficients are calculated. This routine involves evaluating the corresponding local absorption coefficient using a relation calculated by Jansen et al.[13]:

$$\mu_a(T) = \mu_{a,o} + \beta*(T-T_o) \qquad (4)$$

where β = -0.00661 (1/mm/$^\circ$C), $\mu_{a,o}$ = 2.982 1/mm, and T_o is 23 $^\circ$C.

It is often assumed that the main chromophore in egg white at λ = 2.12 μm is water. This is evidenced by the fact that albumen - which is 86% water[17] - has an absorption coefficient (2.55 1/mm)[7] which is 85% that of water (3.0 1/mm) [13]. The index of refraction is 1.4. Albumen thermal properties are listed in Table 1.

Table 1: Thermal properties of albumen[17, 18]

k	0.56 W/m/$^\circ$C
ρ	997 kg/m^3
c_p	4180 J/kg/$^\circ$C
E_a	3.8 x 10^{57} J/mole
A	3.85 x 10^5 1/s

In the first set of simulations, laser parameters corresponding to those specified in the study by Asshauer et al. were implemented so as to perform a comparison with the literature: τ_p = 1.0 ms, beam diameter of 0.6 mm, flat top beam profile, and dynamic optical properties. The radiant exposure level was varied. The second set of simulations involved simulation of the laser parameters used in the experimental portion of this study: τ_p = 250 μs, beam diameter of 0.5 mm. Simulations were performed for (a) a flat top spatial beam profile and dynamic μ_a , (b) a Gaussian profile and dynamic μ_a and (c) a flat top profile and constant μ_a.

3. RESULTS

3.1 Verification of model

Simulations were performed using parameters similar to those employed in two previous studies, so as to provide verification against data from the literature. A comparison of final coagulation depth measured by Asshauer et al.[7] and our modeled data for a 0.6 mm diameter beam, pulse duration of 1.0 ms and radiant exposures between 10 and 45 J/cm² is shown in Figure 4. For the model, a uniform beam profile was assumed and the standard definition of coagulation as $\Omega > 1.0$ was used. Although there is a discrepancy in the threshold radiant exposure and depth of coagulation at lower radiant exposures, the predicted coagulation depths are in general agreement with the experimental data.

A comparison of data regarding the transient increase in depth of coagulation for radiant exposures (H) of 15.5 and 41.7 J/cm² are shown in Figure 5. The data sets show good agreement for time lesion onset as well as depth of coagulation growth during and within a few milliseconds after the pulse. Significant disagreement begins to occur well after the laser pulse, leading to a final discrepancy in coagulation depth of about 50 µm for both cases. The onset of coagulation for the 41.7 J/cm² case occurs after about 0.5 ms whereas for the 15.5 J/cm² case, onset occurs at the end of the 1.0 ms laser pulse. The simulated increase in coagulation depth after the laser pulse was approximately 150 µm for both cases.

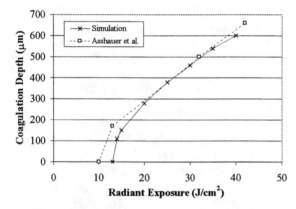

Figure 4: Final depth of coagulation at the center of the laser beam as a function of radiant exposure. Data from optical-thermal simulations (solid line, X) are presented alongside experimental data) from Asshauer et al.[7] (dashed line, □) Laser parameters: beam diameter = 0.6 mm, τ_p = 1.0 ms.

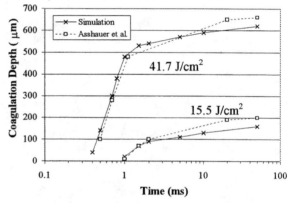

Figure 5: Transient increase in coagulation depth at the center of the laser beam. Data predicted by the optical-thermal model (solid line, X) are graphed with experimental data from Asshauer et al.[8] (dashed line, □) Laser parameters: beam diameter = 0.6 mm, τ_p = 1.0 ms, and H = 15.5, 41.7 J/cm².

3.2 Fast flash videography

A set of images documenting the transient development of the region of highly scattering denatured albumen for a radiant exposure of 18.3 ± 1.0 J/cm^2 is presented in Figure 6. The maximum depth of coagulation is graphed as a function of time with corresponding simulated data in Figure 7. Note that the last experimental data point in Figure 7 (50 ms) actually corresponds to a time delay of several seconds. Onset of coagulation occurred 200 µs after the beginning of the laser pulse. Coagulation depth increased at a decreasing rate, with the vast majority of the lesion formed well after the pulse was over. Irregularities in the distribution of damage are apparent, particularly during the first few milliseconds of lesion growth. These irregularities tended to become smoothed or blurred as the lesion growth slows and stops. The final image shown in Figure 6, taken several seconds after the laser pulse, shows a more rounded damage profile.

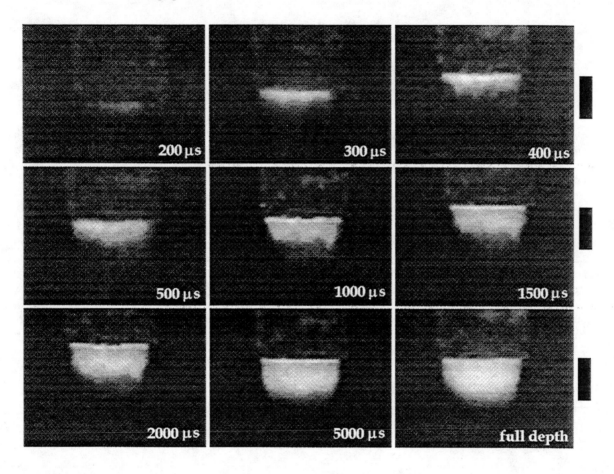

Figure 6: Fast flash videography images documenting coagulation development in albumen. Laser parameters: beam diameter = 0.5 mm, τ_p = 250 µs, H= 18.3 J/cm^2. Vertical length of black bar corresponds to 0.25 mm.

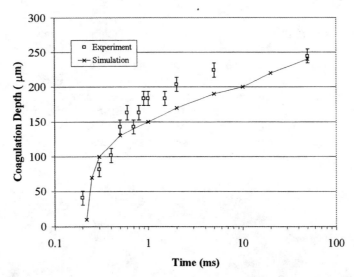

Figure 7: Transient increase in coagulation depth at the center of the laser beam. Experimentally determined (□) and simulation results (X) are presented. Final experimental data point (shown as 50 ms) was taken at full lesion depth, several seconds after laser pulse. Laser parameters: beam diameter = 0.5 mm, τ_p = 250 μs, H = 18.3 J/cm^2.

3.3 Optical-thermal simulations

The second set of simulations involved implementation of the laser parameters used in the fast flash videography experiment. Figure 7 shows the predicted transient changes in maximum coagulation depth which always corresponded to the center of the beam. The simulated data is in good agreement for the first millisecond after the onset of the pulse, less so for 1-10 milliseconds. The predicted final coagulation depth agrees well with the experimental data. The predicted extent of the thermal damage lesion is shown in two dimensions at several time delays in Figure 8. This graph provides another view of the rate of increase in coagulation, particularly the smoothing effect seen in the change in coagulation profile from 5 to 50 ms. Simulated temperature distributions vs. depth below the center of the laser beam are shown in Figure 9 for several points in time. Temperature is an exponential function of depth during the laser pulse, whereas tens of milliseconds after the laser pulse there is a decrease in temperature near the surface and a small increase for deeper regions. By 50 ms, the temperature has fallen significantly in and around the coagulated region. For example, at a depth of 0.24 mm, the temperature is 80.5 °C at 0.25 ms, 81.0 °C at 20 ms and 75.6 °C at 50 ms.

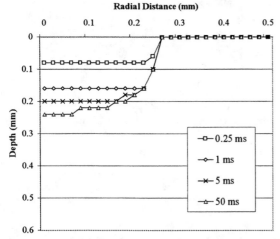

Figure 8: Predicted transient development of coagulation (Ω>1). Laser parameters: beam diameter = 0.5 mm, τ_p = 250 μs, H = 18.3 J/cm^2.

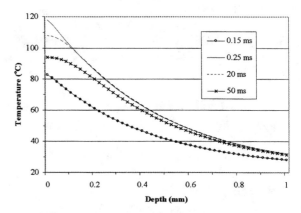

Figure 9: Axial temperature distribution for region directly below the beam center at 0.15, 0.25, 20 and 50 ms after onset of laser pulse. Laser parameters: beam diameter = 0.5 mm, τ_p=250 μs, H = 18.3 J/cm^2.

The effect of a change in beam profile from flat top beam to Gaussian ($1/e^2$ radius, $\omega_o = 0.25$ mm; $H_{max} = 36.6$ J/cm^2) was investigated using the numerical model. Total beam energy remained the same. The predicted extent of the coagulated is shown for several points in time in Figure 10. The final coagulation depth at the center of the beam was 500 μm, about twice that of the uniform beam. The final width of the lesion was about 0.2 mm at the fiber, tapering gradually to the lesion tip. Although the lesion size increased greatly, its shape changed little during the simulation.

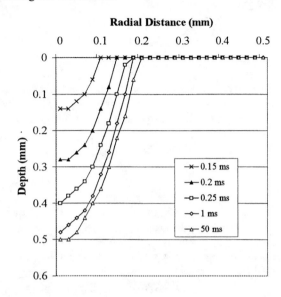

Figure 10: Predicted transient development of coagulation ($\Omega > 1$) for irradiation with a Gaussian beam profile ($\omega_o = 0.25$ mm; $H_{max} = 36.6$ J/cm^2). Total energy and other laser parameters were the same as that used for the data in Figure 8.

Simulations were performed using dynamic and constant μ_a models for radiant exposures of 18.3 and 36.6 J/cm^2. The temperature distributions at the end of the laser pulse (Figure 11a) show higher values for the dynamic μ_a simulation at the surface, and lower values for depths greater than about 0.3 mm. The disparities between the two models are more significant for the 36.6 J/cm^2 case. Similar trends are seen in extent of thermal damage (Figure 11b). For the 18.3 J/cm^2 case, the two models predict similar coagulation (log $\Omega > 0$) depths, whereas for the 36.6 J/cm^2 case, the dynamic μ_a model predicts a coagulation depth 0.04 mm larger than the constant μ_a model.

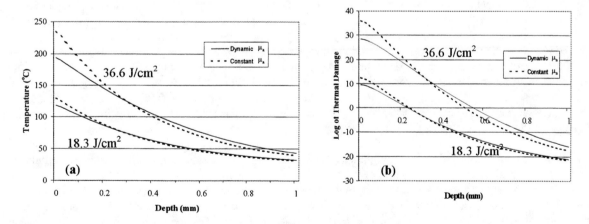

Figure 11: Comparison of data from dynamic μ_a (dashed line) and constant μ_a (solid line) models vs. depth at the beam center for radiant exposures of 18.3 and 36.6 J/cm^2. Graphs show (a) temperature distribution at the end of the laser pulse and (b) final thermal damage distribution. Laser parameters: beam diameter = 0.5 mm, τ_p = 250 μs.

4. DISCUSSION

The good agreement between modeled and experimental results indicates that the basic optical and thermal mechanisms involved in sub-vaporization, Ho:YAG laser-albumen interaction are, for the most part, well understood.

The primary optical mechanism is Beer's Law energy absorption, since light scattering in native albumen is negligible. As temperature rise occurs, the absorption coefficient of albumen decreases, thus allowing light to penetrate deeper into the tissue. However, the effect of dynamic changes in μ_a do not appear to significantly affect coagulation depth until higher radiant exposures approach the vaporization threshold ($\sim$45 J/cm^2). Another dynamic optical property mechanism - the increase in scattering caused by thermal damage - was also observed and predicted. The Beers law-based optical model does not accurately estimate the light propagation/absorption process in highly scattering tissue, however, onset of coagulation before the end of the laser pulse did not appear to affect the model's ability to predict coagulation depth. Further investigation of the effect of scattering at 2.12 μm is necessary, particularly for processes in which denaturation occurs towards the beginning of the laser pulse.

After energy absorption is complete, thermal mechanisms slowly take over. Initially, thermal confinement is observed in the model's prediction of temperature distributions which decrease exponentially with depth (following Beer's Law). Tens of milliseconds after the laser pulse ends, heat diffusion becomes significant. The thermal gradient established through energy absorption drives the conduction process, reducing the temperature near the surface, and slightly raising deeper temperatures. The increase in temperature is not large enough to significantly affect thermal damage. The heat diffusion that has occurred by 50 ms after the laser pulse is enough to lower temperatures by several degrees. In the case of a flat top or irregular beam profile, thermal diffusion smoothes sharp temperature gradients. This diffusion effect is in turn seen in the smoothing of the coagulation profile. After approximately 50 ms, temperature decrease has affected the entire region around the lesion to a point where further growth does not occur. It should be noted that for this process, two dimensional time constant analysis was only moderately useful in estimating the time (63 to 108 ms) over which minimal thermal diffusion occurred[19].

Temperature rise also leads to the denaturation of proteins in albumen, following the Arrhenius rate process relationship. Although the good agreement between modeled and experimental data strongly suggests that the Arrhenius relation holds for the pulsed laser regime, true verification requires experimental data regarding the temperature history in the albumen. The coagulation that occurred during and soon after the pulse was a result of high temperature denaturation. Given the specified thermal damage coefficients, coagulation requires exposures such as 0.04 ms at 105 °C or 1.1 ms at 95 °C. The deepest coagulation occurred at lower temperatures - around 85 °C - which requires an exposure of 35.5 ms. The fact that a large portion of the damage occurred while temperatures were relatively constant indicates that the thermal damage process involves time as well as temperature. The most significant disagreement between modeled and experimental data tended to occur during the millisecond time domain. The model consistently underestimated the depth of coagulation by up to 50 μm. The fact that this disparity occurred for the case of 15.5 J/cm^2 in Figure 5 indicates that this was not due to changes in scattering coefficient during the laser pulse. Agreement during the initial lesion growth phase indicates that inaccurate specification of the beam profile is not a problem, either. Further research is required to investigate this discrepancy.

The laser beam profile at the fiber tip should be a flat top, changing to a Gaussian profile. However, simulations employing the assumption of a flat top beam were much more accurate in predicting coagulation. The long, tapered profile predicted in the Gaussian beam simulation was not noted during the present experiments. The comparison of uniform and Gaussian beam profiles indicates that there is a strong correlation between the beam profile and the distribution of coagulation. Thus, the influence of irregularities in beam profile should be significant. Experimental data suggests that the coagulation profile in the sub-millisecond time domain corresponds to the beam profile. However, after tens of milliseconds, heat diffusion causes micron-scale nonuniformities in the thermal damage lesion to expand and blend together, forming a smoother, more continuous profile.

5. CONCLUSIONS

This study has combined experimental and numerical techniques to analyze the transient development of thermal damage in albumen during pulsed Ho:YAG laser irradiation. Fast flash photography was used to document the development of coagulation in albumen and thus demonstrate the effect of heat conduction and the rate process characteristics of thermal damage. Experimental data from this study and from the literature has been used to demonstrate that the optical-thermal dynamic optical property numerical model presented here is accurate. The agreement between predicted and observed coagulation regions provides strong evidence that the Arrhenius relation is valid for the pulsed laser regime. Simulations and experiments show delayed onset of coagulation and two phases of thermal damage: an initial high rate of increase in depth of coagulation within milliseconds of the beginning of the laser pulse and a slower increase in lesion size primarily due to lower temperature (85 °C) coagulation. The model predicts that dynamic changes in absorption become more significant as radiant exposure increases, leading to decreased surface temperature, increased laser penetration depth, and an increase in coagulation depth. The spatial beam profile is shown to play a significant role in the shape and depth of coagulation. A flat top profile leads to a flatter, rounded lesion, whereas a Gaussian profile leads to a longer, tapered lesion. Irregularities in the beam profile are seen during formation of the lesion, but tend to be minimized by conductive effects after tens of milliseconds.

6. ACKNOWLEDGEMENTS

Funding for this research was provided in part by grants from the Office of Naval Research Free Electron Laser Biomedical Science Program (N00014-91-J-1564) and Department of Energy Center of Excellence for Medical Laser Applications (DE-FG03-95ER 61971) and the Albert W. and Clemmie A. Caster Foundation. The authors wish to thank Jennifer and Andrew Barton and their hens Lady Godiva (Leghorn) and Ginger (Buff Orpington), for contributions of albumen.

7. REFERENCES

1. van Gemert, M.J.C., A.J. Welch, J.W. Pickering, and O.T. Tan., "Laser Treatment of Port Wine Stains", in *Optical-Thermal Response of Laser-Irradiated Tissue*, A.J. Welch and M.J.C. van Gemert, eds., Plenum Press, New York, 1995.
2. Smithpeter, C., E. Chan, S. Thomsen, H.G. Rylander III, A.J. Welch, "Corneal photocoagulation with continuous wave and pulsed holmium:YAG radiation", *J Cataract Refract Surg*, **21**, p.258-267, 1995.
3. Oz, M.C., L.S. Bass, H.W. Popp, R.S. Chuck, J.P. Johnson, S.L. Trokel, and M.R. Treat, "In Vitro Comparison of Thulium-Holmium-Chromium:YAG and Argon Ion Lasers for Welding of Biliary Tissue", *Las Surg Med*, **9**, p. 248-253, 1989.
4. Moritz, A.R., and F C Henriques, "Studies in thermal injury II. The relative importance of time and surface temperature in the causation of cutaneous burns", *Am J Pathol*, **23**, p. 695-720, 1947.
5. Pearce, J. and S. Thomsen, "Rate Process Analysis of Thermal Damage", in *Optical-Thermal Response of Laser-Irradiated Tissue*, A.J. Welch and M.J.C. van Gemert, eds., Plenum Press, New York, 1995.
6. Halldorsson, T., J. Langerholc, L. Senatori and H. Funk, "Thermal action of laser irradiation in biological material monitored by egg-white coagulation", *Appl Opt*, **20**(5), p. 822-825, 1981.
7. Asshauer, T., G.P. Delacretaz, S. Rastegar, "Photothermal denaturation of egg white by pulsed holmium laser", *Proc. SPIE*, **2681**, p.120-124, 1996.
8. Asshauer, T., G. Delacretaz, S. Rastegar, "Observation of delayed coagulation during egg white denaturation by pulsed holmium laser", *Proc. CLEO*, paper no. CtuN2, 167-168, 1996.
9. Sankaran, V., and JT Walsh, "An Optical, Real-time Measurement of Collagen Denaturation", *Proc. SPIE*, **2975**, p.34-42, 1997.
10. deBoer, J.F., T.E. Milner, M.J.C. van Gemert, and J. S. Nelson, "Two-dimensional birefringence imaging in biological tissue by polarization-sensitive optical coherence tomography", *Optics Letters*, **22**(12), p. 934-936, 1997.
11. Brinkmann, R., N. Koop, G. Droge, U. Grotehusmann, A. Huber, R. Birngruber, "Investigations on Laser Thermokaratoplasty", *Proc. SPIE*, **2079**, p.120-130,1994.

12. Brinkmann, R., J. Kampmeier,U. Grotehusmann, A. Vogel, N. Koop, M. Asiyo-Vogel, R. Birngruber, "Corneal collagen denaturation in laser thermokeratoplasty", *Proc. SPIE*, **2681**, p.56-63, 1996.

13. Jansen, E., T G van Leeuwen, M Motamedi, C Borst, and A J Welch, "The effect of temperature on the absorption coefficient of water for holmium:YAG laser light", *Proc. SPIE*, **2077**, p.195-201, 1994.

14. Walsh, J., and J P Cummings, "Effect of the dynamic optical properties of water on mid-infrared laser ablation", *Lasers Surg Med*, **15**, p.295-305, 1993.

15. Gebhart, B., "Heat Conduction and Mass Diffusion," McGraw-Hill, 1993.

16. Henriques, F.C.and A.R. Moritz, "Studies in thermal injury I. The conduction of heat to and through skin and the temperature attained therein. A theoretical and experimental investigation", *Am J Pathol*, **23**, p. 531-549, 1947.

17. Yang, Y., A. J. Welch, and H.G. Rylander, "Rate Process Parameters of Albumen", *Las Surg Med*, **11**, p.188-190, 1991.

18. Orr, C.S., and R.C. Eberhart, "Overview of Bioheat Transfer", in *Optical-Thermal Response of Laser-Irradiated Tissue*, A.J. Welch and M.J.C. van Gemert, eds., Plenum Press, New York, 1995.

19. van Gemert, M.J.C. and A.J. Welch, "Approximate Solutions for Heat Conduction", in *Optical-Thermal Response of Laser-Irradiated Tissue*, A.J. Welch and M.J.C. van Gemert, eds., Plenum Press, New York, 1995.

Ultrashort pulse laser ablation of biological tissue

B.-M. Kim, M. D. Feit, A. M. Rubenchik, D. M. Gold, B. C. Stuart, L. B. Da Silva

Lawrence Livermore National Laboratory
Livermore, CA 94550

ABSTRACT

Temperature and shock wave propagation in water (as a model of tissue) irradiated by sub-picosecond and nanosecond pulses were modeled. The high temperature and pressure generated during sub-picosecond irradiation did not penetrate deeply into the water due to quickly ejected plasma while significant pressure and temperature increases were observed in deep regions with nanosecond pulses. Knowing that the sub-picosecond pulses are effective for tissue ablation, additional studies were done to examine the effect of short pulse widths (< 20 ps). Ablation threshold, temperature rise and ablation crater quality on human dentine were investigated for different pulse widths in the range of 150 fs - 20 ps. The ablation threshold fluence was approximately 4 times higher with 20 ps pulses than with 150 fs pulses but the quality of the ablation craters were not significantly different in this pulse width range .

Keywords: ultrashort pulse lasers, tissue ablation, laser-tissue interaction modeling, pulse width effect

1. INTRODUCTION

Biological tissue ablation using ultrashort pulse laser (USPL, < 1 ps) has drawn much attention due to its high ablation efficiency and minimal collateral damage[1,2]. Also, many possible clinical applications were proposed including ophthalmology[3,4], dentistry[5,6], neurosurgery[7], etc. This paper reports both theoretical and experimental results. The advantages of using sub-ps pulses in tissue ablation are demonstrated by computer modeling. Experiments were performed to test if these advantages hold for pulses as long as tens of picoseconds.

USPL ablation in dielectrics does not depend on linear absorption of the incoming light by specific chromophores but on optical breakdown by multiphoton ionization and following electron avalanche[8-10]. The optical breakdown generates plasma during the laser pulse that reflects and absorbs the incoming light energy, which prevents deeper light penetration. The plasma does not have any strong bond with the material anymore and it is quickly ejected. Absorbed laser energy increases the ejection velocity of the plasma rather than increasing the temperature of the surrounding material. This plasma-mediated ablation process for USPL and ablation for nanosecond pulse are investigated by numerical simulation and the effects are compared.

The drawbacks of USPL system for clinical use are its high cost, relatively large size, and the inability to use optical fiber delivery due to optical damage and pulse dispersion. A solution to some of these problems may be to use a slightly longer pulses than 1 ps because it is easier and cheaper to build ps lasers than sub-ps lasers. Also, it might be possible to use optical fibers in that slightly longer pulse width region. Therefore, the purpose of this study is to analyze the ablation quality for the pulse width range of 150 fs - 20 ps by measuring ablation threshold, temperature rise and micro-morphologic changes in the ablation craters.

B.-M. K. (correspondence) : E-mail : kim12@llnl.gov; Telephone : 510-423-3262; FAX : 510-424-2778

2. SIMULATION RESULTS

Fig. 1 shows the temperature and pressure buildup during and shortly after the USPL. In this simulation water was illuminated by 1 μm pulse of duration 500 fs and the energy density was 1.5 J/cm². The immediate temperature rise following USPL irradiation reaches 20 eV (1 eV = 11600 °K) and the pressure increases up to near 1 Mbar. However, later this high temperature rise does not affect deeper regions because energy is rapidly carried away by the ejected material and there is little shock heating as shown in Fig. 2(a). On the other hand, the temperature rise caused by longer pulse (Fig. 2(b)) is significant in deep regions and the high temperature remains much longer indicating that much greater thermal damage will be induced in the surrounding material. The energy density for 5 ns pulses (25 J/cm²) were chosen because it removes similar amount of material as in USPL ablation (500 fs, 1.5 J/cm²). Similarly, the shock wave caused by USPL decays quickly and plasma is ejected in an extremely short time. The pressure at the shock wave front decreases to less than several kbars at depth of 10 μm as shown in Fig. 3(a). Fig. 3(b) shows how shock wave propagation using ns pulses creates high pressures in deeper regions which causes serious mechanical damage to the material. Detailed description of the simulation schemes can be found in reference 8 and 9.

3. PULSE WIDTH STUDIES

Our ultrashort pulse laser ablation system is equipped with two pumping lasers, an oscillator, and a regenerative amplifier. An 82 MHz Ti-Sapphire actively mode-locked oscillator (Spectra Physics, Model # 3960) is pumped by a 5 W, frequency doubled Nd:YAG laser (Spectra Physics Model : Millenia) running at 532 nm. The oscillator pulse has duration of 100 fs (FWHM) at 790 nm. Its pulse is amplified by a Ti-Sapphire regenerative amplifier (Positive Light, Model : Spitfire) through a chirped pulse amplification (CPA) process. This amplifier is pumped by a 10 W, 527 nm Nd:YLF laser (Positive Light, Model : Merlin). The shortest final pulse duration is about 150 fs running at 1 kHz and its amplified energy is more than 1 mJ/pulse at 790 nm. Longer pulse widths were obtained by changing the light path in the compressor. The ablation rate is approximately 1 mm/s using a 1 kHz beam train. The focused beam size was approximately 100 μm (FWHM) with TEM$_{00}$ mode. Human teeth were collected from local dentists and they were cut and polished to make slices with various thickness.

Fig. 4 shows the ablation threshold in the pulse width range of 150 fs - 20 ps. The criteria for ablation was "any morphologic change" on the surface as seen with an optical microscope. The ablation threshold at 5 ps is about two times higher than that at 150 fs and it becomes four times higher as the pulse width is extended up to 20 ps. These numbers are consistent with previous results[5,11]. The rate of increase in threshold with increasing pulse width becomes high after 5 ps as predicted in previous report[8,12]. Below 5 ps the increase is moderate. Theoretical simulations were performed assuming that the ablation threshold corresponds to the energy density to create critical density of free electrons by multiphoton ionization and subsequent avalanche. This curve was calculated for general large band-gap dielectric such as fused silica because of the uncertainty with tooth parameters. It implies that the human dentine can be treated as a ceramic similar to fused silica.

The peak temperature rise at the back side of the tooth slice (thickness = 600 μm) were measured for different pulse width as shown in Fig. 5. The Gaussian beam diameter was approximately 100 μm (FWHM) and the power density was 2.5 times threshold for each pulse width. The exposure time was 2 seconds for 1 kHz beam train and 20 seconds for 100 Hz during which the temperature rise reaches a peak and decreases afterwards because the high temperature plasma cannot be generated after the ablation crater stalls out which is typical for USPL ablation craters[2]. The ablation crater stalls in less than 1000 shots. The peak temperature rise was only 2.5 - 4 °C for 1 kHz and 0.8 - 2 °C for 100 Hz. Is was expected that the temperature rise would be higher for higher repetition rate because the plasma from individual pulses interacts and the heat is accumulated during pulse train. The peak temperature did not increase significantly with increasing pulse width even if the actual threshold was four times higher for 20 ps than that for 150 fs as seen in Fig. 4.

Fig. 6 shows scanning electron microscopy (SEM) pictures of ablation craters drilled by pulses with different pulse widths. The rep rate was 1 kHz and the beam size was 100 μm for each picture. The exposure time was 1 sec. All the craters were generated using power density of 2.5 times higher than threshold, therefore, the power density for 20 ps crater was approximately 4 times high than that for 150 fs crater. From these figures, it is shown that the mechanical cracks or charring are not observed from any of the pictures which are normally seen in longer pulse ablation craters. The original tubules in the dentine are intact on the crater walls formed by 1 ps and shorter pulses. Melting of the dentine is observed at the edge of craters formed by 5 ps or longer pulses.

4. DISCUSSION

Two major factors contribute to low collateral damage for USPL ablation. First, the ablation threshold is significantly reduced for shorter pulses as demonstrated in this study and other literature[5,8,11]. The power density of ultrashort pulses is so large that it is easy to generate critical number of free electrons by multiphoton ionization. Loss of incoming energy by plasma reflection and absorption is minimized also because the energy deposition is so fast and the plasma does not propagate further to the free surface during pulse separating the absorbing plasma and ablation surface. Secondly, the shock wave is quickly reduced due to fast pressure release by plasma ejection and due to dispersion of narrow pressure pulse.

It seems that from Fig. 4 the ablation threshold does not increases sharply with longer pulse width up to ~ 5 ps. The temperature rise from the back surface of the 600 μm thick tooth slice was limited to less than 4 - 5 °C for entire pulse width range (150 fs - 20 ps). Especially, the ablation crater quality was not significantly different for each pulse width even if the slightly sharp edge started to show from 5 ps or longer craters. There were no mechanical cracks or thermal charring observed in this range. As a conclusion, the ablation of biological tissues performed at several ps pulses might be comparable with that by 150 fs pulses.

5. ACKNOWLEDGMENTS

This work was performed at Lawrence Livermore National Laboratory under the auspices of the U.S. Department of Energy under contract No. W-7405-ENG-48.

6. REFERENCES

1. A. A. Oraevsky, L. B. Da Silva, A. M. Rubenchik, M. D. Feit, M. E. Glinsky, M. D. Perry, B. M. Mammini, W. Small,, and B. C. Stuart, "Plasma mediated ablation of biological tissues with nanosecond-to-femtosecond laser pulses: Relative role of linear and nonlinear absorption," *IEEE J. Selected Topics in Quantum Electronics*, **2**, no. 4, pp. 801-809, 1996.

2. L. B. Da Silva, B. C. Stuart, P. M. Celliers, T. D. Chang, M. D. Feit, M. E. Glinsky, N. J. Heredia, S. Herman, S. M. Lane, R. A. London, D. L. Mattews, J. Neev, M. D. Perry, and A. M. Rubenchik, "Comparison of soft and hard tissue ablation with sub-ps and ns pulse lasers," *SPIE*, **2681**, pp. 196-200, 1996.

3. T. Juhasz, G. A. Kastis, C. Suárez, Z. Bor, and W. E. Bron, "Time-resolved observations of shock waves and cavitation bubbles generated by femtosecond laser pulses in corneal tissue and water," *Lasers Surg. Med.*, **19**, pp. 23-31, 1996.

4. M. H. Niemz, T. Hoppeler, T. Juhasz, and J. F. Bille, "Intrastromal ablations for refractive corneal surgery using picosecond infrared laser pulses," *Lasers Light Ophthalmol.*, **5**, pp. 145-152, 1993.

5. J. Neev, L. B. Da Silva, m. D. Feit, M. D. Perry, A. M. Rubenchik, and B. C. Stuart, "Ultrashort pulse lasers for hard tissue ablation," *IEEE J Selected Topics in Quantum Electronics*, **2**, no. 4, pp. 790-800, 1996.

6. J. Neev, D. S. Huynh, C. C. Dan, J. M. White, L. B. Da Silva, M. D. Feit, D. L. Mattews, M. D. Perry, A. M. Rubenchik, and B. C. Stuart, "Scanning electron microscopy and ablation rates of hard dental tissue using 350 fs and 1 ns laser pulses," *SPIE*, **2672**, pp. 250-261, 1996.

7. B.-M. Kim, M. D. Feit, A. M. Rubenchik, B. M. Mammini, and L. B. Da Silva, "Optical feedback signal for ultrashort laser pulse ablation of tissue," *Applied Surface Science*, 1998 (in press).

8. B. C. Stuart, M. D. Feit, S. Herman, A. M. Rubenchik, B. W. Shore, and M. D. Perry, "Nanosecond-to-femtosecond laser-induced breakdown in dielectric," *Physical Review B*, **53**, pp. 1749-1761, 1996.

9. M. D. Feit, A. M. Rubenchik, B.-M. Kim, L. B. Da Silva, and M. D. Perry, "Physical characterization of ultrashort laser pulse drilling of biological tissue," *Applied Surface Science*, 1998 (in press).

10. A. Vogel, K. Nahen, D. Theisen, and J. Noack, "Plasma formation in water by picosecond and nanosecond Nd:YAG laser pulses-Part I: Optical breakdown at threshold and super threshold irradiance," *IEEE J Selected Topics in Quantum Electronics*, **2**, pp. 847-860, 1996.

11. F. H. Loesel, M. H. Niemz, J. F. Bille, and T. Juhasz, "Laser-induced optical breakdown on hard and soft tissues and its dependence on the pulse duration: Experiment and model," *IEEE J of Quantum Electronics*, **32**, pp. 1717-1722, 1996.

12. B. C. Stuart, M. D. Feit, A. M. Rubenchik, B. W. Shore, and M. D. Perry, "Laser-induced damage in dielectrics with nanosecond to subpicosecond pulses," *Phys. Rev. Lett.*, **74**, pp. 2248-2251, 1995.

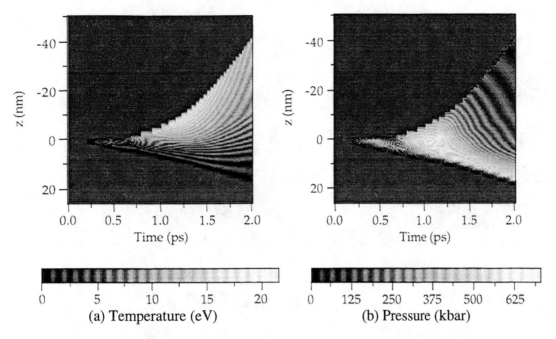

(a) Temperature (eV)

(b) Pressure (kbar)

Fig. 1. Temporal and spatial evolution of (a) temperature and (b) pressure on water irradiated by 500 fs pulse. The wavelength is 1 μm and energy density is 1.5 J/cm².

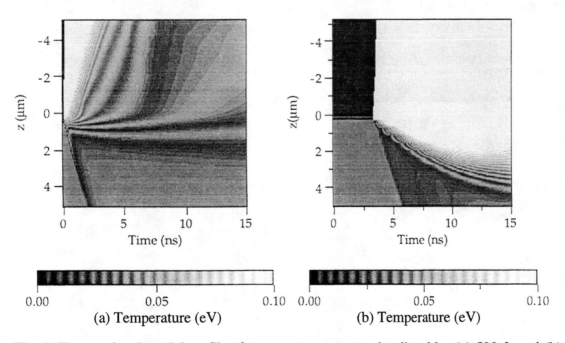

(a) Temperature (eV)

(b) Temperature (eV)

Fig. 2. Temporal and spatial profile of temperature on water irradiated by (a) 500 fs and (b) 5 ns. Calculations were performed using fluences 1.5 J/cm² and 25 J/cm² for 500 fs and 5 ns pulses respectively because they create approximately the same amount of volume removal. Note that the time and depth scales are much larger than those in Fig. 1.

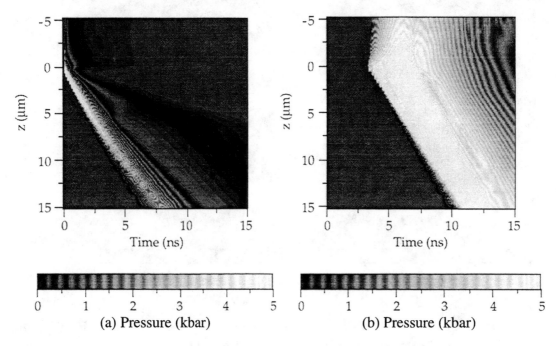

Fig. 3. Temporal and spatial profile of pressure on water irradiated by (a) 500 fs and (b) 5 ns. Same parameters were used as in Fig. 2.

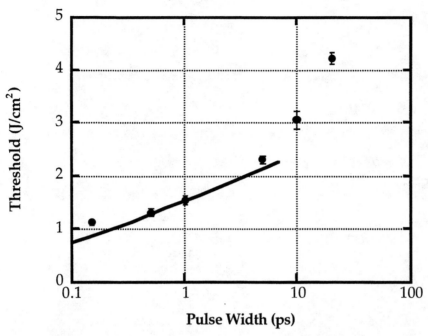

Fig. 4. Ablation threshold for dentine. The criteria for ablation is "any morphologic changes" on the surface as seen under optical microscopy. Solid line is the calculated threshold.

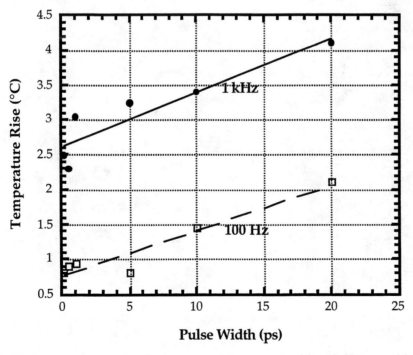

Fig. 5. Peak temperature rise for measured from back side of 600 μm thick dentine slice. Beam size was 100 μm and energy density is 2.5 times higher than threshold as shown in Fig. 4.

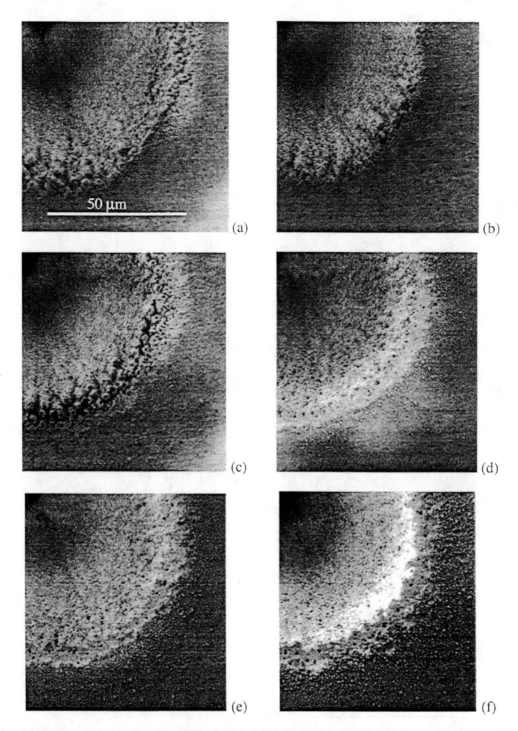

Fig. 6. Ablation craters on dentine drilled with (a) 150 fs, (b) 500 fs, (c) 1 ps, (d) 5 ps, (e) 10 ps, and (f) 20 ps pulses for 1 second. The diameter on the surface is approximately 100 μm for each hole.

Synthetic thrombus model for *in vitro* studies of laser thrombolysis

Robert E. Hermes and Keti Trajkovska

Los Alamos National Laboratory, MST-7 @ E549, Los Alamos, NM 87545 USA

ABSTRACT

Laser thrombolysis is the controlled ablation of a thrombus (blood clot) blockage in a living arterial system. Theoretical modeling of the interaction of laser light with thrombi relies on the ability to perform *in vitro* experiments with well characterized surrogate materials. A synthetic thrombus formulation may offer more accurate results when compared to *in vivo* clinical experiments. We describe here the development of new surrogate materials based on formulations incorporating chicken egg, guar gum, modified food starch, and a laser light absorbing dye. The sound speed and physical consistency of the materials were very close to porcine (arterial) and human (venous) thrombi. Photographic and videotape recordings of pulsed dye laser ablation experiments under various experimental conditions were used to evaluate the new material as compared to *in vitro* tests with human (venous) thrombus. The characteristics of ablation and mass removal were similar to that of real thrombi, and therefore provide a more realistic model for *in vitro* laser thrombolysis when compared to gelatin.

Keywords: thrombolysis, laser, gelatin, egg, thrombus, guar, starch

1. INTRODUCTION

A Cooperative Research and Development Agreement (CRADA) between the Los Alamos National Laboratory (operated by the University of California), the Oregon Medical Laser Center [OMLC] (Providence St. Vincent Hospital and Medical Center, Portland, OR) in association with Palomar Medical Technologies[1] (Beverly, MA) was established to provide an understanding of the fundamental mechanism(s) responsible for effective laser thrombolysis. Theoretical calculations were performed by several other team members,[2-5] which used input from experiments performed at the Oregon Medical Laser Center,[2] and the gelatin experiments described here.

As the materials science part of the multidisiplinary laser thrombolysis team, we developed surrogates which were used in the *in vitro* laser thrombolysis experiments described below. Although our main objective was to reproduce the gelatin/dye mixture used at the Oregon Medical Laser Center,[2] we also provided the important material properties needed by the team members responsible for the theoretical code development. They were primarily interested in the density and the speed of sound through the material. Their work relied upon the gelatin/dye material as being the most convenient choice for simplifying the parameters in the initial theoretical code development. However, the gelatin/dye material neither had the appearance of, nor behaved like a thrombus under the conditions established in our *in vitro* laser thrombolysis studies.

We realized there would eventually be a need for a more complex surrogate that would have the general physical characteristics of a real thrombus, and behave similarly under the laser thrombolysis conditions studied here. One practical requirement was that the material had to be stable enough to withstand several minutes under water (and contrast fluid), without breaking up or dissolving. After several unsuccessful attempts at using crosslinking agents for the gelatin/dye mixture, we began investigating several other bioderived gums such as xanthan, guar, and acacia in combination with egg white (both powdered and liquid), egg yolk, and/or gelatin. Interestingly, we found that one of our best surrogate materials (a combination of gelatin, egg yolk and red dye), was irreproducible in that chicken eggs obtained from New Mexico worked fine, but those obtained in Oregon did not set up under the conditions established in New Mexico.

2. EXPERIMENTAL

2.1 Materials

Regular tap water was used where indicated. The X-ray contrast fluid MD-76 from Mallinckrodt Medical, Chesterfield, MO, was kindly provided to us by the Oregon Medical Laser Center, and diluted 1:1 with tap water prior to use. Porcine gelatin, ~175 bloom, and gum guar were used as received from Aldrich Chemical Company, Milwaukee, WS. Normal octane was purchased from J. T. Baker Chemical Company, Phillipsburg, NJ, and the mineral oil (USP) was obtained from Paddock Laboratories, Inc., Minneapolis, MN. The laser energy absorbing Direct Red 81 dye was obtained from Sigma Chemical Company, St. Louis, MO. The laser dye Rhodamine 575 was used as received from Exciton Chemical Company, Dayton, OH. Grade AA chicken eggs were purchased at the local grocery store. The 1-cm path length plastic cuvettes (clear path on all four sides), and polypropylene disposable pipets were obtained from VWR Scientific, San Francisco, CA. Vanilla flavored JELLO® Stir 'n Snack™, Kraft Foods, Inc., White Plains, NY, was purchased at the local grocery store. This latter component is comprised of sugar, modified food starch, sodium phosphates (for thickening), glycerine, salt, polysorbate 60, artificial color, artificial flavor, yellow 5, yellow 6, and natural flavors in undetermined amounts. The human thrombus was obtained by drawing venous blood into a siliconized tube and allowing the blood clot to coagulate at close to body temperature.

2.2 Sample Preparation

Gelatin/dye samples were prepared from the formulation previously developed at OMLC.[2] Porcine gelatin (3.5 grams) was gradually added to rapidly stirred boiling water (100 milliliters) in a 250 milliliter capacity beaker until dissolved. Upon cooling, clear gels were prepared by carefully pipetting the liquid into cuvettes to a level of about half full, then refrigerated for about 30 minutes for gellation to occur. The gelatin/dye mixture was prepared similarly, except Direct Red 81 (0.15 grams) was added during the mixing step. Hot water was introduced to the top of each cold gel and placed into a freezer for a few minutes. When decanted and rinsed with cold water, this had the effect of leveling the gel in each cuvette by removing the miniscus. This was important in order to obtain acceptable electronic photographs through the cuvette. These samples were also used as the base material for the other samples. The gelatin/dye mixture was added to a level of approximately 1 millimeter on top of the clear gel, and refrigerated. This is called OMLC clot in the photographs.

The surrogate thrombus was prepared by mixing vanilla flavored JELLO® Stir 'n Snack™ (8.0 grams) with gum guar (3.0 grams), Direct Red 81 dye (1.0 gram) and the contents of one chicken egg (~51 grams, 50 milliliters). This mixture was blended for 30-40 seconds in a stainless-steel cup, using the low speed position on a Waring™ blender. Pipetting was performed immediately because of the fast set-up time of this mixture. One or two drops were carefully introduced to the flattened top of the clear gels, and refrigerated. This sample type is called LANL clot in the photographs.

The human thrombus was carefully sliced into several samples (2 millimeter thick) having a radial diameter of 1 centimeter. These were rinsed with water just prior to placing them on the surface of the clear gels used for the experiments. These are called Venous Clot in the photographs.

2.3 Apparatus Description

A Palomar Medical Technologies Model 3010 dye laser was kindly provided by Palomar,[1] and was equipped with a fiber optic delivery device (multimode fiber, 300 micron diameter). We used Rhodamine 575 laser dye and the appropriate laser controls to deliver 50-mJ from the fiber tip in a single shot mode. The tip was generally centered in the cuvette, and held to 1 millimeter above the test surface. The pulsewidth (FWHM) was nominally 1-microsecond (system specifications, not measured). A 400 milliwatt continuous wave doubled Nd:YAG Verdi™ laser, Coherent Laser Group, Santa Clara, CA, was used for back illumination of the samples during each experiment. Time resolved images were obtained with a gated electronic framing camera, model 486, Hadland Photonics, Cupertino, CA, with each frame having an exposure time of 500 nanoseconds. The first frame was timed close to the laser pulse and considered to be T=0. The other seven frames were recorded at the following times: 25, 90, 100, 150, 300, 500, and 800 microseconds. A data set of eight images was obtained for each laser pulse. Experiments were run in triplicate with each test material, but in a different location for each shot. Each test was also videotaped through a magnifying lens using a videocassette recorder connected to a camera.

2.4 Laser Thrombolysis Experimental Procedure

The test cuvettes were removed from refrigeration, and allowed to reach room temperature prior to each experiment. In each case, the test liquid was added to the top of the solidified material within a few minutes of testing. The cuvette was placed into a special holder while the fiber optic tip was adjusted to 1 millimeter from the surface of the test material. The laser and camera were simultaneously triggered to obtain the laser thrombolysis record.

3. RESULTS AND DISCUSSION

Throughout these experiments, we attempted to provide time-resolved data that demonstrates the utility of our new synthetic thrombus model for *in vitro* laser thrombolysis. The driving factor was the need to evaluate several operational conditions using liquids of various density above the samples. The liquids were chosen from those previously studied at OMLC: water, 1:1 mixture of MD-76:water, and mineral oil. Addtitionally, we tried octane, which has a lower density and much lower boiling point than that of mineral oil. The differences in the bubble dynamics obtained with each liquid and matrix were to be evaluated and emulated using the data for the theoretical calculations. As materials scientists, we were attempting to answer the questions - can we make a material that is stable enough to withstand several liquids? have the look and feel of a "standard" thrombus? and will the surrogate perform under laser thrombolysis conditions similar to that of a real thrombus? The examples shown in this paper were chosen to address these issues.

3.1 Description of Figures

The figures on the following pages were taken from the data files generated by the Hadland camera. They are viewed starting from the first frame in the top left corner, then down to frame two, back up and to the right for frame three, then down, and repeating until frame eight is on the far bottom right. For simple comparison, three photographs are included in each figure, with the OMLC Clot on top, the LANL Clot in the middle, and the Venous Clot on the bottom. In all cases, we compared the first two sets of photographs with the results obtained from the laser thrombolysis of the Venous Clot. Figure 1 shows the first set having water on top. Figure 2 shows the 1:1 MD-76:water. Figure 3 shows mineral oil, and figure 4 shows octane. Observations include the size of the bubble in each respective time frame (generally 2-5), and whether jetting of material occurs at similar times in the sequence (usually frames 6-8). The OMLC Clot data shows typical behavior for bubble formation and collapse, and conveniently includes a visually acceptable view of the bubble below the surface. Unfortunately, the others do not display such behavior, even though the test material was also prepared on top of the clear gelatin.

Figure 1. *in vitro* laser thrombolysis using OMLC, LANL, and Venous Clot materials under water

OMLC clot

LANL clot

Venous clot

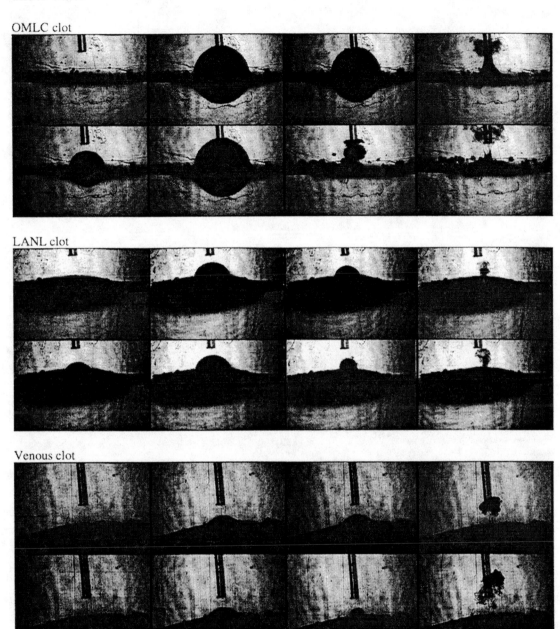

Figure 2. *in vitro* laser thrombolysis using OMLC, LANL, and Venous Clot materials under MD-76:water

OMLC Clot

LANL Clot

Venous Clot

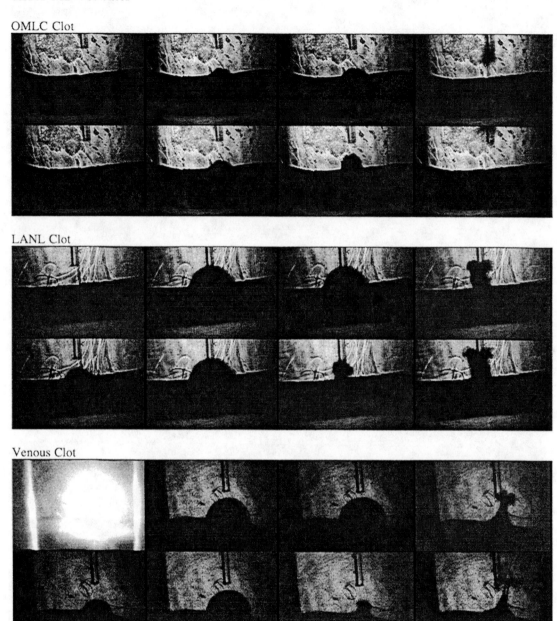

Figure 3. *in vitro* laser thrombolysis using OMLC, LANL, and Venous Clot materials under mineral oil

OMLC Clot

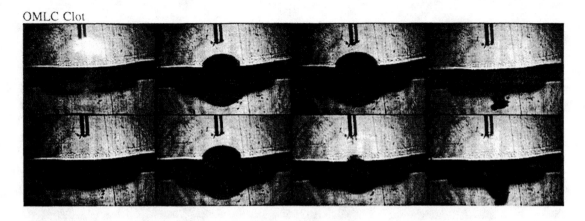

LANL Clot

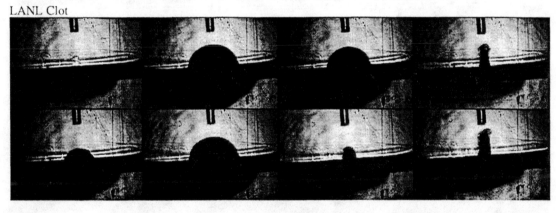

Venous Clot

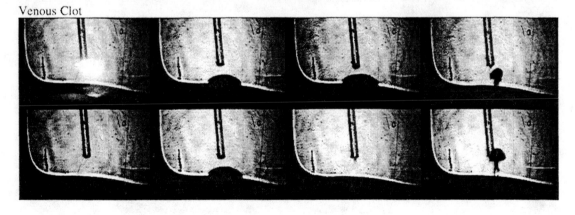

Figure 4. *in vitro* laser thrombolysis using OMLC, LANL, and Venous Clot materials under octane

OMLC Clot

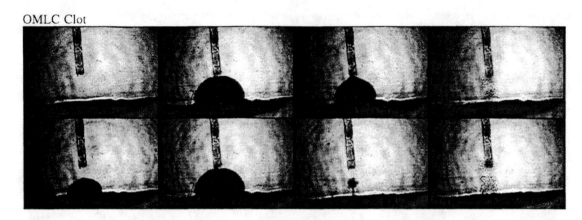

LANL Clot

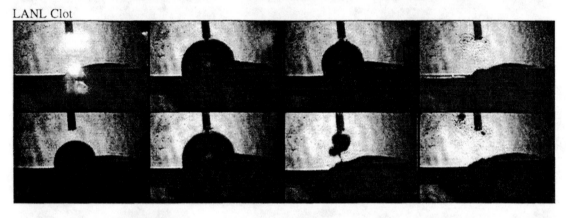

Venous Clot

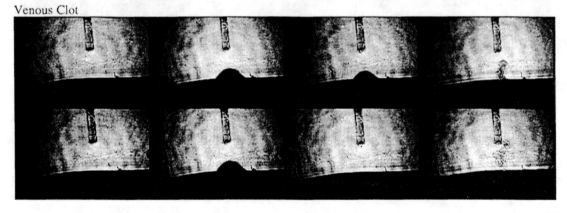

3. RESULTS AND DISCUSSION, continued

3.2 Under water

In Figure 1, a comparison between all three clots shows a great similarity between the apparent diameter of the bubble in the LANL Clot and the Venous Clot, especially in frames 3-6. However, the bubble on the Venous Clot is somewhat obscured by the surface facing the camera, and makes for a difficult measurement. A nice particulate jet is evident in the last frame of the Venous Clot, as well as the LANL Clot. The OMLC Clot shows the typical behavior in a uniform system.

3.3 Under MD-76:water

This was perhaps the most important series because Figure 2 was performed with the conrast fluid used in *in vivo* laser thrombolysis experiments. The bright flash in frame 1 of the Venous Clot was due to the framing camera catching the laser pulse. It is clear that the performance of the LANL Clot is virtually identical to that of the Venous Clot. Although it may not be perfect, this result was the best we have ever witnessed.

3.4 Under mineral oil

Figure 3 displays a unique phenomenon, particularly when comparing the OMLC Clot and the LANL Clot. Although the density of mineral oil is below that of both materials, one can clearly see that the jet reverses direction in the OMLC Clot (into the gel matrix), and appears to provide a normal direction for the ejecta in the LANL Clot. Apparently, the majority of the bubble in the OMLC Clot was below the interface, and just the opposite in the LANL Clot. The good news was that the ejecta in the Venous Clot was also above the interface.

3.5 Under n-octane

Figure 4 proved to be very interesting. Hardly any response was observed for the Venous Clot but it still produced a jet. The LANL Clot had a much larger bubble formation, and was shown to blow expanding microbubbles, as evident in the change from frame 7 to frame 8. Both the OMLC Clot and the LANL Clot displayed radically different behavior when compared with the Venous Clot.

4. CONCLUSIONS

After several iterations of trying to make a synthetic thrombus material that looks, feels, and performs like a real venous thrombus (Venous Clot) under *in vitro* laser thrombolysis, we believe we have succeeded in preparing a simple mixture that met the performance criteria established by the experimental procedures studied here. In particular, the performance of the LANL Clot was nearly identical to that of the Venous Clot, expecially under the contrast fluid. The results achieved under mineral oil and octane are left for the theoretical types to ponder. The authors recognize that a Venous Clot is not the best model for the thrombi usually associated with coronary disease or stroke.

5. ACKNOWLEDGEMENTS

The authors gratefully acknowledge the assistance of Scott Prahl of OMLC in helping to define the scope of our work. We also thank U. Sathyam and H. Shangguan for their expert knowledge in the preparation of the OMLC gelatin/dye surrogate. Alan Shearin and Henry Aldag of Palomar were instrumental in providing both technical assistance and the laser used for these experiments. Dennis Paisley and David Stahl of Los Alamos National Laboratory were responsible for the optical set-up and laser testing, without which our experiments could not have been performed.

This CRADA was supported by the U.S. Department of Energy under Contract W-7405-ENG-36.

6. NOTES AND REFERENCES

1. The medical laser division of Palomar Medical Technologies, Inc. has recently been purchased by Physical Sciences Inc., Andover, MA.
2. U. S. Sathyam, A. Shearin, E. A. Chasteney, and S. A. Prahl, "Threshold and Ablation Efficiency Studies of Microsecond Ablation of Gelatin Under Water," Lasers in Surgery and Medicine 19, 397, 1996.
3. E. J. Chapyak, R. P. Godwin, S. A. Prahl, and H. Shangguan, "A comparison of numerical simulations and laboratory studies of laser thrombolysis," in *SPIE Proceedings of Diagnostic and Therapeutic Cardiovascular Interventions VII* , K. Gregory, ed., Vol. 2970A, presented at Bios'97, February 1997, San Jose, CA, SPIE, Bellingham, WA.
4. R. P. Godwin, E. J. Chapyak, S. A. Prahl, and H. Shangguan, "Laser mass ablation efficiency measurements indicate bubble-driven dynamics dominates laser thrombolysis," in *SPIE Proceedings of Diagnostic and Therapeutic Cardiovascular Intervcentions-VIII* , K. Gregory, ed., Vol. 3245A, presented at Bios'98, January 1998, San Jose, CA, SPIE, Bellingham, WA.
5. E. J. Chapyak and R. P. Godwin, "Physical mechanisms of importance to laser thrombolysis," in *SPIE Proceedings of Diagnostic and Therapeutic Cardiovascular Intervcentions-VIII* , K. Gregory, ed., Vol. 3245A, presented at Bios'98, January 1998, San Jose, CA, SPIE, Bellingham, WA.

Acoustic spectroscopy of Er:YAG laser ablation of skin
– first results –

Kester Nahen[a] and Alfred Vogel[a]

[a]Medical Laser Center Lübeck, Peter-Monnik-Weg 4, D-23562 Lübeck, Germany

ABSTRACT

We investigated the acoustic signal of Er:YAG laser ablation in a gaseous environment. The high absorption coefficient of water at the laser wavelength of 2.94 μm leads to a small penetration depth of the Er:YAG laser pulses into tissue. The deposition of laser energy in a thin layer at the tissue surface causes a rapid evaporization of tissue water. The resulting tissue removal is used, for example, in laser skin resurfacing. The explosive evaporation of the tissue leads to an acoustic signal. We investigated the generation process of the signal caused by free-running laser pulses and its characteristic parameters in the time and frequency domain in correlation to the tissue and laser parameters with the aim to identify different tissues or tissue layers by analyzing the acoustic signal. Porcine skin and gelatin probes were ablated. Acoustic signals up to 1 MHz were measured using a condenser microphone and a piezoelectric airborne transducer. Schlieren photography was performed simultaneously to the acoustic investigations to visualize gaseous and condensed ablation products. We found that the high frequency content of the acoustic spectrum is due to shock waves created by each of the first laser spikes. Later in the laser pulse the acoustic signal is dominated by lower frequency components, because the generation of the high frequency components is inhibited by the interaction of the radiation with the ablation plume. The acoustic signature of free-running Er:YAG laser ablation seems to be particulary tissue specific during the first part of the laser pulse when the radiation interacts directly with the tissue.

Keywords: photoablation, acoustic spectroscopy, Er:YAG laser

1. INTRODUCTION

Infrared laser ablation in gaseous environment is used for example in skin resurfacing[1] and for the removal of burned skin in reconstructive burn surgery.[2,3] Previous investigations by Bende et al.[4] showed promising results with regard to tissue differentiation during Excimer laser ablation. For a selective removal of tissue layers an online control of the ablation process is needed. The aim of our investigations is to realize a feedback system using acoustic spectroscopy of the ablation noise.

We used Schlieren laser flash photography to get an understanding of the kinetics of the ablation process generating the ablation noise. The acoustic measurements covered the frequency range from 6.5 Hz to 1 MHz. In contrast to the investigations of Bende et al.[4] who were only able to measure frequencies up to 150 kHz using a condenser microphone, we extended the detecable frequency range to 1 MHz by using a piezoelectric airborne transducer. Time and frequency domain analysis were performed to characterize the acoustic signal.

2. METHODS

2.1. Laser Irradiation

We used a free-running Er:YAG laser (LISA Laser Products) delivering pulses with a maximum pulse energy of 400 mJ and 300 μs pulse duration. The laser was operated at 10 Hz repetition rate. The Er:YAG laser radiation was combined with a He:Ne laser beam using a dichroic mirror (Fig. 1). To perform single shot experiments a shutter was used. The laser pulse shape was detected by a GaAs photodiode (EG&G Judson J125AP-R02M) connected to an oscilloscope (TEK TDS-540). The laser energy could be varied by means of two rotatable quartz plates which were mechanical coupled to rotate in opposite direction. This allows an energy variation without changing the pump energy which would otherwise alter the pulse duration and beam profile. The pulse energy was measured using a

Send correspondence to
K. Nahen: E-mail: nahen@mll.mu-luebeck.de; WWW: http://www.mll.mu-luebeck.de/english/nahen_e.htm;
Telephone: +49-451-5006513; Fax: +49-451-505486

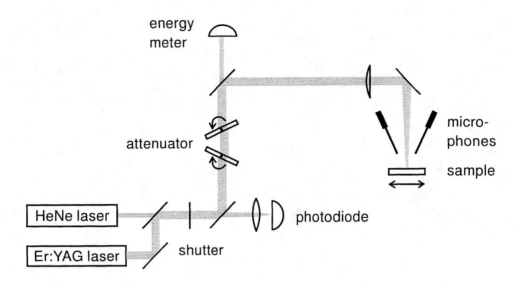

Figure 1. Experimental setup for Er:YAG laser ablation.

pyroelectric probe (DigiRad P-444) calibrated against a second energy meter located in place of the sample. The laser beam irradiated the probe in vertical direction. It was focussed with a 100 mm planoconvex lens to a spot diameter of 450 μm.

2.2. Laser flash photography

We performed laser flash photography using a dark field Schlieren arrangement to investigate the dynamics of the ablation process (Fig. 2). For illumination we used 6 ns-pulses from a frequency doubled Nd:YAG laser pumping a dye laser (Rhodamin 6G). The dye laser was employed to achieve spectral broadening leading to reduced speckle. Spatial frequency filtering was performed using a wire blocking out the image of a slit located in the illumination beam path. Wire and slit are orientated perpendicular to the sample surface giving a maximum sensitivity to refractive index changes parallel to the sample surface and total insensitivity to variations perpendicular to the sample surface. Photographs with different delays between the Er:YAG laser pulse and the illuminating laser pulse were taken on photographic film.

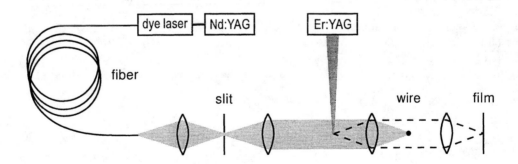

Figure 2. Dark field Schlieren arrangement for laser flash photography.

2.3. Acoustic investigations

The ablation noise was detected using a condenser microphone with a bandwidth of 6.5 Hz – 140 kHz (±2 dB), and a piezoelectric airborne transducer with a bandwidth of 5 kHz – 1 MHz. The microphone signals were recorded with a digital oszilloscope (TEK TDS 540) and read out into a PC to perform signal analysis. Time window FFT analysis was implemented using IDL (Interactive Data Language). All measurements were performed simultaneously with both microphones. The microphones were oriented under an angle of 35° to the optical axis of the laser beam in a distance of 30 mm to the probe surface.

2.4. Irradiated Samples

In vitro measurements were performed using porcine skin and gelatin samples. We used porcine skin from the ear of freshly slaughtered animals, kept for a maximum of 8 hours. To inhibit desiccation of the skin, the ears were stored in a closed plastic bag at 7 °C until use. The gelatin samples containing 90% water were stored in a refrigerator until use. The experiments were performed within 20 minutes after exposing the samples to room temperature in order to minimize the effect of gelatin liquification.

3. RESULTS AND DISCUSSION

3.1. Laser flash photography

Figure 3 shows laser flash photographs of the Er:YAG laser ablation of gelatin and porcine skin at various times after the first laser spike. The ablation was performed using a pulse energy of 33 mJ and a focus diameter of 450 μm, corresponding to a radiant exposure of 21 J/cm^2.

The picture of gelatin ablation taken 4 μs after the first laser spike shows the emission of a spherical shock wave. The part of the shock wave oriented parallel to the sample surface could not be detected because the spatial filtering in the Schlieren setup was performed with a wire oriented in vertical direction (section 2.2). The picture taken after 7 μs shows the radial propagation of the shock wave. In addition we see a second shock wave which was generated by the second laser spike as demonstrated in figure 4. Besides the shock wave, a 1 mm thick layer of ablation products is visible 500 μm above the surface in the picture taken 4 μs after the beginning of the laser pulse. These particles are probably droplets of a liquid film evaporated from the sample surface. This film arises probably from the liquification of the gelatin which takes place when the sample is exposed to room temperatur during the measurement series. Seven microseconds after the first laser spike the ejection of ablation material is much more pronounced and a crater begins to form in the sample surface. The ejected particles are round and stringlike shaped droplets, and some irregularly shaped gelatin fragments can also been seen.

After 80 μs, a large ablation plume of gaseous and condensed material is visible. A hump has appeared which is probably a wall formed around the crater in the sample surface from which the material is ejected. Near the ablation site, the stringlike droplets are oriented in a direction perpendicular to the surface, but in a greater distance they show no preferential orientation. This phenomenon can be explained by fluid dynamic processes leading to turbulences during the evolution of the ablation plume. Besides the focused images of ablation products we can also see blurred images of particles located outside the object plane, and the turbulent flow of the hot water vapor in the plume. The further growth of the ablation plume occures mainly in direction of the incident laser beam as seen on the picture taken 164 μs after the beginning of the laser pulse; hardly any lateral expansion is observed. Near the ablation crater, the particle density is decreasing already during the laser pulse. This can be explained by the absorption of the incident laser beam in the upper parts of the ablation plume which hinders the energy deposition at the sample surface (Sec. 3.2.1) .

The picture series taken from the ablation of skin do not show a shock wave. Already 4 μs after the first laser spike, a hump is visible at the sample surface. The rupture of the sample surface occures earlier than in the case of gelatin. The particles ejected from the skin sample are smaller and more rugged than in the case of gelatin, with less variations in size. The condensed ablation products of skin are mainly solid, whereas they are in the liquid phase in the case of gelatin.

Our photographic observations are consistent with the description of Er:YAG laser ablation given previously by Walsh et al.[5,6] and Venugopalan et al.[7]: The ablation is viewed as an explosive process driven by the rapid heating, vaporization, and subsequent high pressure expansion of irradiated tissue. The expansion of the plume is preceeded by a shock front, both moving at supersonic velocity.

The differences in the ablation dynamics and appearence of the ablation products of gelatin and skin are caused by the different physical properties of the samples. The low melting temperature of gelatin (50 °C) causes the generation of a liquid film on the sample surface before complete evaporation of a superficial gelatin layer occurs. Each laser spike causes a superficial evaporation of the liquid which generates a radial flow inside the liquid layer.[8] The rapid radial flow is probably responsible for the creation of the hump around the ablation crater as well as for the ejection of liquid particles. Fig. 3 shows that the hump formed during skin ablation is less prominent than in the case of gelatin during the first 80 μs of the ablation process. This can be explained by the higher stability of the tissue matrix which better withstands the radial forces in the ablation crater. The liquidlike appearance of the ablation products of gelatin is also caused by the low melting point of gelatin. In the case of skin the condensed ablation products are probably components of the tissue matrix with a high melting and evaporation temperature driven by the evaporation of other components having a lower evaporation temperature.

Our photographic investigations showed that the difference between the ablation dynamics of gelatin and skin is most pronounced during the initial part of the ablation process. It can therefore be assumed that the specificity of the acoustic signal is also greater during this phase, whereas it is later obscured by the interactions between the incident laser beam and the ablation plume.

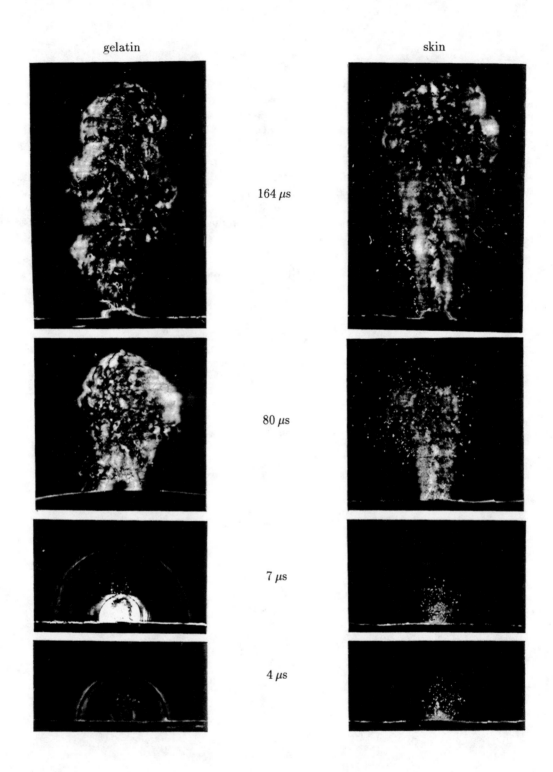

Figure 3. Laser flash photographies of Er:YAG laser ablation of gelatin and porcine skin. The photographs were taken with a dark field Schlieren technique at various times after the first laser spike (Laser pulse energy 33 mJ, focus diameter 450 μm (├──┤ = 1 mm).

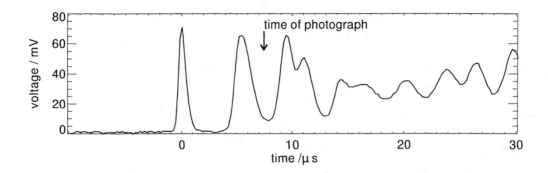

Figure 4. Pulse shape of the laser pulse used for the gelatin ablation shown in figure 3. The arrow indicates the time (7 μs) at which the second frame of the picture series was taken.

3.2. Acoustic spectroscopy

3.2.1. Time domain

Figure 5 shows the Er:YAG laser pulse and the microphone signals of the ablation noise measured for skin ablation with pulse energies of 20 mJ (a) – (c) and 100 mJ (d) – (f). The duration of the microphone signals is similar to the laser pulse duration. At high pulse energies, the signal amplitude decreases significantly during the first 50 μs of the laser pulse. This is partly due to less signal generation at the tissue surface because of the increasing light absorption in the ablation plume, and also partly a result of the strong damping of pressure waves by the ablation plume. The effect is less pronounced with small pulse energies where the ablation plume is more transparent. The absorption coefficient, α in vapor water is approximately 2.7 cm^{-1} for 100 atm at 3,000° K,[9] corresponding to an optical penetration depth of $1/\alpha \approx 3.7$ mm. The ablation plume reaches a hight equal to $1/\alpha$ approximately 40 μs after the beginning of the laser pulse. Assuming a constant conversion factor from optical to acoustic energy the amplitude of the pressure signal should drop to 36% at this time compared to the maximum pressure at the beginning of the laser pulse. The experimental data confirm this assumption with an accuracy of better than 10% even though the ablation plume does not only consist out of water vapor but also of condensed matter having a higher absorption coefficient.

The maximum pressure values measured by the piezoelectric transducer are about a factor 4.5 higher than the values detected with the condenser microphone. This discrepancy is due to the different temporal resolution of the transducers. The actual duration of the pressure spikes is probably similar to the duration of the laser spike ($\leq 1\mu$s, FWHM) and thus shorter than the rise time of either microphone. The corresponding distortion of the signal amplitude[10] is larger for the condenser microphone, because its rise time is longer. The distortion is most pronounced during the first part of the laser pulse where the ablation leads to the generation of shock waves (Fig.4). The comparison between the transducers shows that a lot of information is lost using the condenser microphone, and that it would be desirable to have an even better resolution than that achieved with the airborne piezoelectric transducer.

The flash photographs of tissue and gelatin ablation showed maximum differences during the beginning of the laser pulse when the radiation interacts directly with the sample. Tissue specific information in the ablation noise will therefore be mainly contained in the first part of the laser pulse. In the following we pay particular attention to this part of the acoustic signals. Figure 6 shows the first 30 μs of a laser pulse and the corresponding acoustical signal of the piezoelectric transducer. To facilitate a comparison between the signals, they are aligned for coincidence of the fifth acoustic signal with the fifth maximum of the laser spike. The peaks in the time signals show a one to one correlation. This indicates that each individual laser spike causes a seperate ablation event leading to the generation of a pressure pulse. The acoustic transients produced by the first two laser spikes appear shifted to earlier times with respect to the laser spikes. These transients are shock waves (Fig. 3) traveling faster than the speed of sound because of their high pressure amplitude. The intensity of the first laser spike in figure 6 (a) is higher than the second one leading to a higher pressure and thus to a higher velocity of the first shock wave (Fig. 6 (b)). The pressure difference is not reflected in the microphone signal. This could be due to a smaller width of the first pressure pulse which would lead to a larger distortion of its amplitude by the slow rise time of the microphone.

223

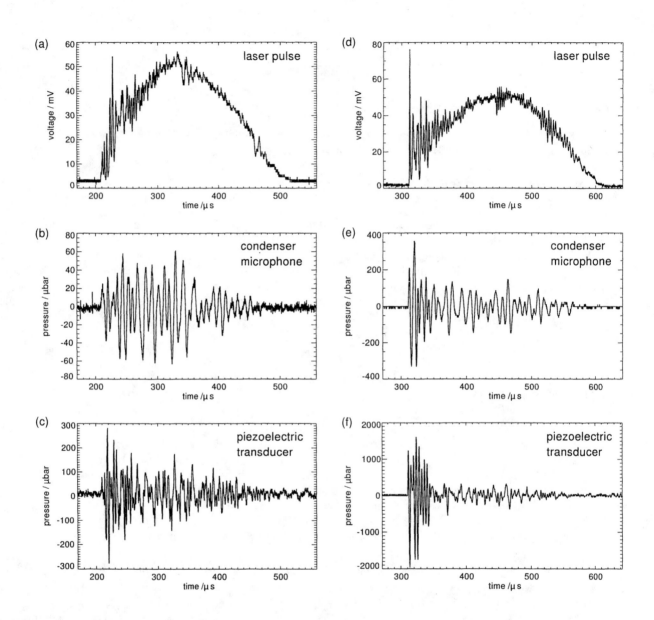

Figure 5. Er:YAG laser pulse and corresponding microphone signals for skin ablation with pulse energies of 20 mJ (a) – (c) and 100 mJ (d) – (f). The pressure signals refer to a distance of 30 mm from the source. They were measured simultaneously with both microphones.

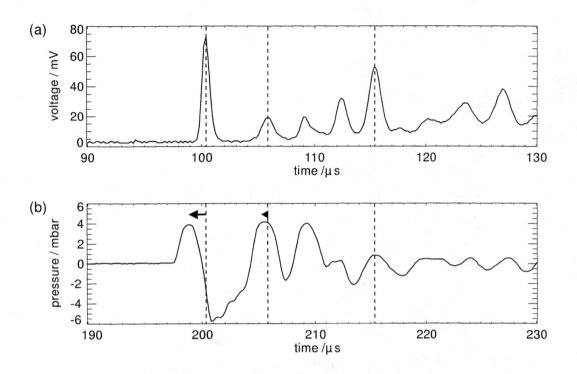

Figure 6. Initial part of the laser pulse (a) and the acoustical signal measured with a piezoelectric transducer (b). The signals are aligned for coincidence of the fifth maximum of the acoustic signal with the fifth laser spike.

Our observations agree qualitatively with the results of Frenz et al.[11,12] who investigated Er:YAG laser ablation of gelatin and tissue at radiant exposures 5 times higher as applied in this study. By means of Schlieren flash photography they observed shock wave generation during the first $10\,\mu s$ of the laser pulse, and by monitoring the deflection or interruption of a HeNe probe laser, they could show a correlation between material ejection and the individual laser spikes during the first $40-70\,\mu s$ of the laser pulse. Similar observations by means of a pump-probe arrangement were also reported by Walsh and Deutsch.[6] The similarity between the microphone signals detected in this study and the probe beam signals analyzed previously suggests that the probe laser signals were due to a diffraction of the laser beam by the pressure waves created during ablation (rather than to a beam interruption by the ablation products). Detection of the acoustic signals with a microphone is, however, simpler and better suited for an online analysis in a clinical surrounding.

3.2.2. Frequency domain

Algorithms for a FFT analysis[13] of arbitrary time windows of the acoustic signal and the laser pulse were implemented in IDL (Interactive Data Language). Hanning windows with a bandwidth of 20 kHz were scanned over the selected window of the time signals. Figure 7 (c) shows spectra of the microphone signals in figure 7(a) and (b) which were calculated for a time window covering the whole laser pulse duration. The spectrum of the piezoelectric transducer signal shows frequency components of up to 500 kHz in the ablation noise. The condenser microphone is unable to detect the high frequency components because of its limited bandwidth. The piezoelectric transducer makes it possible to investigate the high frequency components of the ablation noise which means a progress compared to earlier experiments by Bende et al.[4] performed with a condenser microphone. Our further analysis will therefore focus on the signals provided by the piezoelectric transducer.

The FFT analysis for different time windows in figure 8 shows that the high frequency components are predominantly produced during the first part of the laser pulse, whereas low frequencies are mainly generated at the end of the laser pulse. This agrees with our photographic observations that fast processes like shock wave emission take place only at the beginning of the laser pulse (section 3.1).

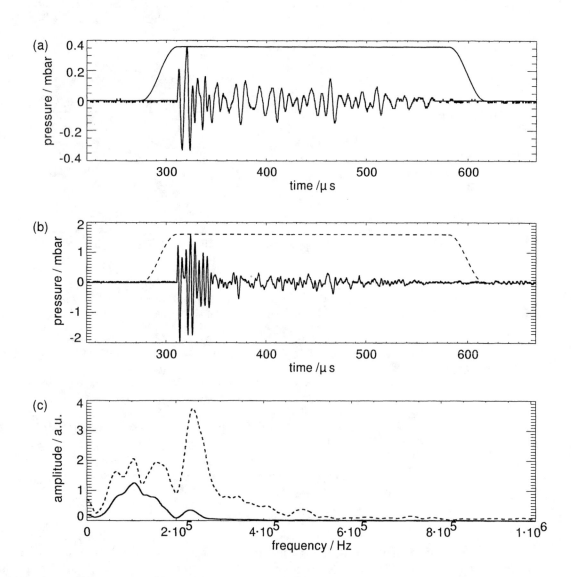

Figure 7. Time window FFT analysis of acoustical signals during Er:YAG laser ablation of skin. (a) Condenser microphone, (b) piezoelectric transducer, (c) frequency spectra for the time windows shown in (a) and (b). Pulse energy 100 mJ. The signal of the piezoelectric transducer contains considering more information than that of the condenser microphone.

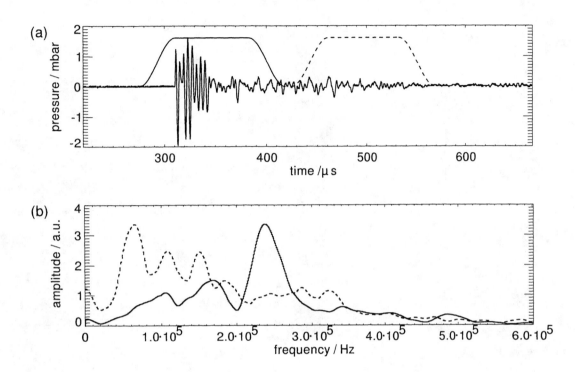

Figure 8. Time window FFT analysis of different time windows of a piezoelectric transducer signal during Er:YAG laser ablation of skin. (a) Acoustic signal, and (b) frequency spectra for the time windows shown in (a). Spectra are normalized with in respect to their maximum amplitude. Pulse energy 100 mJ. The high frequency content of the spectrum decreases during the laser pulse.

Figure 9 compares the spectrum of the piezoelectric transducer and the photodiode signal of the laser pulse for a time window at the beginning of the laser pulse to obtain information about the origin of the maxima observed in the acoustic spectrum. The maxima in both spectra coincide very well in the frequency range of 100 – 450 kHz. A detailed analysis of the time signal of the laser pulse shows that these frequency components in the spectrum are due to the time constants of the spiking sequence. This explains that the spiking sequence of the laser pulse is driving the acoustic signal. Further investigations need to concentrate on the transfer function between the spectra of the laser pulse and the acoustic signal. This function consists of the transfer function between the laser pulse and the acoustic signal which carries the tissue specific information, and of the transfer function of air and of the microphone which tend to obscure this information. Detailed knowledge of all three steps is required to retrieve the tissue specific information from the acoustic signal.

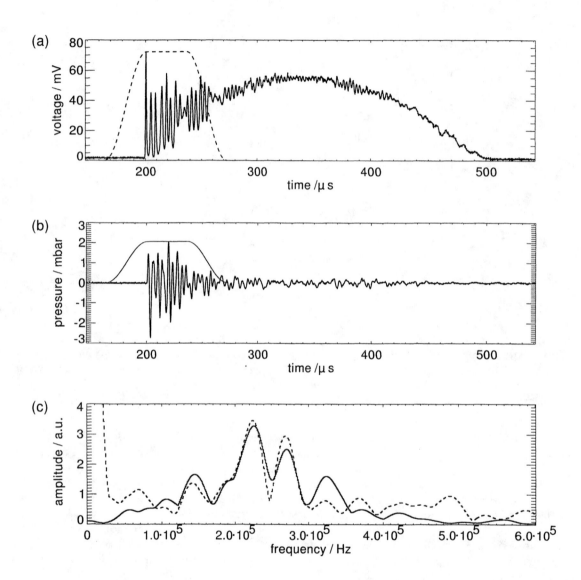

Figure 9. Time window FFT analysis of the laser pulse and of a acoustic signal during Er:YAG laser ablation of skin. (a) Photodiode, (b) piezoelectric transducer, and (c) frequency spectra for the time windows shown in (a) and (b). Pulse energy 100 mJ. The peaks in the acoustic spectrum are strongly correlated with the time constants in the spiking sequence.

4. SUMMARY AND CONCLUSIONS

We performed photographic investigations in conjunction with microphone measurements to correlate the acoustic ablation noise with the underlying ablation dynamics. We found that high frequency components produced by the direct interaction of the laser with the tissue are produced mainly at the beginning of the laser pulse. The major differences in the ablation dynamics of skin and gelatin appear also in this phase of the ablation process. This observation suggests that characteristic information about the ablated tissue can be found in the first $50\,\mu s$ of the acoustic signal. The larger bandwidth of the piezoelectric transducer is essential for these investigations. For the complete resolution of the shock waves, even faster piezoelectric transducers or optical techniques are needed. To take the pulse to pulse fluctuations in the free-running laser pulse into account, one has to perform a pulse to pulse analysis of both the acoustical signal and the laser pulse.

5. ACKNOWLEDGEMENT

The authors appreciate helpful discussions with J. Noack. The research was supported by a grant of the state of Schleswig-Holstein, Germany.

REFERENCES

1. T. S. Alster and D. B. Apfelberg, *Cosmetic laser surgery*, John Wiley & Sons, 1996.
2. H. A. Green and Y. D. amd N. S. Nishioka, "Pulsed carbon dioxide laser ablation of burned skin: In vitro and in vivo analysis," *Lasers Surg. Med.* **10**, pp. 476–484, 1990.
3. H. A. Green, E. E. Burd, N. S. Nishioka, and C. C. Compton, "Skin graft take and healing following 193-nm excimer, continuous-wave carbon dioxide (CO_2), pulsed CO_2, or pulsed holmium:YAG laser ablation of graft bed," *Arch. Dermatol.* **129**, pp. 979–988, 1993.
4. T. Bende, M. Matallana, B. Kleffner, and B. Jean, "Noncontact photoacoustic spectroscopy during photoablation: a step towards the smart laser?," in *Ophthalmic Technologies V*, vol. 2293, pp. 111–119, SPIE, 1995.
5. J. T. Walsh, T. J. Flotte, and T. F. Deutsch, "Er:YAG laser ablation of tissue: Effect of pulse duration and tissue type on thermal damage," *Lasers Surg. Med.* **9**, pp. 314–326, 1989.
6. J. T. Walsh and T. F. Deutsch, "Measurement of Er:YAG laser ablation plume dynamics," *Appl. Phys. B* **52**, pp. 217–224, 1991.
7. V. Venogopalan, N. S. Nishioka, and B. B. Mikic, "Thermodynamic response of soft biological tissue to pulsed infrared-laser irradiation," *Biophysical Journal* **70**, pp. 2981–2993, 1996.
8. A. D. Zweig, M. Frenz, V. Romano, and H. P. Weber, "A comparative study of laser tissue interaction at $2.94\,\mu m$ and $10.6\,\mu m$," *Appl. Phys. B* **47**, pp. 259–265, 1988.
9. J. S. Young, "Evaluation of nonisothermal band model for H_2O," *J. Quant. Spectrosc. Radiat. Transfer.* **18**, pp. 29–45, 1977.
10. A. Vogel and W. Lauterborn, "Acoustic transient generation by laser-produced cavitation bubbles near solid boundaries," *J. Acoust. Soc. Am.* **84**(2), pp. 719–731, 1988.
11. M. Frenz, V. Romano, Y. D. Zweig, and H. P. Weber, "Instabilities in laser cutting of soft tissue," *J. Appl. Phys.* **66**(9), pp. 4496–4503, 1989.
12. M. Frenz, A. D. Zweig, V. Romano, H. P. Weber, N. I. Chapliev, and A. S. Silenoc, "Dynamics in laser cutting of soft tissue," in *Laser-Tissue Interaction*, vol. 1202, pp. 22–33, SPIE, 1990.
13. R. B. Randall, *Frequency Analysis*, Brüel & Kjaer, 1987.

SESSION 8

Ablation II

Hard Tissue Ablation Simulations using the LATIS Computer Code

D. S. Bailey, R. A. London and W. E. Alley

Lawrence Livermore National Laboratory
Livermore, California   94550

ABSTRACT

A simulation code for analyzing laser matter interactions is described in the context of short pulse laser ablation of hard tissue. Some experimental results on short pulse laser absorption are presented and used to motivate employing such systems for ablating biological tissues. Results of simulations of hard tissue drilling are given, including hydrodynamic response and ablation efficiency.

Keywords: ablation, hard tissue, simulation, short-pulse lasers

1. INTRODUCTION

In order to efficiently design and analyze laser-matter experiments, the laser-fusion program at LLNL has made use of computer modeling from the inception of the program. Using simulations allows one to explore a much wider parameter space (e.g., laser wavelength, pulse length, and pulse energy) than is feasible experimentally. It also gives more rapid convergence to an optimal set of parameters than would undirected experiments. We describe in this paper the use of such simulations to design experiments using short pulse lasers to produce ablation of hard biological tissue as an example of the application of such laser systems in a medical context.

To be useful in laser-matter interaction modeling, a computer program must treat the important physical processes involved. For medical applications, the three main categories are photo-chemical, photo-mechanical, and photo-thermal. To calculate these effects, one must consider laser light propagation, material changes due to photo-chemistry and coagulation, hydrodynamic motion, and thermal heat transport, as discussed in detail in a recent textbook.[1] We have developed a computer code named LATIS (for laser-tissue interaction) to realistically model these physical processes. This gives us a tool to accurately predict results of proposed experiments and to analyze the results of such experiments.

In this paper we give a short introduction to the capabilities of the LATIS program, and demonstrate its use in an application to ablation of hard biological tissues.

2. LATIS PROGRAM

LATIS is a two-dimensional, time-dependent simulation program based on more than twenty years experience modeling high-intensity laser-matter interactions for fusion research with the LASNEX[2] program. LATIS assumes cylindrical symmetry, with coordinates (r, z), on a logically connected quadrilateral (k, l) mesh. The positions and velocities are node centered, while the material quantities such as mass and energy are zone centered. Physical properties are modeled by partial differential equations, analytic formulas, and interpolated tables. The partial differential equations are solved by either finite-difference or finite-element methods, or in the case of laser propagation, with a Monte-Carlo method. For further information on LATIS, see a recent LLNL paper.[3] Here we will give some details on two newer packages not discussed in that paper, namely, an electromagnetic wave solver and a material strength package.

2.1. Electromagnetic wave solver

The wave solver[4] treats one-dimensional plane wave propagation for both S and P polarizations. It integrates the Maxwell equations through the problem mesh, with an option that uses a WKB method in low density zones ($\ll$ critical density), to permit zone sizes in such regions much larger than a laser wavelength (e.g., the plasma blow-off region). As a part of the solution, the phase of the electromagnetic wave is tracked and the total absorbed energy is calculated.

To get an accurate solution, it is important to have a good frequency dependent conductivity. The conductivity used here is obtained from solving the Boltzmann equation in the relaxation time approximation, including degeneracy

SPIE Vol. 3254 • 0277-786X/98/$10.00

effects at high density. It is designed to be correct in the quantum limit $h\nu/<\epsilon> \geq 1$ for high energy photons. There is also an option to include the effects of a band resonance, which is important for some metals (e.g., gold), and many dielectrics.

For dielectric breakdown, the Keldysh[5] ionization model is employed. This generates the initial electrons via multi-photon and tunneling processes. The further development is followed by integrating rate equations for the avalanche breakdown in the laser electric field. For the calculations presented here, the avalanche process saturated at one electron per atom. In reality, recombination processes limit the final electron density. We are in the process of adding recombination to the rate equations, since they decrease the rate of ionization as well as changing the steady-state electron density.

2.2. Material strength

To include material strength effects, we have added to LATIS a package the generalizes the scalar pressure hydrodynamic equations to a stress tensor for isotropic materials. This adds an extra constitutive parameter to the equations, beyond the bulk modulus supplied by the equation of state, namely the modulus of elasticity, μ. This parameter is specified by an analytic formula or table, and must be explicitly given by the user. To increment the stresses, a generalized form of Hooke's law is used, $\dot{s} = \mu(\rho, T, s, \ldots)\dot{\epsilon}$, where s and ϵ are the deviatoric stress and strain, and the dot denotes a time derivative. This permits a model for the elasticity coefficient that can include the effects of melting and material failure.

In order to obtain tensile restoring forces, special equations of state are required that allow negative pressures in some regions below solid or liquid density (i.e., in non-equilibrium, thermodynamically). However, in damaged or melted zones that don't have strength, one should use an equilibrium solution across the two-phase region that always maintains positive pressure. This is accomplished by using the well-known Maxwell construction. For room temperature solids, we use tables generated by the QEOS[6] program that can be set to have extra resolution near solid density and other regions important for the problem at hand. This permits quite good accuracy for the bulk modulus and sound speed near solid conditions, and can provide enhanced resolution along the melt curve at the cost of larger tables. For the particularly well known case of water, which is very important in biological simulations, we use the analytic NIST[7] fits to experimental data. These are much more accurate for the complicated phase system of water than would be possible for the analytic Cowan ion model used by QEOS.

There are several mechanisms available for treating material failure. An isotropic von Mises stress limit is used to treat plastic flow, which unloads to a state of finite strain. Static strain limits for both tensile and stress induced are provided, but there are options that allow for quite general yield limits, including rate dependence, if desired. Finally, if the damage index exceeds the specified limit, the stresses are relaxed to zero, with an optional healing mechanism which is used for a material such as water that can regain strength.

3. SHORT PULSE ABSORPTION

Understanding how the laser interacts with biological tissues is essential to model experiments involving such tissues. In particular, we need to understand the absorption process. Since we are proposing the use of short pulses to minimize collateral damage, some recent LLNL experiments,[8] (see Fig. 1) are relevant. At a laser intensity of 10^{13} W/cm^2 they show a moderate 25% absorption for normal metals like aluminum, but $\geq 40\%$ for others such as gold. For dielectrics, the absorption is over 85%. The explanation for the enhanced absorption in both cases is believed to be an optical band resonance (that gives gold its color), which in the dielectric case is at a much lower energy than the band gap. This is discussed in a paper by Arnold and Cartier.[9] As illustrated in Fig. 2, we then obtain two absorption regions in such a case: the normal metallic plasma of ≈ 1000 Å, and a bulk region (due to the band absorption) that is comparable to the laser wavelength in extent. The bulk heating, aside from increasing the laser absorption, ensures that the deeper region (if not melted directly), can be more easily removed by the subsequent shock wave. Since the deep absorption stops once the electron density becomes overcritical for the laser, knowing the relevant ionization and recombination rates is very important in order to predict the overall laser absorption and how the energy is distributed below the surface.

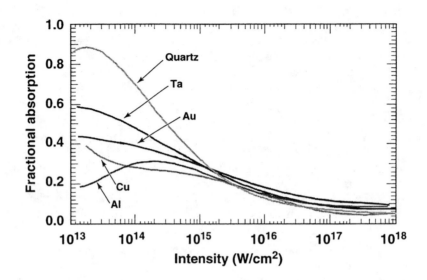

Figure 1. LLNL short pulse absorption results

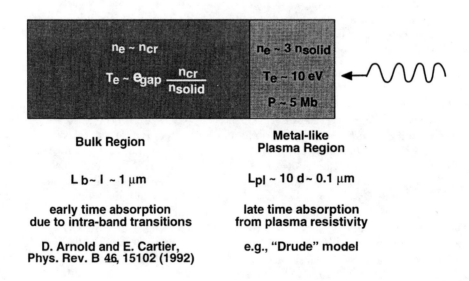

Figure 2. Skin depth and bulk absorption regions

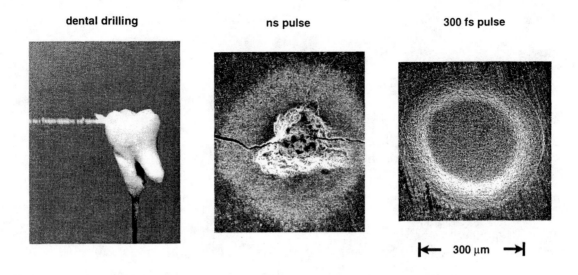

dental drilling **ns pulse** **300 fs pulse**

$\longmapsto$ 300 μm $\longrightarrow|$

Figure 3. Comparison of long and short pulse ablation results

4. HARD TISSUE ABLATION

As shown in Fig. 3, from Ref. 10,the use of short pulse laser ablation leads to much cleaner drilling of hard tissue. Similar results have been achieved in soft tissue experiments at LLNL, as discussed in Ref. 10. We want to discuss some details of how the ablation process occurs in hard tissue experiments. First, we delineate the time scales involved, since the various processes involved separate into three distinct classes:

1. laser propagation and absorption

   - $t \approx t_{pulse} \approx$ 300 fs
   - $r_{spot} \gg l_{abs} \Rightarrow$ 1-D wave propagation

2. hydrodynamic ablation

   - $t \approx l_{abs}/c_s \approx$ 30 ps
   - $r_{spot} \gg l_{abs} \Rightarrow$ 1-D hydrodynamics

3. whole tooth thermal calculation

   - $t \approx r_{spot}^2/\kappa \approx$ 1 sec
   - $r_{spot} \approx l_{thermal} \Rightarrow$ $\geq$ 2-D thermal transport

We will only consider the first two regimes in this paper. For the simulations done here, Fig. 4 illustrates the problem setup, and indicates that we need much finer (sub-micron) zones near the surface for the propagation calculation than is needed for the hydrodynamics.

4.1. Laser absorption

We used the parameters shown in Table 1 to calculate the laser absorption with the wave solver. Since we did not have recombination effects included in the rate equations, the intra-band transitions did not enhance the total absorption. This was due to the rapid rate of ionization, which raised the electron density above critical before the extra absorption could make an effect. This is illustrated in Fig. 5, which shows the time history of the surface electron density and absorption compared to the laser pulse. The spatial distribution of the absorbed energy is shown in Fig. 6, which clearly shows a small surface region heated to a few eV, and a larger bulk region at a much lower temperature. The absorption values given in Table 1 show an increasing trend with shorter wavelengths.

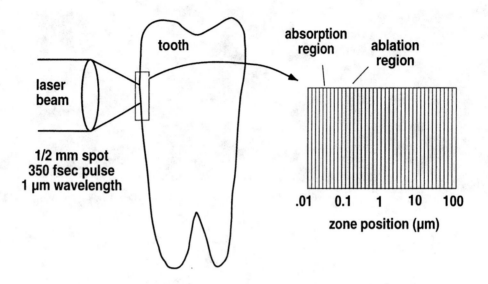

Figure 4. Problem zoning for laser drilling simulation

Table 1. Input parameters and laser absorption results

Laser intensity	$\approx 10^{13}\ W/cm^2$
Pulse width	300 fs
Band gap	5 eV
Melt temperature	.15 eV
Resonance oscillator strength	10.5
Resonance energy	3.8 eV
Resonance width	2.3 eV

Absorption results

Wavelength	$3\ \mu m$	$1\ \mu m$	$.1\ \mu m$
Average	18%	24%	34%
Maximum	28%	44%	63%

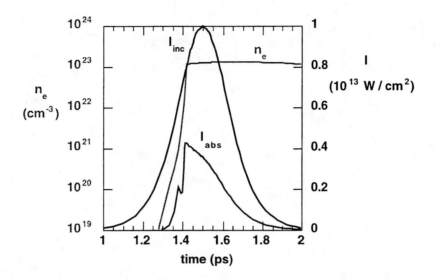

Figure 5. Time history of laser pulse, electron density and absorption

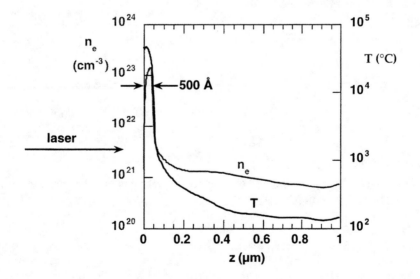

Figure 6. Spatial distribution of absorbed laser energy

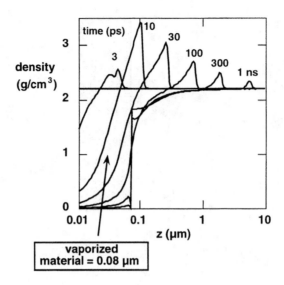

Figure 7. Density profiles at several times

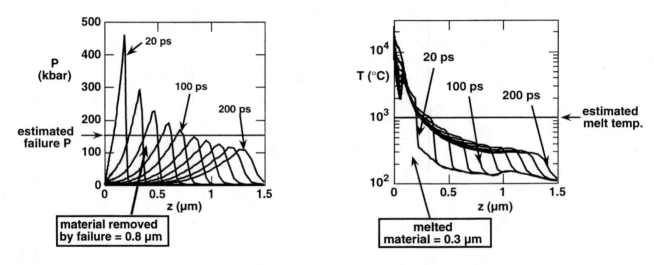

Figure 8. Damage due to over-pressure and melting

4.2. Hydrodynamic response

The high temperatures of a few eV at the surface produce high pressures at solid density, reaching several hundred kilobars. This drives a strong shock into the bulk region, as the surface plasma blows off. This shock wave both compresses and heats the bulk region, causing material failure. The effects on density are shown in Fig. 7, where the density is plotted versus space at several times much later than the laser pulse. To estimate the amount of damaged material, we show in Fig. 8, the amount of material removed due to over-pressure effects and material melting. The limits shown are estimates, and need to be validated by more experiments, but the magnitude is a large fraction of a micron, which is the canonical value quoted by the experimentalists for a single laser pulse. The very clean holes shown in Fig. 3 lead us to believe that the damaged region was melted.

4.3. Ablation efficiency

The efficiency of the ablation process is defined as the ratio of the material removed to the absorbed laser energy. We desire high efficiency to lower the required laser energy (and therefore cost), but also to limit the collateral damage.

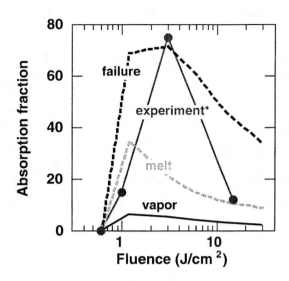

Figure 9. Material removal efficiency versus fluence

In a medical context, extra energy means excess heat, which damages more tissue than desired. To show the efficiency trend versus fluence, we plot in Fig. 9, the results based on the damage estimates in Section 4.2, compared to some experimental results of Neev.[11] The simulation results show the same efficiency trend as the experimental ones, but are lower, and being based on early damage estimates need refinement. It is very clear the vaporized surface material cannot explain the results, some extra damage mechanism is required.

5. SUMMARY

We have presented our current picture of short pulse laser ablation. To summarize the paper, we list the status and future improvements.

The fundamental mechanisms have been identified:

Laser absorption is due to a multi-photon initiated plasma and is enhanced by optical intra-band transitions.

Mechanical coupling is a result of the plasma generated shock wave propagating into the bulk material.

Mass removal at the surface is vaporization, while in the bulk melting and material failure are the causes.

Thermal coupling is driven by the bulk heating in the under-dense plasma and the subsequent enhancement from the shock passage.

Experiments are needed to improve model:

The amount of absorbed and reflected energy for each material of interest is needed to calibrate the absorption parameters.

Pressure and temperature measurements are desirable to check damage limits and thermal conductivities.

Accurate equations of state are important since their results determine the hydrodynamic response and the magnitude of thermal effects.

Desired improvements to model:

We want a self-consistent melting and failure model which will include phase change effects..

We are in the process of adding the effects of recombination on ionization balance.

The intra-band absorption model needs to be refined by the inclusion of collisional coupling to the free electrons.

We remain confident that short pulse laser ablation will prove a useful tool in biomedical applications that require accurate drilling with minimal collateral damage.

ACKNOWLEDGMENTS

This work was performed under the auspices of the U. S. Department of Energy by the Lawrence Livermore National Laboratory under Contract No. W–7405–Eng–48.

REFERENCES

1. A. J. Welch and M. J. C. Van Gemert, *Optical-Thermal Response of Laser-Irradiated Tissue*, (Plenum, New York, 1995)

2. G. B. Zimmerman and W. L. Kruer, "Numerical simulation of laser-initiated fusion", *Commun. Plasma Phys. Controlled Fusion*, **11**, pp 51-61 (1975)

3. R. A. London, M. E. Glinsky, G. B. Zimmerman, D. S. Bailey, D. C. Eder, and S. L. Jacques, "Laser-tissue interaction modeling with LATIS", *J. Appl. Optics*, **36**, pp 9068-9074 (1997)

4. W. E. Alley, "A Maxwell equation solver for the simulation of moderately intense ultrashort pulse laser experiments", *UCRL-LR-105821-92-4 (LLNL, Livermore, CA)*, pp 160-165 (1992)

5. L. V. Keldysh , "Ionization in the field of a strong electromagnetic wave", *Sov. Phys. JETP*, **20**, pp 1307-1314 (1965)

6. D. A. Young and E. M. Corey , "A new global equation of state for hot, dense matter", *J. Appl. Physics*, **78**, pp 3748-3755 (1995)

7. L. Haar, J. S. Gallagher, and G. S. Kell, *NBS/NRC Steam Tables*, (Hemisphere, Washington D.C., 1984)

8. D. F. Price, R. M. More, R. S. Walling, R. L. Shepard, R. E. Stewart, and W. E. White, "Absorption of ultrashort laser pulses by solid targets heated rapidly to temperatures 1-1000 eV", *Phys. Rev. Lett.*, **75**, pp 252-255, (1995)

9. D. Arnold and E.Cartier, "Theory of laser-induced free-electron heating and impact ionization in wide-band-gap solids", *Phys. Rev.*, **B46**, pp 15102-15115, (1992)

10. L. B. Da Silva et al, "Comparison of soft and hard tissue ablation with sub-ps and ns pulse lasers",in *Laser-Tissue Interaction VII*, Steven L. Jacques, Editor., Proc. SPIE **2681**, pp 196-200, (1996)

11. J. Neev, L. B. Da Silva, M. D. Feit, M. D. Perry, A. M. Rubenchik, and B. C. Stuart, "Ultrashort pulse lasers for hard tissue ablation", *IEEE Sel. Topics in Quantum Elect.*, **2**, pp 790-800, (1996)

Fabrication of biosynthetic vascular prostheses by 193 nm excimer laser radiation

W. Husinsky[a], C.Cseköö[a], A. Bartel[a], M. Grabenwöger[b], F. Fitzal[b] and E. Wolner[b]

[a]Institut für Allgemeine Physik, University of Technology Vienna, Wiedner Hauptstraße 8-10, A-1040 Wien, Austria
[b]Department of Cardio-Thoracic Surgery, University of Vienna, Währinger Gürtel 18-20, A-1090 Wien, Austria

ABSTRACT

This study was undertaken to investigate the feasibility of transmural capillary ingrowth into the inner surface of biosynthetic vascular prostheses (Omniflow™) through perforations created by an excimer-laser, thus inducing an endothelial cell coverage. The biosynthetic vascular prostheses (10 cm length, 6 mm $\varnothing$) were perforated with an excimer laser ($\varnothing$ of the holes 50-100 µm, distance 4 mm) and implanted into the carotid arteries of 8 sheep. The laser tissue interaction process of 193 nm radiation ensures minimal thermal damage to the prostheses. They were compared to untreated Omniflow™ prostheses implanted at the contralateral side. 3 month after implantation the prostheses were explanted and evaluated by gross morphology, histological examination and scanning electron microscopy. Scanning electron microscopy showed endothelial cells in the midgraft portion of all perforated prostheses, whereas collagen fibers, fibrin meshwork and activated platelets formed the inner layer in 6 out of 8 untreated Omniflow™ prostheses. It can be concluded, that spontaneous endothelialization of biosynthetic vascular prostheses can be achieved by transmural capillary ingrowth through perforations in the wall of the prostheses in an experimental sheep model.

Keywords: Laser Ablation, UV-Lasers, Non-thermal Ablation, Cardio-Thoraic Surgery, Biosynthetic vascular grafts - Endothelialization -transmural capillary ingrowth

1. INTRODUCTION

Long-term patency of synthetic peripheral vascular prostheses is still not satisfying, especially when small diameters and long length are required [1]. The superior performance of autologous vein bypasses as compared to synthetic graft materials is due to the thromboresistance of the autologous material which is provided by a layer of endothelial cells [2].

In order to establish a biologically active, thromboresistant endothelial cell layer on the inner surface of prosthetic grafts, one-stage endothelial cell seeding techniques as well as two-stage "in-vitro endothelialization" procedures were developed [3, 4]. Until now these very time-consuming and difficult techniques failed to enter the clinical practice.

The most obvious way to obtain an endothelial cell layer on the inner surface of vascular grafts would be the spontaneous endothelial cell ingrowth. Poor biocompatibility of the prostheses as well as the long distance from the host artery are suggested to be responsible for the lack of endothelial cells in the midgraft region. Transmural capillary ingrowth from the surrounding tissue through the wall of vascular grafts may provide a source of endothelial cells at the inner graft surface [5, 6].

We have performed studies to evaluate the feasibility of transmural capillary ingrowth through perforations in the wall of biosynthetic vascular prostheses (Omniflow™) in order the achieve an endothelial cell coverage of the inner graft surface. The perforations have been produced by 193 nm excimer laser radiation. The non-thermal character of UV - laser ablation with laser light at this wavelength [7-10] offers the possibility to perforate the grafts with high precision and minimal damage of the non-perforated material. Methods to study the nature of laser ablation processes in more detail are for example laser postionization combined with time of flight (TOF) mass analysis.

2. NON - THERMAL LASER ABLATION

2.1 CLASSIFICATION OF ABLATION MECHANISMS AND THEIR CHARACTERISTICS

Studies on model systems as well as measurements of tissue ablation have established three different mechanisms for how the energy deposited by the laser photons into electronic transitions of the tissue molecules can be converted into kinetic energy of the desorbing molecules. The specific characteristics of these mechanisms then critically determine the damage induced in the tissue surrounding the interaction zone of the laser light with the tissue.

„Thermal" ablation is observed whenever the photon flux is sufficiently high to heat the tissue by conversion of electronic excitations into vibrational energy. An explicit threshold flux for ablation and strong damage induced in the surrounding tissue is characteristic for this process. For practical use, situations in which thermal ablation occurs should be avoided. „Photochemical (non-thermal) ablation", on the other hand shows extremely low damage, due to the strong localization of the energy. The direct conversion of electronic energy into fragmentation happens on a time scale short enough to avoid thermalization and does not create vibrating („heated") molecules. This process in its pure form should not exhibit a flux-threshold for ablation. However, it is not quite understood whether the fragmentation can happen only at the topmost layer or whether bond-breaking in several layers of the tissue can take place accompanied by immediate ejection of the molecules. In all cases rather low ablation rates are expected. This seems to be confirmed by experimental data, if one compares the ablation rates with those achieved by other mechanisms. However, typical ablation rates of a few μm/pulse demand the bond-breaking to evolve in a corresponding large volume of the tissue.

A third mechanism has also been experimentally identified, which is basically of thermal nature, but differs from the conventional thermal ablation in that it requires extremely high heating (energy deposition), resulting in „explosive ablation" of the irradiated material. The main difference of this mechanism as compared to the thermal situation is the fast time scale in which the energy is transformed to kinetic energy, not allowing the unwanted thermal energy transfer to not-irradiated tissue. This makes this mechanism interesting for practical applications.

Ultra-short-pulse lasers at visible wavelength may be a potential alternative to excimer lasers for non-thermal tissue ablation. The use of lasers with visible wavelengths would have substantial advantages over far-UV lasers if a damage zone in the same or, even better, in a smaller range can be achieved. Moreover, wavelengths in the visible and near UV range would make glass or quartz fibers applicable, thus facilitating surgical use. The processes involved in femto-second ablation are still not fully understood, but multiphoton processes might play a substantial role [11, 12].

2.2. INVESTIGATIONS OF ABLATION MECHANISMS

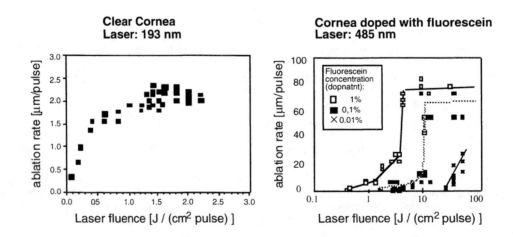

Fig. 1: Typical Ablation rate vs. Laser Fluence curves for two different ablation mechanisms

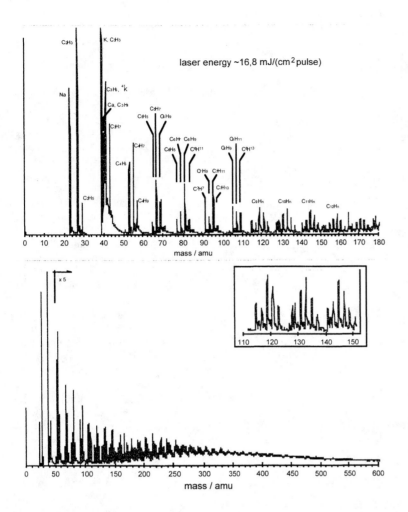

In this context only a short summary of various possibilities to investigate the nature of laser ablation mechanisms can be given. It should also be stated, that in spite of intensive investigations over the last couple of years, the understanding is still very rudimentary and a detailed model not available. The major type of investigations are represented by measurements of the *ablation rates vs. laser intensity* for different parameters. These investigations have been performed for many materials and many laser wavelengths. The obtained ablation rates are fundamental for many applications, since most of them rely on them as fundamental input parameter. Furthermore, the particular shape of the ablation curves (i.e. threshold, slope) yield important information concerning the ablation mechanism. An example is given in Fig. 1. The ablation rate for ablation of corneal tissue with 193 nm laser light is characterized by a low threshold and low ablation rates, which is typical for photochemical ablation. On the other hand, ablation of corneal tissue with light at 485 nm can only be achieved, if special absorbers are introduced into the tissue (in this case fluorescein dye). The resulting explosive ablation, which by the way can also be achieved by light around 3µm and water as absorbing medium, is cha–racterized by high ablation rates and a distinct ablation threshold.

Measurements of the total ablation rate, as described above, are relatively easy to perform, but the information obtained about the details of the processes involved in the ablation is limited. More detailed information can be obtained by measuring the partial ablation rate (*individually ablated masses*) and their energy. Only few investigations of this kind have been performed so far [13]. The following difficulties arise in connection with experiments of this kind: a) the measurements have to be performed in vacuum, b) most of the ablated particles are neutral. In our laboratory we have recently started with investigations, measuring the mass distribution of sputtered particles from biological samples for laser ablation and ion bombardment [14]. In a first step ablated ionic and neutral particles have been measured for interaction of 193 nm laser light with bone- and cartilage-tissue. The measurements have been performed with a time-of-flight system described elsewhere [15]. As an example, in Fig. 2 the mass spectrum of ions ablated from bone tissue during interaction with 193 nm laser radiation is shown. It is interesting to observe, that the mass spectrum for laser ablated ions is quite similar to the mass spectrum of ions „sputtered" under ion bombardment. Since the energy deposited per volume is of the same order of magnitude, we can conclude that both types of radiation must result in comparable inelastic excitations, which cause the particle removal. Since the majority of ablated particles are, however, neutral it is important to measure the neutral particles as well. For this purpose, laser postionization [16-18] can be used. The mass spectrum in Fig. 2 implies that it is important to avoid fragmentation of molecules by the laser radiation in order to obtain useful information. We have shown that using conventional laser radiation from an excimer laser would result in severe fragmentation of the molecules. We, therefore, plan to use femto-second laser pulses to minimize fragmentation [19-21] in the near future.

Fig. 2: Mass Spectrum of ionic particles ablated from bone tissue by 193 nm laser radiation.

243

3. EXPERIMENTAL SET-UP

3.1 PERFORATION OF GRAFTS

The outline of the experimental arrangement of the „Computer controlled Excimer Laser Biograft Ablation System" is shown in Fig. 3. The details of the beam delivery system in Fig. 4. Since the spatial intensity distribution of an excimer laser is not ideally gaussian and, furthermore, exhibits hotspots and a rectangular shape, it turned out to be essential to use an unstable resonator configuration in the Lambda Physics excimer laser. A system was developed which allows to use excimer laser (Lambda Physik, EMG 53 MSC) ablation at 193 nm for the perforation of the prostheses. The grafts themselves were mounted on a teflon rod which was rotated by a computer controlled stepper motor. A second stepper motor was installed for the movement of the graft in the horizontal axis. These two stepper motors (VEXTA PK 264-OlA, motorcontroler from AML) ensured the exact positioning of the excimer laser beam on the prostheses. A computer program controlled the entire perforation procedure. The system allows to perforate the biosynthetic vascular prostheses, which have typically a length of 10-15 cm more or less automatically. During the procedure the grafts can be moisturized to prevent drying. The pattern (number of holes per length and radius of the grafts) and the size of the holes can be varied. The diverging laser beam was spatially reduced by a diaphragm of 1 mm and then focused by a f = 120 mm quartz lens (Fig. 4). A repetition rate of 30 Hz and a laser energy of 100 mJ were used.

Fig. 5 shows the electron micrograph of a typical perforation in a biosynthetic vascular prostheses. The diameter of the holes could be varied from 40 to 70 µm.

3.2. VASCULAR IMPLANTS

In general anesthesia and under sterile conditions glutarldehydetanned ovine collagen composites (Omniflow), which were perforated with an excimer-laser as described above, were interposed end-to-end into the

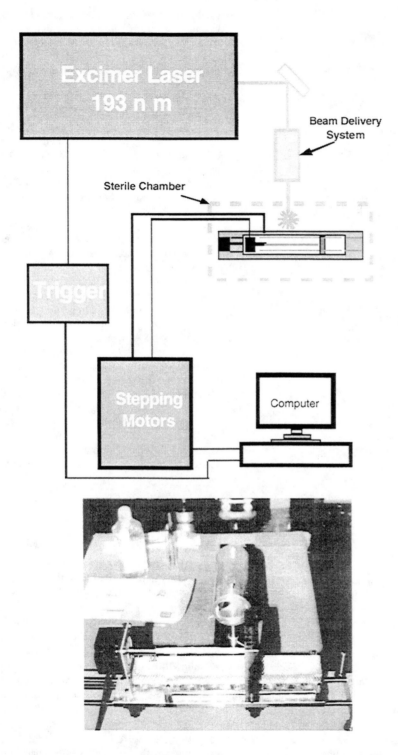

Fig. 3: Schematic of the experimental setup for computer controlled perforation of the vascular grafts. The photo shows the graft mounted during perforation.

carotid arteries of 8 male sheep (50-70 kg body weight). The prostheses were 10 cm in length and exhibit a diameter of 6 mm. On the contralateral side, untreated Omniflow prostheses were implanted as controls. Patency of the prostheses was checked using duplex Doppler sonography in the first and second postoperative week and after one and two month. 3 month after surgery the animals were anesthetized again and after intravenous administration of 20.000 IU heparin the prostheses were explanted, opened longitudinally, and flushed with Ringer s solution. At this point the animals were killed and the explants were subjected to further morphologic evaluation. All experiments were performed according to the Austrian law of animal experimentation.

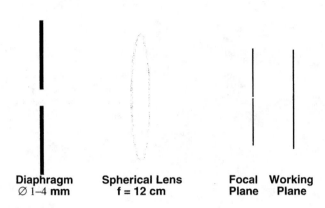

| Diaphragm | Spherical Lens | Focal | Working |
| ⌀ 1–4 mm | f = 12 cm | Plane | Plane |

Fig. 4: Schematic of Beam delivery system.

4. MORPHOLOGIC EVALUATION

Explanted vascular prostheses were rinsed in phosphate buffered saline and photographs were taken from the inner surface of the prostheses. Areas covered with red thrombotic material were evaluated in photographic prints at a magnification of 5x. Results were given as percentage of inner prosthetic surface. Specimens were excised from the proximal and distal anastomosis as well as from the midportion of the graft and prepared for further processing.

For light microscopy, immersion fixation was performed in 3% neutralized formalin. Specimens were routinely dehydrated and embedded in paraffin wax. Serial sections were cut at 6 μm thickness and alternately stained hematoxylin and eosin, Weigert 's resorcin fuchsin for elastic fibers, van Gieson's connective tissue stain for collagen fibers and Masson - Goldner's trichrom staining for connective tissue and smooth muscle cells.

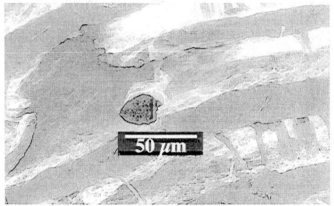

Immunohistochemistry was used to identify the nature of suspected endothelial cells and smooth muscle cells of neo-intimal layers. Sections were dewaxed and brought to water. Endogenous peroxidatic activities were blocked with 3% hydrogen peroxide in methanol. After pre-incubation with 2% goat serum in phosophate - buffered salt solution (PBS) at room temperature for 20 min, incubation with the first antibody solution lasted for 1 h at room temperature.

Fig. 5: Electron Micrograph of a typical perforation in a biosynthetic vascular prostheses.

5. RESULTS

All grafts remained patent after 3 month of implantation. Morphometric evaluation of the thrombus free surface revealed no significant difference between laser-perforated and untreated prostheses. However, scanning electron microscopy of the inner graft surface showed that in both groups the proximal and distal anastomosis were covered by a layer of endothelial-like cells. Cells were oriented in direction of the blood flow and exhibit typical microvilli at the surface. These cells were also observed in the midgraft area of all laser-perforated prostheses as shown in Fig. 6. In 6 out of 8 untreated prostheses collagen fibers of the original prosthesis formed the most inner layer at the midportion of the graft. Small areas were covered by single activated platelets and fibrin meshwork. The border between endothelial cells which spread from the adjacent artery and the "uncovered" midgraft area is shown in Fig. 7. Two untreated prostheses exhibit endothelial cells in the middle of the graft.

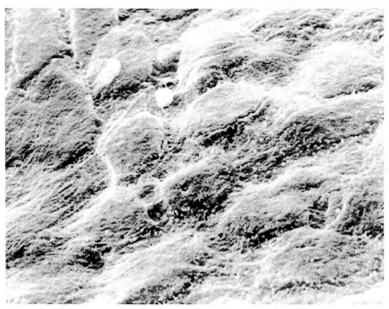

Histologic examination of the explants showed that three layers can be discerned: the adventitial layer, the implant proper and the neo-intimal layer. The adventitial layer was made up of loosely arranged connective tissue and well provided with a microvascular bed. The implant proper was characterized by the meshwork of synthetic fibers and tightly arranged coarse collagen fibers. Grouped macrophages and single foreign body giant cells were regularly seen on the surface of the synthetic fibers. Perforation sites were readily identified in the walls of the prostheses. Although now being filled with granulation tissue, the former channels were clearly defined as straight cylindrical defects in the coarse connective tissue walls. These defects showed straight course and constant width of about 50 to 100 µm. They were filled with highly cellular granulation tissue richly provided with capillaries and capillary sprouts.

Fig. 6: Scanning electron microscopy of perforated prostheses (x 1500). The midgraft area is covered by a layer of endothelial like cells.

6. CONCLUSIONS

This study shows that capillaries derived from granulation tissue surrounding the graft penetrate the wall through laser channels and provide multiple sources of endothelium at the luminal surface of the graft in a sheep model.

The Omniflow prosthesis showed a significant larger extension of neovascularization as compared to e-PTFE grafts. The favorable biocompatibility of Omniflow prostheses is substantiated by our finding of regular endothelial cell proliferation in-vitro. To investigate whether or not spontaneous endothelial cell ingrowth can be promoted in-vivo through the wall of the prosthesis, perforations were created by an excimer-laser. The hypothesis of capillary formation in laser channels is now under evaluation in cardiac surgery.

The perforations, created by the excimer laser used, measured between 50 and 100 µm in diameter. However, these multiple perforation channels never caused bleeding during or after implantation of the graft. Evidently, the channels were rapidly closed by red thrombi and these thrombi were replaced by granulation tissue later on. All perforated grafts showed endothelial cells in the midgraft region. These cells grew on a layer of myofibroblasts and not directly on the inner graft surface. Endothelialization in unperforated prostheses was limited to areas next to the anastomoses (proximal as well as distal anastomes) and microscopic examination failed to reveal endothelialization even in macroscopically smooth areas. The entire length of laser-perforated prostheses was covered with a smooth surface, macroscopically white appearing neo-intimal layer, while such a neo-intima was restricted to anastomotic areas in non-perforated prostheses. We suggest, that the formation of a neo-intimal layer is promoted by cellular components of the granulation tissue that replaces the initial thrombotic clots. Immunohistochemistry showed that neo-intimal layers in the grafts consist of myofibroblasts which most likely resemble

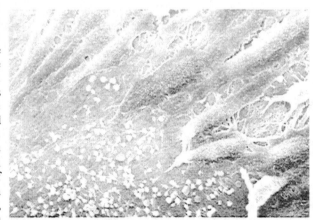

Fig. 7: Scanning electron microscopy of untreated prostheses (X 1000);A: Endothelial cell migration from the anastomotic area towards the midportion of the graft. Note deposition of activated platelets on the "uncovered" graft surface.

descendants of granulation tissue myofibroblasts. This assumption is supported by the observation that such neo-intimal areas are missing in unperforated prostheses. Moreover, the neointimal layer in perforated prostheses was almost entirely endothlialized.

In conclusion the study presented highlights the feasibility of transmural capillary ingrowth through perforations created by an excimer laser, thus supporting endothelial cell coverage of biosynthetic vascular prostheses in sheep.

7. ACKNOWLEDGMENTS

The work was supported by the "Fond zur Förderung der wissenschaftlichen Forschung" grant numbers P 09637 - MED and P 10928 PHY and by the "Ludwig Boltzmann Institute for Cardiosurgical Research".

8. REFERENCES

1.   J.F. Veith, S.K. Gupa, E. Ascer, S. Weith-Flores, R.H. Samson and L.A. Scher, "Six year prospective multicenter randomized comparison of autologous saphenous vein and expanded polytetrafluoroethylene grafts in infreinguinal arterial reconstructions", *J Vasc Surg*, **3**, pp. 104-114, 1986

2.   J.B. Chang and T.A. Stein, "The long-term value of composite grafts for limb salvage", *J Vasc Surg*, **22**, pp. 25-31, 1995

3.   M. Kadletz, H. Magometschnigg and E. Minar, "Implantation of in-vitro endothelialized polytetrafluoroethylene grafts in human beings", *J Thorac Cardiovasc Surg*, **104**, pp. 736-742, 1992

4.   M.B. Herring, A.L. Gardner and J.A. Glover, "A single stage technique for seeding vascular grafts with autologous endothelium", *Surgery*, **84**, pp. 498-504, 1978

5.   A.W. Clowes, T.R. Kirkman and M.A. Reidy, "Mechanism of arterial graft healing", *Am J Pathol*, **123**, pp. 220-230, 1986

6.   A.V. Sterpetti, W.J. Hunter, R.D. Schultz and C. Farina, "Healing of high-porosity polytetrafluoroethylene arterial grafts is influenced by the nature of the surrounding tissue", **111**, pp. 677-682, 1992

7.   W. Husinsky, S. Mitterer, G. Grabner and I. Baumgartner, "Photoablation by UV and Visible Laser Radiation of Native and Doped Biological Tissue", *Applied Physics B - Photophysics and Laser Chemistry*, **49**, pp. 463-467, 1989

8.   W. Husinsky, G. Grabner, I. Baumgartner, F. Skorpik, S. Mitterer and T. Temmel "Mechanisms of Laser-Ablation of Biological Tissue" Desorption Induced by Electronic Transitions, DIET IV, Kranichberg, Austria, 1990.

9.   R. Srinivasan and B. Braren, "Ultraviolet laser ablation and etching of polymethyl methacrylate sensitized with an organic dopant.", *Appl. Phys. A*, **45**, pp. 289, 1988

10. R. Srinivasan, J.J. Wynne and S.E. Blum, "Far-UV photoetching of organic material", *Laser Focus*, **19**, pp. 62, 1983

11. F. Loesel, M. Niemz, J. Bille and T. Juhasz, "Laser-induced optical breakdown on hard and soft tissues and its dependence on the pulse duration - experiment and model", *IEEE Journal of Quantum Electronics*, **32**, 10 pp. 1717-1722, 1996

12. W. Kautek, S. Mitterer, J. Kruger, W. Husinsky and G. Grabner, "Femtosecond-Pulse Laser Ablation of Human Corneas", *Applied Physics A - Solids and Surfaces*, **58**, 5 pp. 513-518, 1994

13. M. Tsunekawa, S. Nishio and H. Sato, "Multiphoton ionization mass spectrometric study on laser ablation of polymethylmethacrylate and polystyrene at 308 nm", *Japanese Journal of Applied Physics Part 1 - Regular Papers Short Notes & Review Papers*, **34**, 1 pp. , 1995

14. A. Bartel, "LSNMS and SIMS for studying the interaction of UV-LAserlight with biological tissue", [Diploma Thesis]. Kepler University; 1997.

15. O. Kreitschitz, W. Husinsky, G. Betz and N.H. Tolk, "Time-of-Flight Investigation of the Intensity Dependence of Laser-Desorbed Positive Ions from SrF2", *Applied Physics A - Solids and Surfaces*, **58**, 6 pp. 563-571, 1994

16. M.J. Pellin, C.E. Young and D.M. Gruen, "Multiphoton ionization followed by time-of-flight mass spectroscopy of sputtered neutrals", *Scanning Microscopy*, **2**, 3 pp. 1353-1364, 1988

17. M.J. Pellin, "Laser ionization of sputtered atoms: trace analysis of samples with atomic dimensions", *Pure & Appl. Chem.*, **64**, 4 pp. 591-598, 1992

18. W. Husinsky and G. Betz, "Fundamental aspects of SNMS for Thin Film Characterization - experimental studies and computer simulations [Review]", *Thin Solid Films*, **272**, 2 pp. 289-309, 1996

19. C. Weickhardt, C. Grun, R. Heinicke, A. Meffert and J. Grotemeyer, "The application of resonant multiphoton ionization by sub-picosecond laser pulses for analytical laser mass spectrometry", *Rapid Communications in Mass Spectrometry*, **11**, 7 pp. 745-748, 1997

20. G. Nicolussi, M. Pellin, K. Lykke, J. Trevor, D. Mencer and A. Davis, "Surface analysis by SNMS - femtosecond laser postionization of sputtered and laser desorbed atoms", *Surface & Interface Analysis*, **24**, 6 pp. 363-370, 1996

21. T. Freudenberg, W. Radloff, H. Ritze, V. Stert, K. Weyers and F.H.I. Noack, "Ultrafast fragmentation and ionization dynamics of ammonia clusters", *Zeitschrift fur Physik D-Atoms Molecules & Clusters*, **36**, 3-4 pp. 349-364, 1996

Characterization of tissue processing with a continuous wave Tm:YAG laser at 2.06 μm wavelength

H. Lubatschowski[1], M. Fiebig[2], P. Fuhrberg[2], H.O. Teichmann[2], H. Welling[1]

[1] Laser Zentrum Hannover e.V., Germany
[2] LISA Laser Products OHG, Germany

ABSTRACT

Laser radiation in the mid infrared region is a promising tool for soft tissue processing due to its strong absorption in water. In this study, a cw Tm:YAG laser emitting at 2.06 μm was used for basic investigations. The laser has a maximum output power of more than 30 W. Fresh pig skin, liver and heart tissue were irradiated at different intensities (up to 65 kW/cm²) and irradiation times (400 ms to 20 s). As a delivery system a 400 μm quartz fiber was used in contact as well as in non-contact mode. The irradiated samples were examined by light and electron microscopy. The ablation efficiency on soft tissue was determined to about 0.3 mg/J. The thermal induced damage covered a region of 100 to 500 μm lateral and 500 to 1000 μm axial to the crater. With regard to its compact dimensions and high efficiency the cw Tm:YAG laser appears to be a promising alternative to the CO_2 laser especially when fiber transmission of the radiation is required.

Keywords: vaporisation, mid infrared, fiber transmission

1. INTRODUCTION

Up to now, the CO_2 laser is the only high power laser source emitting continous wave radiation with strong optical absorption in biological tissue. These features qualify the CO_2 laser for a variety of surgical applications in the field of general surgery, plastic surgery, dermatology, otorhinolaryngology and many other disciplines. However, the advantages of high water absorption, which enables the surgeon to precise micro surgical operations, take along significant problems regarding the delivery system of the laser radiation. At 10 μm wavelength no fiber optics are available, which satisfy all requirements for medical applications.

Looking for other wavelengths with high absorption in biological tissue or rather in water, one will find the erbium lasers at 3 μm wavelength (Fig.1). Cw-operation of erbium lasers was demonstrated by different groups [1,2], but the generation of several 10 W output power requires a great deal of cost. Besides the ZrF_4 optical fibers for radiation transport are very expensive as well and not suitable for applications with direct contact to the tissue.

At 2 μm wavelength where the absorption depth in biological tissue is still around 200 to 600 μm the radiation shows a very good transmission (<0,04 db/m) in conventional fused silica fibers. Beach et al. [3] have demonstrated cw operation at this wavelength with comparable small expenditure. Based on the concept of Beach, a diode pumped Tm:YAG laser system was realized emitting at 2.06 μm wavelength to characterize the effects of cw-2 μm radiation on biological tissue.

---

e-mail address of the author: hl@lzh.de

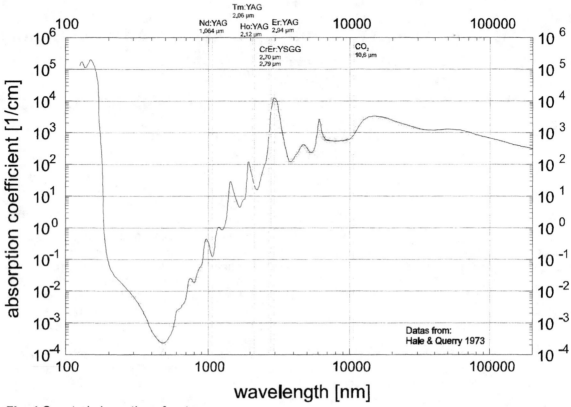

Fig. 1 *Spectral absorption of water*

MATERIAL AND METHODS

The setup of the laser system is shown in Fig. 2. The resonator consists of a 3 mm x 50 mm rod which is HR coated for the 2 µm radiation and AR coated for the 805 nm pump light and a concave mirror which acts as an output coupler. The pump light is focussed on the 805 nm AR coated rod end and guided through the rod by total internal reflection. This pump geometry leads to a homogeneous energy distribution inside the rod and avoids thermal problems.

The slope efficiency of the realized Tm:YAG laser is better than 25% resulting in an output power of more than 30 W. A beam quality of better than 15 mm mrad allows an efficient coupling of the laser energy into fiber optics. To characterize the laser tissue interaction, fresh pig skin, liver and heart tissue were irradiated at different intensities (up to 65 kW/cm²) and irradiation times (400 ms to 20 s).

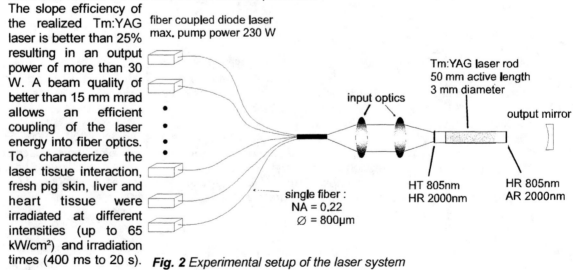

Fig. 2 *Experimental setup of the laser system*

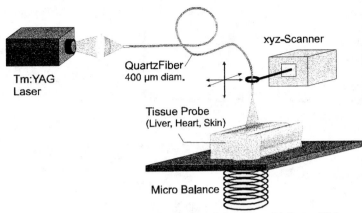

As a delivery system a 400 µm quartz fiber was used in contact as well as in non-contact mode. The distal fiber tip was fixed at a xyz-scanner in order to provide a defined irradiation pattern on the tissue surface.

The mass loss as a function of irradiated laser energy was determined with a micro balance (Fig. 3). The irradiated samples were examined by light and electron microscopy.

Fig. 3 *Experimental setup for determining the ablation efficiency*

RESULTS

Fig. 4 and 5 show the ablated mass as a function of irradiated laser energy on liver tissue at a laser power of 5 W and 10 W. The laser spot size on the tissue was 1.1 mm in diameter which corresponds to an irradiance of 0.5 kW/cm² and 1 kW/cm² respectively. At a scanning speed of 1 cm/s no carbonisation on the tissue was observed. The mass loss is quite linear with increasing deposition of energy for both irradiances with a similar slope which results in a constant ablation efficiency of 0.245 mg/J (see also Fig 6). Merely the onset of ablation is delayed for the lower irradiance.

At significantly higher irradiances the ablation efficiency increases, which is shown as an example for heart tissue in Fig. 7. At a constant laser power of 10 W, the tissue was irradiated once with the bare fiber end at a spot size of 1.1 mm diameter and an irradiance of 1 kW/cm² and second the light was focussed to a spot size of 140 µm in diameter leading to an irradiance of 65 kW/cm². The ablation efficiency increases from 0.238 mg/J at 1 kW/cm² to 0.338 mg/J at 65 kW/cm² but also the threshold for ablation increases 6 times higher from 200 J/cm² to 1200 J/cm².

The increasing ablation efficiency is probably due to the fact that at higher irradiances the ablation process is more disruptive. Larger particles like tissue fragments and water droplets leave the tissue without consuming vaporization energy. However, the higher ablation threshold can more likely be attributed to a geometrical effect. At a tighter focus the

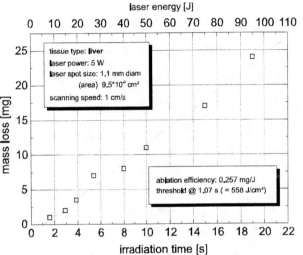

tissue type: liver
laser power: 5 W
laser spot size: 1.1 mm diam
(area) 9.5*10⁻³ cm²
scanning speed: 1 cm/s

ablation efficiency: 0.257 mg/J
threshold @ 1.07 s (= 558 J/cm²)

Fig. 4 *Ablation efficiency on liver tissue at a laser power of 5 W*

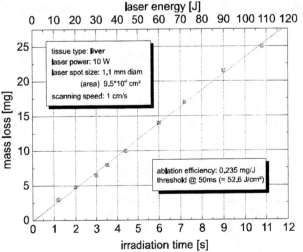

tissue type: liver
laser power: 10 W
laser spot size: 1.1 mm diam
(area) 9.5*10⁻³ cm²
scanning speed: 1 cm/s

ablation efficiency: 0.235 mg/J
threshold @ 50ms (= 52.6 J/cm²)

Fig. 5 *Ablation efficiency on liver tissue at a laser power of 10 W*

relation between the irradiated tissue volume and the surface through which the heat can dissipate into the non irradiated tissue is relatively high. Thus, due to the higher diffusion losses the threshold increases for smaller laser spot sizes.

The extent of thermal damage induced by cw - 2- μm laser irradiation is shown in Fig. 8. Here heart muscle tissue was irradiated with 10 W through a bare 400 μm fiber. The fiber was scanned across the tissue several times to perform a cut of 3 mm depth. The distance between fiber tip and tissue surface was kept constant to about 0.5 to 1 mm. As it can be seen on the histological section, the amount of thermally altered tissue is between 500 and 1000 μm.

Certainly, the collateral thermal damage is significantly reduced when the fiber is used in contact mode. In Fig. 9, a hole drilled in a heart muscle is shown as a histological section in a radial and an axial cut refered to the laser beam axis. The laser power at the end of a 400

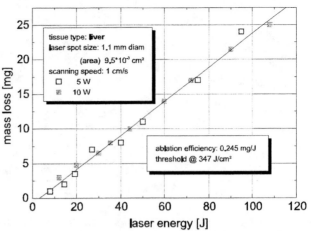

Fig. 6 *Ablation efficiency on liver tissue at a laser power of 5 and 10 W*

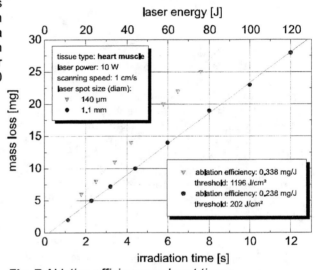

Fig. 7 *Ablation efficiency on heart tissue*

μm fiber was 10 W. The speed of the fiber advancement into the tissue was approx. 0.5 cm/s. This results in a collateral laser induced thermal damage of about 200 to 600 μm.

This damage zone can even be reduced by a faster advancement of the fiber tip which is demonstrated in Fig. 10. Here the fiber tip was put on the tissue's surface with a certain pressure. The pressure was chosen low enough, not to penetrate the muscle without any laser energy. Only during laser operation the fiber penetrates the tissue with a speed of approx. 1 to 2 cm/s. In this configuration the resulting collateral thermal damage is reduced to 100 μm or even less.

On pig skin a distinct shrinking effect was observed when the laser energy was irradiated with subablative fluence. Fig. 11 shows a histological section of skin, irradiated

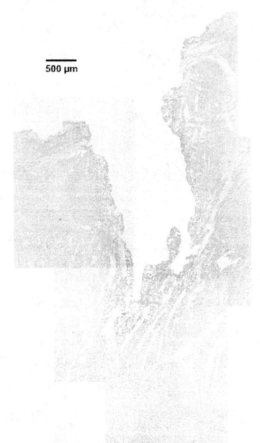

500 μm

Fig. 8 *Histological section of heart tissue irradiated with 10 W through a bare fiber (400 μm)*

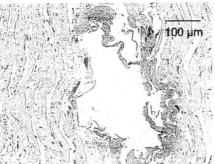

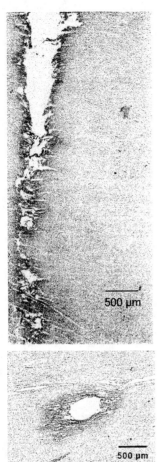

with approx. 300 W/cm² and a scanning speed of 2 cm/s. The collagen of the dermis is coagulated up to a depth of 400 μm.

Fig. 10 Exzision in a heart muscle (axial cut). The laser power at the fiber end (400 μm) was 10 W and the speed of the fiber advancement was approx. 1-2 cm/s.

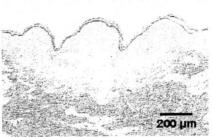

Fig. 11 *Histological section of skin irradiated with approx. 300 W/cm² and a scanning speed of 2 cm/s*

Fig. 9 Exzision in a heart muscle shown in a radial (top) and an axial cut (bottom). The laser power at the fiber end (400 μm) was 10W and the speed of the fiber advancement was 0.5 cm/s

CONCLUSION

The presented cw Tm:YAG laser is a very compact and efficient surgical tool with high output power and a good beam quality. The ablation efficiency of about 0.3 mg/J is comparable to the CO_2 laser radiation when similar laser parameters are applied. However, the thermal induced damage of 100 to 500 μm lateral and 500 to 1000 μm axial is clearly larger compared to CO_2 laser application. But still the cw Tm:YAG laser appears to be a promising alternative to the CO_2 laser especially when fiber transmission of the radiation is required.

Among other applications like cutting and drilling [4] the laser has the potential for a specific coagulation of tissue like tissue welding [5] or defined collagen shrinkage for orthopaedics [6] and skin resurfacing.

ACKNOWLEDGEMENT

This work was supported in part by the Bundesministerium für Bildung, Wissenschaft, Forschung und Technologie FKZ: 13N6548/7.

REFERENCES

1. Jensen T, Diening A, Huber G, Chai BHT; Investigation of diode pumped 2.8 μm $Er:LiYF_4$ lasers with various doping levels; Opt. Lett. 21(8),585-587 (1996)
2. Nikolov S, Daimler Benz AG, Forschung und Technik, Munich, personal communications
3. Beach RJ, Sutton SB, Honea EC, Skidmore JA, Emanuel MA; High power 2 μm diode-pumped Tm:YAG Laser; Proc. SPIE Vol. 2698,168 (1996)
4. Kadipasaoglu KA, Pehlivanoglu S, Conger JL, Sasaki E, de Villalobos DH, Cloy M, Piluiko V, Clubb FJ, Cooley DA, Frazier OH; Lang- and short-term effects of transmyocardial laser revascularisation in acute myocardial ischemia; Lasers Surg. Med. 20,6-14 (1997)
5. Cilesiz I, Thomson S, Welch AJ, Chan EK; Controlled temperature tissue fusion: Ho:YAG laser welding of rat intestine in vivo;Laser Surg.Med. 21,278-286 (1997)
6. Hayashi K, Markel MD, Thabit G, Bogdanske JJ, Thielke RJ; The effect of nonablative laser energy on joint capsular properties; Am.J.Sports Med. 23(4),482-487 (1995)

SESSION 9

Bubbles

A Scaling Model for Laser-Produced Bubbles in Soft Tissue

R. A. London[a], D. S. Bailey[a], P. Amendt[a], S. Visuri[a] and V. Esch[b]

[a] Lawrence Livermore National Laboratory, Livermore CA 94550
[b] Endovasix, Inc., Belmont CA 94004

ABSTRACT

The generation of vapor-driven bubbles is common in many emerging laser-medical therapies involving soft tissues. To successfully apply such bubbles to processes such as tissue break-up and removal, it is critical to understand their physical characteristics. To complement previous experimental and computational studies, an analytic mathematical model for bubble creation and evolution is presented. In this model, the bubble is assumed to be spherically symmetric, and the laser pulse length is taken to be either very short or very long compared to the bubble expansion timescale. The model is based on the Rayleigh cavitation bubble model. In this description, the exterior medium is assumed to be an infinite incompressible fluid, while the bubble interior consists of a mixed liquid-gas medium which is initially heated by the laser. The heated interior provides the driving pressure which expands the bubble. The interior region is assumed to be adiabatic and is described by the standard water equation-of-state, available in either tabular, or analytic forms. Specifically, we use adiabats from the equation-of-state to describe the evolution of the interior pressure with bubble volume. Analytic scaling laws are presented for the maximum size and duration of bubbles as functions of the laser energy and initially heated volume.

1. INTRODUCTION

Laser produced vapor bubbles are important in many fields of laser medicine. They occur in cardiology in the applications of thrombolysis and angioplasty, in ophthalmology in the study of damage threshold, and in urology in lithotripsy, to mention a few applications. The effects of the vapor bubble can be either desired–as in the case of emulsifying clots in thrombolysis or undesired–as in the case of damage to the eye.

Recently, much theoretical and experimental work has been done on elucidating the mechanisms of bubble formation, the dynamics of bubbles, and the effects on ambient soft tissue. In this paper we present a scaling model with the main goal of calculating the maximum bubble size for various input parameter values. The bubble size is of interest, as a characteristic parameter which indicates how much tissue is effected. In some cases we can equate the maximum volume of the bubble to the removed tissue volume.

Our goal is to develop a simple and computationally quick model which enables estimates of the maximum bubble size and bubble duration. This allows us both to understand the bubble dynamics on a fundamental level and to perform quick surveys of parameter space for the purpose of designing systems for various applications. The scaling model which we have developed to attain this goal is intermediate in complexity compared to various theoretical models which have been discussed in the literature.

The simplest model in the literature is the Rayleigh cavitation bubble model[1]. This model describes the expansion and collapse of an empty bubble in an ideal incompressible liquid, given initial conditions. The often used result is the formula for the bubble expansion time (equal to the collapse time):

$$t_m \approx \sqrt{\rho_{ext}/P_{ext}} R_m \qquad (1)$$

where t_m is the expansion time (the m-subscript denotes the maximum bubble size), R_m is the maximum radius, ρ_{ext} and P_{ext} are the density and pressure in the medium external to the bubble. In the Rayleigh model there is no gas and therefore no pressure inside the bubble.

Our analysis extends the Rayleigh model by considering the gas inside the bubble and the pressure which it exerts on the external medium. By using a self consistent description of the creation of this gas by vaporization of liquid by the laser, and by using an accurate equation-of-state (EOS) to describe the evolution of the energy and pressure of the internal gas, we have constructed a model which allows a calculation of the bubble dynamics. In particular we can calculate the maximum bubble size and the time from the deposited laser energy, (Q_L), and the external medium parameters in limiting cases of short and long laser pulse length (t_L).

Many other models have been presented which include internal pressure and other effects in the Rayleigh model. Kirkwood and Bethe, and Plesset[2] have included acoustic emission, and recently Glinsky et al[3] included an improved treatment of acoustic emission as well as material strength and failure.

The most comprehensive models are the computational hydrodynamic simulations done by the Livermore and Los Alamos groups in the last few years[4]. These models include accurate EOSs, acoustic and shock wave emission, non-spherical effects, and most recently, material strength effects. These models serve both to verify simpler models, as well as to compare to and guide experiments. They also allow the study of complicated 2-D effects such as vorticity generation and the creation of jets on bubble collapse.

2. ELEMENTS OF BUBBLE SCALING MODEL

2.1 Assumptions.

Several basic assumptions are made in deriving the scaling model. The geometry is assumed to be 1-dimensional with spherical symmetry. The correspondence to a realistic geometry associated with optical fiber delivery is illustrated in Figure 1. The essence of the approximation is to equate the initial volume of the spherical bubble with the volume into which the laser energy is deposited by the fiber. We also assume that the bubble is created by vaporization of the water, rather than cavitation. This requires a minimum laser energy necessary to bring the heated volume to a temperature above the boiling point of the water.

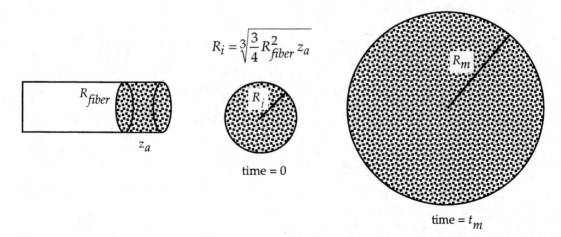

Figure 1. The deposition region for a fiber is approximated by a sphere of equal volume. R_{fiber} is the fiber radius and z_a the absorption length of the laser light in the fluid or tissue. The maximum bubble radius is R_m, reached at time t_m.

Another approximation is the neglect of heat conduction. We estimate that this is valid for heated volumes such that the heat conduction time ($R^2/4D$ where D is the thermal diffusivity) is greater than the Rayleigh time [Eq. (1)]. For properties of water, this occurs for R_i > .06 µm, which include all cases of practical interest. We also ignore acoustic emission, which is valid for moderate laser energy densities (Q_L < 3 kJ/g), but which breaks down for very high laser energy densities[5].

The model is based on two fundamental energy balance conditions, the first law of thermodynamics applied to the gas inside the bubble:

$$dQ = dE - PdV,$$ (2)

and the balance of the kinetic energy acquired by the external fluid with the net work done by the bubble

$$K_{ext} = W \equiv \int (P - P_{ext}) dV.$$ (3)

Here Q is the heat per unit mass, E the internal energy, P the pressure, and V the specific volume of the bubble interior, K_{ext} the kinetic energy of the external fluid, and W the net work done on the external fluid by the bubble. In addition we use an accurate EOS relating the pressure and energy of the internal gas to the temperature and density. This EOS is based on the NIST steam tables[6], and is used as a FORTRAN computer program. This is expected to accurately represent soft tissue, since water is the dominant constituent (75%). The main effect of the tissue is to provide a shear strength which inhibits the growth of the bubble. We include an enhanced external pressure equal to the failure stress of the material. This prescription has been shown to be a an approximate, yet valid way to model the strength of the tissue[3]. For typical soft tissues this value ranges from 1-10 bar.

2.2 Qualitative Behavior for Long and Short Laser Pulses.

We consider two limiting cases of the laser pulse length relative to a pressure equilibration timescale. Schematic illustrations of the bubble evolution are given in Figures 2a and b for the short and long pulse cases. In the case of long pulse, the pressure inside the bubble never greatly exceeds the external pressure, P_{ext}. The bubble grows in a near-equilibrium condition for the duration of the pulse. It reaches its maximum radius at the end of the laser pulse. Since the bubble does not overshoot its equilibrium radius as in the short pulse case, there is no real bubble collapse. The bubble may oscillate a bit about its equilibrium radius, and finally collapse when heat conduction cools the interior gas. In the short pulse case the laser energy is deposited before the bubble can expand very much. The pressure builds up during the laser pulse, typically to a value much larger than the external pressure. The bubble radius begins to grow. As the internal pressure drops below the external pressure, the inertia of the external fluid allows the bubble to continue to grow. The bubble radius overshoots the equilibrium radius achieved in the long pulse case. At a time t_m the bubble comes to rest at its maximum radius and then begins to collapse. The determination of the equilibrium time (t_{eq}) is made self-consistently from the short pulse solution given below.

2.3 Long Pulse Limit: $t_L >> t_{eq}$.

For long pulses we find the maximum bubble size by assuming that the bubble expands at a pressure equal to the external pressure. We also assume that the temperature inside the bubble is equal to the equilibrium boiling temperature, which is 100 °C for P_{ext} = 1 bar, but is somewhat larger for higher external pressure, e. g. 180 °C for P_{ext} = 10 bar. The latter assumption can only hold when the specific laser energy is less than the latent heat at constant pressure. For higher laser energies the temperature will rise above the boiling point. The essence of this derivation is that the laser first heats the water to the boiling point and then the remainder of the energy goes into making water vapor at the boiling point. Given these assumptions, we can integrate Eq. (2) to give:

$$\Delta Q_L = E_m - E_0 + P_{ext}(V_m - V_0) \tag{4}$$

where the subscript "o" indicates conditions before the laser pulse. We use Eq. (4) in conjunction with the EOS to solve for V_0 given Q_L, T_0 (the initial temperature), and P_{ext}. Finally we find the maximum radius from the cube root of the volume. Results are presented in section III.

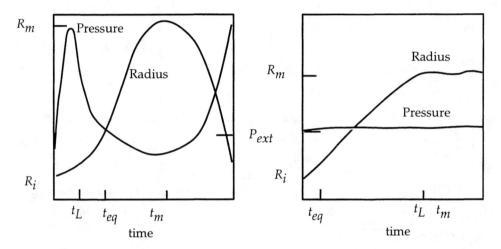

Figure 2a. Schematic representation of the time variation of the bubble radius and internal pressure for the short pulse case.

Figure 2b. Variation of the bubble radius and internal pressure for the long pulse case.

2.4 Short Pulse Limit: $t_L \ll t_{eq}$.

In the short pulse limit, we assume that the laser energy is deposited instantaneously– before the bubble can expand. Since no further heat is added, the following expansion is adiabatic. Before solving for the time-dependent bubble dynamics, we can easily calculate the maximum bubble radius by finding the conditions when the kinetic energy is zero. From Eq. 3, this occurs when the net work is zero:

$$\int (P - P_{ext})dV = 0. \tag{5}$$

We apply the first law (Eq. 2.) to the bubble in two steps. First it is used to equate the bubble internal energy immediately after the pulse to the initial internal energy plus the laser energy. Then it is applied in the adiabatic limit ($dQ = 0$) after the laser pulse up to the time of maximum expansion. The net result is an expression for the first term in the integral in Eq. (5):

$$\int P dV = (E_0 + Q_L) - E_m. \tag{6}$$

The 2nd term in the integral is straightforward since P_{ext} = constant. We express the result of the evaluation of Eq. (5):

$$E_m(V_m) = (E_0 + Q_L) + P_{ext}(V_m - V_0). \tag{7}$$

Equation (7) is used along with the EOS, and the adiabatic condition for $P(V)$, to implicitly solve for the maximum volume and radius. The solution is accomplished by a simple numerical searching method. A graphical picture of the determination of the maximum volume is shown in Figure 3. Since we are considering only the period of bubble growth, the specific volume parameterizes time. We see the monotonic drop in bubble pressure with time. At first the kinetic energy grows in time. This is called the acceleration phase of the bubble dynamics. When the pressure drops below the external pressure, the kinetic energy begins to decrease. This is called the coasting, or overshoot phase. The maximum bubble is reached when K_{ext} drops to zero. After this time the bubble collapses.

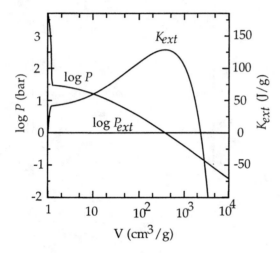

Figure 3. Variation of pressure and kinetic energy with specific volume, for P_{ext} = 1 bar. The curves follow an adiabatic expansion. The maximum bubble size is reached when the kinetic energy drops to zero, at $V = 4 \times 10^3$.

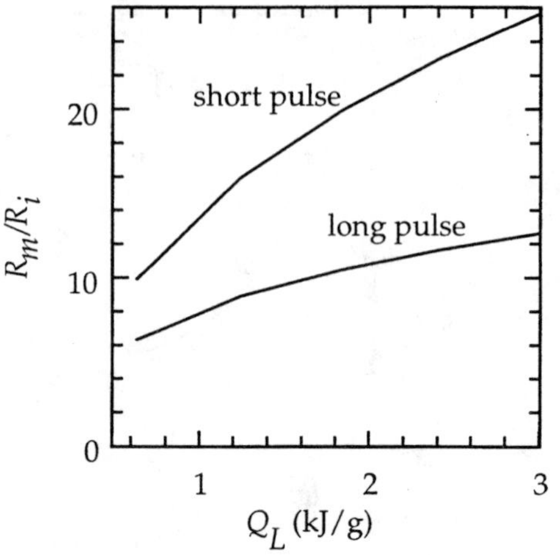

Figure 4. The maximum radius grows with specific laser energy deposition. Short pulses produce larger bubbles than long pulses. All cases have P_{ext} = 1 bar.

In the short pulse limit we can also find the time dependent bubble trajectory and therefrom, the equilibrium time and the time of maximum radius. We follow an analysis of the Rayleigh model extended to include an internal bubble pressure[7]. We first derive the kinetic energy of the external fluid to use in Equation (3). For an incompressible spherical flow in an infinite medium, the fluid velocity decreases as the inverse square of the radius:

$$u = \left(\frac{R}{r}\right)^2 \frac{dR}{dt},$$ (8)

where r is the radial coordinate of a point external to the bubble, and dR/dt is the velocity of the bubble boundary. The kinetic energy is found by integrating:

$$K_{ext} = \frac{1}{2}\rho_{ext}\int_R^\infty u^2 dV = 2\pi\rho_{ext}\left(\frac{dR}{dt}\right)^2 R.$$ (9)

The net work done by the bubble on the external fluid, minus that done by the stationary fluid far from the bubble is:

$$W = \int(P - P_{ext})dV. \tag{10}$$

Equating the kinetic energy to the work we find the following integral expression relating the bubble radius and time:

$$t = \sqrt{2\pi\rho} \int_{R_o}^{R} \left(\frac{R^2}{W}\right)^{1/2} dR. \tag{11}$$

Equation 11 can be evaluated at various radii to give the whole bubble trajectory during the expansion phase. The EOS is used along with the adiabatic condition relating $P(V)$.

3. RESULTS

In Figure 4, we show the maximum bubble radius versus specific laser energy for the long pulse and short pulse cases, using Eqs. (4) and (7) respectively. In both cases the radii grow increasing laser energy. The radii for short pulses are about twice as large as those for long pulses. This is due to the overshoot of the equilibrium radius which occurs in the short pulse.

For short pulses, we can also find the radius versus time, using Eq. (11). Results are shown in Figure 5, for three values of Q_L. The time is expressed in terms of a characteristic timescale, (essentially the Rayleigh time for the initial radius)

$$t_0 = \sqrt{\frac{\rho_{ext}}{P_{ext}}} R_i = 10\,\mu s\left(\frac{R_i}{100\,\mu m}\right)\left(\frac{P_{ext}}{1\,bar}\right)^{1/2}. \tag{12}$$

The equilibrium time t_{eq} is found from the trajectory for the short pulse case, and shown in Figure 6. For all cases it is approximately equal to the characteristic Rayleigh time for the initial heated volume, as given by Eq. (12).

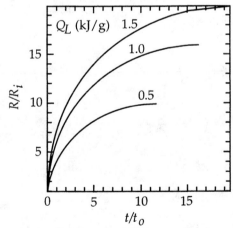

Figure 5. The bubble trajectory up until the time of maximum radius is shown versus time for three specific energy deposition values. All cases are for short pulses and P_{ext}=1 bar.

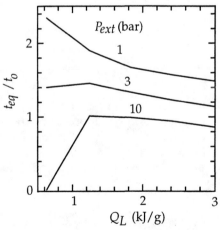

Figure 6. The pressure equilibration timescale is shown versus specific energy deposition for three values of the external pressure.

In Figure 7, we show the model results (R_m, t_m and t_{eq}) in dimensional units, choosing R_i = 50 μm and P_{ext} = 1 bar.

In Figure 8, we show bubble radii calculated with the LATIS[8] hydrodynamic simulation code compared to results of the scaling model in the short and long pulse limits. We see good agreement in both limits. In the short pulse limit the scaling model overpredicts the maximum bubble radius by 15%, probably due to its omission of acoustic radiation, which is included in the hydro model. In the long pulse limit, the hydro simulation oscillates about the scaling model prediction, as expected. Such comparisons give us confidence in the scaling models results for approximate estimates of the bubble radius for a wide range of parameters.

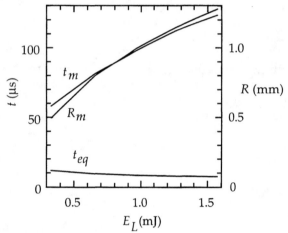

Figure 7. Maximum bubble radius, time of maximum and equilibrium time versus laser energy for a 50 μm radius deposition region.

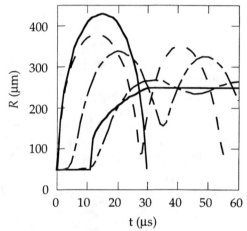

Figure 8. The scaling model compares well with numerical simulations. The dashed lines are LATIS results for laser pulses of 1 ns, 10 μs and 30 μs. The solid lines are the short and long pulse scaling model results

In summary, we have presented a scaling model which provide quick estimates of bubble dynamics. It is based on 1-D spherical geometry. It uses thermodynamic and kinetic energy conservation equations and a realistic equation-of-state. With this model we have identified the short and long pulse limits of bubble dynamics. We have been able to predict the bubble radius and duration for a wide range of input parameters. This model is useful for preliminary designs of laser produced bubble experiments for a wide range of applications.

4. ACKNOWLEDGMENTS

We thank L. B. Da Silva, M. Glinsky, D. Ho, and M. Strauss for helpful conversations concerning this work. This work was performed under the auspices of the U. S. Department of Energy by the Lawrence Livermore National Laboratory under Contract No. W-7405-Eng.-48.

5. REFERENCES

1. L. Rayleigh, "On the pressure developed in a liquid during the collapse of a spherical cavity," *Philos. Mag.*, **34**, p. 94-98, 1917.
2. J. G. Kirkwood and H. A. Bethe, "The pressure wave produced by an underwater explosion, I," OSRD Report No. 588, 1942. M. S. Plesset, "The dynamic of cavitation bubbles," *J. Appl Mech.*, **16**, p. 278-231, 1949.
3. M. E. Glinsky, P. A. Amendt, D. S. Bailey, R. A. London, and M. Strauss, "Extended Rayleigh model of bubble evolution with material strength compared to detailed dynamic simulations," in *Laser-Tissue Interaction VIII*, Ed.: S. L. Jacques, Proc. SPIE **2975**, p. 318-334, (SPIE, Bellingham, 1997).
4. M. Strauss, P. Amendt, R. A. London, D. J. Maitland, M. E. Glinsky, P. Celliers, D. S. Bailey, and D. A. Young, "Computational modeling of laser thrombolysis for stroke treatment," in *Lasers in Surgery VI*, Ed.: R. Anderson, Proc. SPIE **2671**, p. 11-21, (SPIE, Bellingham, 1996). P. Amendt, M. Strauss, R. A. London, M. E. Glinsky, D. J. Maitland, P. M. Celliers, S. R. Visuri, D. S. Bailey, D. A. Young, and D. Ho, "Modeling of bubble dynamics in relation to medical applications," in *Laser-Tissue Interaction VIII*, Ed.: S. L. Jacques, SPIE **2975**, p. 362-373, (SPIE, Bellingham, 1997). E. J. Chapyak, and R. P. Godwin, "A comparison of numerical simulations and laboratory studies of laser thrombolysis," in *Lasers in Surgery VII*, Ed.: R. Anderson, Proc. SPIE **2970**, p. 28-34, (SPIE, Bellingham, 1997).
5. A. Vogel, K. Nahen, J. Noack, S. Busch, U. Parlitz, and R. Birngruber , "Energy balance of optical breakdown in water," in in *Laser-Tissue Interaction IX*, Ed.: S. L. Jacques, Proc. SPIE **3254**, in press (SPIE, Bellingham, 1998).
6. L. Haar, J. S. Gallagher, and G. S. Kell, *NBS/NRC Steam Tables*, (McGraw-Hill, NY, 1984). An updated version by S. Klein and A. Harvey is available from NIST at: srdata@nist.gov.
7. R. T. Knapp, J. W. Daily, and F. G. Hammitt, *Cavitation*, Chap. 4, (McGraw Hill, New York, 1966).
8. R. A. London, M. E. Glinsky, G. B. Zimmerman, D. S. Bailey, D. C. Eder, and S. L. Jacques, "Laser-Tissue Interaction Modeling with LATIS," *Appl. Optics*, **36**, 9068-9074, 1997.

Simulations of shock waves and cavitation bubbles produced in water by picosecond and nanosecond laser pulses

Richard J. Scammon, Edward J. Chapyak, and Robert P. Godwin

Los Alamos National Laboratory
Los Alamos, NM 87545

Alfred Vogel

Medizinisches Laserzentrum Lübeck GmbH
D-23562 Lübeck, Germany

ABSTRACT

We compare numerical simulations of bubble dynamics in water with experiments performed at the Medizinisches Laserzentrum Lübeck. Spatial and temporal features of the laser beam were modeled. Plasma growth was predicted using a moving breakdown model. We compare the measured and calculated positions of the shock front and the bubble wall as a function of time after optical breakdown in water. Nd:YAG laser pulses of 30-ps 1-mJ and 6-ns 10-mJ were simulated. We have extended previous work in which picosecond deposition was modeled as temporally instantaneous and spatially uniform[1].

Keywords: bubble dynamics, cavitation, experimental and numerical hydrodynamics, shocks, laser medical applications

1. INTRODUCTION

Bubble dynamics and its associated shock waves, acoustic waves, and jetting, are important mechanisms in laser medical applications. The dynamics produce both intended medical effects and undesirable collateral effects. Multidimensional Eulerian compressible hydrodynamics codes are capable of modeling the shock waves and highly distorted flows associated with these applications. Combined with appropriate laser absorption models, material equations of state (EOS), tissue dynamics and tissue failure models, such codes can aid in understanding and optimizing clinical protocols in which bubble dynamics are an important consideration.

Vogel et al.[2-4] used time-resolved photographic methods to investigate shock wave and cavitation bubble expansion after optical breakdown in water using Nd:YAG laser pulses of 30-ps and 6-ns duration (full width at half-maximum) with energies typical of medical applications. They measured the position of the shock front and bubble wall position as a function of time with temporal resolution ~1-ns and spatial resolution ~4-μm. These high-resolution measurements provide excellent data for quantitative comparison with numerical simulations. Selected photos from the Medizinisches Laserzentrum Lübeck (MLL) experiments are reproduced in Figs. 1 and 2. The laser light is incident from the right.

In previous work by Chapyak et al.[1] the Los Alamos National Laboratory code MESA-2D was used to examine the MLL picosecond experiments assuming that the energy deposition was temporally instantaneous and spatially uniform. These assumptions worked well because there is little dynamic motion of the target material during energy delivery for the short pulse width. The excellent agreement of the calculations with the experimental data serves to validate both the numerical hydrodynamics of the MESA-2D code and the water equations of state used in the simulations.

SPIE Vol. 3254 • 0277-786X/98/$10.00

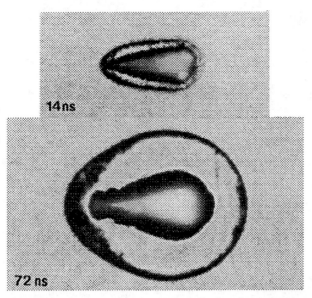

Fig. 1. Photographic records of the shock wave and bubble wall after the optical breakdown in water by a 6-ns, 10-mJ laser pulse in the MLL experiments. (The photos are not reproduced to the same scale.)

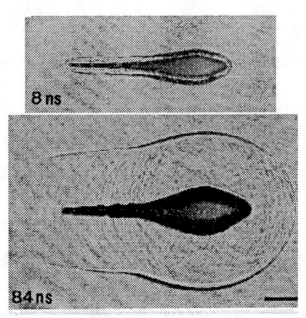

Fig. 2. Photographic records of the shock wave and bubble wall after the optical breakdown in water by a 30-ps, 1-mJ laser pulse in the MLL experiments. (The photos are not reproduced to the same scale.)

The principal purpose of the present calculations is to extend the previous work to include the 6-ns MLL experiments. For these experiments there is significant dynamic response of the target material during the laser pulse and we could no longer make the assumption that the energy deposition is temporally instantaneous and spatially uniform. In order to accomplish the simulation we modeled the temporal and spatial features of the laser beam, plasma ignition, plasma growth, and the deposition of the laser energy in the plasma. Relatively straightforward models were employed which are easy to implement and use but which ignore the detailed plasma physics. Plasma ignition and growth is predicted using a moving breakdown model while the laser energy deposition in the plasma is treated as an exponential function.

2. MESA-2D ENERGY DEPOSITION MODEL

In order to treat the temporal and spatial aspects of the laser energy deposition it was necessary to add a new model to the MESA-2D user-defined subroutines. The model accounts for the pertinent aspects of the laser experiments presented in Ref. 2; i.e., the beam focusing angle, Gaussian radial energy distribution and the experimentally determined energy rate.

The laser beam energy is tracked using constant-energy beam segments based on the Eulerian mesh at the beam focal plane and includes the Gaussian radial energy distribution. These "constant energy" segments are projected back toward the laser and used to follow the incoming energy. The model follows the beam out to 1.5 times the $1/e^2$ radius and thus tracks 98.9 % of the beam energy under the assumption that it is Gaussian.

Ionization is predicted using the moving breakdown model discussed in Refs. 3 and 4. It assumes that breakdown occurs independently at each location as soon as the irradiance of the electrical field surpasses the threshold value. At each time step in the calculation the energy irradiance is calculated as a function of time, and spatial location in the beam, with the result checked against the ignition threshold.

Energy deposition in the plasma is treated as exponential, as a function of distance from the leading edge of the plasma. No energy is deposited in cells that are below the breakdown threshold and laser energy is either absorbed or lost via transmission. Only minimal energy reflection was measured in the experiments[4] and thus none is included in the model. The model keeps track of the energy absorbed and lost.

References 3 and 4 report the ignition thresholds and absorption coefficients that were derived from experimental data. These were used as input parameters for the energy deposition model and are listed in Table I. Both values are treated as constants. The temporal evolution of the laser power P_L is described as a $\sin^2$ function with duration τ (full-width at half-maximum), and total duration 2τ.

$$P_L = P_{LO} \sin^2\left(\frac{\pi}{2\tau} t\right), \quad 0 \le t \le 2\tau$$

Table I. Laser parameters derived from experiments

	30-ps laser	6-ns laser
Breakdown irradiance threshold [3]	6.3×10^{11} W/cm^2	5.1×10^{10} W/cm^2
Exponential absorption coefficient [4]	360 cm^{-1}	900 cm^{-1}

Several alternative energy deposition options are included in the general model. All use the moving breakdown model to predict ionization but differ in the way in which the energy is distributed within the plasma. Options include uniform energy deposition in the plasma as a function of cell volume, or mass. Another option deposits energy as a function of volume in each beam segment but retains the Gaussian radial energy distribution across the beam segments. These options allow investigation, in a general sense, of the affects of energy redistribution within the plasma.

3. CONDITIONS FOR THE SIMULATIONS

The pertinent laser parameters for the experiments, as defined in Ref. 2, are listed in Table II. We used the same LANL SESAME[5,6] tabular water equation of state (EOS) that was used in the previous work. Identified as SESAME #7150, it is an equilibrium, Maxwell construction EOS that includes the effects of both phase changes and ionization. The simulations do not include the effects of viscosity or surface tension.

Table II. Laser experiment definition[2]

	30-ps laser	6-ns laser
Laser frequency	1064 nm	1064 nm
Laser energy	1 mJ	10 mJ
Laser energy at working volume	0.66 mJ	8.2 mJ
Energy lost in transmission[4]	14%	3%
Beam focusing angle [a]	14°	22°
Radius of spot at focal plane ($1/e^2$)	2.9 μm	3.8 μm
Radial energy distribution	Gaussian	Gaussian

[a] The full angle defined by the $1/e^2$ value of the intensity.

For the 6-ns case the computational zones (or cells) in the plasma region are uniform in size and square with $\Delta r = \Delta z = 0.5$ μm. This provides reasonable resolution of the energy deposition details with a little over 7 cells inside the $1/e^2$ radius at the focal plane. Outside of the plasma region the cell size is expanded geometrically by a multiplicative factor (or rezone ratio) of 1.03. The total number of computational cells is 1.23×10^5. The problem takes several hours to run on a CRAY Y-MP. A slightly finer mesh in the plasma region resulted in little change in the results with the exception of slightly smoother contour plots and significantly longer run times. Sensitivity of the results to the rezone ratio will be discussed below.

For the 30-ps case the computational zones in the region of the plasma are uniform in size and square with $\Delta r = \Delta z = 0.375$ μm. Again this provides a little over 7 cells inside the $1/e^2$ radius at the focal plane with the cell size outside of the plasma region expanded geometrically by a multiplicative factor of 1.1. The total number of computational cells is 1.7×10^5. The problem takes several hours to run on a CRAY Y-MP.

4. COMPUTATIONAL RESULTS AND COMPARISONS TO EXPERIMENT

As discussed above, the primary purpose of the present work was to simulate the 6-ns experiment where there is significant material motion during the laser pulse. In addition to the long pulse-width simulation we reran the 30-ps case using the new model to include the time dependent plasma dynamics and energy deposition.

The computed and measured maximum radial shock wave and bubble wall locations for the 6-ns, 10-mJ case are plotted as a function of time in Fig. 3. The shock wave location for the simulation was defined as the location of the 0.1 kbar pressure contour while the bubble wall was defined as coincident with the 0.98 g/cm^2 density contour. Agreement is reasonably good with the velocity of both the shock and bubble wall being a little higher than the experiment at the end of the calculation. The discrepancy of the starting position could be caused by differences between what is apparent in the photos versus what was selected as the edit in the code simulation.

Selecting the element size for the computational mesh is always a trade off, particularly for multidimensional simulations. Finer zones result in finer resolution at the cost of computer time that can result in run times that are cumbersome (long turn around) or prohibitive (cost or resources). The present calculation is a good demonstration of this and of how the velocity of the shock can be adversely affected by the mesh. As discussed previously, in order to minimize the total number of elements in the problem the cell size outside of the plasma volume is increased using a multiplicative factor. The original factor for this problem was 1.1. The resulting mesh tended to spread out the wave front resulting in apparent shock velocities that were unrealistically high. Switching to a rezone ratio of 1.03 more than doubled the computational time but resulted in more realistic shock velocities. The logical next step of further refining the mesh has not been done.

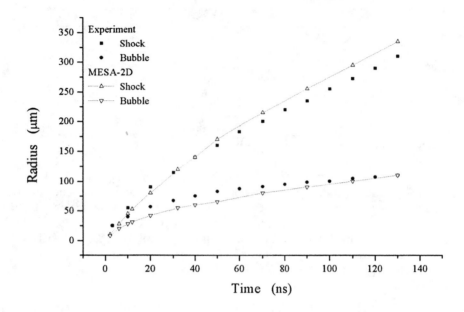

Fig. 3. Measured and computed locations of the shock wave and bubble wall as a function of time for the 6-ns case.

The energy distribution computed by MESA-2D is plotted in Fig. 4. The initial energy in the simulation is defined as zero for the purpose of the plot, it is not zero in the calculation. Figures 5 and 6 are the computed pressure and density as a function of the radius, at the plane of the maximum shock wave and bubble wall radius. The pressure profile at 90-ns shows considerable spreading of the shock front which is probably a function of the increasing mesh size even with the revised rezone ratio. Hydrocodes normally must spread the shock front over several cells to maintain calculational stability. The calculations can not handle an infinitely steep shock front. The density plot shows a high density region following the shock wave with a sharp decrease in density at the bubble wall.

Figures 7 and 8 are contour plots of the bubble wall (density = 0.98 g/cm^3) and the shock front (pressure = 0.1 kbar). These are roughly the computational equivalent of the experimental photos in Fig. 1. There are similarities but also a number of obvious differences in shape. The steps in the bubble contour in Fig. 7 are related to the beam segments used in the energy deposition calculation. The numerical instability or noise in the shock contour in Fig. 8 is essentially inherent in the computational process. It is not a function of the energy deposition model and does not affect the results. It is possible that refining the mesh would eliminate it but since the results are not affected, and considering the increased run time, this was not pursued.

A limited number of calculations were run to examine the sensitivity of the results to various input parameters and the optional energy deposition models. None of calculations resulted in a significant improvement however there are still a number of options to be investigated.

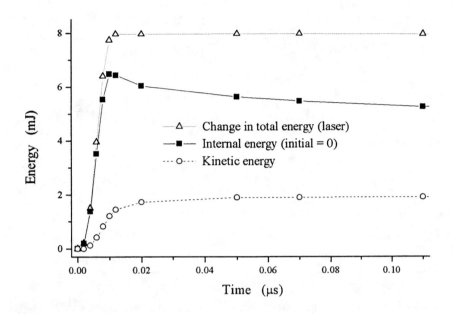

Fig. 4. Computed energy distribution as a function of time for the 6-ns case.

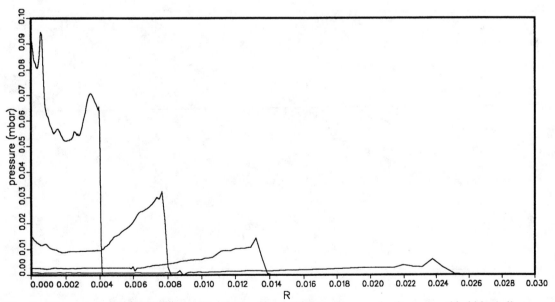

Fig. 5. Computed radial pressure profile, in the plane of the maximum shock wave and bubble wall radius, at 10, 20, 40 and 90-ns for the 6-ns case.

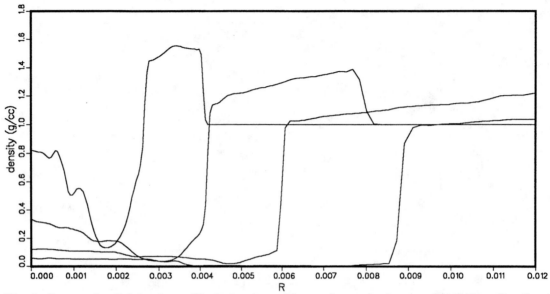

Fig. 6. Computed radial density profile, in the plane of the maximum shock wave and bubble wall radius, at 10, 20, 40 and 90-ns for the 6-ns case.

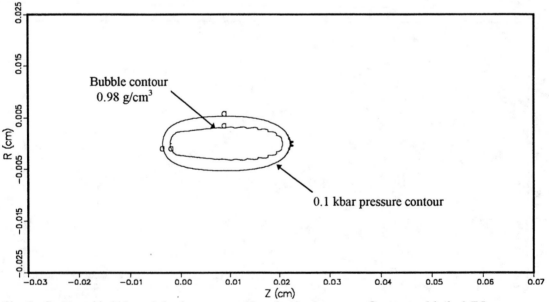

Fig. 7. Computed bubble and shock contour at 12-ns for the 6-ns case. Compare with the MLL photographs in Fig. 1.

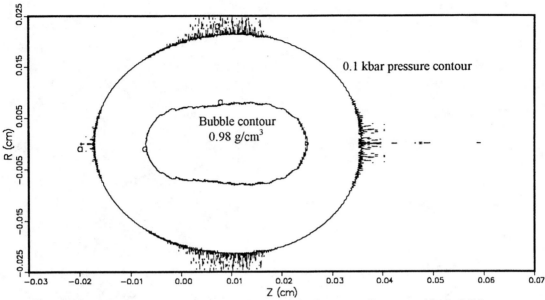

Fig. 8. Computed bubble and shock contour at 70-ns for the 6-ns case. Compare with the MLL photographs in Fig. 1.

The computed and measured maximum radial shock wave and bubble wall location for the 30-ps, 1-mJ case are plotted as a function of time in Fig. 9. Again the shock location for the simulation was defined as the location of the 0.1 kbar shock front while the bubble wall was defined as being coincident with the 0.98 g/cm² density contour. Agreement is quite good for the position and velocity of the shock front. However, there is rather poor agreement between measured and computed bubble wall position and velocity.

The reason for this discrepancy remains unclear. The model works for the 6-ns case and checks of the model as incorporated in the code have not revealed any problems. A limited input parameter study, including the various energy deposition options, did not result in marked improvement. The simulation plotted in Fig. 9 used the uniform-mass energy deposition option that distributes energy uniformly throughout the plasma volume as a function of cell mass at the time the energy is deposited. It provided marginally better results than the standard exponential deposition option. The lack of agreement may indicate that our relatively simple model is not an adequate representation of the laser-matter interactions in this experiment.

The energy distribution computed by MESA-2D is plotted as a function of time in Fig. 10. Figures 11 and 12 present the computed pressure and density as a function of the radius at the plane of the maximum shock wave and bubble wall radius. Again the pressure profile at 90-ns shows considerable spreading of the shock front. The density plot shows the low density region starting at the outside of the plasma region and working its way inward as the pressure is relieved.

Figures 13 and 14 are contour plots of the bubble wall and the shock front. These are roughly the computational equivalent of the experimental photos in Fig. 2. In this case the differences between the computed contours and the photos are more pronounced. Most obvious is the lack of a down-stream tail in the calculated contours. The tail is probably due to self-focusing in the medium in conjunction with self-defocusing inside the plasma. This cannot be modeled with the present energy deposition scheme. In the calculation, essentially all of the laser energy is absorbed in the plasma from the focal plane forward with none left to cause ionization down stream from the focal plane. The steps in the bubble contour in Fig. 13 are a consequence of the resolution of the beam segments used in the energy deposition calculation.

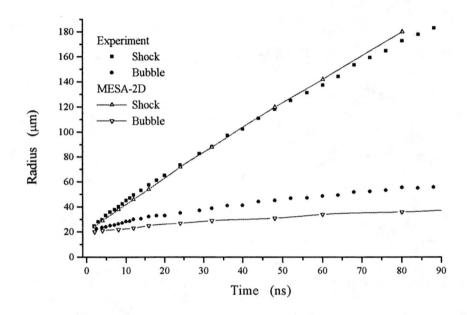

Fig. 9. Measured and computed locations of the shock wave and bubble wall as a function of time for the 30-ps case.

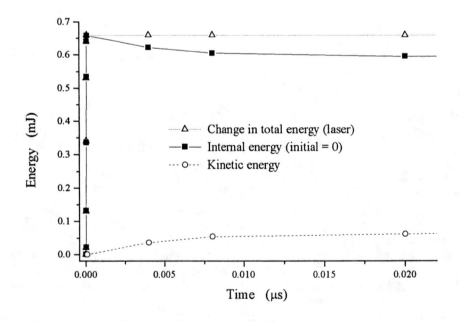

Fig. 10. Computed energy distribution as a function of time for the 30-ps case.

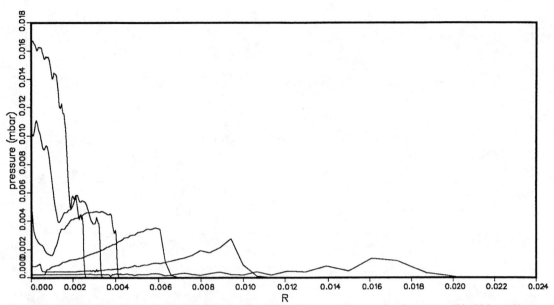

Fig. 11. Computed radial pressure profile, in the plane of the maximum shock wave and bubble wall radius, at 2, 6, 10, 22, 42 and 90-ns For the 30-ps case.

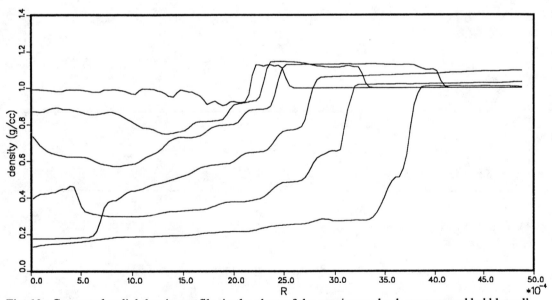

Fig. 12. Computed radial density profile, in the plane of the maximum shock wave an and bubble wall radius, at 2, 6, 10, 22, 42 and 90-ns for the 30-ps case.

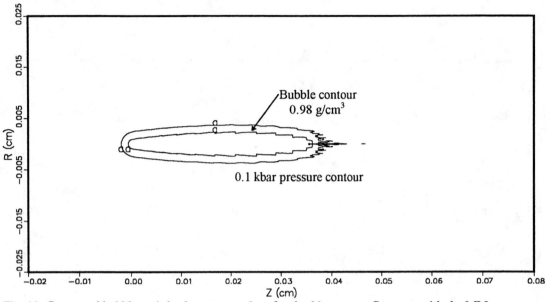

Fig. 13. Computed bubble and shock contour at 8-ns for the 30p-s case. Compare with the MLL photographs in Fig. 2.

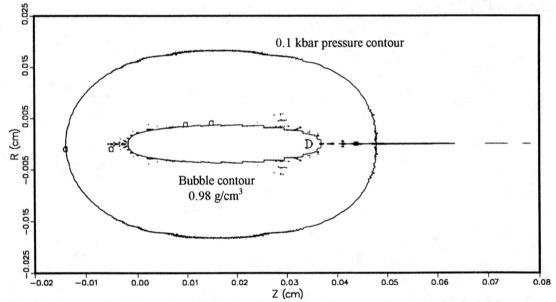

Fig. 14. Computed bubble and shock contour at 80-ns for the 30p-s case. Compare with the MLL photographs in Fig. 2.

5. CONCLUSIONS

We have simulated the dynamics produced by both 6-ns 10-mJ and 30-ps 1-mJ laser pulse plasma breakdown in water. The computed shock wave and bubble wall locations for the 6-ns case are in reasonable agreement with the measurements made at MLL. For the 30-ps case the shock wave predictions agree quite well with the measurement but there is a problem with the bubble size and bubble wall velocity. It is not clear if the discrepancy can be corrected by further work with the existing model or if the relatively simple model is not adequate to describe the physics associated with the 30-ps experiment. Both simulations would benefit from additional effort.

6. ACKNOWLEDGMENTS

A DOE Cooperative Research and Development Agreement (CRADA) between Los Alamos National Laboratory, Oregon Medical Laser Center, and Palomar Medical Technologies supported R. J. Scammon, E. J. Chapyak and R. P. Godwin.

7. REFERENCES

1. E. J. Chapyak, R. P. Godwin and A. Vogel, "A Comparison of Numerical Simulations and Laboratory Studies of Shock Waves and Cavitation Bubble Growth Produced by Optical Breakdown in Water," Laser Tissue Interaction VIII. *Proc. SPIE* **2975**, 335-342, 1997.
2. A. Vogel, S. Busch and U. Parlitz, "Shock wave emission and cavitation bubble generation by picosecond and nanosecond optical breakdown in water," *J. Acoust. Soc. Am.* **100**(1), 148-165, July 1996.
3. A. Vogel, K. Nahen, Dirk Theisen and J. Noack, "Plasma Formation in Water by Picosecond and Nanosecond Nd:YAG Laser Pulses - Part I: Optical Breakdown at Threshold and Superthreshold Irradiance," IEEE Journal of Selected Topics in Quantum Electronics, Vol. 2, No. 4, December 1996.
4. K. Nahen and A. Vogel, " Plasma Formation in Water by Picosecond and Nanosecond Nd:YAG Laser Pulses - Part II: Transmission, Scattering and Reflection," IEEE Journal of Selected Topics in Quantum Electronics, Vol. 2, No. 4, December 1996.
5. K. S. Holian, "T-4 Handbook of Material Properties Data Bases," Los Alamos National Laboratory report LA-10160-MS, 1984,
6. "SESAME: The Los Alamos National Laboratory EOS Data Base," S. P. Lyon and J. D. Johnson, Editors, LA-UR-92-3407, 1992.

Fluorescence-Based Temperature Measurement in Laser-Induced Vapor Bubbles

Kin Foong Chan[a], T. Joshua Pfefer[a], Daniel X. Hammer[a], E. Duco Jansen[b],
Martin Frenz[c], Ashley J. Welch[a]

[a]University of Texas at Austin, Austin, TX 78712
[b]Vanderbilt University, Nashville, TN 37235
[c]University of Berne, CH-3012, Switzerland

ABSTRACT

A fluorescence-based temperature probe (optrode) was designed to measure temperature within laser-induced vapor bubbles. The optrode consisted of a 400-μm optical fiber with a rhodamine B-doped polyurethane film attached to the fiber tip. The film exhibited a fluorescence decay time of 4 ns, and the measured fluorescence yield was temperature dependent in the range from 20 to 110 °C. A Ho:YAG laser ($\lambda = 2.12$ μm, $\tau_p = 250$ μs) with a pulse energy of 256 ± 7 mJ delivered through a fiber was used to produce the vapor bubbles. The bubbles reached maximum expansion 200 μs after the onset of the laser pulse and had an average lifetime of 350 μs. The temperature was measured by positioning the optrode within the vapor bubble and exciting its fluorescent film-coated tip with a nitrogen dye laser ($\lambda = 540$ nm, $\tau_p = 500$ ps). At maximum expansion, the temperatures in the vapor bubbles were approximately 61 °C, indicating sub-atmospheric saturated vapor pressures. The vapor pressure at maximum expansion was confirmed by Rayleigh's equation.

Keywords: Fluorescence-based temperature probe, optical fiber, rhodamine B, polyurethane film, pulsed Ho:YAG laser, nitrogen dye laser, Rayleigh's equation, mid-infrared pulsed laser-induced vapor bubble, fast-flash photography, bubble dynamics.

1. INTRODUCTION

The primary objective of this research was to quantify the transient temperature within pulsed ($\tau_p \sim$ ns to μs) infrared laser-induced vapor bubbles[1]. Previous studies suggested that the photomechanical mechanism was the major cause of laser-induced tissue damage in many clinical applications of nanosecond and microsecond pulsed mid- to far-infrared lasers. Unfortunately, dependent variables such as temperature, pressure, volume[1], work done, etc., of fast transient vapor bubbles were not investigated extensively. Even though several theoretical models of this combined photothermal and photomechanical mechanism were proposed, thermodynamic parameters were not confirmed.

It has been speculated that temperatures within pulsed mid-infrared laser-induced vapor bubbles are below the boiling point of water. The lowest temperature of the saturated vapor is expected at maximum expansion within pulsed laser-induced bubbles. This is mainly due to the overshoot of the expanding vapor volume from the 1 atm equilibrium pressure, as a result of intense initial pressure or momentum at the onset of bubble formation. As will be explained later, cavitation bubble theory best fits bubbles produced by short laser pulses (< 1 μs), where laser radiation is not present after the onset of bubble formation.

---

[a]Author contact information:
Kin Foong Chan, kfchan@ccwf.cc.utexas.edu
Department of Electrical and Computer Engineering, University of Texas at Austin, ENS 610; Austin, TX 78712, U.S.A.

The process of designing a temperature measurement system required consideration of various advantages and disadvantages of measurement configurations. Vapor bubble lifetimes in the range of 100 to 400 μs, and maximum bubble diameters on the order of 1 mm to 4 mm were produced by fiber optic delivery of Ho:YAG Q-switched and long pulse Ho:YAG with pulse energy from 100 mJ to 1 J. Small thermocouples (50-μm diameter) with a rise-time of 0.5 to 1.0 ms are not fast enough to follow rapid temperature changes expected inside an expanding bubble.

On the other hand, a 8-12 μm thermal camera cannot measure temperature within the vapor bubble because this device only measures IR surface radiation[2]. Other non-contact methods such as spatial filtering of thermal fields[3] leads to unacceptable signal-to-noise ratios, limited spatial resolution of the filters, and averaging of measured temperature in a one- or two-dimensional plane. An *in-vivo* method, utilizing laser-induced release of liposome-encapsulated dye[4] provides a possible means of point measurement, but requires long acquisition time from 40 ms to 5.5 s, and a limited operating temperature range between 40 °C and 62 °C. An optically-induced phosphorescence procedure[5,6] offers adequate intensity and high spatial resolution, but its time resolution is limited to about 200 μs due to the slow decay of electrons from a triplet excited state.

In this study, a rhodamine B-doped polyurethane fluorescent film was used for temperature measurement in laser-induced vapor bubbles[7]. The fluorescence decay time for rhodamine B was determined to be approximately 4 ns[7]. This temperature measurement technique provided high-speed temperature sensing at the tip of an optical fiber. The main disadvantage was the relatively large optrode dimension; the 400-μm fiber core diameter limited the spatial resolution. The rise-time of the sensor was limited by the thermal mass and resistance of the sensor at the tip of the optical fiber The fluorescent film used several chemical components[7]. Once the film was made, it was placed on an optical fiber tip. The fiber diameter defined the spatial resolution of the temperature optrode. The system setup of this temperature measurement technique, and the construction and performance of this temperature optrode are discussed in section 3.

2. THEORY

Rayleigh's derivation[8] on the collapse of spherical cavitation bubbles has been applied extensively to predict the pressure within pulsed laser-induced vapor bubbles[9,10,11,12,13]. However, the computation has been inconclusive due to difficulties in realizing an ideal experimental setup for producing spherical vapor bubbles without interference from the solid boundary introduced by the delivery fiber and/or long laser pulses that causes complications in the bubble dynamics. For these reasons, several theoretical and experimental attempts have been made to correct Rayleigh's equation[14,15]. Such corrections of Rayleigh's derivation will not be introduced in this work. Instead, the original equation is applied to analyze the experimental data. Further improvement or correction of the equation may be investigated in the future.

The pressure during maximum expansion of a vapor bubble induced by pulsed mid-infrared laser irradiation as given by Rayleigh's derivation[8] is,

$$P_v = P_o - \frac{\rho_o}{\left[\dfrac{t_c}{0.915 R_{max}}\right]^2} \tag{1}$$

where, P_v is the vapor pressure at maximum expansion, P_o is the pressure in the water at the bubble wall (101.5 kPa ~ 1 atm), ρ_o is the density of water (998 kg/m^3), t_c is the collapse/expansion time of the vapor bubble, and R_{max} is the bubble radius at maximum expansion. The only unknowns are the bubble collapse time and the maximum radius.

In our experiments, pulsed Ho:YAG laser irradiation was used to induce vapor bubbles. Several assumptions were made for comparison of the experimental results with the theoretical model. First, the theoretical model assumed an ideal spherical vapor bubble, and that the existence of vapor did not affect the outcome of the calculation. Second, it was assumed that there were minimum distortions of the bubble geometry and the thermal field due to the insertion of a temperature optrode. Third, the expansion time and the collapse time were assumed to be the same. Finally, it was assumed that the vapor pressure was uniform inside the bubble.

From previous studies of Q-switched Ho:YAG laser-induced vapor bubbles having a pulse duration of 500 ns[16], the expansion or collapse time was measured to be approximately 100 μs, while the maximum radius was around 891 μm. The study was conducted with an incident laser energy of 14 mJ that was delivered with a 200-μm fiber. For reasons to be discussed later, the ratio t_c/R_{max}, of vapor bubbles induced by a Q-switched mid-infrared laser at a specific wavelength, having a corresponding absorption coefficient in water, was found to be independent of the incident energy, or the radiant exposure. Hence, the ratio t_c/R_{max}, using previous experimental data, was calculated to be approximately 0.11 s/m for Ho:YAG irradiation in water. Substituting this value into equation (1), the pressure within the vapor bubbles at maximum expansion, P_v, was computed to be about 35.11 kPa.

The vapor pressure at maximum expansion can be related to the vapor temperature by introducing the gas equation[17].

$$T_v = \frac{P_v V_v^{\gamma}}{nR} \tag{2}$$

where, V_v is the vapor volume at maximum expansion, n is the amount of vaporized water in mole, R is the universal gas constant (8.31 J/mol.K), γ is the ratio C_v/C_p; C_v is the molar heat capacity at constant volume (J/mol.K), and C_p is the molar heat capacity at constant pressure (J/mol.K).

When saturated vapor occupies the bubble, the corresponding vapor temperature can be referred from the steam table[18] by the calculated vapor pressure from equation (1), without any need for further computation. The vapor temperature, T_v, at maximum expansion within the pulsed Ho:YAG laser-induced bubble was predicted to be between 69 °C to 75 °C.

For this experiment, a free-running pulsed Ho:YAG laser irradiation was used. The laser provided pulse durations (FWHM) from 200 μs to 300 μs, with adjustable output energies (< 2 J). Pulses delivered to water via an optical fiber resulted in an elongated vapor bubble (see 'Moses effect'[19]) rather than a spherical vapor bubble often produced by a Q-switched experiment. Although the free-running Ho:YAG laser did not provide the same t_c/R_{max} value as in the case of a Q-switched Ho:YAG laser, long pulses were applied due to a number of reasons. Since Q-switched pulse induced shock waves during bubble expansion and collapse[10,13], it was feared that the magnitude of these pressure waves (> 100 bars) may damage the temperature optrode. With limited resources to implement this fluorescence-based technique[7] for the first time, we were reluctant to take the risk. In addition, the free-running Ho:YAG modality was justified by two major assumptions stated below.

(i) Since the t_c/R_{max} value is independent of the amount of radiant exposure but specific to the laser wavelength, it can be taken from previous experimental results[16] performed using Q-switched Ho:YAG irradiation.

(ii) Temperature differences in the radial proximity of the free-running mode and the Q-switched mode-induced vapor bubbles are negligible for mid infrared radiation (we do not have evidence to support this assumption). This radial proximity can be identified as the highlighted regions in Figure 1.

Finally, it was presumed that the vapor bubble exhibits radial symmetry in either experimental modality discussed above.

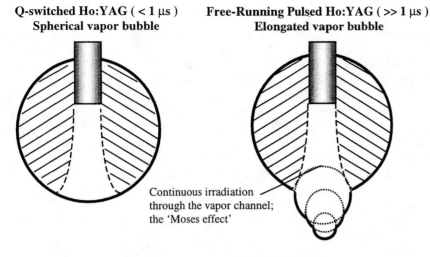

Q-switched Ho:YAG (< 1 μs)
Spherical vapor bubble

Free-Running Pulsed Ho:YAG (>> 1 μs)
Elongated vapor bubble

Figure 1. Experimental modalities of a Q-switched and a free-running Ho:YAG irradiation of water. Highlighted regions of the vapor bubbles are assumed to exhibit minimal differences in temperature.

Continuous irradiation through the vapor channel; the 'Moses effect'

3. METHODS

Fluorescence-based Temperature Probe

A rhodamine B-doped polyurethane fluorescent film, with a thickness of 1.4 μm (± 20 %) adherent to an aluminum substrate of 500 nm in thickness, was placed onto a 400-μm optical fiber tip with non-fluorescing glue, and sealed from harsh external environment with a thin layer (~ 10 μm) of epoxy on the fiber periphery. The coated tip was left exposed to the sensing environment to maximize temporal and spatial response of this optrode. The aluminum substrate, while acting as a protective layer, also optimized reflectance of fluorescence in its return path to the avalanche photodiode (Hamamatsu Module C5460 Series). The excitation source for the probe was a pulsed nitrogen-dye laser (λ = 540 nm; Laser Photonics LN1000 and LN102) with a pulse duration of approximately 500 ps/pulse operating below 2.0 Hz (the repetition rate was adjusted during the experiments, but during calibration of the probe the same repetition rate was used). The fluorescent film at the optrode was previously determined to exhibit a short fluorescence decay time of 4 ns[7], and the emitted fluorescence was centered at λ = 583 nm as shown in Figure 2. The optrode exhibited a linear decrease in fluorescence yield with increasing temperature (R^2 ~ 0.9852) in the range of 20 °C to 110 °C [20]. A schematic diagram of the temperature optrode is shown in Figure 3.

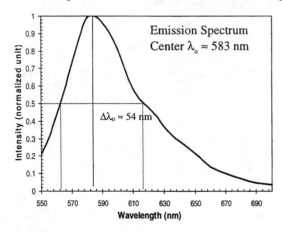

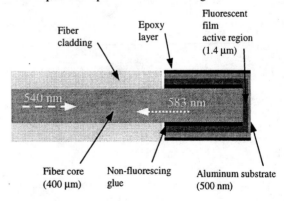

Figure 2. Measured emission spectrum of rhodamine B doped polyurethane fluorescent film and its full-width-half-maximum (FWHM) spectral bandwidth, $\Delta\lambda_o$, of 54 nm.

Figure 3. A schematic diagram of the fluorescence-based temperature probe (optrode).

Fast Flash Photography and Temperature Measurement System

Figure 4 illustrates the optical and electronic setup of the temperature measurement system for conducting statistical point measurements in laser-induced vapor bubbles. Through a GPIB communication bus, the computer was used to program the pulse generator (Stanford Research DG535) to send a series of eight trigger pulses to the Ho:YAG pulsed infrared laser (2.12 μm; Schwartz-Electro-Optics, Laser 1-2-3) in the free-running mode. Pulse energy was set above threshold for inducing a vapor bubble. Seven warm-up Ho:YAG laser pulses were launched to achieve thermal equilibrium in the laser cavity for reproducible pulse energy. Then, a final Ho:YAG laser pulse, triggered at time T_o, was directed through the fiber (400-μm diameter) to induce a vapor bubble in the water bath. At $T_o+\tau$, a trigger pulse was sent to the nitrogen-dye pulsed (540 nm) laser to provide excitation light for the temperature optrode. The excitation pulse also acted as a flash lamp for bubble imaging with a CCD camera. It was experimentally demonstrated that the flash lamp pulse did not interfere with the fluorescent film on the optrode since the fiber tip/fluorescent film was enclosed by an aluminum layer. The Ho:YAG irradiation created a fast transient vapor bubble in the water bath, while the temperature optrode, excited at delay time, τ, with respect to the rising edge of the infrared laser pulse, measured the temperature during the duration of the nitrogen-dye pulse. The temperature dependent fluorescence intensity, I_f, and the nitrogen-dye laser reference, I_r, were collected by an avalanche photodiode (APD) and an ultra-fast photodiode (PD; Hamamatsu S1722-02), respectively, and displayed on the 500 MHz digital oscilloscope (Tektronix TDS 640A). The GPIB communication bus then retrieved the signals over a period or time span of 500 ns.

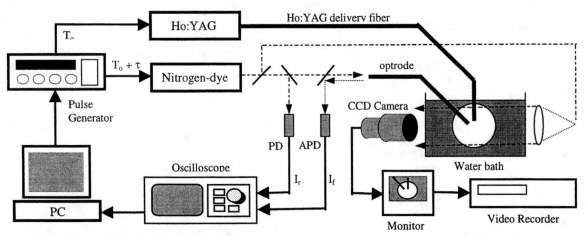

Figure 4. The fluorescence-based temperature measurement system setup. The computer-based software commands the pulse generator to trigger the Ho:YAG laser and the nitrogen-dye laser at difference delay times. The Ho:YAG laser generates a fast transient vapor bubble within the water bath, while the nitrogen-dye laser excites the florescent film at the optrode at the preferred delay time. The fluorescence yield is coupled to an avalanche photodiode via a dichroic beam splitter, and the signal-to-noise ratio is determined with respect to the reference photodiode. The computer retrieves the information and fits the data onto a calibration curve before outputing the measured temperature value. The nitrogen-dye laser also acts as the flash lamp for the fast flash photography system, where images are taken simultaneously with temperature measurements.

4. RESULTS

Bubble Dynamics by Fast-Flash Photography

Figure 5 illustrates the progress of vapor bubble formation by the free-running pulsed infrared Ho:YAG laser. In this experiment, the temperature optrode was placed at a 30-degree angle with respect to the infrared delivery fiber at a horizontal distance of 250 μm from the center of the delivery fiber core, and 200 μm below the fiber exit. The energy delivered was 256 ± 7 mJ, with a radiant exposure of 2.03 ± 0.06 J/mm^2, and an irradiated power of 792 ± 22 W. As can be seen in the figure, the temperature optrode was comparable in size to the delivery fiber, with a spatial resolution of 400 μm, measuring temperature over an area of 0.126 mm^2. As the vapor bubble expanded, the vapor-water boundary passed the temperature optrode tip 50 μs to 75 μs after the creation of the bubble or the time after initiation of the Ho:YAG laser pulse. The vapor bubble reached maximum expansion around 200 μs, after which it began to collapse. At about 300 μs, the vapor-water boundary once again passed the temperature optrode tip during the collapsing phase. The lifetime of the primary vapor bubble was between 325 μs and 350 μs.

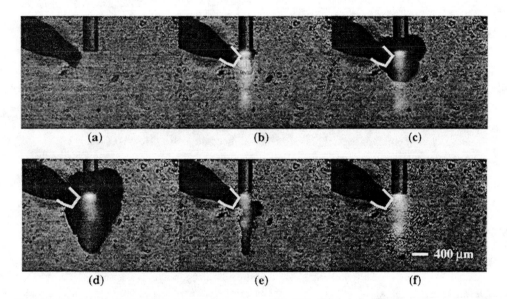

Figure 5. Fast-flash photography of events after the onset of pulsed Ho:YAG laser irradiation, where the vapor bubble expands and collapses. (a) control: no Ho:YAG irradiation (b) 25 μs: bubble expands at high initial pressure (c) 75 μs: expanding vapor-water boundary passes optrode sensing tip (d) 175-200 μs: maximum expansion (e) 300 μs: collapsing vapor-water boundary passes optrode sensing tip (f) 500 μs.

Transient Temperature Distribution at Fixed Location

Transient temperatures were measured simultaneously with fast-flash photography at various delay times, τ, with respect to the rising edge or initiation of the infrared pulsed laser irradiation. Ten measurements were made at each delay time. Figure 6 shows the results of the experiment. The overall standard deviation of this set of experimental data was calculated to be ± 2.24 °C, with a maximum standard deviation of ± 3.28 °C at 700 μs, and a minimum of ± 1.29 °C at 250 μs. The temperature remained near room temperature for times below 50 μs, but ascended rapidly after 75 μs. The temperature saturated between 61 °C and 65 °C, and prevailed until 300 μs, after which the temperature declined slowly over a period of 10 ms before settling at room temperature.

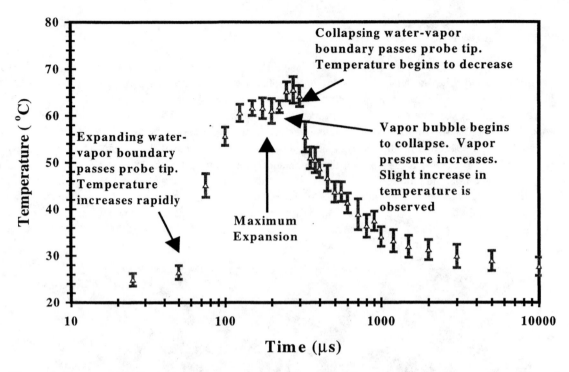

Figure 6. Temporal distribution of temperature measured at a fixed location. The time was measured from the creation of the bubble or the initiation of the pulsed Ho:YAG laser.

5. DISCUSSION

Bubble Dynamics

By utilizing fast-flash photography, snapshots of bubble formation, expansion, and collapse have been captured with an exposure time of 500 ps using collimated nitrogen-dye laser pulses. Previous studies[1] have indicated that superheating of water directly under the infrared delivery fiber at the onset of laser-irradiation created hot filaments related to changes in the liquid's index of refraction. This thermal effect resulted in partial vaporization of water (strictly has only been demonstrated for Q-switched pulses), forming micro-vapor bubbles at nucleation sites[1]. These bubbles were formed at high pressure (> 1 atmosphere) or by bipolar stress waves (with negative component due to acoustic diffraction following ablative recoil)[21] within a very small confined region immediately below the infrared delivery fiber. These micro-vapor bubbles coerced to form one large vapor bubble. Newtonian physics dictate that under such high pressure the resultant force was radially outward, thus the vapor bubble began to expand as shown in Figure 5(b).

The initial radial expansion velocity was estimated in Figure 7 to be about 0.01 mm/μs, slower than sound velocity in water (1.5 mm/μs) by more than two orders of magnitude[22]. Since this event occurred outside the stress confinement region, no shock wave was observed. At 75 μs, as shown in Figure 5(c), the vapor-water boundary passed the optrode's sensing tip. The bubble continued to expand to its maximum volume. Figure 7 indicates a maximum expansion at around 150 μs. However, snapshots by fast-flash photography imply a later maximum expansion at about 175-200 μs, as illustrated in Figure 5(d). The discrepancy was due to curve-fitting error in Figure 7. Also, the radial expansion velocity in Figure 7 was only measured in the preferential collapse direction of the bubble. The expansion velocity decreased as the bubble expands due to a loss of kinetic energy. The vapor bubble maximum expansion may overshoot the vapor-water phase pressure and temperature equilibrium resulting in sub-atmospheric pressure in the bubble. Rayleigh's equation[8] predicted sub-atmospheric pressure within a spherical bubble, assuming a uniform distribution of pressure. In pulsed Ho:YAG laser-induced vapor bubbles in water, the pressure has been calculated to be approximately 35.11 kPa.

When the vapor bubble reached its maximum expansion; that is, when all the initial momentum has been converted from kinetic energy to potential energy, the vapor bubble began to collapse after 200 μs. Due to continuous Ho:YAG laser irradiation (τ_p ~ 322.8 μs), the existing vapor bubble, with lower absorption coefficient, provided an open channel for infrared ablation of water at the base of the vapor bubble, causing formation of a pear-shape bubble. Because of this 'Moses effect'[19], the bubble collapse was more apparent in the horizontal than the vertical direction. Hence, as the bubble collapsed, it appeared to have an elongated arrow-head. This potentially beneficial consequence for tissue treatment, especially in the case of orthopedic surgery, has been widely investigated by Frenz et al.[23,24,25]. They have used a combination of erbium and holmium laser irradiation, with a controlled time delay of firing between these two pulsed lasers to optimize ablation while reducing pressure waves.

By 300 μs (Figure 5(e)) the collapsing vapor-water boundary passed the temperature optrode once again. Due to this asymmetric but elongated collapse, the vapor bubble converged on various points of singularities centered along the vertical axis. This nature of convergence produced scattered and weaker collapse pressures compared to a perfectly spherical vapor bubble, which only has one convergence point[23]. The spread of energy of these multiple-point collapses regenerated bubbles of asymmetric and scattered nature. Notice that the elongated bubble in Figure 5(d) and 5(e) is caused by the 'Moses' effect[19].

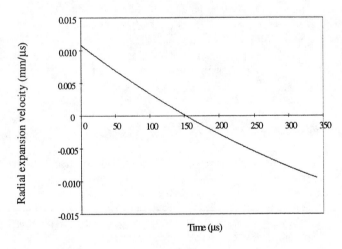

Figure 7. Radial expansion velocity of the primary vapor bubble as a function of time. The expansion velocity was curve-fitted in mm/μs. Notice that the maximum absolute expansion velocity was much slower than the velocity of sound in water (1.5 mm/μs).

Bubble Temperature Distribution

The physical interpretation of the temporal temperature profile at a fixed location was such that the temperature remained near room temperature until the vapor-water boundary passed the optrode sensing tip at about 75 μs. The temperature then increased rapidly as shown in Figure 6. The measured temperature rose to between 61 and 65 °C during maximum expansion. The saturation of temperature has two important implications. First, the underestimation of the actual vapor temperature due to a relatively large optrode thermal mass that prolonged the heat diffusion time, and a low value of thermal conductivity in the vapor phase. This low vapor temperature may also be a result of condensation and other dynamics in the vapor bubble. Second, the pressure in the vapor at that instant and location was indeed lower than an atmospheric pressure of 1 atm due to an overshoot of the vapor bubble volume from its vapor-water pressure equilibrium caused by the immense initial momentum generated during the bubble formation. This temperature measurement was in good agreement with the predicted vapor pressure of 35.11 kPa using Rayleigh's equation in (1), of which the corresponding temperature of saturated vapor was found to be between 69 °C and 75 °C based on the gas equation of (2). This vapor temperature, T_v, and the corresponding vapor pressure, P_v, at maximum expansion as defined in section 2, were independent of the radiant exposure, H_o, or the absorption coefficient, μ_a, if either were held constant[26]. Therefore, the measured vapor temperature agreed well with the theoretical prediction of vapor pressure and temperature based on Rayleigh's derivation and the steam table of saturated vapor[18].

In the collapsing phase after maximum expansion, when the probe tip was still submerged in the vapor bubble, a slight increase in temperature was observed. This slight increase was in accordance with the anticipated increase in pressure during the bubble collapse. When the vapor-water boundary once again passed by the optrode's sensing tip during the collapsing phase, at 300 μs, the temperature began to decrease. The temperature decline was considerably slower than the earlier temperature increase. The amount of time it took for the temperature to reduce to room temperature was approximately three orders of magnitude longer than the temperature rise. This was because of a warm and localized region in the water surrounding the delivery fiber just after the infrared irradiation was turned off. It took 10 or 20 ms before the temperature reduced to room temperature because of the relatively slow heat diffusion time in water and along the temperature optrode.

The fact that the measured temperature distribution was below the boiling temperature of 100 °C (at 1 atm) has profound implications in the understanding of vapor bubble dynamics. Assuming that underestimation of the temperature data occurred, the discrepancies must be more significant around the vapor-water boundary where a fast transient temperature gradient, $(\partial T/\partial r)/\partial t$, did not permit enough diffusion time for the temperature probe to "see" or settle at the real temperature.

On the other hand, the overall sub-100 °C implied that the vapor pressure must have a sub-atmospheric value due to overshooting of the vapor bubble volume from its vapor-water pressure equilibrium. This studies is still in the preliminary phase and requires more theoretical efforts and experimental trials. The immediate tasks are to improve the performance of the optrode to smaller spatial resolution (< 250 μm) and enhance accuracy (< 1 °C). To better match experimental data with theoretical model, a Q-switched experiment should be conducted in the near future, while a robust micro-device is highly desirable for pressure measurement within the vapor bubble.

6. CONCLUSION

The concept of partial vaporization based on the fraction of radiant exposure in actual superheating of nucleation sites was first mentioned in 1963 by Askar'yan et al.[27]. It was also suggested that a non-shock wave compression during boiling is determined by the vapor pressure of the liquid at the temperature of local heating[27]. This initial pressure can far exceed normal atmospheric pressure, a definite condition for momentum built-up allowing overshoots of vapor bubble maximum volume beyond the vapor-water pressure equilibrium. Therefore, it is suggested in this study that the vapor pressure, P_v, within the laser-induced bubble at maximum expansion may well be at sub-atmospheric pressure, and therefore the corresponding saturated vapor temperature, T_v, must be of sub-100 °C.

First, Rayleigh's derivation was presented to propose that in laser-induced vapor bubbles, the vapor pressure at maximum expansion is similar to that within cavitation bubbles. By predicting the vapor pressure, P_v, the vapor temperature within the bubble may be estimated using the gas equation in (2) or from the steam table for saturated vapor[18]. With Rayleigh's derivation in equation (1), the vapor pressure was calculated to be approximately 35.11 kPa, yielding vapor temperatures around 69 to 75 °C. Our measurements of vapor bubble temperatures, based upon the assumptions made in the experimental modalities discussed in section 2, yielded values ranging from 61 to 65 °C (average standard deviation ~ ± 2.24 °C), which are in fairly good agreement with the prediction.

7. ACKNOWLEDGEMENTS

Funding for this research was provided in part by grants from the Office of Naval Research Free Electron Laser Biomedical Science Program (N00014-91-J-1564) and the Albert W. and Clemmie A. Caster Foundation. *Paper # 3254A-36*

8. REFERENCES

[1] E. Duco Jansen, Ton G. van Leeuwen, Massoud Motamedi, Cornelius Borst, and Ashley J. Welch, "Partial Vaporization Model for Pulsed Mid-Infrared Laser Ablation of Water," J. Appl. Phys. 78(1), pp. 564-570, 1995.

[2] Jorge H. Torres, Thomas A. Springer, Ashley J. Welch, and John A. Pearce, "Limitations of a Thermal Camera in Measuring Surface Temperature of Laser-Irradiated Tissues," Lasers in Surgery and Medicine, vol. 10, pp. 510-523, 1990.

[3] Rudolf M. Verdaasdonk, "Imaging Laser-Induced Thermal Fields and Effects," SPIE, vol. 2391, pp. 165-175, 1995.

[4] S. Mordon, T. Desmettre, and J. M. Devoisselle, "Laser-induced Release of Liposome-Encapsulated Dye to vol. Monitor Tissue Temperature: A Preliminary *In Vivo* Study," Lasers in Surgery and Medicine, 16, pp. 246-252, 1995.

[5] Paul Kolodner and J. Anthony Tyson, "Microscopic Fluorescent Imaging of Surface Temperature profiles with 0.01°C Resolution," Appl. Phys. Lett., 40(9), pp.782-784, 1982.

[6] Paul Kolodner and J. Anthony Tyson, "Remote Thermal Imaging with 0.7 μm Spatial Resolution Using Temperature-Dependent Fluorescent Thin Film," Appl. Phys. Lett., 42(1), pp. 117-119, 1983.

[7] V. Romano, A. D. Zweig, M. Frenz, and H. P. Weber, "Time-Resolved Thermal Microscopy with Fluorescent Films," Applied Physics B, vol. 49, pp. 527-533, 1989.

[8] Lord Rayleigh, "On the Pressure Developed in a Liquid During the Collapse of a Spherical Cavity," Philosophical Magazine, vol. XXXIV, pp. 94-98, 1917.

[9] Martin Frenz, Hans Pratisto, Flurin Konz, E. Duco Jansen, Ashley J. Welch, and Heinz P. Weber, " Comparison of the Effects of Absorption Coefficient and Pulse Duration of 2.12 μm and 2.79 Radiation on Laser Ablation of Tissue," IEEE Journal of Quantum Electronics, vol. 32, no. 12, 1996.

[10] Tibor Juhasz, George A. Kastis, Carlos Suarez, Zsolt Bor, and Walter E. Bron, "Time-Resolved Observations of Shock Waves and Cavitation Bubbles Generated by Femtosecond Laser Pulses in Corneal Tissue and Water," Lasers in Surgery and Medicine, vol. 19, pp. 23-31, 1996.

[11] Alfred Vogel, Werner Hentschel, Joachim Holzfuss, and Werner Lauterborn, "Cavitation Bubble Dynamics and Acoustic Transient Generation in Ocular Surgery with Pulsed Neodymium:YAG Lasers," Ophthalmology, vol. 93, no. 10, pp. 1259-1269, 1986.

[12] A. Vogel, W. Lauterborn, and R. Timm, "Optical and Acoustic Investigations of the Dynamics of Laser-Produced Cavitation Bubbles near a Solid Boundary," J. Fluid Mech., vol. 206, pp. 299-338, 1989.

[13] A. Vogel, S. Busch, and M. Asiyo-Vogel, "Time-Resolved Measurements of Shock-Wave Emission and Cavitation-Bubble Generation in Intraocular Laser Surgery with ps- and ns-pulses and Related Tissue Effects," SPIE vol. 1877, pp. 312-322, 1993.

[14] Milton S. Plesset and Richard B. Chapman, "Collapse of an initially spherical vapour cavity in the neighbourhood of a solid boundary," J. Fluid Mech., vol. 47, part 2, pp. 283-290, 1971.

[15] W. Lauterborn and H. Bolle, "Experimental investigations of cavitation-bubble collapse in the neighbourhood of a solid boundary," J. Fluid Mech., vol. 72, part 2, pp. 391-399, 1975.

[16] E. Duco Jansen, Thomas Asshauer, Martin Frenz, Massoud Motamedi, Guy Delacretaz, and Ashley J. Welch, "Effect of Pulse Duration on Bubble Formation and Laser-Induced Pressure Waves During Holmium Laser Ablation," Lasers in Surgery and Medicine, vol. 18, pp. 278-293, 1996.

[17] Robert Resnick and David Halliday, *PHYSICS Part I*, John Wiley & Sons, Third Edition, 1977.

[18] Sonntag and van Wylen, Introduction to Thermodynamics - Classical and Statistical, John Wiley & Sons, pp. 630-631, Third Edition, 1991.

[19] Isner JM, "Blood," in Isner JM, Clarke R (eds.), Cardiovascular Laser Therapy, Raven Press, pp.39-62, New York, 1989.

[20] Kin F. Chan, Master's Thesis, the University of Texas at Austin, 1997.

[21] G. Paltauf, M. Frenz, and H. Schmidt-Kloiber, "Laser-induced micro bubble formation at a fiber tip in absorbing media: Experiments and theory," SPIE, vol. 2624, pp. 72-82, 1996.

[22] Ton G. van Leeuwen, E. Duco Jansen, Massoud Motamedi, Cornelius Borst, and A.J. Welch, "Pulsed Laser Ablation of Soft Tissue," Optical-Thermal Response of Laser-Irradiated Tissue, Plenum Press, New York, 1995.

[23] Martin Frenz, Hans Pratisto, Michael Ith, Flurin Konz, and Heinz P. Weber, "Effects of simultaneously fiber transmitted Erbium and Holmium radiation on the interaction with highly absorbing media," SPIE, vol. 2391, pp. 517-524, 1995.

[24] Hans Pratisto, Martin Frenz, Michael Ith, Hans J. Altermatt, E. Duco Jansen, and Heinz P. Weber, "Combination of fiber-guided pulsed erbium and holmium laser radiation for tissue ablation under water, " Applied Optics, vol. 25, no. 19, pp. 3328-3337, 1996.

[25] Hans Pratisto, Martin Frenz, Flurin Konz, Hans J. Altermatt, and Heinz P. Weber, "Combination of erbium and holmium laser radiation for tissue ablation," SPIE, vol. 2681, pp. 201-206, 1996.

[26] Ton G. Van Leeuwen, E. Duco Jansen, Ashley J. Welch, and Cornelius Borst, "Excimer Laser Induced Bubble: Dimensions, Theory, and Implications for Laser Angioplasty," Lasers in Surgery and Medicine, vol. 18, pp. 381-390, 1996.

[27] G. A. Askar'yan, A. M. Prokhorov, G. F. Chanturiya, and G.P. Shipulo, "The Effects of a Laser Beam in a Liquid," J. Exptl. Theoret. Phys. (U.S.S.R.), vol. 17, no. 6, pp. 1463-1465, 1963.

Laser thrombolysis using a millisecond frequency-doubled Nd-YAG laser

John A. Viator, Scott A. Prahl

Oregon Graduate Institute, Portland, OR 97291
Oregon Medical Laser Center, Portland, OR 97225

ABSTRACT

A frequency-doubled Nd:YAG laser at 532 nm with pulse durations of 2, 5, and 10 ms was used to ablate blood clot phantoms. The clot phantoms were prepared with 3.5% (175 Bloom) gel and Direct Red 81 dye to have an absorption coefficient of 150 cm^{-1}. Ablation thresholds were determined by a fluorescent technique using flash photography to detect the gel surface. The threshold was 15±2 mJ/mm^2 and corresponded to calculated temperatures of 80±10°C. Ablation efficiency experiments were conducted at 20 mJ. Ablation efficiencies were approximately 1.7±0.1 μg/mJ for the millisecond pulses and were comparable to previously published efficiencies for ablation of clot with a 1 μs pulsed dye laser.

Keywords: ablation, threshold, ablation efficiency, clot, stroke

1. INTRODUCTION AND BACKGROUND

Laser thrombolysis is the selective removal of clot from an occluded artery by directed laser energy. Laser thrombolysis was originally performed in coronary arteries with a 1 μs pulsed dye laser to clear thrombosed arteries, but conventional therapies (e.g., balloon angioplasty) are very successful. Current work centers around proving the safety and efficacy of laser thrombolysis as a treatment for stroke. A large number of stroke cases are ischemic, caused by a clot occluding a cerebral artery. Laser thrombolysis has been used clinically for coronary arteries, but deploying a catheter into the cerebral arteries requires the use of a small, flexible optical fibers. The laser pulse energy required to ablate clot depends on the spot size, but is roughly 10 mJ. The irradiances reached when coupling 10 mJ into a 100 μm fiber in 1 μs approach the optical breakdown threshold for quartz. Reducing the irradiance by using a longer laser pulse would mitigate this problem. If ablation threshold and efficiencies for longer pulses are comparable to the microsecond pulses, then the long pulse laser would be a more suitable device for laser thrombolysis. Additionally, the compact, efficient, self-contained solid state millisecond lasers currently available would be more manageable in a clinically setting than the microsecond pulsed dye laser.

With a pulse duration in the millisecond realm, thermal confinement becomes a concern. Thermal confinement is determined by the thermal diffusivity of the material and the initial distribution of the laser energy. It can be described as

$$\tau_{th} = \frac{\delta^2}{\kappa}$$

where τ_{th} is the time of thermal confinement, δ is the absorption depth, and κ is the thermal diffusivity of the material. For the gel used in these experiments, κ=0.0014 cm^2/s and $\delta = 0.007$ cm. This gives a thermal confinement time of about 30 ms, which, though longer than the pulses used in these experiments, it is close enough that thermal confinement must be considered.

These experiments use a frequency-doubled Nd-YAG laser at 532 nm, to ablate a clot phantom. The ablation threshold and ablation efficiency are compared to those for the 1 μs pulses published previously.[1] Clot phantoms are confined in 3 mm diameter tubes and a 300 μm fiber is positioned above the phantom for the ablation experiments.

The results show that ablation threshold and efficiency for the 2, 5, and 10 ms pulses are comparable to the 1 μs pulses.

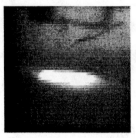 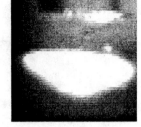 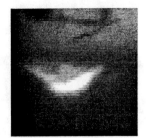

| Pre-Ablation | Ablative Event | Post-Ablation |

Figure 1. The subthreshold pulse has fluorescence indicating the undisturbed gel surface (left). The ablative pulse (middle). A subsequent subthreshold pulse indicates a lower surface due to ablation (right).

2. MATERIALS AND METHODS

2.1. Laser Parameters

The laser used for these experiments was a frequency-doubled Nd-YAG laser (Coherent VersaPulse) operating at 532 nm. The laser energy was delivered from the laser cavity through an optical fiber delivery system with focusing optics that produced a spot of 2–10 mm at the focal point. The 2 mm setting was used in all experiments. This spot was launched into a 300 μm fiber through additional focusing optics.

The pulse duration of the laser was set to 2, 5, and 10 ms. The pulse shapes were observed with a photodiode (Thorlabs DET-200) with a rise time of 1 ns. The pulse shapes were true square waves with no spikes or unusual features. The repetition rate was 1 Hz. The energy through the fiber was 20 mJ and all ablation efficiency experiments were performed at this clinically appropriate energy. A series of absorbing neutral density filters were used to reduce the laser pulse energy in the threshold level studies.

2.2. Target Preparation

A gel preparation was used to model thrombus that consisted of 3.5% 175 Bloom gelatin (Sigma Chemical) in water, 0.18% Direct Red 81 (Sigma Chemical) was added to produce a thrombus phantom with an absorption coefficient of 150 cm^{-1} at 532 nm (comparable to bulk whole blood absorption at this wavelength). The gel was drawn into 3 mm diameter silicone tubes (Patter Products) and set overnight. The tubes were approximately 6 cm in length with the center occupied by 2 cm of gel.

2.3. Threshold Detection

The pulses were monitored with a flash photography set up. A CCD camera (Motion Analysis, CV-251) was coupled to a video monitor (Panasonic PVM-1271Q). The laser pulse was detected by a photodiode (Thorlabs, DET-200) which triggered a flashlamp (EG&G, MVS-2601) and the CCD. The moment of image capture was set by a delay generator (Stanford Research Instruments, DG 535). A filter for the 532 nm light was used to prevent the CCD from being blinded by the laser pulse.

The ablation threshold for the microsecond pulses was determined by visual detection of bubble formation in the gel within the 3 mm tubes. A 100 μm fiber was positioned 500 μm above the gel surface to produce a spot size of 190 μm. Spot size was determined by irradiating black ablation paper under water. Four gel ablation threshold trials were conducted.

The ablation threshold for the millisecond pulses was detected by using the fluorescence of the thrombus phantom (Figure 1) The initial gel surface was visualized using a subthreshold pulse that caused the surface to fluoresce during the time of the laser pulse. A subsequent pulse of higher energy was emitted as an ablative attempt. The subthreshold pulse was again used to examine the gel surface. This process was repeated at successively higher energies until ablation was detected. The spot size was measured directly by evaluation of the subthreshold fluorescent spot.

The radiant exposure of the 1 μs pulsed dye laser was continuously varied, but the experimental apparatus used with the millisecond laser required using neutral density filters to change the radiant exposure from the nominal

20 mJ. The smallest increment of absorbance was 0.1, resulting in a change in energy by a factor of 1.25. This is a small loss in precision of measurement, although the loss is not so great when considering that the pulsed dye laser energy varied on the order of 5–10% between pulses.

2.4. Ablation Efficiency

Ablation efficiency experiments were conducted at four laser pulse durations, $1\,\mu s$, $2\,ms$, $5\,ms$, and $10\,ms$. The tubes containing the thrombus phantoms were set in a rigid frame which allowed insertion of a flushing catheter containing a $300\,\mu m$ fiber for delivery of laser energy. The catheter was connected to a syringe pump (Syringe Infusion Pump 22, Harvard Apparatus) which flushed $2\,ml/min$ of deionized water around the fiber to clear and collect ablated material. The fiber was positioned $500\,\mu m$ above the gel surface. The ablated mass was collected in a standard spectroscopy cuvette for later measurement. The flow was continued for about 90 seconds after the last pulse to ensure that all ablated mass was collected. This procedure was repeated without firing the laser to provide control samples to determine the amount of mass removed from the target by the flow of water alone. The mass was determined by a spectrophotometric means.[2] Five samples and controls were used for each data point.

The microsecond ablation efficiencies were determined at 1.5, 5.0 and 7.5 mJ. One hundred pulses at 1 Hz were used for each sample. The pulse energies were measured with a Joule meter (Molectron). The millisecond ablation efficiencies used 30 pulses at 1 Hz and 20 mJ. The pulse energies were measured with a calorimeter (Scientech).

3. RESULTS

3.1. Ablation Threshold

All four microsecond ablation thresholds resulting in threshold detection at 0.6 mJ. This translates to a threshold radiant exposure of $21\,mJ/mm^2$.

Ablation threshold for the $1\,\mu s$ pulse from the pulsed dye laser is compared to the thresholds for the 2, 5, and 10 ms pulses in the top graph in Figure 2. The ablation threshold for the $1\,\mu s$ pulse is $21\,mJ/mm^2$ which agrees with the calculated threshold to bring the gel temperature to 100°C. The threshold for the 2 ms pulse is $15\pm2\,mJ/mm^2$ which indicates ΔT of 52 ± 15°C. The initial temperature was 25°C. The threshold for the 5 ms pulse was $16\pm2\,mJ/mm^2$ which indicates ΔT of 56 ± 6°C. The threshold for the 10 ms pulse was $12\pm1\,mJ/mm^2$ which indicates a ΔT of 43 ± 5°C.

3.2. Ablation Efficiency

Ablation efficiency for the $1\,\mu s$ pulse from the pulsed dye laser is compared to the thresholds for the 2, 5, and 10 ms pulses in bottom graph in Figure 2. The ablation efficiencies are 1.5 ± 0.1, 1.7 ± 0.1, and $1.9\pm0.1\,\mu g/mJ$ for the 2, 5, and 10 ms pulses, respectively.

4. DISCUSSION

Previous work by Sathyam *et al.* has investigated the effects of variations of energy, spot sizes, pulse repetition rate, and wavelength on ablation threshold and efficiency.[2] This work shows that changing the pulse duration by five orders of magnitude (from $1\,\mu s$ to $10\,ms$) has very little effect upon the ablation of gelatin.

4.1. Ablation Threshold

The ablation threshold is slightly higher for the $1\,\mu s$ pulse than for the millisecond pulses. The data agree with the radiant exposure ($21\,mJ/mm^2$) necessary to raise the surface temperature of a $150\,cm^{-1}$ gel at 25°C to 100°C. This is also consistent with previous ablation threshold studies.[4]

4.2. Ablation Efficiency

The ablation efficiency shows excellent agreement between the $1\,\mu s$ data and the millisecond data. It agrees with previous work[2,4,5] indicating that the ablation mechanism for the millisecond pulse is also derived from mechanical action of the vapor bubbles.

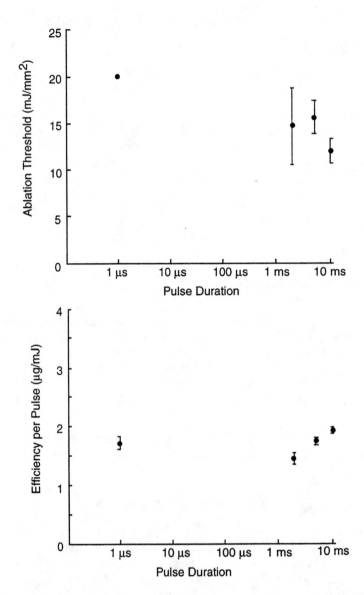

Figure 2. (Top) The ablation thresholds for microsecond and the millisecond pulses. (Bottom) The ablation efficiencies for the microsecond pulse and the millisecond pulses. The average and standard deviations of five samples at each millisecond pulse duration are shown.

5. CONCLUSION

The use of a solid state, millisecond pulse laser for stroke treatment can be a preferred alternative to the microsecond pulsed dye lasers. Reliable, clinically proven solid state lasers are currently available. These lasers are compact, portable, and are self-contained. Additionally, the efficacy of the laser as a treatment for ischemic stroke also lies in its suitability for launching into small fibers. The millisecond pulse avoids optical breakdown at the fiber face and has comparable clot phantom ablation properties. Since good correlation has been shown in the ability to ablate clot phantoms and clots,[2] the solid state, millisecond pulse laser is suitable as a clinical device for laser thrombolysis for stroke.

6. ACKNOWLEDGEMENTS

We would like to acknowledge Dr. R. Godwin and Dr. J. Chapyak of Los Alamos National Laboratory for conversations on long pulse ablation. I would also like to thank the Department of Dermatological Surgery at the Oregon Health Sciences University for the use of the Coherent VersaPulse laser.

REFERENCES

1. U. S. Sathyam and S. A. Prahl, "Limitations in measurement of subsurface temperatures using pulsed photothermal radiometry," *J. Biomed. Opt.* **2**, pp. 251–261, 1997.

2. U. S. Sathyam, *Laser Thrombolysis: Basic Ablation Studies.* PhD thesis, Oregon Graduate Institute of Science and Technology, 1996.

3. B. S. Amurthur and S. A. Prahl, "Acoustic cavitation events during microsecond irradiation of aqueous solutions," in *SPIE Proceedings of Diagnostic and Therapeutic Cardiovascular Interventions VII*, R. R. Anderson *et al.*, eds., vol. 2970, pp. 4–9, 1997.

4. U. S. Sathyam, A. Shearin, E. A. Chasteney, and S. A. Prahl, "Threshold and ablation efficiency studies of microsecond ablation of gelatin under water," *Lasers Surg. Med.* **19**, pp. 397–406, 1996.

5. J. A. Viator, U. S. Sathyam, A. Shearin, and S. A. Prahl, "Ablation efficiency measurements of soft materials with a small optical fiber," *Lasers Surg. Med.* **S9**, p. 4, 1997 (abstract).

SESSION 10

Optoacoustic Imaging and Sensing

Axial resolution of laser optoacoustic imaging:
Influence of acoustic attenuation and diffraction

Rinat O. Esenaliev [1], Herve Alma [2], Frank K. Tittel [2], and Alexander A. Oraevsky [3*]

[1] Biomedical Engineering Center, Department of Physiology and Biophysics,
The University of Texas Medical Branch, Galveston, TX 77555

[2] Department of Electrical and Computer Engineering, Rice University, Houston TX 77005

[3] Biomedical Engineering Center, Department of Ophthalmology and Visual Sciences,
The University of Texas Medical Branch, Galveston, TX 77555
phone: (409)-772-8348, FAX: (409)-772-0751, e-mail: <alexander.oraevsky@utmb.edu>

ABSTRACT

Laser optoacoustic imaging can be applied for characterization of layered and heterogeneous tissue structures *in vivo*. Accurate tissue characterization may provide: (1) means for medical diagnoses, and (2) pretreatment tissue properties important for therapeutic laser procedures. Axial resolution of the optoacoustic imaging is higher than that of optical imaging. However, the resolution may degrade due to either attenuation of high-frequency ultrasonic waves in tissue, or/and diffraction of low-frequency acoustic waves. The goal of this study was to determine the axial resolution as a function of acoustic attenuation and diffraction upon propagation of laser-induced pressure waves in water with absorbing layer, in breast phantoms, and in biological tissues. Acoustic pressure measurements were performed in absolute values using piezoelectric transducers. A layer or a small sphere of absorbing medium was placed within a medium with lower optical absorption. The distance between the acoustic transducer and the absorbing object was varied, so that the effects of acoustic attenuation and diffraction could be observed. The location of layers or spheres was measured from recorded optoacoustic pressure profiles and compared with real values measured with a micrometer. The experimental results were analyzed using theoretical models for spherical and planar acoustic waves. Our studies demonstrated that despite strong acoustic attenuation of high-frequency ultrasonic waves, the axial resolution of laser optoacoustic imaging may be as high as 20 μm for tissue layers located at a 5-mm depth. An axial resolution of 10 μm to 20 μm was demonstrated for an absorbing layer at a distance of 5 cm in water, when the resolution is affected only by diffraction. Acoustic transducers employed in optoacoustic imaging can have either high sensitivity or fast temporal response. Therefore, a high resolution may not be achieved with sensitive transducers utilized in breast imaging. For the laser optoacoustic imaging in breast phantoms, the axial resolution was better than 0.5 mm.

Key words: thermal stress, laser ultrasound, acoustic transducer, cancer detection, tissue characterization.

1. INTRODUCTION

Applications of optical imaging for detection and localization of diseased tissues have been intensively investigated for the last decade (see, for instance, SPIE and OSA Proceedings[1,2]). Optical imaging is based on differences in optical properties between normal and abnormal tissues. The contrast in optical properties is greater than contrast in acoustic properties. However, the sensitivity and the resolution of optical imaging are limited by the light scattering in tissues.

Ultrasound imaging is a widely used clinical technique for tissue characterization[3]. It is based on reflection of ultrasonic waves from acoustic inhomogeneities in tissues. Ultrasonic waves can propagate in tissues significantly deeper with minimal attenuation and distortion compared with optical waves[4]. Resolution of ultrasound imaging is often acceptable, especially when performed at higher frequencies. The major limitation of the ultrasonic imaging is its low contrast in soft tissues.

Laser optoacoustic imaging combines advantages of optical and ultrasound imaging in one technology[5]. It is based on optical contrast and time-resolved detection of laser-induced ultrasonic waves. The laser-induced ultrasonic waves in tissues are generated by the thermoelastic mechanism and resembles profile of thermal energy distribution in the irradiated volume (see, for example, [6,7]). Laser optoacoustic imaging system can operate in two modes, suitable for deep (up to 7 cm) and subsurface (up to 4 mm) imaging[5,8]. Application of sensitive acoustic transducers allows detection of millimeter-sized optical inhomogeneities in strongly scattering media simulating biological tissues[9]. Recently, detection of a small (2 mm) phantom tumors was demonstrated with the use of the laser optoacoustic imaging system (LOIS) at the depth of 60-mm within a breast phantom ($\mu_{eff} = 1.0$ cm^{-1})[10].

Resolution limits for the laser optoacoustic imaging has been studied, but not thoroughly[11,12]. In general, theoretical limit of z-axial (in depth) resolution is defined by the temporal response of acoustic transducers and the detection system, and by the laser pulse duration. However, resolution of LOIS may also be limited due to distortion of ultrasonic pulses by the following processes (1) diffraction of acoustic waves that occurred upon propagation in tissues and in acoustic detectors, and (2) attenuation of acoustic waves in tissues. Diffraction and attenuation may widen the ultrasonic pulses and shift their positions in measured pressure profiles. Therefore, location and dimensions of the objects or layers in optoacoustic images will be measured inaccurately. The goal of this study was to understand the influence of acoustic diffraction and attenuation on z-axial resolution of laser-optoacoustic imaging, i.e. on accuracy of localization and dimension measurements.

2. THEORETICAL BACKGROUND

2.1. Generation and detection of laser-induced acoustic waves.

Two different cases of laser optoacoustic imaging were considered in this study: (1) optoacoustic imaging utilizing detection of spherical waves and (2) optoacoustic imaging utilizing detection of plane waves. Spherical acoustic waves can be emitted by small acoustic sources such as deeply located tumors in the breast, brain, and other organs. In this case, laser irradiation and acoustic wave detection are usually performed from opposite sides of the investigated organ. This type of imaging is called imaging in forward mode because detected acoustic waves propagate along the direction of incident laser radiation (Fig. 1a, b). The optoacoustic imaging in forward mode was used in this study to detect model tumors in breast phantom.

Plane acoustic waves can be emitted by subsurface tissue layers in the skin, arteries, or hollow organs. Both the laser irradiation and acoustic wave detection can be performed *in vivo* at one and the same side of the investigated organ. This type of imaging is called optoacoustic imaging in backward mode because detected acoustic waves propagate in the direction opposite to the direction of incident laser radiation (Fig. 1c).

Detection of plane acoustic waves in the forward mode can be used in the cases of (1) thin tissues *in vivo*, (2) tissues *in vitro* which can be prepared as thin slices, and (3) in model experiments. In this study plane waves from tissues *in vitro* and from a phantom tissue layer (optical filter) were detected in the forward mode.

Maximal contrast, resolution and sensitivity of laser optoacoustic imaging can be obtained, if the irradiation conditions of temporal stress confinement are satisfied[6]. In this case, maximal efficiency of thermoelastic pressure waves is achieved and distribution of laser-induced acoustic sources resembles distribution of absorbed energy deposition. Laser radiation with nanosecond pulses is usually applied to satisfy the irradiation conditions of temporal stress confinement in the irradiated volume.

Generated pressure wave. A pressure rise distribution P(r) upon stress-confined irradiation condition is expressed as:

$$P_{gen}(\mathbf{r}) = \Gamma(\mathbf{r})\mu_a(\mathbf{r})F(\mathbf{r}) \tag{1}$$

where $\Gamma(\mathbf{r})$ is the Grüneisen coefficient which is dependent on mechanical and thermophysical parameters of tissue, $\mu_a(\mathbf{r})$ is the absorption coefficient, and F(**r**) is the fluence distribution in the tissue. This general formula is valid for any type of laser optoacoustic imaging.

Detected pressure wave. An amplitude of detected pressure wave is dependent on tissue type and detection geometry. In case of an absorbing sphere deeply located within the irradiated tissue, it can be calculated by the formula[13]:

$$P_{\mathrm{det},sph} = \frac{P_{gen}}{2}\frac{r_o}{R} \tag{2}$$

where r_0 is the sphere radius, R is the distance between the sphere and acoustic detector. The ratio r_0/R is due to spherical propagation of acoustic waves from the source. The pressure pulse from the spherical source will have a bipolar N-shaped profile[14, 15].

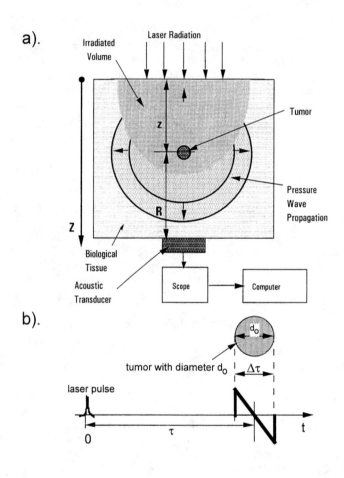

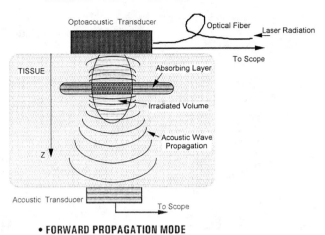

c). • BACKWARD PROPAGATION MODE

• FORWARD PROPAGATION MODE

Figure 1. Schematics of optoacoustic imaging utilizing spherical wave detection in forward mode (a); Pressure profile from a spherical source (b); Schematics of optoacoustic imaging utilizing plane wave detection in forward and backward modes (c).

In the case of an acoustic source emitting plane waves, the detected pressure amplitude is expressed by the formula:

$$P_{\det,pl} = P_{gen}/2 \qquad (3)$$

where factor 1/2 is due to propagation of two plane waves in two opposite directions from the source. Formulae (2) and (3) are valid if acoustic diffraction and attenuation are negligible.

Distance between acoustic source and transducer. It is necessary to measure the distance between an acoustic source and a transducer to localize the source and reconstruct its image. For any type of optoacoustic imaging this distance is given by the formula:

$$R = c_s\tau \qquad (4)$$

where c_S is the speed of sound and τ is the temporal delay between the laser pulse and the signal from the source.

Dimensions of acoustic source. The dimensions of acoustic sources can be calculated by the formula:

$$d_0 = c_s\Delta\tau \qquad (5)$$

where d_0 is either the sphere diameter in case of a spherical source, or the layer thickness in case of a layered source, and $\Delta\tau$ is the duration of acoustic pulses emitted by the source.

2.2. Distortion of acoustic waves.

Profile of laser-induced pressure waves can be distorted due to their diffraction and attenuation in tissue[6, 15, 16]. This may decrease the accuracy of dimension measurements and measurements of the distance between the source and detector. Therefore, the resolution of laser optoacoustic imaging may be influenced by these processes.

Influence of acoustic wave diffraction. Acoustic wave diffraction can substantially change profile of detected pressure[15, 16]. The pressure profile at the depth, z, distorted due to diffraction and detected perpendicular to the axis of propagation of the acoustic wave, $P(z,\tau,r_\perp = 0)$ and generated pressure profile, $P_{gen}(t)$, are related by the following expression[15]:

$$P_{diffr}(z, t, r_{\perp} = 0) = P_{gen}(t) - \int\limits_{-\infty}^{t} w_D exp(-w_D(t - t))P_{gen}(t)dt \qquad (6)$$

where $\omega_D = 2c_S z/a_L^2$ is the diffraction frequency, and a_L is the laser beam diameter. Using (6), the generated pressure profile can be calculated by the formula:

$$P_{gen}(t) = P_{diffr}(t) + \int\limits_{-\infty}^{t} w_D P_{diffr}(\tau)d\tau \qquad (7)$$

Therefore, the generated pressure profile can be reconstructed from the measured profile taking into account the diffraction effect.

Influence of acoustic wave attenuation. It is well known that acoustic attenuation coefficient, $\alpha(f)$, increases with the increase of frequency. The following relation is valid for tissues in a wide range of acoustic frequencies[17]:

$$\alpha(f) = af^b \qquad (8)$$

where a and b are factors that depend on tissue composition and structure. Typical value of b ranges between 1 and 2 for soft tissues.

Laser-induced acoustic waves have a wide frequency spectrum. Their spectral maximum is defined by the dimension of optoacoustic source, d_0, and estimated as:

$$f_{max} \sim c_S / d_0 \qquad (9)$$

Therefore, high-frequency acoustic waves (10 to 100 MHz) are generated in soft tissues, if the dimension of the acoustic source is of the order of 10 to 100 μm. The acoustic attenuation coefficient for these high-frequency waves may vary significantly (0.1 to 100 cm^{-1}) depending on tissue type[17].

The acoustic source with this dimensions can be either an absorbing volume (or layer) surrounded by other tissues with low absorption or a strongly absorbing tissue with high optical attenuation coefficient, μ_{eff}, of the order of 100 - 1000 cm^{-1}. Such high optical attenuation results in generation of pressure only in a thin subsurface layer with the thickness of the order of 10 - 100 μm.

High-frequency component of the generated pressure pulse will be attenuated stronger than the low-frequency component as depicted by expression (8). The acoustic attenuation can widen sharp edges of the pressure pulse with high-frequency spectrum. Therefore, attenuated pulse will be wider than the initially generated one. Furthermore, the amplitude of the high-frequency pressure pulse will decrease significantly. If pressure pulse propagates longer distances, the distortion of the pulse will be stronger.

Resolution of optoacoustic imaging will be decreased due to the pressure pulse broadening, because accuracy of localization and dimension measurement will be lower. The longer the propagation distance the lower the resolution.

Influence of acoustic detector dimension. The dimension of acoustic detectors may influence the profile of detected ultrasonic pulses and decrease resolution of optoacoustic imaging. For instance, if the distance between a spherical acoustic source and detector is comparable to the detector aperture, the detected pressure profile will be different from the pressure profile detected at a distance much greater than detector aperture.

3. MATERIALS AND METHODS

3.1. Laser sources.

Experiments on breast phantoms were performed with a Q-switched Nd:YAG laser with the following parameters: wavelength - 1064 nm, pulse duration - 10 ns, pulse energy - 50 mJ, diameter of laser spot - 8 mm, fluence - 100 mJ/cm^2. Third harmonic of a Q-switched Nd:YAG laser was used for experiments on acoustic diffraction. The parameters of laser radiation were: wavelength -532 nm, pulse duration - 12 ns, pulse energy - 5 mJ, diameter of laser spot - 8 mm, laser fluence - 10 mJ/cm^2.

Experiments on acoustic attenuation were performed with an ArF-laser with the following parameters: wavelength - 193 nm, pulse duration - 11 ns, pulse energy - 100 mJ, laser beam diameter - 6.2 mm. Incident pulse energy was attenuated and equal to 0.118 mJ providing incident fluence of 0.39 mJ/cm^2.

Irradiation with these parameters can not induce any thermal or mechanical damage to the samples, because maximal temperature and pressure rise were less than 0.5° K and 5 bar, respectively.

3.2. Sample preparation and measurement procedures.

Breast phantoms were made of 10%-gelatin and had dimensions of 100 x 97 x 57 mm. The breast phantom that resemble optical properties of human breast and the phantom preparation procedure were previously described[10,16]. Attenuation coefficient in the phantoms was 1.0 cm^{-1} which is equal to the attenuation coefficient of the human breast *in vivo* in the in the near-infrared spectral range[20-21]. Polystyrene spheres or milk were used as scatterers. Bovine hemoglobin was used as an absorber to make spheres with enhanced absorption. Diameter of the spheres was varied from 2 to 6 mm. The sphere diameters and distance between them and acoustic transducer were calculated by the formulas (4) and (5), respectively, and compared with actual ones measured with a caliper. Irradiation scheme of the phantoms is presented in Figure 1a.

(a)

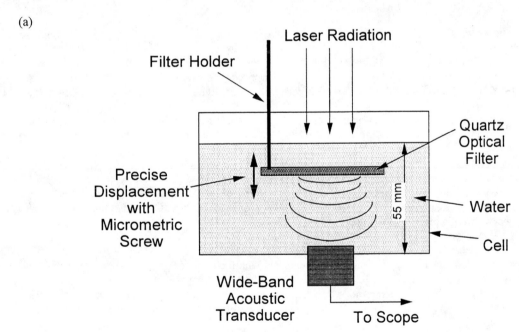

(b)

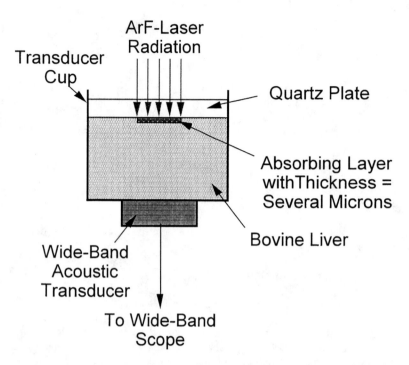

Figure 2. Experimental set up to study: (a) diffraction of optoacoustic waves, (b) attenuation of high-frequency optoacoustic waves in tissues.

A neutral density optical filter (thickness = 2 mm, μ_a = 32 cm^{-1} at λ = 532 nm) was used as a source of optoacoustic plane waves in the experiment on acoustic diffraction (Fig. 2a). The filter was embedded in water. The distance between the water surface and the transducer was 55 mm. Displacement of the filter was performed by a micrometric screw with the displacement accuracy of 1 μm. This allowed monitoring the distance between the irradiated filter surface and the transducer with the accuracy of 1 μm. Flat and smooth surface of the filter provided generation of optoacoustic wave with a planar front.

Optoacoustic signals were recorded at various distances between the filter and the transducer. This distance was calculated from the measured optoacoustic pressure profiles using formula (4) and compared with the distance determined with the micrometric screw.

Bovine liver slabs 50 x 50 mm with thickness from 0.060 to 5.0 mm were used in the acoustic attenuation experiment (Fig. 2b). The slabs were placed between a quartz plate and an acoustic transducer. The quartz plate surfaces were aligned parallel to the transducer surface and perpendicular to the incident laser beam. Optical quality of the quartz plate surface and fine alignment allow generation of a plane acoustic wave in the liver samples.

Typical attenuation coefficient in tissues is about several thousand cm^{-1} at the ArF-laser wavelength yielding penetration depth of several microns. Therefore, a thin subsurface layer with the thickness of several microns was an acoustic source in this case. Acoustic propagation time in this source was equal to several nanosecond which is less than laser pulse duration. That means that the conditions of temporal stress confinement are not satisfied. In this case the duration of the generated ultrasonic pulses is equal to the laser pulse duration[6] yielding acoustic wave frequency of the order of 100 MHz.

3.3. Acoustic transducers and detection systems.

High sensitivity of acoustic wave detection was required for the experiment on the breast phantoms. The profiles of laser-induced acoustic waves may be measured employing either piezoelectric transducers[18] or optical detection[19]. Our study utilized the piezoelectric detection. A specially designed sensitive acoustic transducer LBAT-14 (sensitivity - 2.5 V/bar, bandwidth - 2.5 MHz) with pre-amplifier was used in this experiment.

Broad-band acoustic transducers and detection system were needed for the acoustic diffraction and attenuation experiments. An acoustic transducer WAT-12 (Science Brothers Inc., Houston, TX) with sensitivity of 12 mV/bar and bandwidth of >100 MHz was used for the experiment on acoustic diffraction. High-frequency acoustic transducer WAT-04 (sensitivity - 10 mV/bar, bandwidth - 300 MHz) was applied for the experiment on acoustic attenuation. Signals from the transducer were recorded by a Tektronix scope (500 MHz bandwidth) and processed with a personal computer.

4. RESULTS

4.1. Breast phantom experiment.

Several different breast phantoms were used for this experiment. One of the pressure profiles obtained upon irradiation of the breast phantom with 2-mm and 4-mm spheres is presented in Figure 3. The first peak is caused by absorption of laser radiation in the acoustic transducer. It is used as a reference signal. The second signal is the signal from the 4-mm sphere. It has two maxima and one minimum. The next signal is signal from the 2-mm sphere. It has bipolar N-shaped profile typical for spherical sources.

The upper x-axis represents depth, z, from irradiated surface. The sharp edge at z=0 is caused by reflection of the laser-induced acoustic waves from gelatin-air interface. It indicates position of the surface. Wavelet filtering was used to increase of signal-to-noise ratio. The wavelet-filtered signal is also presented in the plot. Exponential slope representing background optoacoustic pressure was automatically subtracted from raw experimental signals by this filtering procedure.

Both diameter of the spheres and distance between the spheres and transducer were calculated from the measured profiles using formula (4) and (5). The calculated values were compared with the actual ones measured with a caliper. Table 1 represents the calculated and actual values of the distance between the spheres and transducer. The calculated and actual values of the sphere diameter are shown in the Table 2.

4.2. Acoustic diffraction experiment.

Pressure profiles recorded from the filter positioned at various distances from the transducer are presented in Figure 4. If the filter was at the distance of 5 mm to the transducer, the detected pressure profile is bipolar. It indicates that the diffraction is negligible and the pressure wave is planar. The second maximum appears with the increase of the distance between the filter and transducer. The diffraction is significant at the distance of 30 - 50 mm. The pressure profiles are plotted so that their first maxima coincide. In this case, the pressure pulse distortion due to diffraction is clearly seen.

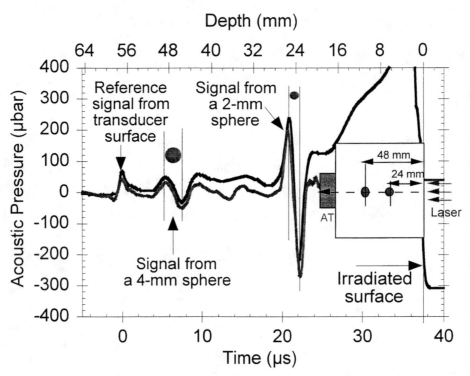

Figure 3. Optoacoustic signals from small spheres in the breast phantom (upper curve) and the same signal after wavelet processing (lower curve).

Table 1. Accuracy of localization of small spheres in the phantom.

Sphere Diameter (mm)	Measured Distance (mm)	Actual Distance (mm)	Δ (mm)	Δ/R (%)
2.0	39.2	39.0	0.2	0.5
4.0	74.3	74.0	0.3	0.4
6.0	76.5	76.0	0.5	0.7

Table 2. Accuracy of dimension measurement for small spheres in the phantom.

Sphere Diameter (mm)	Measured Diameter (mm)	Δ (mm)	Δ/do (%)
2.0	2.16	0.16	8.0
4.0	3.5	0.5	12.0
6.0	5.5	0.5	8.3

Figure 5 depicts the acoustic arrival time, τ, as a function of distance between the irradiated surface of the filter and the transducer. The right y-axis represents this distance calculated from optoacoustic pressure profiles using the formula (4). There is a good agreement between the calculated and the actual distance. The location of the absorbing layer was determined with an accuracy of about 10 μm at the distances of 30 to 50 mm.

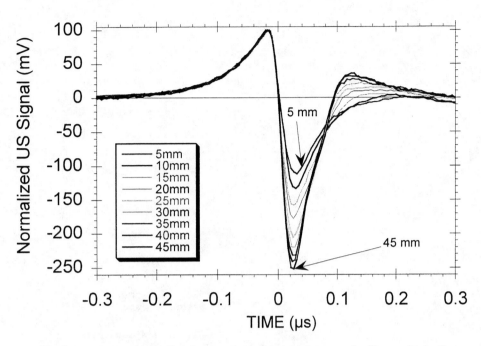

Figure 4. Optoacoustic signals at various distances between the filter and transducer.

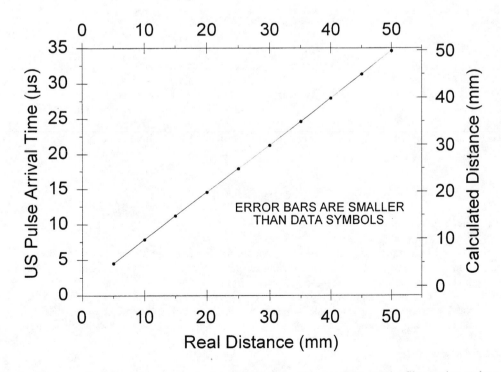

Figure 5. Acoustic arrival time and calculated distance vs. distance between the filter and transducer.

4.3. Acoustic attenuation experiment.

Pressure profiles from the liver samples with the thickness of 0.06 and 3.9 mm are presented in Figure 6. The pressure profile from the 0.06-mm liver sample has a duration of 11 ns which equals the laser pulse duration. The pressure profile amplitude from the 3.9-mm sample is substantually less than that measured from the thin sample. Furthermore, its duration increased to 23 ns. The distortion of initial acoustic pulse was significant. The change in ultrasonic pulse shape indicates an influence of the acoustic attenuation on pressure profiles.

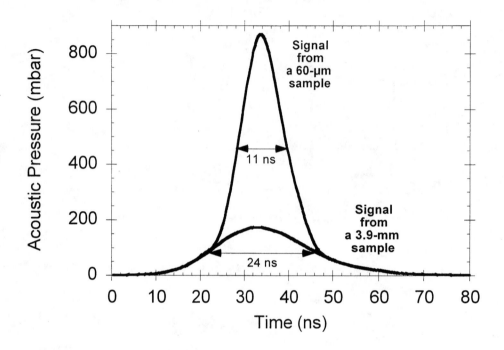

Figure 6. Optoacoustic pressure profile measured from bovine liver with different thickness.

Figure 7 shows pressure amplitude as a function of liver thickness. A strong acoustic attenuation was observed, when acoustic pulses propagated first several hundred microns in the liver samples. A lower attenuation was observed if the pulses propagate longer distance. The experimental data were fit with a function representing a sum of two exponents. The fit determined the attenuation coefficient of 7.1 mm^{-1} within the fraction of millimeter and 0.26 mm^{-1} for the distances of several millimeters.

5. DISCUSSION

5.1. Breast phantom experiment.

The accuracy of localization and diameter measurement was in the range of a fraction of millimeter for the spherical acoustic sources in the breast phantoms. Therefore, z-axial resolution was equal to a fraction of millimeter in this case. It is limited by the temporal response of the acoustic transducer. This resolution is enough for accurate localization of spherical sources and measurements of their dimensions at the distance of several centimeters . This statement is valid, if the distance between the spherical sources and the transducer is greater than the characteristic dimensions of the transducer. If the distance is comparable to the transducer dimensions, the resolution is lower due to pressure pulse distortion.

5.2. Acoustic diffraction experiment.

The experiment on diffraction demonstrated that z-axial resolution can be up to 20 μm even for strongly diffracted signals. It is very close to the z-axial resolution for ideal plane wave limited by the temporal response of acoustic transducers and the electronic detection system, and the laser pulse duration. We demonstrated that measurements of dimensions and location of tissue layers are insignificantly influenced by diffraction effects. Application of diffraction correction algorithms are not necessary in case when only z-axial resolution is concerned.

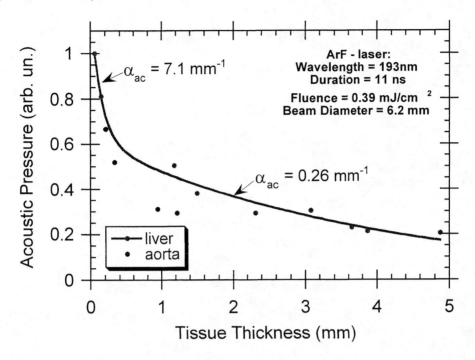

Figure 7. A ultrasonic pulse pressure amplitude as a function of thickness for a liver slab and an aorta wall. Two major ultrasonic frequency components may be delineated in the curve (exp fit is shown for the liver slab only).

5.3. Acoustic attenuation experiment.

The data on acoustic attenuation demonstrated strong attenuation of high-frequency component in the pressure pulses at distances of the order of 100 μm. A low-frequency component was attenuated at the distances of the order of several millimeters. These data are consistent with the fact that the acoustic attenuation coefficient for high-frequency waves is greater than that for low-frequency ultrasonic waves.

The position of the irradiated tissue surface can be calculated using the formula (4) from the position of the maximum in the pressure profiles. The axial resolution for thin samples was about 15 μm as defined by a longest of threee times: the temporal resolution of the transducer, the response of detection system, and the laser pulse duration. The ultrasonic pulse propagated through a 3.9-mm liver sample was 13-ns wider that the initially generated pulse. Therefore, resolution was 20 μm in this case.

The generated pressure profiles can be reconstructed from the detected one if acoustic attenuation is known at different frequencies. This can decrease acoustic attenuation effects and improve z-axial resolution of laser optoacoustic imaging.

6. CONCLUSION

This study demonstrated that acoustic diffraction decreases insignificantly the z-axial resolution of the laser optoacoustic imaging. The accuracy of dimensions measurement in laser optoacoustic imaging is defined by the widening of ultrasonic pulses upon propagation in tissues due to a stronger attenuation of high ultrasonic frequencies. The thickness of an absorbing layer within our phantom was measured with a 20-μm precision. The axial resolution was approximately 0.5 mm in breast phantoms with characteristic dimension of 10 cm.

Acoustic transducer aperture may also decrease the resolution, if it is comparable to the distance between the spherical source and the transducer. In the case of spherical sources located far from the transducer, the resolution is not influenced by its aperture and defined by its temporal response and bandwidth of detection system.

7. ACKNOWLEDGMENTS

This work is supported in part by grants from the Whitaker Foundation and the Advanced Technology Program of the Texas Higher Education Coordinating Board.

8. REFERENCES

1. "Optical Tomography, Photon Migration, and Spectroscopy of Tissue and Model Media: Theory, Human Studies, and Instrumentation," *Proc. SPIE* **2389**, 1995; "Optical Tomography and Spectroscopy of Tissue: Theory, Instrumentation, Model and Human Studies," *Proc. SPIE* **2979**, 1997.
2. *"OSA Proceedings on Advances in Optical Imaging and Photon Migration,"* (R. R. Alfano, ed.), **21**, 1994; *"OSA Trends in Optics and Photonics on Advances in Optical Imaging and Photon Migration,"* R. R. Alfano and J. G. Fujimoto, eds. (OSA, Washington, DC), **2**, 1996.
3. R.C. Sanders: "Clinical (ultra)sonography: a practical guide", Little & Brown, Boston, 1991
4. F. A. Duck, *"Physical properties of tissue: A comprehensive reference book"*, Academic Press, San Diego, 1990.
5. A.A. Oraevsky, R.O. Esenaliev, S.L. Jacques, F.K. Tittel: Laser Opto-Acoustic Tomography for medical diagnostics: principles, *Proc. SPIE* 1996; **2676**: 22-31.
6. A.A. Oraevsky, S.L. Jacques, F.K. Tittel: Determination of tissue optical properties by time-resolved detection of laser-induced stress waves. *Proc. SPIE* 1993; **1882**: 86-101.
7. A.A. Oraevsky, S.L. Jacques, F.K. Tittel: Measurement of tissue optical properties by time-resolved detection of laser-induced transient stress, *Applied Optics*, 1997; **36**(1): 402-415.
8. A.A. Oraevsky: Laser optoacoustic imaging for cancer diagnosis, *LEOS NewsLetter* 1996; **12**: 17-20.
9. R.O. Esenaliev, A.A. Oraevsky, S.L. Jacques, F.K. Tittel: Laser Opto-Acoustic Tomography for medical diagnostics: experiments with biological tissues, *Proc. SPIE* 1996; **2676**: 84-90.
10. R.O. Esenaliev, F.K. Tittel, S.L. Thomsen, B. Fornage, C. Stelling, A.A. Karabutov, and A.A. Oraevsky: Laser optoacoustic imaging for breast cancer diagnostics: Limit of detection and comparison with X-ray and ultrasound imaging, *Proc. SPIE* 1997; **2979**: 71-82.
11. A. A. Oraevsky, R. O. Esenaliev, S. L. Jacques, and F. K. Tittel: "Lateral and z-axial resolution in laser optoacoustic imaging with ultrasonic transducers", *Proc. SPIE*, **2389**, pp. 198-208, 1995.
12. C.G.A. Hoelen, R.Pongers, G. Hamhuis, F.F.M. deMul, J. Greve: Photoacoustic blood cell detection and imaging of blood vessels in phantom tissue, Proc. SPIE 3196: 142-153, 1997.
13. G. J. Diebold and T. Sun. "Properties of optoacoustic waves in one, two, and three dimensions", *Acustica*, **80**, pp. 339-351, 1994.
14. A. A. Oraevsky, R. O. Esenaliev, S. L. Jacques, F. K. Tittel, and D. Medina: "Breast Cancer Diagnostics by Laser Opto-Acoustic Tomography", *OSA Trends in Optics and Photonics on Advances in Optical Imaging and Photon Migration,"* R. R. Alfano and J. G. Fujimoto, eds. (OSA, Washington, DC), **2**, pp. 316-321, 1996.
15. V. E. Gusev and A. A. Karabutov. "Laser Optoacoustics", AIP Press, New York, 1993.
16. A.A. Karabutov, N.B. Podymova, V.S. Letokhov: "Time-resolved laser optoacoustic tomography of inhomogeneous media", *Applied Phys. B* vol. **63**: 545-563, 1996.
17. S. A. Goss, R. L. Johnston, and F. Dunn. "Comprehensive compilation of empirical ultrasonic properties of mammalian tissues", *J. Acoust. Soc. Am.*, **64**(2), pp. 423-457, 1978.
18. M.W. Sigrist: Laser generation of acoustic waves in liquids and gases, J. Appl. Phys. 60: R83-R121, 1986.
19. G. Paltauf, H. Schmidt-Kloiber, H. Guss: Light distribution measurement in absorbing materials by optical detection of laser-induced stress waves, Appl. Phys. Lett. 69: 1526-1528, 1996.
20. J. Kolzer, G. Mitic, J. Otto, and W. Zinth. "Measurements of the optical properties of breast tissue using time resolved transillumination", *Proc. SPIE*; **2326**, pp. 143-152, 1994.
21. K. Suzuki, Y. Yamashita, K. Ohta, M. Kaneko, M. Yoshida, and B. Chance. "Quantitative measurement of optical parameters in normal breasts using time-resolved spectroscopy: *in vivo* results of 30 Japanese women", *J. Biomed. Optics,* **1**(3), pp. 330-334, 1996.

Non-contact detection of laser-induced acoustic waves from buried absorbing objects using a dual-beam common-path interferometer.

S. L. Jacques[a], P. E. Andersen[b], S. G. Hanson[b], L. R. Lindvold[b]

[a]Oregon Medical Laser Center, [b]Risø National Laboratory (Denmark)

Abstract

The feasibility of a noncontact all-optical probe for surface detection of laser-induced acoustic waves generated in buried absorbing objects was investigated. The goal is to detect subsurface optically absorbing objects, such as hemorrhages or vascularized tumors, which generate acoustic waves when slightly heated by a Q-switched laser pulse transported to an internal object by light diffusion within a turbid tissue. A dual-beam common-path interferometer was constructed to provide sensitive time-resolved detection of surface movements. Arrival of a pressure wave at one surface beam irradiation site before arrival at the other beam site caused a differential surface movement and a pathlength difference detected by the interferometer. The dynamic range of linear measurement was about 20 mbar - 200 bar at 20 mV/bar. The sensitivity (20 mV/bar) and noise level (10-30 mbar) of the interferometer matched or exceeded the performance of a lithium-niobate piezoelectric transducer. The point spread function of response was studied in liquid phantoms which demonstrated a null plane of no response in the plane symmetrically between the two beams. The ability to image an absorbing object at a depth of 11 mm within an aqueous phantom medium was demonstrated illustrating sub-mm resolution.

Key words: photoacoustic imaging, optoacoustic, stress waves, laser, interferometry, optical diagnostics, medicine, biology

1. INTRODUCTION

Photoacoustic imaging uses a Q-switched pulsed laser to generate a slight temperature rise in an absorbing object buried within a tissue, for example a hemorrhage or the vasculature of a tumor. The temperature rise elicits thermoelastic expansion on a time scale which allows stress confinement, hence maximal pressures are generated in the object. This pressure distribution then propagates to the tissue surface as acoustic stress waves at the speed of sound. Their time of arrival at a surface site of detection indicates the distance the wave has traveled and hence the detected signal can be backprojected into the tissue. Superposition of such backprojected signals from an array of surface detectors can locate objects and provides a means for image reconstruction.

This paper investigates the performance of a noncontact detection system based on a dual-beam common-path interferometer which is sensitive to surface movements caused by arriving stress waves [1]. We characterize the sensitivity and point spread function of response and demonstrate the ability for edge detection for an absorbing object submerged in aqueous phantoms.

Further author information:
S.L.J.: Email: sjacques@ece.ogi.edu; WWW: http://ece.ogi.edu/omlc; Telephone: 503-216-4092; FAX: 503-216-2422
P.E.A.: Email: peter.andersen@risoe.dk; http://www.risoe.dk/ofd; Telephone: (+45) 46 77 45 55; FAX: (+45) 46 77 45 65

2. MATERIALS AND METHODS

2.1 Experimental Setup

A common path interferometer was assembled as shown in Fig. 1. The source (a linearly polarized HeNe laser at 632.8 nm rotated 45°) was passed through a beam splitter, through a Wallaston prism to divert the polarized components of the HeNe beam into two beams diverging at different angles, through a lens (12 cm F.L.) to recollimate the beams as two parallel beams separated by 9 mm, and reflected by a 90 degree mirror down onto the phantom to be measured. Reflected light from the phantom surface returned through the same optical path to the beam splitter which diverted the returned coaxial beams toward a pinhole in front of a photodiode detector. The beams passed through a polarizing filter oriented at 45° so that a parallel or perpendicular component of each beam was sampled to yield two co-aligned beams with common polarization to provide for interference. The beams were passed through an interference filter to reject any 532-nm Q-switched laser light (see 2.3 below). A lens focused the beams through a pinhole to reach the detector. The two beams interfered at the detector causing the photodiode to yield a DC current with an AC modulation due to interference of the two beams. Differential movement of the phantom surface at one beam versus the other beam caused fluctuation of the interference. The modulation (AC/DC current) was 87%. The signal was preamplified. Under usual operation, the signal was AC coupled and attenuated by a high-pass filter (100 Hz cutoff frequency) to decrease sensitivity to persistent low-frequency surface waves on the liquid phantoms used in the study. The signal was AC coupled to the 1-MOhm input of a digitizing scope (200-MHz bandwidth).

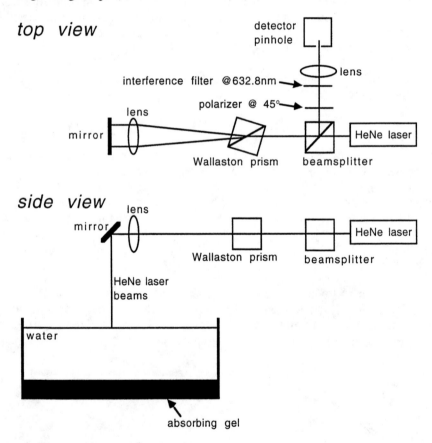

Fig. 1. Experimental setup. (TOP VIEW) The two polarization components of a linearly polarized HeNe laser beam are split by a Wallaston prism into two angles to yield two beams which are collimated by a lens and turned by a mirror down onto a liquid phantom. The reflected light from the phantom surface returns the two beams back through the Wallaston prism, off the beamsplitter, through a polarizer at 45°

to equally sample both components of the two reflected polarized beams, through an interference filter to reject any Nd:YAG laser radiation (532 nm), and focused by a lens through a pinhole to reach a photodiode detector. The two beams interfere at the photodiode yielding a signal which is sensitive to the differential total pathlength of photons after reflection off the phantom surface. (SIDE VIEW) The two beams are reflected by the phantom surface.

2.2 Phantoms

Phantoms were prepared in a 10-cm-diameter 5-cm-deep glass petri dish. The phantom consisted of water with or without added scatterer (coffee whitener). Absorbing objects were prepared using 4% (g/cm^3) gelatin which contained India ink at a 1% (vol/vol) concentration which yielded an absorption coefficient of 18.6 cm^{-1} at 532 nm. In the experiments investigating the point spread function of response (section 3.2), a 2-cm layer of absorbing gel was placed on the bottom of the dish and the YAG laser irradiation was delivered down through the water to reach the gelatin which deposited energy to create a pressure source. In the imaging experiments (section 3.3), a 2-mm layer of absorbing gel was placed in the dish and the Nd:YAG laser irradiation was delivered from below to directly irradiate the gel.

2.3 Laser irradiation

Stress waves were generated by a Q-switched pulsed second-harmonic Nd:YAG laser (532 nm, 10 ns, 16 mJ, 10 Hz repetition rate; Continuum Inc.) which will be referred to as simply the YAG laser. The beam was focused by a 30-cm focal-length lens and directed by an adjustable mirror down onto the phantom at an angle of 20 degrees off the axis normal to the surface as a 2-mm diameter spot. The spot size did not significantly vary during adjustment of the spot position using the adjustable mirror, nor when the height of the phantom surface was adjusted relative to the focal plane of the lens.

2.4 The interferometric signal

The signal was sensitive to any movement of the surface which caused a differential optical pathlength, $\Delta L = 2\Delta h$, for the round trips of the two beams in the interferometer, where Δh is the difference in the relative heights of the phantom surface at the irradiation sites of the two beams. The signal, S, would oscillate around its DC value, S_{DC}, with an amplitude S_{AC} as a function of the differential pathlength ΔL between the two beams:

$$S = S_{DC} + S_{AC}\cos(2\pi\Delta L/\lambda + \phi) \qquad \text{Eq. 1}$$

where ϕ was a slowly varying phase associated with the mechanical instabilities of the setup which was measured to be a two-minute cycle using a mirror as the surface. For measurements of the surfaces of liquid phantoms, the S_{DC} and S_{AC} values were 3.02 V and 2.62 V, respectively. The incremental signal response to an incremental change, d(Δh), in the Δh between the sites of beam reflectance depended on the derivative dS/d(Δh) which is here called the gain factor:

$$dS/d(\Delta h) = -(4\pi S_{AC}/\lambda)\sin(4\pi\Delta h/\lambda + \phi) \qquad \text{Eq. 2}$$

The maximum gain factor had a magnitude of $4\pi S_{AC}/\lambda$, or 52 mV/nm, which was only realized under two conditions: (1) when the interferometer was operating at the condition for optimum response, $4\pi\Delta h/\lambda + \phi = \pm\pi/2$, and (2) when the deflection d(Δh) was very small. For example, to achieve linearity within 95% of ideal, d(Δh) must be small such that $4\pi d(\Delta h)/\lambda <$ arcsin(0.95), or d(Δh) < 63 nm. Larger d(Δh) will move the calibration factor out of the optimum response condition and saturate the detector. Very large d(Δh) will cause dS to vary cyclically. The typical dS values recorded in response to laser-induced stress waves were $\pm$ 10-1000 mV. The response would be linear for signals of (52 mV/nm)(63 nm) or 3276 mV which is well above the range of typical stress waves recorded. Hence, the signal response dS was linear with a differential surface movement $d(\Delta h)$. Henceforth, we shall refer to $d(\Delta h)$ as simply Δh such that a measured change ΔS occurs in response to a change in the net surface movement $\Delta h = \Delta h_1 - \Delta h_2$ where the surface movement at the site of beam #1 is Δh_1 and the surface movement at the site of beam #2 is Δh_2.

2.5 Signal processing

Low-frequency surface waves on the liquid phantom surface imposed a time-varying Δh value on the time scale of 100 μs - 1 s. Slow variations in the ϕ associated with the interferometer system occured on the scale of minutes which also contributed to variation. These variations caused a random sampling of the argument $4\pi\Delta h/\lambda + \phi$ and hence a random sampling of the gain factor. Eq. 2 indicates that the gain factor could be either positive or negative, depending on the current values of Δh and ϕ. This behavior was observable. Laser pulses sometimes elicited positive ΔS and sometimes negative ΔS in the AC coupled signal.

Figure 2 shows a typical response. The arrival of the pressure wave at beam #1 caused a negative ΔS, and subsequent arrival of the pressue wave at beam #2 caused a positive ΔS. The signal was acquired by taking a running 32-data average of the square of ΔS, $\langle mV^2 \rangle$, so that a positive value was always obtained and an average accumulated. The square root of the $\langle mV^2 \rangle$ value was taken to return the signal to units of [mV] which was linearly related to surface displacement.

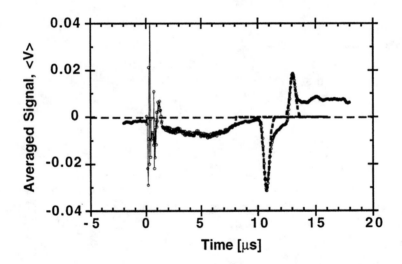

Fig. 2: Typical trace of signal vs time acquired by a digitizing oscilloscope at 10-Hz pulse repetition rate averaging 32 pulses. YAG laser irradiation was delivered down through 11.5 mm of water and heated an absorbing gel which generated a stress wave that propagated back to surface toward the pair of probe beams. The stress wave reached the first beam at $t_{arr} \approx 10.8$ ms and the second beam at $t_{arr} \approx 13.1$ μs. In this example, the bias of the interferometer was such that surface movement at the first beam created a negative shift in signal, and surface movement at the second beam created a positive shift in signal. The peaks of the arriving stress wave transients were discernible above a more slowly varying background signal. Dashed lines show approximate fits using a Gaussian function:
$$\text{constant} \times \exp(-(t - t_{arr})^2/\tau^2)$$
where $\tau = 0.33$ μs and $c_s\tau = 0.49$ mm is the apparent 1/e half-width of the stress wave.

The above data acquisition protocol was flawed. A random sampling of a $\sin^2$ term would yield an average calibration factor of 1/2 the $4\pi S_{AC}/\lambda$ term. Unfortunately, in these preliminary experiments a true random sampling was not conducted. Rather, we attempted to record the peak signal from an ensemble of measured values. Consequently, our data was subject to variation due to unreliable sampling of the slowly varying gain factor. This was a major source of variation in the data presented in this preliminary paper. We are now developing a method which will detect the combination of two quadrature signals, $\sin^2(4\pi\Delta h/\lambda + \phi)$ and $\sin^2(4\pi\Delta h/\lambda + \phi + \pi/2)$, to yield a signal whose gain factor is invariant with any drift in ϕ or change in Δh.

2.6 Theoretical Analysis

The initial pressure (P_0) deposited in the incremental volume at the surface of the absorbing gel after pulsed YAG laser irradiation was calculated:

$$P_0 = 10\Gamma\mu_a H \quad [bar] \qquad Eq. 3$$

where Γ is the Grueneisen coefficient ($\Gamma = 0.14$ at 25°C) which is the dimensionless fraction of the total energy deposition that couples into pressure, μ_a is the gel absorption coefficient ($\mu_a = 18.6$ cm^{-1}), and H is the radiant exposure (H = (16 mJ/pulse)/(π 0.12^2 cm^2) = 0.51 J/cm^2 per pulse). The factor 10 accounts for a pressure of 1 J/cm^3 corresponding to 10 bar. The product μ_aH was 9.5 J/cm^3 which induced a 2.3 °C temperature rise in the gel. The product $10\Gamma\mu_a$H equaled 13.3 bar. The absorbing gel strongly attenuated the laser beam with a 1/e distance of $1/\mu_a = 0.54$ mm. A more careful analysis would consider the spatially distributed pressure generation by the distributed energy deposition in the gel. But for this preliminary paper, we simplify the analysis by just considering P_0.

The propagation of a point source of pressure as a spherical stress wave follows a 1/r dependence. One should consider the transition from the near-field pressure distribution due to the spatially distributed source to the far-field traveling pressure wave, however in this preliminary paper the propagation is approximated:

$$P(r, t) \approx P_0 \frac{a}{c_s t} \exp\left(-((r - c_s t)/c_s\tau)^2\right) \qquad Eq. 4$$

where a is the apparent 1/e half-width of the source along the vector toward the detection beam site, r is the distance from the center of the spot of laser deposition to the point of observation, t is the time of observation, c_s is the sound velocity (1.494 mm/μs), and the exponential is a spreading function (Gaussian) which approximates the apparent width of the stress wave arriving at the observation point. Eq. 4 says that when $c_s t = a$, the pressure at $r = a$ is P_0 which is the initial laser-induced pressure. However, the equation is applied at much longer times t and distant positions r. The width of the stress wave as it reaches the detection site is a function of the initial spatial distribution of energy deposition and any diffraction effects arising by propagation from this distribution. These issues are not considered in this paper but are characterized empirically by the factor $c_s\tau$ in Eq. 4 as the apparent half-width of the stress wave arriving at a detection site.

The movement of the phantom surface is modeled as being linearly related to the pressure of the arriving stress wave: pressure = force/(unit area) = $-\cos(\theta)$(spring constant)Δh/(unit area), where θ is the angle of stress wave propagation relative to the surface normal (see Fig. 3). Also recall that the gain factor $dS/d(\Delta h)$ describes the change in intensity of the interference pattern observed by the photodiode and recorded in mV in response to a change in the net Δh. We combine the factors (spring constant)/(area) and dS/d(Δh) into one calibration constant called A [mV/bar]. The absolute value of the signal change ΔS, or |ΔS| [mV], is expressed:

$$|\Delta S| = A \ |\cos(\theta_1)\Delta h_1 - \cos(\theta_2)\Delta h_2| \qquad \text{Eq. 5}$$

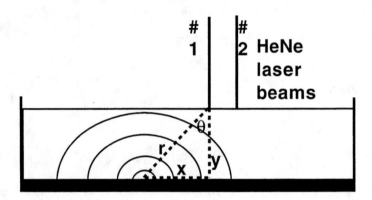

Fig. 3: Geometry of arriving pressure waves originating a distance x from the closest HeNe laser beam. The water layer has a height y above the absorbing gel. The angle of arrival is θ. The distance of propagation is r.

In summary, the measured signal |ΔS| [mV] depends on the various parameters according to the following approximate expression:

$$|\Delta S(t)| = A \ P_0 \frac{a}{c_s t} \ |\cos(\theta_1)\exp\left(-((r_1 - c_s t)/c_s\tau)^2\right) - \cos(\theta_2)\exp\left(-((r_2 - c_s t)/c_s\tau)^2\right)| \qquad \text{Eq. 6}$$

where r_1 and r_2 are the distances from the pressure source at the submerged absorbing gel to beamsite #1 and beamsite #2, respectively, on the phantom surface. θ_1 and θ_2 are the angles of arrival at the beamsites.

3. EXPERIMENTAL RESULTS

3.1 Detector response vs distance above surface of test medium

The dual-beam common-path interferometer had a maximum sensitivity when the surface of the phantom was located one focal length from the imaging lens that essentially focused the output of the Wallaston prism onto the phantom surface.

Figure 4 shows measurements of a standard laser-induced signal for various heights of the phantom surface. A normal distribution is shown to approximately characterize the height-dependent response: peak at the focal plane (h = 0 cm), full-width half-max ~1.5 cm. All subsequent experiments were conducted with the phantom surface at the optimal height h.

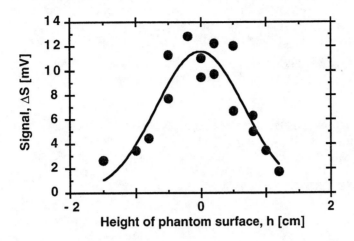

Fig. 4: Response (ΔS) vs height (h) of phantom surface relative to the imaging lens. Maximum response occured when the surface of phantom was located at h = 0 cm which was one focal length from the imaging lens (see Fig. 1) that focused the beams leaving the Wallaston prism onto the phantom surface.

3.2 Point spread function of response for interferometer

How well does Eq. 6 describe the response of the dual-beam vibrometer to pressure sources generated as a function of depth and lateral position? To answer this question, the position of the laser-induced pressure source was varied to map the point spread function of response. Experimental measurements of the signal $|\Delta S|$ were compared with the predictions of Eq. 6 using A and τ as free parameters for fitting. Hence, a preliminary calibration of the measurement system (specifying A) was obtained.

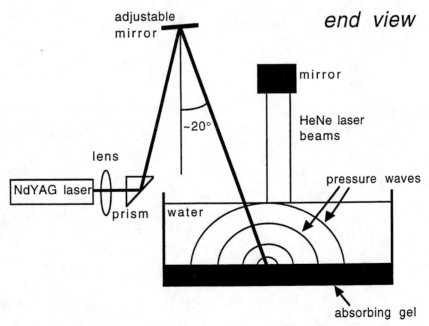

Fig. 5: Experimental setup. Laser irradiation was down through the clear water. An adjustable mirror varied the site of laser irradiation of the absorbing gel.

As shown in Fig. 5, the YAG laser pulse was directed to different positions on the absorbing gel by an adjustable mirror. The sites of irradiation were placed along a line connecting the two beams which was perpendicular to the midplane between the two beams. The time of arrival (t_{arr}) of the pressure wave at the closest beam site was used to establish the distance from signal source to closest beam, $r = t_{arr}c_s$.

Knowing the gel-to-surface distance y, the lateral position x was calculated: $x = \sqrt{r^2 - y^2}$, (see Fig. 3). Two experiments were conducted, one with y = 17.8-mm of water over the gel and the second with y = 11.5-mm of water.

Figure 6 shows the response as a function of distance from the sensing beams. The two figures show two heights of water above the absorbing gel. The x axis in each figure is position parallel to the line joining the two beams and perpendicular to the midplane between the two sensing beams. The position x is zero at the midpoint between the two beams. A null plane is evident between the two beams where the stress wave arrives at both beams simultaneously and hence there is no net $d(\Delta h)$ to be sensed.

The data sets were fitted by a calibration factor, A [mV/bar]. The timespread of the arriving waves, τ in Eqs. 4 and 6 was assigned the value 0.33 μs based on Fig. 2, corresponding to a 0.49-mm 1/e half-width of the stress wave . The calibration factor A equaled 40 mV/bar in Fig. 6A and 70 mV/bar in Fig. 6B. The calibration factor A should have been a common constant. The 1.8-fold discrepancy is not understood and is likely to be simply due to the preliminary nature of this work and the uncertainty in how we were sampling the gain factor $dS/d(\Delta h)$ in Eq. 2, as discussed above.

Approximate values for A, P_0, a, and τ used in these experiments were 30-70 mV/bar, 13 bar, 1 mm, and 0.33 μs, respectively. The noise level for measurements of $|\Delta S|$, based on the peak value of ΔS^2 using a 32-point average, was about 1 mV or 10-30 mbar of pressure.

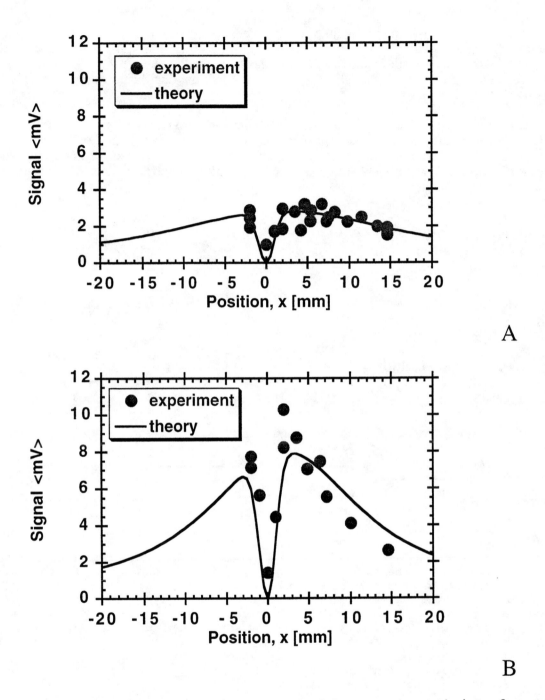

A

B

Fig. 6: Point spread function of response for dual-beam common-path interferometer. Measurements were made along a line connecting the two laser beam irradiation sites which was perpendicular to the null plane between the two beams at x = 0. The distance from midplane to point of energy deposition is x [mm]. Solid lines are the analytic expression, Eq. 6, fitting for A and τ. The value of τ was 0.33 μs which implies an apparent width of arriving stress wave is $c_s(0.3 \ \mu s) = 0.49$ mm. (A) Height of water above absorbing gel is 17.8 mm. Calibration was 40 mV/bar. (B) Height of water above absorbing gel is 11.5 mm. Calibration was 70 mV/bar.

3.3 Demonstration of imaging buried objects

To demonstrate the resolution possible for an object buried within a phantom, the setup in Fig. 7 was prepared allowing irradiation from below the phantom. This setup allowed precisely localized generation of pressure waves despite addition of scatterer to the water medium above the gel. The experiment tested whether scattering particles in the phantom medium affect the dual-beam interferometer's detection of arriving pressure waves.

The absorbing object was a long thin bar of absorbing gel (20 mm long x 10 mm wide x 2 mm thick). In one experiment the phantom was clear water and in a second experiment a scatterer (coffee whitener) was added to the water. For the clear phantom, the signal depended on the specular reflectance from the water surface. For the scattering phantom, the signal depended on the both the specular surface reflectance and the scattering from lipid droplets in the scattering phantom.

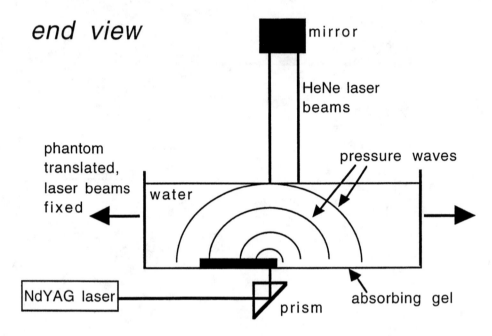

Fig. 7: Experimental setup. The liquid phantom was held in a clear glass container. The absorbing object was a collagen gel phantom with India ink (20 mm long x 10 mm wide x 2 mm thick). The object was submerged in water 11 mm from the surface. The Nd:YAG laser irradiated the absorbing object from the bottom (3-mm-dia. spot) and the two HeNe laser detection points impinged on the top surface of the phantom. Pressure waves generated in the gel propagated to the surface for detection by the HeNe laser beams. The YAG laser pulse was aligned with one of the beams of the interferometer to optimize sensitivity. The phantom containing the absorbing object was translated to vary the relative position of the object while keeping the YAG laser and HeNe laser beams in a fixed relationship. Measurements were made along a line perpendicular to the long axis of the object.

Figure 8 shows the measured signal vs position of the interrogating laser detection system. The data demonstrated that the edge of the object could be detected with sub-mm resolution. The edge response of the system was a linear curve extending from -1 mm to 0.7 mm, where the object edge was at 0 mm. The half-max midpoint of this edge response was within 0.15 mm of the true edge, comparable to the apparent width, $c_s\tau$, of the pressure wave arriving at the HeNe beams.

The results in Fig. 8 for the clear water vs scattering medium were similar. The resolution of the dual-beam interferometer response was not degraded in the scattering medium due to any subsurface scattering that might contribute to the signal.

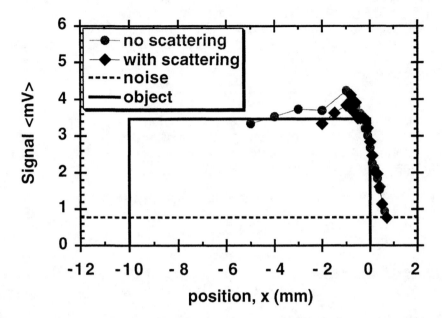

Fig. 8: Edge detection for an absorbing gel object submerged 11 mm in an aqueous phantom. The phantom assembly with gel object (2 mm thick x 10 mm wide) was moved past the immobile detection system. The signal <mV> is plotted versus the position on the phantom that was irradiated from below by the YAG laser (3-mm-dia. beam) and detected from above by one of the HeNe laser beams. The object edge was located at x = 0. The object was submerged in either clear water (circles) or water plus a scatterer (diamonds). The object position is indicated by the rectangular solid line. The noise level is indicated by the dashed horisontal line.

4. DISCUSSION

This paper has demonstrated that a noncontact measurement of laser-induced pressure waves arriving at a tissue surface from a buried absorbing object can be implemented using a dual-beam vibrometer based on a common-path interferometer. The calibration factor for the device was tentatively about 30-100 mV/bar. For comparison, the calibration factor for a lithium niobate piezoelectric transducer has been reported by Oraevsky et al. [2] to be 100 nV/Pa, or 10 mV/bar. Therefore, the interferometer is tentatively 3-10-fold more sensitive than the piezoelectric transducer.

The noise threshold was about 1 mV (10-30 mbar). Oraevsky et al. used the third-harmonic Q-switched Nd:YAG laser (355-nm, 3-mm-dia. spot, energy = 5 mJ, exposure = 4.4 mJ/cm^2) and K_2CrO_4 solutions to test the linearity of their lithium niobate transducer. Their lowest measurement was for μ_a = 6.5 cm^{-1} which with their laser exposure would yield a pressure of 40 mbar. The noise threshold quoted in the manufacturer's literature is 20-40 mbar. Hence, the interferometer appears to have a noise threshold comparable to the piezoelectric detector.

The maximum signal that still retained 95% linearity was estimated to be 3276 mV or 33-100 bar. Hence, the vibrometer provides a dynamic range of 1-3300 mV. In comparison, the maximum absorption coefficient measured by Oraevsky et al. was $\mu_a = 1000$ cm^{-1}, which with their laser exposure would correspond to 6 bar. Probably the piezoelectric transducer can detect much larger pressures, however in practical experiments involving laser-induced temperature jumps much less than 100°C it is difficult to attain higher pressures. Higher absorption coefficients have such thin depths of attenuation that it is difficult for a 10-ns laser pulse to attain stress confinement in the object. Also, the high acoustic frequencies associated with thin depths of attenuation are strongly attenuated in most media, especially tissues. So from a practical matter, the upper limit of detector response is not usually utilized in photoacoustic imaging. The interferometer appears to have sufficient upper dynamic range to provide linear responses for photoacoustic imaging applications.

5. CONCLUSION

In conclusion, this work demonstrates the priniciple of an all-optical noncontact method for measuring laser-induced acoustic pressure waves. The point spread function of response for the system has been measured and the system performance, in terms of figures of merit, compares favorably with the previous experience with a lithium-niobate piezo-electric transducer. Finally, the potential for sub-mm resolution imaging of buried absorbing objects in aqueous phantoms based on pressured waves induced by absorption of Q-switched Nd:YAG pulsed laser radiation has been demonstrated.

6. REFERENCES

1   Hanson, S.G.; Lindvold, L.R.; Hansen, B.H., Industrial implementation of diffractive optical elements for nondestructive testing. *SPIE Proceedings* 2868:216-224, 1996, *Vibration measurements by laser techniques: Advances and applications. 2.* International conference on vibration measurements by laser techniques, Ancona (IT), 23-25 Sep 1996. Tomasini, E.P. (ed.), (The International Society for Optical Engineering, Bellingham, WA).

2   A.A. Oraevsky, S.L. Jacques, F.K. Tittel, "Measurement of tissue optical properties by time-resolved detection of laser-induced transient stress," *Applied Optics* 36:402-415, 1997.

Comparison with transient measurements of infrared radiation and stress wave

for the practical ablation monitoring during Photorefractive Keratectomy

Miya Ishihara, Tsunenori Arai, Makoto Kikuchi,
Hironori Nakano*, Satoko Kawauchi*, Minoru Obara*

Dept. of Medical Engineering, National Defense Medical College, Tokorozawa, Saitama, 359, Japan

*Dept. of Electric Engineering, Keio University, Yokohama, Kanagawa Pref., 223, Japan

Abstract

We compared infrared radiation measurement with stress wave measurement for real-time ablation monitoring during photorefractive keratectomy (PRK). We estimated temperature elevation which may be one of the most effective parameter for PRK monitoring, because the ablation mechanism is mainly attributed to thermal kinetics. The temperature elevation of ablated cornea was evaluated by the infrared radiation and the stress wave. The thermal radiation from irradiated cornea was detected by a MCT detector. The measured signal increased sharply just after the laser irradiation and decreased quasi-exponentially. We could calculate the temperature elevation by observed signal using Stefan-Boltzmann radiation law. In the case of the gelatin gel (15%wt) ablation in vitro, the temperature elevation was 97deg. at $208mJ/cm^2$ in the laser fluence. We also measured transient stress wave by the acoustic transducer which was made by polyvinylidene fluoride (PVDF) film. The temperature elevation could be calculated from the peak stress amplitude based on the short pulsed laser ablation theory. The good agreement on the temperature elevation was obtained between the infrared and the stress based estimations. Due to non-contact and non-invasive method, our infrared measurements for temperature elevation monitoring may be available to accomplish the feedback control on the PRK.

Key words: ArF excimer laser, photorefractive keratectomy(PRK), ablation, temperature

Further author information

M.Ishihara: Email:kobako@ndmc.ac.jp, Telephone:+81-429-95-1211, Fax:+81-429-96-5199

1. Introduction

Photorefractive Keratectomy (PRK) with ArF excimer laser ablation has been developed as a innovative therapy in order to alter the corneal curvature for refractive error correction. The ArF excimer laser is capable of ablating cornea tissue with little damage to surrounding tissue because penetration depth at this wavelength (193nm) for cornea is less than 1μm. Variables demonstrated results of precise cornea ablation by ArF excimer laser[1],[2].

However, There are still some problems on PRK. Discrepancies between planned and actual refractive correction in eyes undergoing PRK may still occur[3]. Another PRK problem is anterior stromal haze which was caused by new collagen production was found in 92% of those undergoing[4].

All procedure during PRK laser ablation should be computed feedback-control due to precise and safety PRK. The real-time monitoring during the ArF excimer laser ablation requires for computed feed-back control. Some reports have studied techniques to monitor the ablation site in real-time during PRK[5].

The effective monitoring subject for the ablation control has to be related to the cornea ablation mechanism by the ArF excimer laser. Regarding to the ablation mechanism, much attentions has been paid[1],[2],[6],[7]. The ArF excimer laser corneal ablation may be attributed to not only photochemical interaction, but also thermal interaction. The mass removal by the ArF excimer laser ablation is mainly attributed to the thermal interaction although photochemical interaction plays a primary role in the ablation.

One is the most effective parameter for laser ablation monitoring might be considered "temperature elevation". The temperature evaluation has already measured during excimer laser corneal ablation by M.S.Kitai et al.[6], T.Bende et al.[8]. In their experimental conditions, time-constants were about 40-200ms. The precise temperature elevation should be measured in higher time-resolution because the maximum temperature elevation by the 13ns pulsed irradiation might occur within several ten nanoseconds.

Our aim of this study is to monitor the temperature elevation with rapid time-resolution during the ArF excimer laser corneal ablation. We demonstrated non invasive thermal radiation measurements. We observed stress wave which is well-understanding, conventional tool for the ablation measurements. The temperature elevation was calculated as follows, the observed infrared radiation was applied to Stefan-Boltzman law and the peak stress amplitude was to the short pulsed laser ablation theory[9]. We compared the calculated temperature elevation by infrared and stress measurements and discussed on the future design, that is, the feedback control on PRK by real time temperature monitoring.

2. Materials & Method

A pulsed ArF excimer laser (C3470, Hamamatsu Photonics Co. Ltd., Shizuoka, Japan) of which wavelength was 193nm and pulse width was 13ns was used. The laser beam was irradiated to samples at the laser fluences of 10-320mJ/cm^2 and repetition rate of 10Hz. Our experimental setup for infrared radiation measurements is illustrated in Fig.1. The thermal radiation from the irradiated surface was collected by Au concave mirror. The gathered thermal radiation detected by cooled MCT(Marcury Cadmium Telluride) detector (P3257, Hamamatsu Photonics Co. Ltd., Shizuoka, Japan) with Ge lens of which detectable wavelength was in excess of 3 μm (Nippon infrared industries Co. Ltd., Kawasaki,

Japan). The MCT detector's rise time is 1 μs. The MCT detector could detect 7-14 μm in wavelength. The measured infrared radiation was about 10% of all radiation from the sample surface. The MCT detector output was documented by the digital storage oscilloscope (7854, Textronics Inc., OR, USA.). The power change of observed signal originated in temperature elevation of the irradiated sample surface.

The stress wave was measured by handmade acoustic transducer which was placed behind the sample. The acoustic transducer consisted of PVDF (polyvinylidene fluoride) piezoelectric film of which thickness was 40 μm and 7mm thickness acoustic absorber. The acoustic transducer had about 18ns rise time which was restricted by the thickness of the PVDF film. The acoustic transducer was enclosed with a metal box in order to decrease noise. The electrical output from the transducer was documented by the digital storage oscilloscope. The measured stress amplitude was given by Eq.(1) using output voltage by the transducer.

Eq.(1): $F(t) = V(t) * (Cd + Cp)/d_t$

where $F(t)$ is detected stress at the transducer, $V(t)$ is output voltage of the transducer, Cd is loading capacitance of the oscilloscope, Cp is capacitance of the transducer, d_t is strain constant for PVDF.

We performed experiments described above using model medium. The organic material of cornea belongs to collagen. Boiling in water converts collagen into gelatin. Gelatin gel at a concentration of 15% in weight and thickness of 5mm was used as our model medium because the concentration of the collagen contents in cornea is about 15% in weight.

3. Results

(1) Infrared radiation measurements

Transient waveform obtained by our infrared radiation measurements system at the laser fluence of 148mJ/cm^2 and the repetition rate of 10Hz is shown in Fig.2. This waveform indicates the time course of the infrared radiation intensity from irradiated gelatin gel surface. The signal increased sharply just after the ArF excimer laser start. The peak of the waveform was at 1μs which was restricted by the rise-time of the MCT detector. The signal decreased quasi-exponentially. The decay time which was defined as the time from the peak to the 1/e (e ≒ 2.718) of the intensity was about 1ms. The peak amplitude of the MCT detector output was increased from 0.1mV to 20mV when the irradiation fluence was varied from 10mJ/cm^2 to 320mJ/cm^2. The decay of the observed waveform did not related to the irradiation fluence. Therefore, the decay of the waveform may be attributed to the heat conduction in the gelatin gel. The increase part of the waveform might be governed by the deposit laser energy.

(2) Stress wave measurements

Transient stress waveform measured by the handmade acoustic transducer at the laser fluence of 152 mJ/cm^2 and the repetition rate of 10Hz is shown in Fig.3. The waveform started 3.5μs after the laser pulse. This delay was agreed with the transit time for the stress wave by sound speed through the gelatin gel whose thickness was about 5mm. The observed waveform differed from thermoelastic wave which consisted of compression and rarefaction wave. It suggested the appearance of recoil momentum from the ablation products. The stress produced by laser ablation was calculated by observed signal using Eq.(1). The peak stress was from 40 to 650MPa when the irradiation laser fluence was varied from 60mJ/cm^2 to 320mJ/cm^2.

4. Discussion

Our observed infrared radiation originated from the temperature elevation by ArF excimer laser irradiation. The maximum temperature elevation during the laser irradiation was estimated from the peak intensity of the observed infrared radiation waveform using the Stefan-Boltzman law. Our calculation was included detective efficiency which is the rate of gathered radiation to all radiation from the sample surface and the calibrated spectral responsibility of the MCT detector as shown in Eq.(2).

Eq.(2): $W = \varepsilon^* \eta^* T_E^{\,4}$

$$W = V / R / \kappa / s$$

where W is infrared radiation power density, ε is emissivity of the sample, η is the Stefan-Boltzman constant, T_E is temperature elevation, V is the MCT detector output voltage, R is calibrated spectral responsibility, κ is detective efficiency and s is irradiated area.

The calculated temperature elevation was indicated in Fig.4. The temperature elevation are plotted versus the laser fluence. The temperature elevation was governed by the laser fluence and reached 75deg. at the laser fluence of $106mJ/cm^2$. The sample temperature reached 373K at the fluence since the sample initial temperature was 298K in our experiments. The increase of the temperature elevation was slow from $106mJ/cm^2$ to $189mJ/cm^2$. Over the fluence of $166mJ/cm^2$, the temperature elevation was significant again.

According to the short pulsed laser ablation theory[9], the maximum temperature elevation(T_E) by pulsed laser irradiation was described as Eq.(3) if two conditions described below were satisfied. The first condition was scattering coefficient $\mu(s)$ was much smaller than absorption coefficient $\mu(a)$. The other condition was the laser pulse duration $\tau(p)$ was much shorter than the heat conduction time $\tau(hd)$. The heat conduction time $\tau(hd)$ is defined the time which takes for heat to diffuse into the sample. The heat conduction time $\tau(hd)$ is indicated as follows, $\tau(hd)=1/4^*\chi^*\mu(a)$, where χ is thermal diffusivity.

Eq.(3): $T_E = \mu(a)^* F / d^* Cv$

where F is laser fluence, d is density of the sample, Cv is specific heat at constant volume. There occurs an instantaneous rise of the pressure P in proportion to the temperature elevation as described Eq.(4)

Eq.(4): $P = \beta^* d^* Vs^{2*} (Cv/Cp)^* T_E$

where β is coefficient of volume expansion, Vs is sound speed, Cp is the specific heat at constant pressure.

We calculated the temperature elevation by applying our experimental data of stress wave measurements to Eq.(4). The temperature elevation was calculated 63deg. when the irradiation fluence of the ArF excimer laser was $139mJ/cm^2$. The temperature elevation was also calculated 101deg. at the laser fluence of $208mJ/cm^2$ and 175deg. of $316mJ/cm^2$.

The comparison of the temperature elevation showed the good agreements with infrared radiation measurements and stress wave measurements. In the case of the irradiation fluence of the ArF excimer laser was $316mJ/cm^2$, the temperature elevation was 180deg. from the infrared measurements and 175deg. from the stress wave measurements. The temperature elevation was 97deg. from the infrared measurements and 101deg. from the stress measurements at the laser fluence of $208mJ/cm^2$.

5. Conclusion

We measured infrared radiation by the MCT detector and stress wave by handmade acoustic transducer during ArF excimer laser cornea ablation. The temperature elevation could be obtained by each transient measurements. The infrared radiation measurements were applied to Stefan-Boltzman radiation law. The temperature elevation was 97deg. at 208mJ/cm^2 in the laser fluence in the case of the gelatin gel ablation. The stress wave measurements which were well-understanding, conventional tool for ablation monitoring were applied to the short pulsed laser ablation theory to calculate the temperature elevation. The comparison with the two measurements carried out good agreements. In conclusion, in view of non-invasive and non-contact measurement method, the infrared radiation measurements for temperature elevation monitoring may be available to accomplish real-time ablation monitoring.

6. Reference

[1] S.L Trokel, R.Shinivasan, B.Braren, "Excimer laser surgery of the cornea.", American Journal of Ophthalmology, 96, 710, 1983

[2] R.Srinivasan, P.E.Dyer, B.Braren, "Far-Ultraviolet laser ablation of the cornea: photoacousitc studies." Lasers in Surgery and Medicine, 6,514-519,1987

[3] N.Rosa, G.Cennamo, A.Pasquariello, F.Maffulli, A.Sebastiani, "Refractive outcome and corneal topographic studies after Photorefractive Keratectomy with different-sized ablation zones.", Ophthalmology, 103(7), 1130, 1996

[4] D.S.Gartry, M.G.K.Muir, J.Marshall, "Excimer laser photorefractive keratectomy, 18-month follow up." Ophthalmology, 99(8), 1209, 1992

[5] J.M.Frantz, J.J.Reidy, M.B.McDonald, "A comparison of surgical keratometers." Refractive & Corneal Surgery, 5,409, 1989

[6] M.S.Kitai, V.L.Popkov, V.A.Semchishen, A.A.Kharizov, "The physics of UV laser cornea ablation.", IEEE J.of Q.E. 27(2), 302, 1991

[7] G.H.Pettit, M.N.Ediger, "Corneal-tissue absorption coefficients for 193- and 213-nm ultraviolet radiation.", Appl.Optics, 35(19), 3386, 1996

[8] T.Bende, T.Seiler, J.Wollensak, "Side effects in excimer laser corneal surgery.", Graefe's Archive Ophthalmology, 226, 277, 1988

[9] R.O.Esenaliev, A.A.Oraevsky, V.S.Letokhov, A.A.Karabutov, T.V.Malinsky, "Studies of acoustical and shock waves in the pulsed laser ablation of biotissue.", Lasers in Surgery and Medicine, 13, 470, 1993

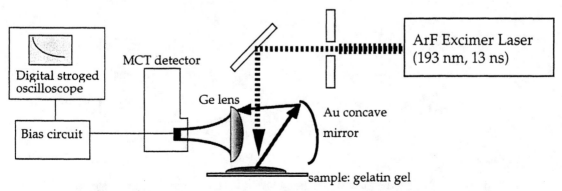

Fig.1 Experimental setup for infrared radiation measurements

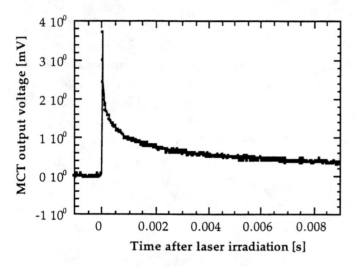

Fig.2 Transient waveform obtained by infrared
radiation measurements system.
laser fluence: 148mJ/cm²

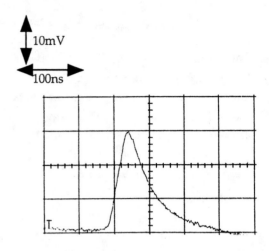

Fig.3 Transient stress waveform obtained
by handmade acoustic transducer
laser fluence: 152mJ/cm²

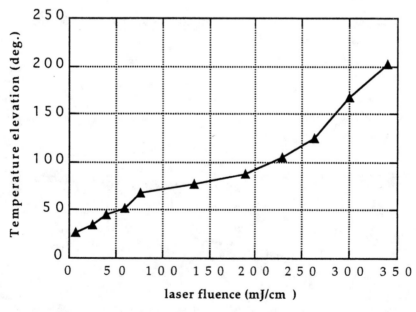

Fig.4 Temperature elevation calculated from infrared radiation results.

Recent Development in Photoacoustic Image Reconstruction

Pingyu Liu

Department of Radiology, Indiana University School of Medicine,
Indianapolis, IN 46202-5111, U.S.A.

ABSTRACT

Photoacoustic phenomenon has been investigated. An experimental protocol using photoacoustic principle has been proposed to image the regional distribution of electromagnetic energy absorption density in an object. This paper presents a rigorous method for photoacoustic image reconstruction. It is proved that photoacoustic image reconstruction is intrinsically a three-dimensional (3D) procedure. The spatial smear function (SSF) is introduced.

An example using synthetic data proves the validity of photoacoustic image reconstruction theory proposed by the paper. The example shows that even the first order approximation of photoacoustic image reconstruction gives good agreement with the reality. It is also seen from the example that the accuracy and noise immunity of the reconstruction procedure depend on the experimental arrangement.

Keywords: photoacoustics, electromagnetic energy absorption, image reconstruction.

INTRODUCTION

Photoacoustic phenomena were discovered about a century ago.[1] For a long period photoacoustic investigation was concentrated in gaseous media. With the advent of laser, photoacoustic research has been intensified in liquid and solid materials. All of these early research studies focused mainly on the depiction of the interaction between an electromagnetic field and matters. In recent years the study of photoacoustics has been revitalized by several research groups in the direction of the investigation of optical and electromagnetic absorption properties of biological tissues.[2,3,4] All the research papers dealt with photoacoustic signals generated at different situations. To obtain a regional distribution of electromagnetic absorption within tissue by photoacoustic measurement, a complete photoacoustic image reconstruction theory is required. This paper is a continuation of the author's endeavor for constructing the theory.

A complete reconstruction theory has to address both the forward and inverse problems. For photoacoustic phenomenon the forward and inverse problems are the generation of photoacoustic pressure signals and reconstruction of regional electromagnetic absorption, respectively.

GENERATION OF PHOTOACOUSTIC SIGNALS

In 1996 the author presented a formula to calculate photoacoustic pressure signals assuming a short external electromagnetic pulse and an acoustically and thermally uniform medium confined in a limited volume. The formula states that if at time t=0 the electromagnetically heterogeneous medium is irradiated by the pulse, the pressure signal observed by an ideal pressure transducer at location $R\mathbf{n}$ and time t > 0 is a volume integral:[5]

$$p(R\mathbf{n}, t) = \frac{\beta}{4\pi c} \int \int \int \frac{d\mathbf{r}}{|R\mathbf{n} - \mathbf{r}|} \frac{\partial S(\mathbf{r}, t')}{\partial t'}, \tag{1}$$

where S(r,t) is the heating power density at location $\mathbf{r}$ and time t caused by the external electromagnetic pulse and $t' = t - |R\mathbf{n} - \mathbf{r}|/v$ and v is the speed of sound of the medium. Transducers are located on a spherical surface of radius R which encircle the electromagnetically heterogeneous medium. Parameters c and β are the specific heat and the bulk thermal expansion coefficient, respectively, of the medium. The vector **n** is an unit direction vector. It is seen that the pressure signal will be zero if there is no absorber in the volume.

If there is only one uniform spherical absorber of radius a centered at **r**=0 and the time dependence of the heating function is the Dirac δ-function, i.e.,

$$S(\mathbf{r},t) = \begin{cases} I_0\delta(t) & \text{if } |\mathbf{r}| < a \\ 0 & \text{else} \end{cases}, \qquad (2)$$

then we have a special solution as

$$p_s(R,t) = \begin{cases} \dfrac{\beta I_0 v}{2Rc}\left(\dfrac{R}{v} - t\right) & \text{if } \dfrac{R-a}{v} < t < \dfrac{R+a}{v} \\ 0 & \text{else} \end{cases}. \qquad (3)$$

Figure 1 shows the special solution as a function of time.

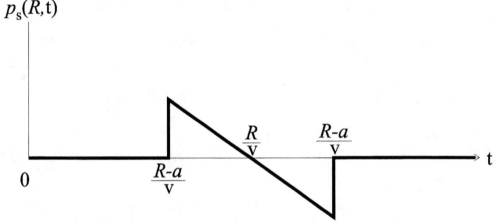

Figure 1. Photoacoustic pressure signal generated by a uniform, spherical absorber irradiated with a very short heating pulse at time zero.

RECONSTRUCTION OF REGIONAL ELECTROMAGNETIC ABSORPTION

Any reconstruction procedure is directly related with how its forward problem is resolved. Therefore, to solve the photoacoustic image reconstruction problem one has to start from its forward solution, i.e., equation (1). If the absorbing object is limited in a finite volume and the time-dependence of the external electromagnetic heating for every point in the object is a square pulse, then equation (1) can be rewritten as

$$p(R\mathbf{n},t) = \frac{\beta}{4\pi c}\frac{\partial}{\partial t}[\frac{1}{t}\iiint A(\mathbf{r})\delta(|R\mathbf{n}-\mathbf{r}|-vt)d\mathbf{r}], \qquad (4)$$

where $A(\mathbf{r})$ is the total heating energy density during the pulse at location **r**. The goal of photoacoustic image reconstruction is to find $A(\mathbf{r})$ from measuring a set of pressure signals, $p(R\mathbf{n},t)$.

It has been proved that the first order approximation to $A(\mathbf{r})$ is $L(\mathbf{r})$: [6]

$$L(\mathbf{r}) = K \iint_{2\pi} d\mathbf{n} \left[t \frac{dp(R\mathbf{n},t)}{dt} + 2p(R\mathbf{n},t) \right] \Bigg|_{t=\frac{|R\mathbf{n}-\mathbf{r}|}{v}} , \tag{5}$$

where $K = \dfrac{-c}{\pi\beta v^2}$. The relationship between $A(\mathbf{r})$ and $L(\mathbf{r})$ is [6]

$$L(\mathbf{r}) = \iiint S(\mathbf{r},\mathbf{r}') A(\mathbf{r}') d\mathbf{r}' , \tag{6}$$

where $S(\mathbf{r},\mathbf{r}')$ is called the spatial smear function (SSF) and defined as a whole phase space integral

$$S(\mathbf{r},\mathbf{r}') = \iiint e^{2\pi i v(|R\mathbf{n}-\mathbf{r}'|-|R\mathbf{n}-\mathbf{r}|)} d\vec{\mathbf{v}} . \tag{7}$$

All that equation (5) poses is a 3D Fredholm integral equation of the first kind with a real, symmetric integral kernel $S(\mathbf{r},\mathbf{r}')$ and a known free-term $L(\mathbf{r})$. This feature makes the integral equation solvable by the Schmidt-Hibert theory. [7]

Equation (5) requires an infinite number of transducers located on a hemisphere of radius R. In practice, it is impossible to have an infinite number of transducers. It is often more likely to have a limited number, say N, of transducers evenly distributed in a 2π-stereoangle. Assuming that each transducer occupies a stereoangle of $\Delta\Omega$ and considering the discretized space, equation (5) will be replaced by

$$L(\mathbf{r}) = K\Delta\Omega \sum_{i=1}^{N} \left[t \frac{dp(R\mathbf{n}_i,t)}{dt} + 2p(R\mathbf{n}_i,t) \right] \Bigg|_{t=\frac{|R\mathbf{n}_i-\mathbf{r}|}{v}} , \tag{8}$$

where $\mathbf{n}_i$ is the unit vector from the origin to the i-th transducer. Figure 2 shows the configuration of real apparatus. Equation (8) is the most important result since when R is much larger than the dimension of the reconstructed object $L(\mathbf{r})$ is very close to $A(\mathbf{r})$.

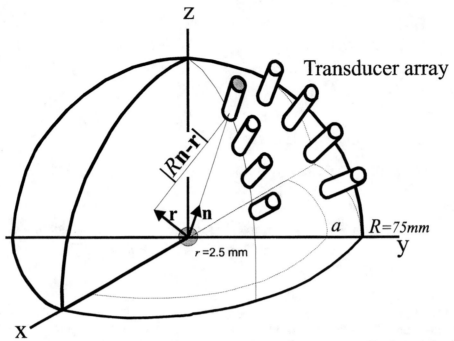

Figure 2. Photoacoustic measurement setup. Transducers, not all shown in the figure, are distributed on the hemisphere surface with y grater than zero. The hemisphere's radius is R. An uniform absorber with radius of 2.5 mm, marked with grey color, is located at the center of the transducer hemisphere of radius of 75 mm. One transducer, which is highlighted with a darker bottom, has the position vector $R\mathbf{n}$.

COMPUTER SIMULATION AND DISCUSSION

As an example to show the validity of the photoacoustic image reconstruction procedure proposed by the paper, let's consider an uniform spherical absorber of radius r=2.5 mm surrounded by infinite, non-absorbing medium. For simplicity it is assumed that the center of the absorber coincides with the center of the hemisphere of the transducer array, as shown in Figure 2. The radius of the transducer hemisphere is R=75 mm. Since R is much larger than r, only the first order approximation of $A(\mathbf{r})$, i.e., $L(\mathbf{r})$, is reconstructed.

To produce photoacoustic pressure signals a short external radiation pulse of 0.5 microsecond(μs) is applied. The photoacoustic pressure signal seen by a transducer of the array can be calculated for the simple model, by integrating equation (3) from 0 to 0.5 μs. In calculation the speed of sound in both the sphere and medium is assumed to be v=1.5 mm/μs. The total number of transducers is $1+N^2$.

Computer simulation of photoacoustic image reconstruction has been carried out for two cases: N=8 and 32, corresponding to 65 and 1025 transducers, respectively. Image reconstruction of the relative absorption density is based on equation (8) using the synthetic pressure data. To exhibit the noise immunity of the approach a random noise is added to pressure signals. The magnitude of the noise is 10% of the maximum signal. Figures 3(a) and (b) show the reconstructed relative absorption density in a center area of 50x50 mm^2 of plane z=0 for the two cases. Figures 3(c) and (d) are the relative absorption density distributions along the line z=y=0. In this simplified example it is appreciated that the photoacoustic image reconstruction procedure proposed by the paper does provide desired information of the relative absorption density distribution, even only the first order approximation, $\mathbf{L(r)}$, is performed. The reconstructed distribution of relative absorption density using 1025 transducers agrees with the true distribution much better than using 65 transducers. The case using 1025 transducers also shows a better noise immunity than using 65 transducers.

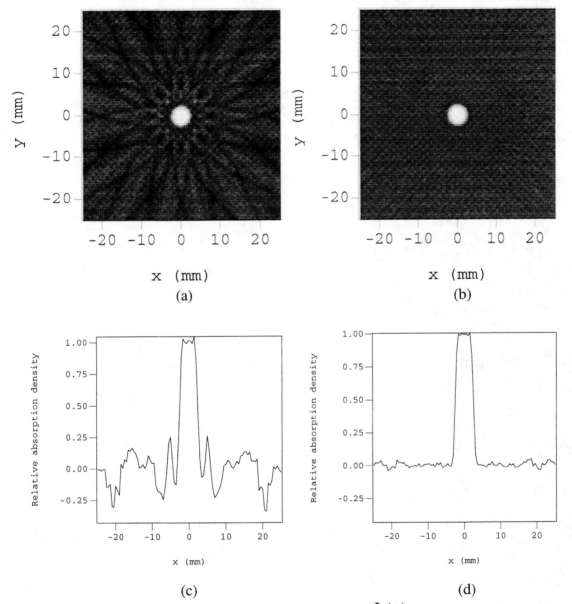

(a)

(b)

(c)

(d)

Figure 3. Reconstructed relative absorption density, $\mathbf{L(r)}$, in plane of z=0. (a) and (b) show the reconstructed relative absorption density in plane of z=0 for cases using 65 and 1025 transducers, respectively. The object is an uniform absorber of radius 2.5 mm at the center of a reconstructed area of 50x50 mm^2. (c) and (d) are the relative absorption density distributions along the line of z=y=0 for cases using 65 and 1025 transducers, respectively.

Photoacoustic imaging mechanism is very unique and different from other imaging mechanisms by its 3D nature. Other image modalities, such as x-ray CT and MRI, may use less data to reconstruct a 'slice' of image than a 'volume' of image. But for photoacoustic image reconstruction one cannot use less data acquisition to make a 'slice' than a 'volume' image for the same object and same resolution. In this sense we say that photoacoustic image reconstruction is intrinsically a 3D procedure. The author proposed a new mathematical tool to treat photoacoustic image reconstruction which is called the P-transform. [6]

ACKNOWLEDGMENT

This work was in part supported by NIH grant 1-R01-CA65744. The author is very grateful to Dr Robert Kruger for his generous support.

REFERENCES

1. A. G. Bell. *Am J Sci* **20**, 30, 1880.
2. T. Bowen. "Radiation-induced thermoacoustic soft tissue imaging," *Proc IEEE Ultrasonics* 817-822, 1981.
3. A. A. Oraevsky A A, S. L. Jacques and F. K. Tittel. "Determination of tissue optical properties by piezoelectric detection of laser-induced stress waves," *Laser-Tissue Interaction SPIE* **1882,** 82-101, 1993
4. R. A. Kruger. "Photoacoustic ultrasound," *Medical Physics* **21,** 127-131, 1994.
5. P. Liu. "Image reconstruction from photoacoustic pressure signals," *Laser-Tissue Interaction SPIE* **2681** 285-296, 1996.
6. P. Liu. "The P-transform and photoacoustic image reconstruction," (Accepted by *Physics in Medicine and Biology*).
7. J. Mathews and R. L. Walker. *Mathematical Methods of Physics* (Menlo Park CA: Benjamin/Cummings,) pp 305-311, 1970.

SESSION 11

Optics I

Measurement of tissue optical properties and modeling of optimal light delivery for tumor treatment

Lihong V. Wang, Ph.D.[a]

Guillermo Marquez, B. S.

Optical Imaging Laboratory, Biomedical Engineering Program

Texas A&M University, College Station, Texas 77843-3120, USA

Robert E. Nordquist, Ph. D.

Wound Healing of Oklahoma, Inc.

3939 N. Walnut Street, Oklahoma City, OK 73105

Wei R. Chen, Ph. D.

Oklahoma School of Science and Mathematics

1141 North Lincoln Boulevard, Oklahoma City, OK 73104

Department of Physics and Astronomy, University of Oklahoma, Norman, OK 73109

ABSTRACT

Oblique-incidence reflectometry was used to measure the optical properties of rat tumors with injected absorption-enhancement dye. The measured optical properties were used to model light delivery into the tissues for optimal therapeutic effects. The goal was to efficiently deliver the maximum amount of optical power into buried tumors being treated while avoiding potential damage to normal tissue caused by strong optical power deposition underneath the tissue surface illuminated by the laser beam. The distribution of power deposition was simulated for single beam delivery and multiple beam delivery as well. The simulated results showed that with an appropriate dye enhancement and an optimal laser delivery configuration, a high selectivity for laser treatment of tumors could be achieved.

KEY WORDS

Monte Carlo, light delivery, optical therapy, turbid media, biological tissues.

(a)   Corresponding author. E-mail: LWang@tamu.edu. URL: http://biomed.tamu.edu/~lw.

INTRODUCTION

Laser-tissue interactions and their therapeutic applications is a fast growing research area. Biological tissues are turbid media, in which light attenuates rapidly because of light absorption augmented by strong light scattering. As a consequence, deeply buried tumors usually receive much less optical power than the subsurface normal tissues, which hampers efficacious optical treatment of tumors. By maximizing the power delivered to the target tumors while avoiding damaging subsurface normal tissues, laser treatments may be improved in several aspects. First, the absorption coefficient of tumors may be significantly increased by infusing dyes into the tumors. Secondly, the wavelength of the laser light may be selected to maximize the ratio between the absorption of the tumor and that of the surrounding normal tissue. Thirdly, the light delivery scheme may be optimized to maximize the power absorption by the target tumors. We will concentrate on the third approach in this paper.

In our work reported in this paper, the optical properties of rat tumors were measured with oblique-incidence reflectometry and Monte Carlo simulations were used to investigate the effect of multiple beam delivery compared with single beam delivery under the condition that the location of the buried tumor was known and the absorption of the tumor was enhanced. Compared with our previous work along this line,[1] this paper covers more recent work based on the actual optical properties of tumors.

METHOD

The optical properties of tumors with photosensitizer were measured using oblique-incidence reflectometry.[2-4] The tumor model was the DMBA-4 metastatic mammary tumor in Wistar Furth female rats. Naive rats (6 to 8 weeks) were inoculated with 100,000 viable tumor cells at both inguinal areas. The tumor cells were injected subcutaneously into the fat pads. Within ten days, the primary tumors became palpable and the metastases to axillary areas through lymphatics appeared within 20 days.

The measurement was performed when the primary tumors reached a size of 4 to 8 cm^3, and the metastases 0.4 to 0.8 cm^3. Following sedation, the hair on the skin overlying the tumors was removed. For dye-enhanced absorption, 200 ml of 0.25% indocyanine green (ICG) solution was injected into the center of the tumors 2 hours prior to measurement. The tumor was exposed and measured using a 3 mm probe based on oblique-incidence reflectometry. The measured absorption and reduced scattering coefficient of the tumor at the 805 nm wavelength were used as input parameters for the subsequent Monte Carlo simulations.

Monte Carlo simulations of light transport in tissues have been implemented previously for simple tissue geometry.[5-9] To compute light distributions according to the tissue geometry and optical properties, including refractive index n, absorption coefficient μ_a, scattering coefficient μ_s, and anisotropy factor g, we have written a Monte Carlo program in C for tissues with buried objects. We used the delta-scattering technique[10] for photon tracing to greatly simplify the algorithm because this technique allows a photon packet to be traced without directly dealing with photon crossings of interfaces between different types of tissues. This technique can be used only for refractive-index-matched tissues, although it allows the ambient clear media (e.g., air) and the tissue to have mismatched refractive indices.

We assume that the tissue system has multiple tissue types with identical refractive indices. The interaction coefficient of the ith tissue type, defined as the sum of μ_a and μ_s, is denoted by μ_i. The technique is briefly summarized as follows.

1.   Define a majorant interaction coefficient μ_m, where $\mu_m \geq \mu_i$ for all i.

2.   Select a step size R between two consecutive interactions based on the majorant interaction coefficient,

$$R = - \ln(\xi) / \mu_m, \tag{1}$$

where ξ is a uniformly distributed random number between 0 and 1 $(0 < \xi \leq 1)$. Then, determine the tentative next collision site $\mathbf{r}_k'$ by:

$$\mathbf{r}_k' = \mathbf{r}_{k-1} + R\,\mathbf{u}_{k-1}, \tag{2}$$

where $\mathbf{r}_{k-1}$ is the current site and $\mathbf{u}_{k-1}$ is the direction of the flight.

3.   Play a rejection game:

    a. Get a random number η, which is a uniformly distributed random number between 0 and 1 $(0 < \eta \leq 1)$.

    a. If $\eta \leq \mu_i(\mathbf{r}_k')/\mu_m$, i.e., with a probability of $\mu_i(\mathbf{r}_k')/\mu_m$, accept this point as a real interaction site $(\mathbf{r}_k = \mathbf{r}_k')$.

    b. Otherwise, do not accept $\mathbf{r}_k'$ as a real interaction site but select a new path starting from $\mathbf{r}_k'$ with the unchanged direction $\mathbf{u}_{k-1}$ (i.e., set $\mathbf{r}_{k-1} = \mathbf{r}_k'$ and return to Step 2).

The treatment of photon tracing after step 3 is similar to that in Ref. 9 and will not be repeated here.

The validity can be easily understood by introducing an imaginary interaction event that changes neither the weight nor the direction of the photon. This definition implies that such imaginary interactions are not physically observable, i.e., they can be introduced with any interaction coefficient at any point. We may assume that the majorant interaction coefficient μ_m is a sum of the real μ_{re} and imaginary μ_{im} interaction coefficients, where the real interaction coefficient is μ_{re} is $\mu_i(\mathbf{r}_k')$. In the procedure outlined above, a fraction of the interactions,

$$1 - \mu_{re}/\mu_m = \mu_{im}/\mu_m \tag{3}$$

are imaginary interactions. From another point of view, it is easy to see that on the average, for every μ_m total interactions, there will be μ_{re} interactions accepted as real interactions. The mean free path for the majorant interactions in the delta-scattering method is $1/\mu_m$, and the mean free path for the real interactions in the direct method is $1/\mu_{re}$. Therefore, the photon will move to the correct interaction site using the delta-scattering technique as it would using the direct method because

$$\mu_m(1/\mu_m) = \mu_{re}(1/\mu_{re}), \qquad (4)$$

where the left-hand side means the average distance traveled by the photon packet with μ_m total steps or with μ_{re} real interactions in the delta-scattering method, and the right-hand side means the average distance traveled with μ_{re} real interactions in the direct method.

During the tracing of each weighted photon,[9] the light absorption, reflection, or transmission were correspondingly scored into different arrays according to the spatial positions of the photon. Multiple photons are traced to achieve an acceptable statistical variation. For this study, 100,000 photons were traced.

This Monte Carlo program was used to simulate power deposition for tissue configurations as shown in Fig. 1. Fig. 1(a) shows a single beam delivery scheme to a tissue slab with a tumor buried in the center. The lateral dimensions in the xy-plane was considered optically infinite, i.e., much greater than the penetration depth of light. Fig. 1(b) illustrates a multiple beam delivery scheme to a tissue cube with a tumor buried in the center.

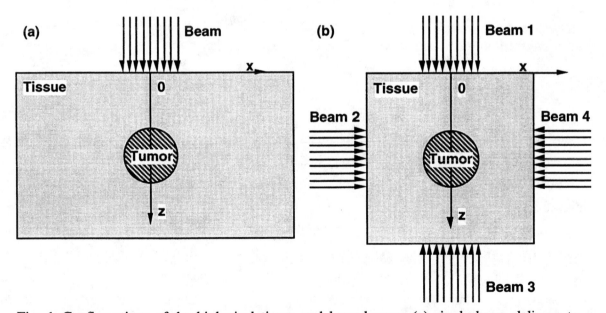

Fig. 1. Configurations of the biological tissue and laser beams: (a) single beam delivery to a wide tissue slab and (b) multiple beam delivery to a tissue cube. The tumor was a sphere that was centered in the background tissue and aligned with the center of the laser beam. In both cases, the optical properties of the background tissue were: absorption coefficient $\mu_a = 0.1$ cm^{-1}, scattering coefficient $\mu_s = 100$ cm^{-1}, anisotropy $g = 0.9$. The optical properties of the tumor were: variable μ_a, $\mu_s = 140$ cm^{-1}, $g = 0.9$. The diameter of the tumor was 1 cm. The thickness of the tissue slab in (a) and the side of the tissue cube in (b) were both 3 cm.

RESULTS and CONCLUSIONS

The absorption coefficient and reduced scattering coefficient of the tumor containing ICG were measured to be 5 cm^{-1} and 14 cm^{-1}, respectively. Assuming the scattering anisotropy g of the tumor was 0.9, we calculated the scattering coefficient to be 140 cm^{-1}. For energy deposition far from the source, the choice of scattering anisotropy g was not important as long as the reduced scattering coefficient was conserved because the energy transport had entered diffusion regime. The optical properties of the normal tissue surrounding the tumor were not measured in this experiment because there was not enough tissue to measure on the rats. We used a typical set of optical properties for the surrounding tissue for the model, where the absorption coefficient, the scattering coefficient, and anisotropy were 0.1 cm^{-1}, 100 cm^{-1}, and 0.9, respectively.

An optimal radius of the laser beam was calculated based on the following expression[1]

$$r_o = \sqrt{\delta\,(2d_t - 2L_t' + \delta)} \qquad (5)$$

where d_t was the distance between the center of the tumor and the upper tissue surface, and δ was the penetration depth. The calculated optimal radius was 1.4 cm, which was used for this modeling.

The energy deposition in tissue was modeled using various values of absorption coefficient for the tumor for single-beam delivery (Fig. 2). As can be seen, the energy deposition in the tumor became comparable with the subsurface energy deposition when the absorption coefficient of the tumor was raised to 1 cm^{-1}. With an further increased absorption coefficient for the tumor, the center and bottom of the tumor received relatively less light because more light was absorbed by the top of the tumor.

The energy deposition in tissue was modeled using various values of absorption coefficient for the tumor for multiple-beam delivery as well (Fig. 3). As the absorption coefficient of the tumor was increased, the surface of tumor received more and more light energy. But the center of the tumor received less and less light energy because much of the light was absorbed by the tumor shell and did not penetrate into the center. Therefore, the surface of the tumor may be killed immediately during phototherapeutics. The center of the tumor may be "starved" to death later because the blood supply to the center of the tumor was interrupted around the shell. The four-beam delivery yielded a much more homogeneous and stronger energy deposition into the tumor than the single-beam delivery without increasing the subsurface energy deposit. The energy deposition on the tumor surface was even stronger than that under the tissue surface when the absorption coefficient of the tumor was enhanced enough, which was highly desirable in optical therapeutics.

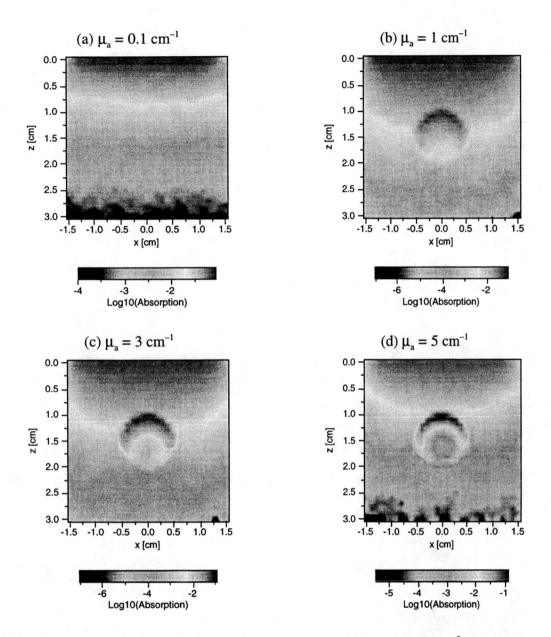

Fig. 2. False-color plots of the deposited power density distribution in W/cm^3 in the tissue in log scale for one-beam delivery when the absorption coefficient of the tumor was set to (a) 0.1 cm^{-1}, (a) 1 cm^{-1}, (a) 3 cm^{-1}, (a) 5 cm^{-1}. The total power of the incident laser beam P_s was set to 1 W.

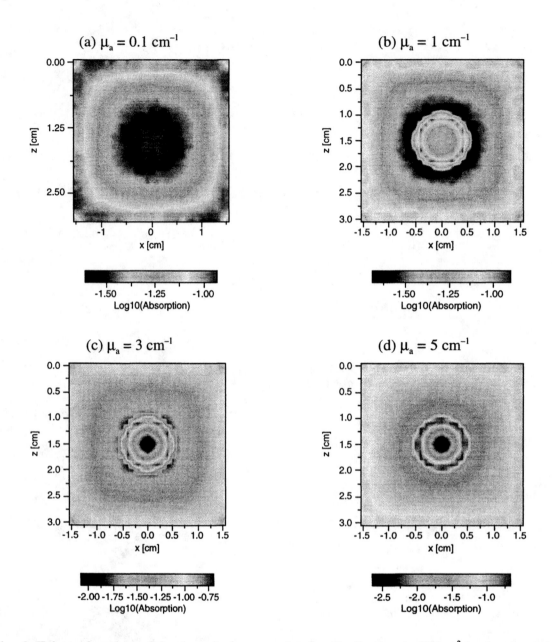

Fig. 3. False-color plots of the deposited power density distribution in W/cm³ in the tissue in log scale for four-beam delivery when the absorption coefficient of the tumor was set to (a) 0.1 cm⁻¹, (a) 1 cm⁻¹, (a) 3 cm⁻¹, (a) 5 cm⁻¹. The total power of each incident laser beam P_s was set to 1 W.

SUMMARY

Oblique-incidence was able to measure optical properties of biological tissues in vivo. Local administration of ICG was found to enhance the absorption coefficient of tumors significantly. Monte Carlo simulations were proved to be a flexible and powerful tool in studying light transport in heterogeneous biological tissues. Four-beam delivery was found superior to single-beam delivery. In the four-beam delivery scheme, the tumor with an ICG-enhanced absorption coefficient was found to absorb more light energy than the surface of the surrounding tissue. However, the center of the tumor received little light and is expected to be killed indirectly in response to lack of blood supply. These results provide guidelines for various laser therapeutics including photothermal therapies, photomechanical therapies, and noninvasive photosensitizer-assisted laser therapies of deep tumors.

ACKNOWLEDGMENT

The project was sponsored in part by The Whitaker Foundation grant and the National Institutes of Health grant R29 CA68562 and R01 CA71980.

GLOSSARY

Absorption coefficient [μ_a, cm^{-1}]	The probability of photon absorption per unit infinitesimal pathlength.
Anisotropy [g]	The average of the cosine value of the deflection angle by single scattering.
Diffusion constant [D, cm]	Linking the gradient of light fluence, $\nabla\phi$, and light current, F, (Fick's law), i.e., $F = -D \nabla\phi$.
Effective attenuation coefficient [μ_{eff}, cm^{-1}]	The decay constant of light fluence far away from light source. $\mu_{eff} = \sqrt{3\,\mu_a/D}$.
Interaction coefficient [μ_t, cm^{-1}]	The probability of photon interaction per unit infinitesimal pathlength, where the interaction includes both absorption and scattering. $\mu_t = \mu_a + \mu_s$. Sometimes, it is also called total interaction coefficient or total attenuation coefficient.
Mean free path [mfp]	The mean pathlength between interactions, which is $1/\mu_t$.
Penetration depth [δ, cm]	$\delta = 1/\mu_{eff}$. It represents decay constant of the light fluence far from the source.
Reduced scattering coefficient [μ_s', cm^{-1}]	$\mu_s' = \mu_s (1 - g)$. Sometimes, it is also called transport scattering coefficient.
Scattering coefficient [μ_s, cm^{-1}]	The probability of photon scattering per unit infinitesimal pathlength.
Transport interaction coefficient [μ_t', cm^{-1}]	$\mu_t' = \mu_a + \mu_s'$.
Transport mean free path [mfp']	$1/\mu_t'$.

REFERENCES

1. L.-H. Wang, R. E. Nordquist, and W. R. Chen, "Optimal beam size for light delivery to absorption-enhanced tumors buried in biological tissues and effect of multiple beam delivery: a Monte Carlo study," Appl. Opt. **36**, 8286-8291 (1997).

2. L.-H. Wang and S. L. Jacques, "Use of a laser beam with an oblique angle of incidence to measure the reduced scattering coefficient of a turbid medium," Appl. Opt. **34**, 2362-2366 (1995).

3. S.-P. Lin, L.-H. Wang, S. L. Jacques, and F. K. Tittel, "Measurement of tissue optical properties using oblique incidence optical fiber reflectometry," Appl. Opt. **36**, 136-143 (1997).

4. G. Marquez and L.-H. Wang, "White light oblique incidence reflectometer for measuring absorption and reduced scattering spectra of tissue-like turbid media," Optics Express **1**, 454-460 (1997).

5. B. C. Wilson and G. A. Adam, "Monte Carlo model for the absorption and flux distributions of light in tissue," Med. Phys. **10**, 824-830 (1983).

6. S. T. Flock, B. C. Wilson, D. R. Wyman, and M. S. Patterson, "Monte-Carlo modeling of light-propagation in highly scattering tissues I: model predictions and comparison with diffusion-theory," IEEE Trans. Biomed. Eng. **36**, 1162-1168 (1989).

7. S. A. Prahl, M. Keijzer, S. L. Jacques, and A. J. Welch, "A Monte Carlo model of light propagation in tissue," Proc. Soc. Photo-Opt. Instrum. Eng. **IS 5**, 102-111 (1989).

8. S. L. Jacques and L.-H. Wang, "Monte Carlo modeling of light transport in tissues," in Optical Thermal Response of Laser Irradiated Tissue, edited by A. J. Welch and M. J. C. van Gemert (Plenum Press, New York, 1995), pp. 73-100.

9. L.-H. Wang, S. L. Jacques, and L.-Q. Zheng, "MCML - Monte Carlo modeling of photon transport in multi-layered tissues," Computer Methods and Programs in Biomedicine **47**, 131-146 (1995). Note: The simulation software package can be downloaded from http://biomed.tamu.edu/~lw.

10. I. Lux and L. Koblinger, *Monte Carlo Particle Transport Methods: Neutron and Photon Calculations* (CRC Press, Boca Raton, 1991).

Novel algorithm to determine absorption and scattering coefficients from time-resolved measurements

Ruikang K Wang, Y Wickramasinghe, Peter Rolfe

Centre for Science and Technology in Medicine, School of Postgraduate Medicine,
Keele University/North Staffordshire Hospital, Thornburrow Drive, Hartshill,
Stoke-on-Trent ST4 7QB, England

ABSTRACT

A novel algorithm is demonstrated to determine the reduced scattering and absorption coefficients from time-resolved reflectance measurements at two positions on the surface of biotissue. The algorithm is very straightforward and fast, in which only some simple mathematical operations are involved, avoiding complicated iterative non-linear fitting to the time-resolved curve. The derived reduced scattering coefficient is not affected by whatever boundary condition is applied. The algorithm was verified using the time-resolved data from the Monte-Carlo model. Both the semi-infinite medium and the turbid slab medium were tested. In contrast to the non-linear fitting method, it is found using this algorithm that both the scattering and absorption coefficients can be determined to a high accuracy.

1. BACKGROUND

During the last decade, the application of diffusion theory to radiative transfer has been vigorously explored, particularly with a view to develop new optical diagnostic method for biological tissue[1]. Photon migration techniques based on diffusion theory have been used to monitor the absorption and scattering coefficient that reflect the physiological state of tissue [2,3]. Time-resolved reflectance measurements have been used to determine the absorption (μ_a) and reduced scattering coefficient (μ_s') of tissue [4,5]. With this technique, a picosecond pulsed light source is used as an input signal and the reflectance is measured as a function of time at a distance of a few centimeters away from the source. Once the time-resolved signal has been obtained, there are several ways to extract the optical properties of the medium. The most accurate one is to compare the experimental data with results from Monte-Carlo (MC) simulations. However, MC simulations are very time consuming. Consequently analysis using an iterative algorithm that compares simulation results with measurements may require several days, a time period that is usually not acceptable in a clinical environment. A much faster way to determine the absorption and scattering coefficient is to fit a diffusion equation curve to the experimental data.

When a semi-infinite medium is assumed and the extrapolated boundary (EPB) condition or zero boundary condition (ZBC) is applied, the reflectance $R(r,t)$ measured at a source-detector separation r and time t is given by [6]

$$R(r,t) = \frac{0.5}{(4\pi Dc)^{\frac{3}{2}} t^{\frac{5}{2}}} \exp(-\mu_a ct) \exp(-\frac{r^2}{4Dct})$$
$$\times \left\{ z_0 \exp(-\frac{z_0^2}{4Dct}) + (z_0 + 2z_b)\exp(-\frac{(z_0 + 2z_b)^2}{4Dct}) \right\} \tag{1}$$

where $D = [3(\mu_s')]^{-1}$ is the diffusion constant, c is the speed of light in the turbid medium, $\mu_s' = (1-g)\mu_s$ is the reduced scattering coefficient. The first term is due to a point source at $z_0 = [\mu_s']^{-1}$ that results from the perpendicularly incident collimated light, and the second term is due to a negative image source at $-z_0 - 2z_b$. For the ZBC z_b is zero, whereas for the EPB

$$z_b = 2D \frac{1 + R_{eff}}{1 - R_{eff}} \tag{2}$$

where R_{eff} represents the fraction of photons that is internally diffusely reflected at the boundary. R_{eff} can be calculated according to Haskell et al [6], from where $R_{eff}=0.470$ for a refractive index of 1.37 which is representative of measured tissue data.

Patterson et al [4] proposed using the asymptotic slope of the logarithm of temporal profile for semi-infinite medium to determine the absorption coefficient. They used the time-resolved reflectance $R(r,t)$ for semi-infinite medium under the ZBC. Log($R(r,t)$) approaches a slope of $-\mu_a c$ when t is sufficiently long enough, therefore it could be possible to determine μ_a from the slope. However, the typical dynamic range of time-resolved experiments based on time-correlated single-photon counting is 10^4;[7] it limits the usage of this method to determine the optical properties of biotissue. Another and obvious method used to determine the tissue optical properties is to fit the diffusion equation curve directly to the experimental data using nonlinear Levenberg-Marquardt or regression fitting method. The nonlinear fitting methods have already delivered some success [7,8] in determining the optical properties of tissue from the measured data, however the complicated procedure and the iterative nature often make them time consuming. To overcome these drawbacks, a simple and fast algorithm is then suggested in this paper for the purpose of deriving the absorption and scattering coefficients, where the time-resolved reflectance measurements at two positions of the biotissue are used to deduce μ_a and μ_s'. The method is so straightforward that only some simple mathematical operations are involved, making it simple to understand and rapid to calculate.

2. BASIC CONCEPTS AND THEORY

For a homogeneous turbid medium, the absorption and reduced scattering coefficient to be determined should be considered to be constants, thus the variables in the solutions of reflectance, or transmittance, will be only the source-detector separation distance r and time t. Eq.(1) can be re-written as a production of the two terms:

$$R(r,t) = f(r,t)f(t) = \left\{ \exp(-\frac{r^2}{4Dct}) \right\} \left\{ \frac{0.5}{(4\pi Dc)^{\frac{3}{2}} t^{\frac{5}{2}}} \exp(-\mu_a ct)f(D,t) \right\} \tag{3}$$

where

$$f(D,t) = \left\{ z_0 \exp(-\frac{z_0^2}{4Dct}) + (z_0 + 2z_b) \exp(-\frac{(z_0 + 2z_b)^2}{4Dct}) \right\} \tag{4}$$

is only related to the boundary conditions applied. It can be seen from Eq.(3) that the function $f(r,t)$ depends on the variables r and t, whereas the usually complicated function $f(t)$ is independent from r. That means, to a certain homogeneous turbid medium, $f(t)$ part in the measured reflectance is the same at any position on the surface of the tissue. The difference observed from the measured reflectance at a different position is only caused by the function $f(r,t)$, which is determined by the source-detector separation distance. Thus it is possible to cancel out the complicated function term of $f(t)$ from the reflectance, i.e. from the measured data $R(r,t)$, if measurements at more than one position are made. Assume that two measurements $R(r_1,t)$ and $R(r_2,t)$ are obtained at the positions r_1 and r_2, it can be seen from Eq.(3) that the term $f(t)$ can be deleted by the operation of $R(r_1,t)/R(r_2,t)$. Thus,

$$\frac{R(r_1,t)}{R(r_2,t)} = \exp(-\frac{r_1^2 - r_2^2}{4Dct}) \tag{5}$$

As $R(r_1,t)$ and $R(r_2,t)$ are the measured data in the experiment, and the distance r_1 and r_2 are known a priori, it leaves only D as an unknown variable. Notice that $D = [3\mu_s']^{-1}$, therefore from Eq.(5),

$$\mu_s' = \frac{4ct}{3(r_2^2 - r_1^2)} \ln[\frac{R(r_1,t)}{R(r_2,t)}] \tag{6}$$

It means that the reduced scattering coefficient, μ_s', can be determined directly from two independent time-resolved measurements, $R(r_1,t)$ and $R(r_2,t)$. Theoretically, from Eq.(6), μ_s' could be obtained from two data at time t from the two different measurements. However, as noise is inevitable in the measurement, a final result should thus be obtained through averaging Eq. (6) for a certain time range in order to improve the accuracy of the determined value of μ_s'. Interestingly, the determination of μ_s', Eq.(6), is totally independent from whatever boundary condition is applied.

Once μ_s' is determined, it can be seen from Eq.(3) that only μ_a leaves unknown, after some mathematical operations:

$$-\mu_a ct + A = \ln[R(r,t)] + \frac{r^2}{4Dct} - \ln[0.5(4\pi Dc)^{-\frac{3}{2}} t^{-\frac{5}{2}}] - \ln[f(D,t)] \qquad (7)$$

where A is a multiplicative factor; it is necessary as relative measurements were often performed. From Eq.(7), it is trivial to determine the value of μ_a using very simple least square fitting technique as the right hand side of Eq.(7) is already made available from the measurement and the determined μ_s' from Eq.(6).

Therefore, from Eq.(6) and Eq.(7), the optical properties, μ_a and μ_s', of a homogeneous medium can be easily extracted rapidly from two time-resolved measurements, avoiding using the complicated nonlinear fitting method. One disadvantage of the proposed technique is that two measurements have to be made instead of one in the nonlinear fitting method.

A technique to determine μ_a and μ_s' has been demonstrated with the straightforward mathematical operations. In contrast to the nonlinear fitting method, it is very simple to understand and very fast in calculation. It should be emphasized that the proposed method is also applicable to the turbid slab case, because the form of reflectance solution of a slab is only different in the function $f(t)$ of Eq.(3) from that of the semi-infinite turbid medium, please see refs [4,10]. Thus the reduced scattering coefficient of a turbid slab can be determined by Eq.(6); and then the determination of absorption coefficient is followed by Eq. (7) where only different part is the last term in the right hand side of Eq.(7) which will be made available after the reduced scattering coefficient is determined.

It was reported that [7], the absorption coefficient can be determined with high accuracy while the scattering coefficient obtained, using nonlinear fitting procedure from the diffusion equations with different boundary conditions, gives a relatively large error. However, it is interesting to find out that this conclusion is not necessarily true if using the proposed technique in this paper. It is found that both the absorption and scattering coefficients can be determined with high accuracy; in particularly, the reduced scattering coefficient so determined is independent from whatever which boundary condition is applied to derive the solution of reflectance from the diffusion equations, see Eq.(6).

3. RESULTS

The validity of the proposed technique for determination of μ_a and μ_s' was verified using the time-resolved results from MC simulations [9] for both the semi-infinite medium and turbid slab medium. The results were compared with those obtained from the iterative non-linear fitting method. In the MC simulations, a δ function pulse is injected into the tissue with given μ_a, μ_s, and g. The reflectance $R(r,t)$, (mm^{-2}ns^{-1}), is recorded as a function of the source-detector separation r and time t. The spatial resolution was 1 mm over a total distance of 5 cm. The time resolution was 10 ps over time period of 3 ns. The MC model accounts for the index mismatch at the air-tissue boundary by calculating the Fresnel reflection [9]. 5 million photons were launched in the simulations; and the refractive index was set to 1.37. The EPB condition was applied to extract the absorption coefficient in both the semi-infinite and slab media in the following demonstrations.

Figure 1(a) shows the results (noise curves) from MC simulations for a semi-infinite turbid medium with given parameters: $\mu_a = 0.001/mm$, $\mu_s' = 0.5/mm$ and $g = 0.9$, where the three noise curves from top to bottom illustrate the time-resolved data at source-detector separation distance $r = 5$ mm, 10 mm, and 20 mm, respectively. When the simulated data from the MC model were used in the proposed technique to extract μ_a and μ_s', the final results are shown in Table I, where for example, the top-left result was obtained from the time-resolved data at $r_1=5$ mm and $r_2=10$ mm. For getting these results, the time-resolved data from the MC model before 100 ps were disregarded in the proposed method as diffusion theory is least accurate for the reflectance at the early times. It can be seen from Table I that the extracted values of μ_a and μ_s', using the current method, are very close to the theoretical values with the relative error less than 7% for μ_a and less than 4% for μ_s'. It should be noted that for r_1=5 mm and r_2=10 mm, the results were still in very good agreement with the theoretical ones with 7% error in μ_a and 3.4% error in μ_s'; it is important as r is often limited in the practical situtation. To better understand the fitting results, μ_a=0.00093 and μ_s'=0.483, obtained from r_1=5 mm and r_2=10 mm, were used in the reflectance equation to draw the predicted time-resolved curve, resulting in the solid-curves in Fig.1 at r=5 mm, 10 mm, and 20 mm respectively which give very good fit to the MC data. For comparison, the results obtained from the non-linear fitting to the MC data at r = 5 mm, 10 mm, and 15 mm respectively, using Leverberg-Marquardt method were also shown in Table I. The different starting times, ranging from 20 ps to 1000 ps [7], were investigated in obtaining μ_a and μ_s' for non-linear fitting, from which the best result was picked up and shown in Table I. It can be seen that the extracted values of μ_a and μ_s' were in large deviation for r less than 10 mm, whereas they were in high accuracy for the present method. Overall, the proposed technique delivers much better results than that from non-linear fitting ones.

Table I: Results of optical properties obtained for semi-infinite medium

	5 mm	10 mm	15 mm
10 mm	μ_a=0.00093 μ_s'=0.483		
15 mm	μ_a=0.00095 μ_s'=0.486	μ_a=0.00094 μ_s'=0.497	
20 mm	μ_a=0.00096 μ_s'=0.490	μ_a=0.00096 μ_s'=0.4954	μ_a=0.00103 μ_s'=0.506
Non-linear fitting	μ_a=0.00114 μ_s'=0.910	μ_a=0.00119 μ_s'=0.436	μ_a=0.00119 μ_s'=0.451

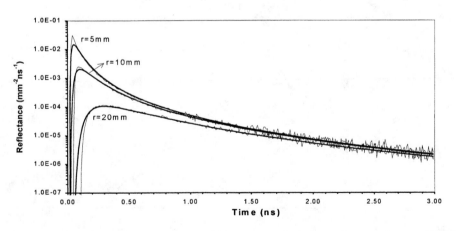

Fig.1, Time-resolved results at r = 5 mm, 10 mm and 20 mm respectively from a homogeneous semi-infinite medium with $\mu_a = 0.001 / mm$, $\mu_s' = 0.5 / mm$ and g = 0.9. Noise curves are from the MC model, and the solid ones are predicted from diffusion equations using the extracted values of μ_a and μ_s' from the proposed method.

The proposed algorithm was also tested using a turbid slab. The infinite slab thickness used in the verification was 20 mm with given parameters: $\mu_a = 0.0045 / mm$, $\mu_s' = 0.6 / mm$ and g = 0.9. The results obtained from the MC simulation at source-detector separation distance $r = 5\ mm$, $10\ mm$ and $20\ mm$ respectively, are illustrated in Fig.2 (noise curves). The EPB condition was applied to derive the solution of reflectance which was used to determine μ_a in the present method. Table II gives the determined μ_a and μ_s' from the simulated data from MC model, where for example the top-left result in the table was obtained from the time-resolved data at $r_1=5\ mm$ and $r_2=10\ mm$. The time-resolved data from the MC model before $100\ ps$ were ignored in getting these results. From Table II, the conclusion is obvious with the relative error less than 5% for μ_a and less than 3% for μ_s'. To illustrate the fitting results, the solid curves in Fig.2 were drawn using $\mu_a =0.00437$ and $\mu_s' =0.596$ that were determined from time-resolved data at $r_1=5\ mm$ and $r_2=10\ mm$. It can be seen that the curves are in very good agreement with the MC simulation. The results obtained from the non-linear fitting at $r=5\ mm$, $10\ mm$, and $20\ mm$ respectively were also shown in the last row of Table II. Although the μ_a determined from non-linear fitting has high accuracy, the values of μ_s' are seen with large deviation; as observed by Hielscher et al [7]. Therefore, the proposed method can also be used to derive the optical properties for the turbid slab case with high accuracy, and delivers a much better performance than the non-linear fitting method.

It should be mentioned that the computation time used in deriving μ_a and μ_s', using the current algorithm was less than 50 ms in all cases.

Table II: Results of optical properties extracted for turbid slab $d = 20mm$

	5 mm	10 mm	15 mm
10 mm	$\mu_a =0.00437$ $\mu_s' =0.596$		
15 mm	$\mu_a =0.00423$ $\mu_s' =0.592$	$\mu_a =0.00427$ $\mu_s' =0.584$	
20 mm	$\mu_a =0.00431$ $\mu_s' =0.593$	$\mu_a =0.00434$ $\mu_s' =0.592$	$\mu_a =0.00461$ $\mu_s' =0.597$
Non-linear fitting	$\mu_a =0.00443$ $\mu_s' =0.681$	$\mu_a =0.00469$ $\mu_s' =0.630$	$\mu_a =0.00423$ $\mu_s' =0.582$

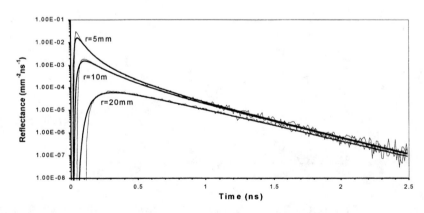

Fig.2, Time-resolved results at $r = 5\ mm$, $10\ mm$ and $20\ mm$ respectively from a homogeneous semi-infinite medium with $\mu_a = 0.0045 / mm$, $\mu_s' = 0.6 / mm$ and $g = 0.9$. Noise curves are from the MC model, and the solid ones are predicted from diffusion equations using the extracted values of μ_a and μ_s' from the proposed method.

4. CONCLUSIONS

We have demonstrated a simple and rapid algorithm to extract optical properties of turbid medium from time-resolved measurements. The calculations were so straightforward that only some simple mathematical operations are involved, making it extremely simple to understand. In contrast to the conclusion drawn from non-linear fitting method [7], it is found, using the proposed method, that the derived values of μ_a and μ_s' were both in high accuracy, particularly where the determined value of μ_s' is independent from whatever which boundary condition is applied to derive the solution of reflectance from the diffusion equations. This is particularly important when only the scattering coefficient is in primarily concern in the clinical applications because the complicated boundary conditions will not be considered; however the boundary condition is a key parameter to determine the optical properties of tissue in other methods. The proposed method was verified by both the semi-infinite and infinite slab media using the time-resolved data from MC model. From the comparison, the proposed method delivers a much better performance than the non-linear fitting method does. Further research is underway to carefully examine this new algorithm for both the semi-infinite medium and slab medium.

5. REFERENCES

1. See, for example, the five special journal issues on biomedical optics: Appl. Opt. **28**(12), (1989); Appl. Opt. **32**(4), (1993); Opt. Eng. **32**(2), (1993); Appl. Opt. **35**(1), (1997); J. Opt. Soc. Am. **A14**(1), (1997).
2. B. Chance, J. Leigh, H. Miyake, D. Smith, S. Nioka, R. Greenfield, M. Finlander, K. Kaufmann, W. Levy, M. Yound, P. Cohen, H. Yodshioka, and R. Boretsky, "Comparison of time-resolved and unresolved measurements of deoxyhemoglobin in brain", Proc. Natl. Acad. Sci. (USA) **85**, 4971-4975(1988).
3. B. Wilson, Y. Park, Y. Hefetz, M. Patterson, S. Madsen, and S.L. Jacques, " The potential of time-resolved reflectance measurements for non-invasive determination of tissue optical properties", Proc. SPIE **1064**, 97-107 (1989).
4. M.S. Patterson, B. Chance, and B.C. Wilson, "Time-resolved reflectance and transmittance for the non-invasive measurement of tissue optical properties", *Appl. Opt.* **28**, 2331-2336 (1989).
5. A.H. Hielscher, H. Liu, L.H. Wang, F.K. Tittel, B. Chance, and S.L. Jacques, *Proc. SPIE* **2136**, 4-15 (1994).
6. R.C. Haskell, L.O. Svaasand, T. Tsay, T. Feng, M.S. McAdams, and B.J. Tromberg, "Boundary conditions for the diffusion equation in radiative transfer", J. Opt. Soc. Am. **A11** 2727-2741 (1994).
7. A. Hielscher, S.L. Jacques, L. Wang, and F.K. Tittel, "The influence of boundary conditions on the accuracy of diffusion theory in time-resolved reflectance spectroscopy of biological tissue", Phy. Med. Biol. **40** 1957-1975 (1995).
8. A. Kienle and M.S. Patterson, "Improved solutions of the steady-state and the time-resolved diffusion equations for reflectance from a semi-infinite turbid medium", J. Opt. Soc. Am. **A14** 246-254 (1997).
9. L.H. Wang, S.L. Jacques and L. Zheng, "MCML - Monte-Carlo modelling of light transport in multilayered tissues" *Comput. Methods Programs Biomed.* **47** 131-146(1995).
10. D. Contini, F. Martelli, and G. Zaccanti, "Photon mogration through a turbid slab described by a model based on diffusion approximation. I: Theory", *Appl. Opt.* **36** (1997, No.7)

Sized-Fiber Array Spectroscopy

S. A. Prahl, S. L. Jacques

Oregon Medical Laser Center, 9205 SW Barnes Rd, Portland, OR 97225

ABSTRACT

Sized-fiber array spectroscopy describes a device and method for measuring absorption and reduced scattering properties of tissue. The device consists of two or more optical fibers with different diameters (comparable to the optical path length in the tissue) that are used to measure the amount of light backscattered into each fiber. Each fiber is used for both irradiation and detection. Only one fiber emits and collects light at a given time. This paper presents Monte Carlo simulations of the sized-fiber device to indicate the behavior of a device with 50 and 1000 μm fiber sizes. Experimental results are presented for a device constructed with 400 and a 600 μm fibers that demonstrate the accuracy of the device in measuring the scattering coefficient of 10%-Intralipid samples over a reduced scattering coefficient range of 1-50 cm^{-1}.

Keywords: Reflectance, Optical Biopsy

1. INTRODUCTION

The determination of the optical properties of materials is important in many fields of medicine. The sized-fiber device described in this paper allows simple and rapid measurement of optical properties by taking advantage of the fact that the amount of light backscattered into an optical fiber is affected by the scattering and absorption properties of the tissue. Furthermore, the sized-fiber array satisfies the medical demands that a clinical device to determine the optical properties of tissue be simple to construct, inexpensive to build, compact in size, and robust in operation.

The sized-fiber device is based on the fact that, generally, tissues with different scattering and absorbing properties will backscatter different numbers of photons into the originating fiber. However, it is possible for two samples (say A and B) with very different optical properties to backscatter the same number of photons back into a particular size fiber, and a single measurement with one fiber would be insufficient to distinguish the two samples from each other. If a measurement is made on samples A and B with a second fiber, having a different diameter from the first, then the two sample will be distinguishable. This is because different sized fibers collect information from different effective volumes of the samples.

This paper begins with Monte Carlo simulations to support this claim. Simulations for a device consisting of a 50 and 1000 μm fiber are presented. This is followed by a description of an experiment to measure the scattering properties of Intralipid. The experimental results indicate that the method is sensitive to changes in reduced scattering from 1 to 50 cm^{-1}.

2. MONTE CARLO SIMULATIONS

A Monte Carlo program was adapted to simulate the light collected by a fiber irradiating a homogenous scattering and absorbing medium.[1,2] A series of simulations were done to demonstrate the feasibility of the sized-fiber method for measuring the optical properties of materials and to interpret experimental the measurements in Intralipid.

Let the axis of the fiber be parallel to the z-axis, and further let this axis be normal to the surface of a semi-infinite scattering and absorbing medium. The face of the fiber is flush against the surface of the medium. The illumination over the face of the fiber is uniform i.e., the photons are launched with equal probability over the entire face of the fiber.

Photons were launched from each point on the fiber face in a direction specified by the direction cosines (ν_x, ν_y, ν_z). The angle $\nu_z = \cos\theta_z$ had a Gaussian distribution that depended on the acceptance angle of the fiber and the other

---

Direct correspondence to S.A.P, prahl@ece.ogi.edu; (503) 216–2197; http://ece.ogi.edu/omlc/

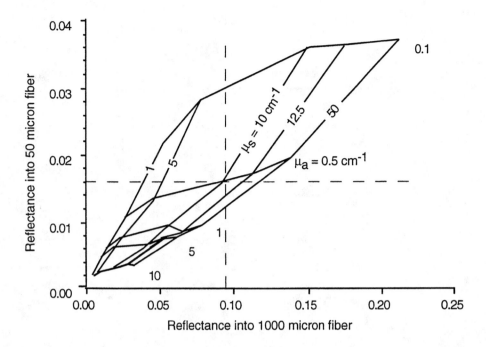

Figure 1. The fraction of light collected by a 50 μm and 1000 μm fiber for various combinations of optical properties. The reduced scattering coefficient is μ_s and the absorption coefficient is μ_a. From this graph it is evident that for a specific reflectance from a 50 μm fiber and from a 1000 μm fiber, a specific optical property is obtained. For example, if $R_{50} = 0.016$ and $R_{1000} = 0.09$ then $\mu_a = 0.05\,\text{cm}^{-1}$ and $\mu'_s = 10\,\text{cm}^{-1}$.

two directions were uniformly distributed. This angular distribution was chosen to simulate the major features of the observed emission by the fibers; it was not directly confirmed experimentally. The distribution of angles that the photon might take was given by the function

$$p(\theta_z)\,d\theta_z = \frac{1}{\sqrt{2\pi}} \exp\left(-\frac{\theta_z^2}{2\theta_a^2}\right)\,d\theta_z$$

where θ_a was the acceptance angle for the fiber. Furthermore, to limit the angles on the shoulders of the distribution, only those values of $\theta_z \leq \theta_a$ were accepted. The other two angles were generated using

$$\nu_x = (1 - \nu_z^2)\cos\phi \qquad \text{and} \qquad \nu_y = (1 - \nu_z^2)\sin\phi$$

where $\phi = 2\pi\xi$ was an azimuthal angle about the z-axis and ξ is a uniformly distributed random number between zero and one. This preserved the all important relation

$$\nu_x^2 + \nu_y^2 + \nu_z^2 = 1$$

The primary statistic collected by the Monte Carlo program was the fraction of light backscattered or reflected back into the fiber. For photons to be counted as reflected they must have exited the surface at a radius that was within the core of the fiber and at an angle that was within the acceptance angle of the fiber. The index of refraction of the core of the fiber was assumed to be 1.46 and the index of the medium was 1.38. Scattering in the medium was assumed isotropic. A total of 20,000 photons were used for each data point.

Figure 1 shows the results of Monte Carlo calculations for a range of optical properties and for a 50 and 1000 μm fiber. The acceptance angle of the fibers were assumed to be 25° in air. As scattering increases from 1 to 50 cm^{-1}, the reflectances into both fibers increase; although less so for the smaller fiber. As the absorption decreases, both reflectances increase, but the effect upon the larger fiber is smaller.

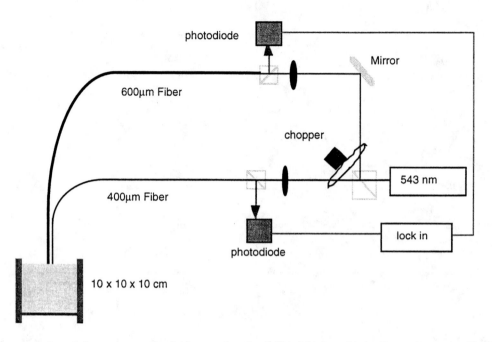

Figure 2. The experimental apparatus used to test the sized-fiber device. Light from the green HeNe is coupled into two fibers with different sizes. Light only travels through one fiber at a time because of the orientation of the chopper blade. The light backscattered into the fibers is detected with large photodiodes and a lock-in amplifier.

3. MATERIALS AND METHODS

The experimental apparatus is shown in Figure 2. The beam from a green He-Ne laser operating at 543 nm was split into two beams with a non-polarizing 50/50 beam splitter. Both beams were modulated at 1 kHz by a single chopper blade (Stanford Research, SR540) in such a way that only one beam was on at a particular instant. Each beam passed through a second beam splitter and were coupled into a $400\,\mu$m and a $600\,\mu$m fiber with acceptance angles in air of 13 and 25° respectively. The distal fiber tips were completely immersed in the Intralipid solutions; this is different from the Monte Carlo simulations, but seemed to make relatively little difference in the measured signals. The light backscattered into the fiber was divided again by the beam splitter and half was collected with a photodiode. The outputs from the photodiodes and chopper were coupled into a lock-in amplifier (Stanford Research, SR510)

The samples measured were dilutions of Intralipid with optical properties from 1 to $50\,\mathrm{cm}^{-1}$. No absorber was added and consequently the absorption coefficient was assumed to be a nominal $\mu_a = 0.01\,\mathrm{cm}^{-1}$.[3]

4. RESULTS

The experimental results for the Intralipid experiments are shown in top graph of Figure 3. In this graph the theoretical Monte Carlo simulation is shown as the solid line. It is not quite straight because only 20,000 photons were used. The numbers beside the line indicate the reduced scattering coefficient for the square nearest the number. The error bars on the measured data are the standard deviation of five measurements.

The graph in the bottom of Figure 3 shows how the measured values taken from top graph compare with the expected values for the various dilutions of Intralipid. The measured values were taken as the nearest point on the theoretical line in the top graph.

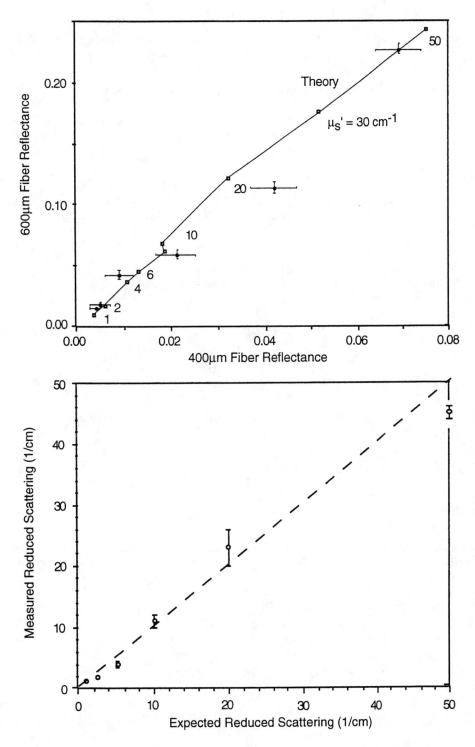

Figure 3. (Top) The fractions of light collected by 400 and 600 μm fibers in various concentrations of Intralipid. (Bottom) A comparison of the expected reduced scattering coefficient with the reduced scattering coefficient determined with the sized fiber device. The dashed line indicates equal values for the measured and expected values of the reduced scattering coefficient.

5. DISCUSSION

The sized-fiber technique is yet another method for measuring the optical properties of materials.[4-6] This particular technique has the advantage that it can be made very small. The accuracy and sensitivity depend on choosing the proper fiber sizes for the material being probed.

What are the limitations of the sized fiber technique? First, scattering must be present in the sample or no light will be backscattered into the fibers. Consequently, the sized-fiber device will not work with absorbing-only media. Second, if the absorption in the sample is very high, then the returned signal becomes very small and the technique works less well. Third, the sizes of the fibers should be comparable to the average reduced scattering pathlength in the sample. Fourth, the conversion of measured values to optical properties remains to be reduced to a simple algorithm.

What are the limitations of this study? The experimental results only determine the scattering coefficients for an assumed absorption coefficient. It remains to be seen how much measurement errors will cause crosstalk in the signals for scattering and absorption. Finally, the choice of fibers for the experiment was poor—the fibers were much too close in size to one another.

What are the advantages to the sized-fiber technique? First, the optical properties are measured over a relatively small area. This is a definite advantage over the measurements made as a function of radius[7] or the oblique incidence technique.[8] Second, this technique can be naturally incorporated into time-domain techniques[9] or into frequency-domain techniques.[10] Another advantage is that the sized-fiber technique are that it can be adapted to very small fibers for possible insertion through a needle. Alternately, the device could be used into a catheter for probing arterial structures or blood flow or into an endoscope for investigating gastro-intestinal structures.

REFERENCES

1. A. N. Witt, "Multiple scattering in reflection nebulae I. A Monte Carlo approach," *Astrophys. J.* **S35**, pp. 1–6, 1977.

2. S. A. Prahl, M. Keijzer, S. L. Jacques, and A. J. Welch, "A Monte Carlo model of light propagation in tissue," in *SPIE Proceedings of Dosimetry of Laser Radiation in Medicine and Biology*, G. J. Müller and D. H. Sliney, eds., vol. IS 5, pp. 102–111, 1989. monte carlo.

3. H. J. van Staveren, C. J. M. Moes, J. van Marle, S. A. Prahl, and M. J. C. van Gemert, "Light scattering in Intralipid-10% in the wavelength range of 400–1100 nm," *Appl. Opt.* **31**, pp. 4507–4514, 1991.

4. B. C. Wilson, M. S. Patterson, and S. T. Flock, "Indirect versus direct techniques for the measurement of the optical properties of tissues," *Photochem. Photobiol.* **46**, pp. 601–608, 1987.

5. W. F. Cheong, S. A. Prahl, A. J. Welch, M. J. C. van Gemert, and C. R. Denham, "Optical properties of bladder tissue and optimal dosage predictions for photoradiation therapy," *Lasers Surg. Med.* **6**, pp. 190–191, 1986.

6. A. J. Welch and M. J. C. van Gemert, *Optical-Thermal Response of Laser Irradiated Tissue*, Plenum Press, 1995.

7. B. C. Wilson, T. J. Farrell, and M. S. Patterson, "An optical fiber-based diffuse reflectance spectrometer for non-invasive investigation of photodynamic sensitizers *in vivo*," in *SPIE Proceedings of Future Directions and Applications in Photodynamic Therapy*, C. J. Gomer, ed., vol. IS 6, pp. 219–232, 1990.

8. L. Wang and S. L. Jacques, "Use of laser beam with an oblique angle of incidence to measure the reduced scattering coefficient of a turbid medium," *Appl. Opt.* **34**, pp. 2362–2366, 1995.

9. S. L. Jacques, "Time resolved propagation of ultrashort laser pulses within turbid tissues," *Appl. Opt.* **28**, pp. 2223–2229, 1989.

10. S. Fantini, M. A. Franceschini, J. B. Fishkin, B. Barbieri, and E. Gratton, "Quantitative determination of the absorption spectra in strongly scattering media: a light-emitting-diode based technique," *Appl. Opt.* **33**, pp. 5204–5213, 1994.

SESSION 12

Optics II

Dependence of light transmission through human skin on incident beam diameter at different wavelengths

Zhong-Quan Zhao and Paul W. Fairchild[a]

ThermoLase Corporation, 10455 Pacific Center Court, San Diego, CA 92129

ABSTRACT

For many skin treatments with light, it is important to have deep photon penetration into the skin. Because of absorption and scattering of photons by skin tissue, both the color and the diameter of the incident beam affect the penetration depth of photons. In this study, the dependence of light transmission through human skin tissues (ear lobs and between the fingers) has been measured *in-vivo* at six wavelengths (532 nm, 632 nm, 675 nm, 810 nm, 911 nm, and 1064 nm). The same measurement was also made on pig skin *in-vitro* for comparison. It was observed that 1) the photons at 1064 nm penetrate deeper than the other colors studied for a given incident beam diameter; and 2) the transmittance at a particular wavelength increases asymptotically with incident beam diameter. For some skin tissues, the transmittance flattens at about 8 mm for 532 nm photons and approaches saturation at about 12 mm for all other colors. The results on pig skin is similar.

Key Words: skin, laser, photon penetration, photon transmittance, beam diameter

1. INTRODUCTION

There has been ever increasing interests in laser-skin interaction in the last a few years propelled by such applications as laser Port Wine Stain treatment, laser hair removal, and laser skin resurfacing. For such applications, a critical photon fluence at a certain depth from the skin surface is necessary to achieve a desired end result. For the case of laser hair removal, high enough laser fluence should be delivered to the hair roots which are typically at about 2-4 mm below the skin surface.

Human skin is optically a very complex turbid medium. The photon transport in the skin is determined by its absorption and scattering properties. Although there are considerable studies on the optical properties of skin[1-6] and photon transport in skin[7], it is still a challenging task to prescribe incident conditions to achieve the necessary fluence at the target because of the complexity of skin and the difficulty of measuring the photon fluence *in-vivo*. Further more, the optical properties of skin also vary from person to person, from anatomic site to anatomic site, and may change dynamically with the environment such as temperature[6]. It was also shown that the optical properties of skin could be altered by pressing the skin[5].

Photons in the wavelength range of about 600 nm - 1200 nm, the so called therapeutic window, penetrate deeper into skin. Photons would travel a few centimeters before being absorbed in dermis. However, because of scattering from centers such as cell membranes and collagen fibers, the photon penetration depth in the skin is only a few millimeters. Photon scatterings would also direct photons back into the incident medium. In the case of illuminating skin from air, as much as 50% of the incident photons could be scattered back into the air[1]. There would also be a photon buildup just blow the skin surface as a consequence of scattering. In the case of an infinite incident beam diameter, the photon fluence distribution with depth can be approximately described as

$$\phi(z) = \phi_0 K e^{-z/\delta} \tag{1}$$

Where ϕ_0 and $\phi(z)$ are the incident photon fluence and photon fluence at depth z with the origin of z at the skin surface; K is the photon buildup factor which is about four for illuminating skin from air with photons in the therapeutic window[8]; δ is the so called effective photon penetration depth which is defined as

---

[a] Further author information-

Z.Q.Z.: Email: zzhao@Thermotrex.com; Telephone: 619-646-5727; Fax: 619-646-5701

P.W.F.: Email: pfairchi@Thermotrex.com; Telephone: 619-646-5714; Fax: 619-646-5701

$$\delta = \frac{1}{\sqrt{3\mu_a(\mu_a+\mu_s(1-g))}} \qquad (2)$$

Where μ_a and μ_s are the absorption and scattering coefficients; g is the anisotropic scattering factor. The effective photon penetration depth δ is about a few millimeters for photons in the therapeutic window.

Because of scatterings, the photon penetration depth would be reduced for finite size beam as seen in the Monte Carlo calculations[8,9]. It is the aim of this study to experimentally reveal that dependence of photon penetration depth on incident beam diameter. The transmittance of photons through human skin between fingers and through ear lobs were measured *in-vivo* at different incident beam diameters.

2. EXPERIMENTAL SETUP

Figure 1 shows systematically the experimental setup. Six lasers at different wavelengths were used in the study. The 532 nm laser (manufactured by ADLAS with a model # DPY 315C) is a CW diode pumped frequency doubled Nd:YAG laser with 100 mw power. The 633 nm laser is a 2 mw CW He-Ne laser. The 675 nm, 807 nm, and 911 nm lasers are CW diode lasers with output powers up to 30 mw, 40 mw, and 50 mw, respectively (All three lasers were bought from SDL Corporation with Model numbers SDL-7311-G1, SDL-202-V3, and SDL-6300-H1 respectively). The 1064 nm laser (LT100 from LORAD Corporation) is a Q-switched Nd:YAG laser with up to 1 J/pulse energy. To avoid detector saturation, the reflected 1064 nm beam from an AR coated wedge was used. The power was further reduced by natural density (ND) filters.

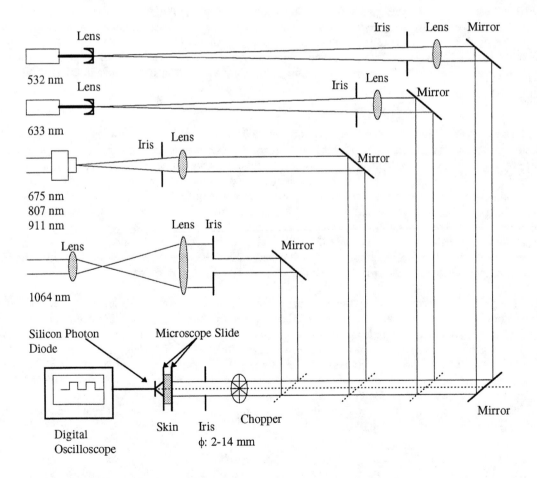

Figure 1. The experimental setup

To obtain uniform flat top intensity beam profiles, all laser beams were expanded and only the central portions of the beams were used. All laser beams were directed to the skin tissue with a mirror which was mounted on a sliding optical rail. The incident beam diameter on the skin is controlled by an iris which was positioned just before the skin and also mounted on the rail. The skin tissues between thumbs and forefingers or the ear lobs were pressed between two microscope slides. The photon detector is a high speed silicon diode (ThorLabs DET2-S1) with a rise time $\leq$ 1 ns, an active area of 1 mm^2, and a peak sensitivity of about 0.5 A/W. The detector was placed right behind the skin tissue at the center of the laser beams and was also mounted on the rail. A chopper (SR 540 from Stanford Research System) operated at 275 Hz was used to chop all CW laser beams. The detector signal was measured with a 500 MHz digital oscilloscope (HP54522A from Hewlett Packard Company). The detector linearity was checked by varying the 675 nm and 911 nm diode laser power. Linear detector response was observed for the power density concerned here (about mw peak power for the pulsed 1064 nm beam and about μw power for all CW lasers falling on the 1mm^2 active detecting area). The incident beam uniformity was measured by stepping the 1 mm detector through the laser beam. The power variation was within 20% in all laser beams.

3. RESULTS

Measurements were done *in-vivo* on the skin tissues between the thumb and forefinger or ear lob. Seven people (two Asians, two African Americans, and three Caucasians) participated in the studies. For comparison, measurements were also carried out on pig skin tissues *in-vitro*.

The measured transmittances at different incident beam diameters and wavelengths on the skin between thumb and forefinger of three people (one Asian, one African American, and one Caucasian), and on the pig skin are presented in figure 2. The pig skin tissue was made of two pieces of skin with little subcutaneous fatty tissue. The skin was first rehydrated and then stacked together back to back. The thickness of the four skin tissues are about the same, about 3.5 mm. The transmittances were obtained by dividing the photon intensities measured with by those without the skin tissues. Note that the photon diode detector was positioned at the center of the beam and the active area of the detector, 1mm^2, is smaller than the cross section of the exit beam from the tissue. Thus the transmittance defined here is related to the photon transmission at the center of the beam. The uncertainty in all *in-vivo* human data is about 20% mainly caused by the movement of the skin during the measurements. The *in-vitro* data on the pig skin should be with better than 20% uncertainty.

Figure 2 shows that the 1064 nm and 532 nm photons are the most and the least penetrating photons, respectively, among the wavelengths studied for all skin types. The absolute values of the transmittance at a given wavelength and incident beam diameter are also about the same for all four skin tissues. While the transmittances at 632 nm, 675 nm, 810 nm, and 911 nm wavelengths at a given incident beam diameter increase monotonically with longer wavelength for the African American skin tissue, they are about the same for the Caucasian skin and slightly different for the Asian skin. The corresponding transmission curves spread out for the African American skin and are almost stacked together for the Caucasian skin. The spread of the transmission curves for the Asian skin falls between the African American and the Caucasian skins. It should be pointed out that the difference in the transmittances among Asian, African American, and Caucasian skins discussed above may not be applied generically. The transmission curves for one Asian skin and one Caucasian skin spread out much like those curves of the African American skin shown in figure 2.

As seen in figure 2, the transmission through skin tissue increases asymptotically with increasing incident beam diameter. The dependency is nearly linear for small values of incident beam diameter. The transmission flattens at larger incident beam diameter. To facilitate comparisons of these transmission curves, the transmittances are normalized and the normalized transmission curves are shown in Figure 3. In general, the shapes of the curves are similar for all skin types and wavelengths studied here. However, small differences do exist. The transmission curves of the 532 nm photons bend earlier, i.e. at smaller incident beam diameter, as clearly seen in the bottom two graphs. It should be pointed out that the curvatures of these photon transmission curves depend also the thickness of the skin tissue. The measured transmittances for a Caucasian skin tissue with 5 mm thickness increase almost linearly with the incident beam diameter up to 12 mm for all the wavelengths concerned in this study.

4. DISCUSSIONS

The transmittance shown in figure 2 is measured through a slab of skin tissue. The solid angle of the field of view of the detector is less than 2π radians. These values should not be used to infer the photon fluence inside a "semi-infinite" thick human skin in which back scattered photons from the tissue below the depth of interest also contribute to the photon fluence. Also, some photons are internally reflected back to the skin tissue from the skin-air interface in the case of slab tissue.

The difference in the spread of the transmission curves for different skin types shown in figure 2 is likely due to variations in the content of skin pigment, i.e. melanin, and the extent of skin pigmentation. Melanin is a generic term describing a group of biopolymers[10]. There are two kinds of melanins in human skin, eumelanin and phaeomelanin. In general, the pigmentation in human skin is a mixture of both kinds of melanins which may vary from one skin type to another and may also change from person to person for the same skin type.

The photon transmission through human skin increases asymptotically with increasing incident beam diameter. For the Caucasian skin shown in figures 2 and 3, the transmittance at 532 nm wavelength reaches saturation at about 8 mm. For all other skin types and wavelengths studied here, the transmittance only approaches flat top at 12 mm, the largest beam incident beam diameter studied here. Therefore for applications requiring deep photon penetration into skin tissue, a large incident beam diameter should be used. However, a more powerful light source is required to deliver the same incident fluence with a larger incident beam diameter. For a given light source power, higher fluence at the center of a beam may be achieved inside the skin for illumination with a small incident beam diameter. For example, when the incident beam diameter is reduced from 8 mm to 4 mm, even though the transmittance through a skin tissue of about 3.5 mm thickness is reduced by about 50% as shown in figures 2 and 3, the exit fluence at the center of beam is increased by about a factor of two because the incident fluence is four times higher when the incident beam diameter is reduced by a factor of two for a given light source power. This conclusion is in agreement with the Monte Carlo calculation on the light distribution in tissue[11].

5. ACKNOWLEGEMENTS

We are grateful to the employees of ThermoLase and ThermoTrex Corporations who participated in the study. We also thank the management of ThermoLase Corporation for allowing us publishing this work.

6. REFERENCES

1. R. Rox. Anderson and John A. Parrish, "The Optics of Human Skin", Selected Papers on Tissue Optics: Applications in Medical Diagnostics and Therapy, Valery V. Tuchin, editor, SPIE Milestone Series, Volume MS 102, pp. 29-35, 1994.

2. M. J. C. van Gemert, Steven L. Jacques, H. J. C. M. Sterenborg, and W. M. Star, "Skin Optics", Selected Papers on Tissue Optics: Applications in Medical Diagnostics and Therapy, Valery V. Tuchin, editor, SPIE Milestone Series, Volume MS 102, pp. 85-93, 1994.

3. Steven L. Jacques, "Origin of Tissue Optical Properties in the UVA, Visible and NIR regions", OSA Trends in Optics and Photonics on Advances in Optical Imaging and Photon Migration, R. R. Alfano and James G. Fujimoto, eds. (Optical Society of America, Washington, DC 1996), Vol. 2, pp. 364-371.

4. Rebecca Simpson, Jan Laufer, Matthias Kohl, Matthias Essenpreis, and Mark Cope, "Near infrared optical properties of ex-vivo human skin and sub-cutaneous tissue using reflectance and transmittance measurements", in Optical Tomography and Spectroscopy of Tissue: Theory, Instrumentation, Model, and Human Studies II, Britton Chance, Robert R. Alfano, Editors, Proceedings of SPIE Vol. 2979, 307-313, 1997.

5. Eric Chan, Brian Sorg, Dmitry Protsenko, Michael O'Neil, Massoud Motamedi, and Ashley J. Welch, "Effects of Compression on Human Skin Optical Properties", in Optical Tomography and Spectroscopy of Tissue: Theory, Instrumentation, Model, and Human Studies II, Britton Chance, Robert R. Alfano, Editors, Proceedings of SPIE Vol. 2979, 314-324, 1997.

6. J. T. Bruulsema, J. E. Hayward, T. J. Farrell, M. Essenpreis, and M. S. Patterson, "Optical Properties of Phantoms and Tissue Measured in vivo from 0.9-1.3 μm using Spatially Resolved Diffuse Reflectance", in Optical Tomography and Spectroscopy of Tissue: Theory, Instrumentation, Model, and Human Studies II, Britton Chance, Robert R. Alfano, Editors, Proceedings of SPIE Vol. 2979, 325-334, 1997.

7. See chapters in " Optical-Thermal Response of Laser-Irradiated Tissue", edited by A. J. Welch and M. J. C. van Gemert, Plenum Press, New York, 1995.

8. Martin J. C. van Gemert, A. J. Welch, John W. Pickering, and Oon Tian Tan, "Laser Treatment of Port Wine Stains", in Optical-Thermal Response of Laser-Irradiated Tissue, edited by A. J. Welch and M. J. C. van Gemert, Plenum Press, New York, pp. 789-829, 1995.

9. Marleen Keijzer, Steven L. Jacques, Scott A. Prahl, and Ashley J. Welch, "Light Distributions in Artery Tissue: Monte Carlo Simulations for Finite-Diameter Laser Beams", Selected Papers on Tissue Optics: Applications in Medical Diagnostics and Therapy, Valery V. Tuchin, editor, SPIE Milestone Series, Volume MS 102, pp. 108-114, 1994.

10. See articles in "Melanin: Its Role in Human Photoprotection", edited by Lisa Zeise, Miles R. Chedekel, Thomas B. Fitzpatrick, Valdenmar Publishing Company, Overland Park, Kansas, 1994.

11. Steven L. Jacques and Lihong Wang, "Monte Carlo Modeling of Light Transport in Tissue", in Optical-Thermal Response of Laser-Irradiated Tissue, edited by A. J. Welch and M. J. C. van Gemert, Plenum Press, New York, pp. 73-100, 1995.

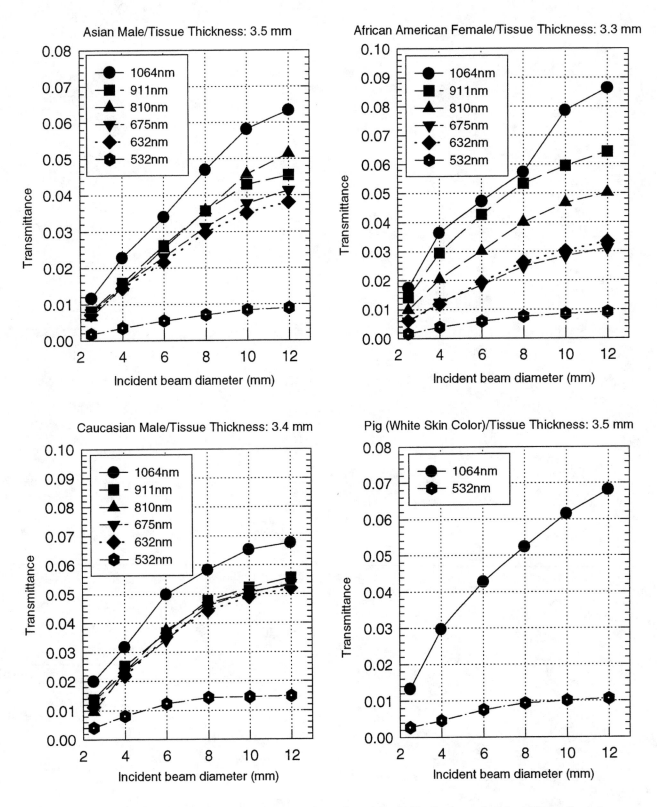

Figure 2. Dependence of photon transmittance through a slab of skin tissue on incident beam diameter at differenent wavelengths

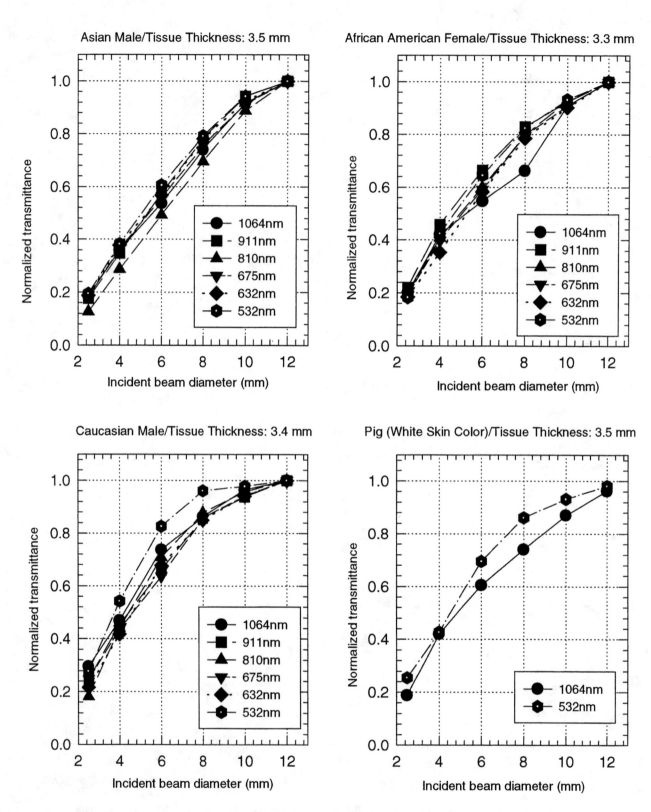

Figure 3. Dependence of normalized photon transmittance through a slab of skin tissue on incident beam diameter at different wavelengths

Changes in the optical properties of laser coagulated and thermally coagulated bovine myocardium

H.-J.Schwarzmaier[1], A.N.Yaroslavsky[2], A.Terenji[2], S.Willmann[2], I.V.Yaroslavsky[2], T.Kahn[3]

[1] German National Research Center for Information Technology,
Schloss Birlinghoven, 53754 St.Augustin, Germany
[2] Department of Laser Medicine, Heinrich-Heine-University,
Universitätsstr.1, D-40225 Düsseldorf, Germany
[3] Department of Diagnostic Radiology, Heinrich-Heine-University,
Moorenstr.5, D-40225 Düsseldorf, Germany

ABSTRACT

The optical properties of seven native, seven laser-coagulated (Nd:YAG $\lambda=1064$ nm, 11W, 15 min, T$\leq$90°C), and seven thermally coagulated (60 min, T$\leq$80°C) samples of bovine myocardium were determined. The absorption coefficient μ_a, the scattering coefficient μ_s, and the anisotropy factor g were obtained in the spectral range from 1000 nm to 1500 nm from double integrating sphere measurements using an inverse Monte Carlo technique. The results indicate that both, laser coagulation and thermal coagulation increase the μ_a and μ_s values by a factor of 2 and 4, respectively, while g is not significantly changed.
Conclusion. Thermal denaturation leads to significant changes in the optical properties of bovine myocardium. The changes are comparable to those induced by laser coagulation.

Keywords: laser coagulation, thermal denaturation, bovine myocardium, absorption, scattering, anisotropy factor, Monte Carlo method, integrating sphere.

1. INTRODUCTION

The optical properties of tissue are essential for light dosimetry in laser medicine. During irradiation the optical properties of biological tissues change[1-5], altering the penetration depth of the laser radiation. Therefore, the knowledge of the laser-induced changes of the optical properties within the irradiated tissue is required. Thermal coagulation in a saline bath is widely used to simulate laser coagulation. There are, however, no reports in the literature making a direct comparison between laser coagulated and thermally coagulated tissue samples in the near infrared spectral range. The present study evaluates validity of this approach by comparing the optical properties of bovine myocardium after thermal denaturation with those obtained after laser coagulation. To determine the optical properties of native, thermally coagulated, and laser coagulated bovine myocardium we used a double-integrating sphere measuring technique in combination with an inverse Monte Carlo algorithm.

2. MATERIALS AND METHODS

2.1. Sample preparation

Three sections (approximately 7x5x5cm) were cut out of fresh bovine heart that was obtained from the slaughter house. The first section was wrapped in an aluminum-foil and slowly heated in a saline bath up to 80°C for 1 hour to simulate laser coagulation. The second section was laser coagulated for 15 minutes using a Nd:YAG laser (λ=1064nm, cw, 11W, T≤90°C). The laser radiation was delivered to the tissue through a specially designed water-cooled applicator (water temperature 8°C) to obtain laser lesions sufficiently large for further analysis. The third section was kept at low temperatures (4°C). From those sections the slices were cut with the thickness of 0.4 mm for the native tissue and 0.1 mm for the laser and saline bath coagulated tissue using a microcryotome. Each tissue slice was then placed on a glass slide. A drop of saline solution was added to prevent the samples from drying. The cover glasses were carefully positioned onto the slices avoiding bubble formation. The gap between the glass slides was sealed with Entellan[TM].

2.2. Integrating sphere measurements

The total transmittance, the diffuse reflectance, and the collimated transmittance were measured using a double-integrating sphere system described previously[6]. The respective sample under investigation was positioned between two integrating spheres (Labsphere Inc. USA). Chopped monochromatic light from a Xenon lamp (Osram, Germany) and with a monochromator (AMKO, Germany) was focused on the sample. The spectral bandwidth of the radiation incident on the sample was 15 nm. Diffusely reflected and transmitted light was detected by sandwich Si/Ge photodiodes (K1713-03, Hamamatsu, Japan). The photodiode currents were A/D converted and measured with lock-in amplifiers (3981, ITHACO, USA). All measurements were performed in the spectral range from 1000 nm to 1500 nm with a step width of 20 nm.

2.3. Data processing

We used an inverse Monte Carlo method[7] to determine the optical properties of the samples from the measured data; i.e., the diffuse reflectance, the total transmittance, and the collimated transmittance. The complete set of optical properties, i.e. the absorption coefficient μ_a, the scattering coefficient μ_s, and the anisotropy factor g, was determined from the experimental quantities using the Henyey-Greenstein approximation of the scattering phase function[8]. We assumed a refractive index of 1.38 for all samples (native and coagulated) and 1.51 for the glass slides.

3. RESULTS

We have measured seven native, seven laser-coagulated, and seven thermally coagulated samples in the spectral range from 1000 nm to 1500 nm with a step width of 20 nm. The optical properties obtained from the measurements with the double integrating sphere set-up using inverse Monte Carlo technique are summarized in Figs.1, 2, 3.

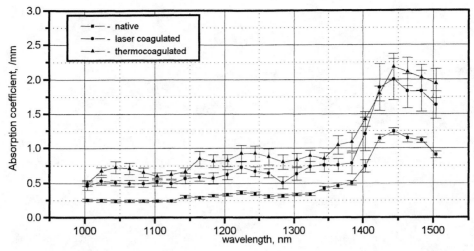

Fig. 1. Absorption coefficient μ_a of the bovine myocardium. Average of 7 samples. Bars - standard errors.

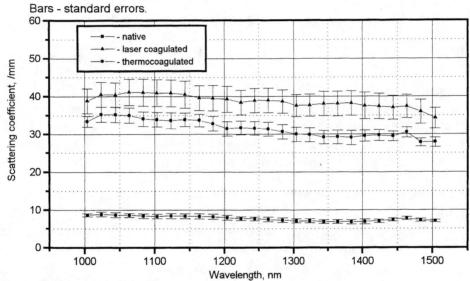

Fig. 2. Scattering coefficient μ_s of the bovine myocardium. Average of 7 samples. Bars - standard errors.

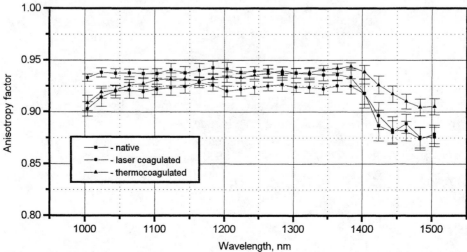

Fig. 3. Anisotropy factor g of the bovine myocardium. Average of 7 samples. Bars -standard errors.

Within the respective spectral range from 1000 to 1500 nm, the μ_a values of the native myocardium samples varied from 0.24 ± 0.05 mm^{-1} to 1.2 ± 0.1mm^{-1}, the μ_s values decreased from 8.7 ± 1.5 mm^{-1} to 6.6 ± 0.9 mm^{-1}, and g was in the range from 0.94 ± 0.02 to 0.88 ± 0.03.

For the laser-coagulated samples μ_a varied from 0.46 ± 0.16 mm^{-1} to 1.8 ± 0.6 mm^{-1}, μ_s decreased from 35 ± 5 mm^{-1} to 26 ± 3 mm^{-1}, and g was in the range between 0.92 ± 0.02 and 0.87 ± 0.03. For the thermally coagulated samples μ_a varied from 0.5 ± 0.10 mm^{-1} to 2.2 ± 0.5 mm^{-1}, μ_s decreased from 41 ± 9 mm^{-1} to 34 ± 8 mm^{-1}, and g varied from 0.94 ± 0.13 to 0.90 ± 0.02.

Thus, laser and thermal coagulation increased μ_a by a factor of 2, μ_s by a factor of 4, while g was not significantly changed.

4. DISCUSSION

Within the NIR spectral range 1000-1500 nm both laser and saline bath coagulated samples yielded an approximate twofold increase in the absorption coefficient compared with the native samples. The increased absorption coefficient of the thermally coagulated myocardium compared with that of native tissue has been reported in Ref. 3,10. An explanation of this phenomenon may be the following. A shrinkage of myofibrils would lead to an increased concentration of the absorbers per unit volume and would be accompanied by an increase of the free water content in the coagulated tissue. For a test of this hypothesis, however, additional investigations are needed.

The scattering coefficient was found to be essentially increased. This can be explained by a disordering of the tissue fibrils and a creation of numerous protein granules from the degeneration of the fibrilar contractile proteins[9] during the coagulation process, causing enhanced scattering. Significant increase of the scattering coefficient due to thermally induced changes in the myocardium was observed by several authors.[1, 3, 10]

The anisotropy factor remained nearly unchanged. One possible explanation besides creation of small protein granules is that an increase of the size of the mitochondrial aggregates in the myocardium tissue could occur when the coagulation temperature increases above 75°C[4]. These oppositely directed structural changes can result in the same anisotropy factor for both native and coagulated tissue.

The comparison of the results obtained for native and coagulated samples of bovine myocardium shows that laser and saline bath coagulation lead to similar - although not identical - changes in the optical properties of the tissue. It is known that protein denaturation and further structural changes in tissues are determined by heating temperature and duration[3]. Hence, a possible reason for the slight differences in the optical properties of laser and saline bath coagulated samples may originate from the differences of the temperature histories of the samples. It should also be mentioned that contrary to the homogeneous temperature distribution during thermal denaturation, the laser-induced temperature distribution has a substantial gradient.

5. CONCLUSION

Thermal coagulation in the saline bath leads to significant changes in the optical properties of bovine myocardium, comparable to those induced by laser coagulation. Therefore, coagulation in the saline bath is a valid technique for investigation and verification of the effects caused by laser thermal coagulation.

6. REFERENCES

1. R.Splinter, R.H.Svenson, L.Littmann, J.R.Tuntelder, C.H.Chung, G.P.Tatsis, M.Thompson, „Optical properties of normal, diseased, and laser photocoagulated myocardium at the Nd:YAG wavelength", *Las.Surg.Med.*, Vol.11, pp.117-124, 1991.
2. J.W.Pickering, P.Posthumus, M.J.C.van Gemert, „Continuous measurement of the heat induced changes in the optical properties (at 1.064 nm) of rat liver", *Las.Surg.Med.*, Vol.15, pp.200-205, 1994.
3. J.W.Pickering, S.Bosman, P.Posthumus, P.Blokland, J.F.Beek, M.J.C.van Gemert, „Changes in the optical properties (at 632,8 nm) of slowly heated myocardium", *Appl.Opt.*, Vol.32, pp.367-371, 1993.
4. S.Bosman, „Heat induced structural alterations in myocardium in relation to changing optical properties", Appl.Opt., Vol. 32, pp.461-463, 1993.
5. H.J.Schwarzmaier, A.N.Yaroslavsky, I.V.Yaroslavsky, Th.Goldbach, Th.Kahn, F.Ulrich, P.C.Schulze, R.Schober, „The optical properties of native and coagulated human brain structures," *Proc.SPIE* Vol.2970, pp.492-499, 1997.
6. A.N.Yaroslavsky, I.V.Yaroslavsky, T.Goldbach, H.-J. Schwarzmaier, „ Optical properties of blood in the near-infrared spectral range", *Proc.SPIE* Vol.2678, pp314-324, 1996.
7. I.V.Yaroslavsky, A.N.Yaroslavsky, T.Goldbach, H.-J.Schwarzmaier, "Inverse hybrid technique for the determination of the optical properties of turbid media," *Appl.Opt.,* Vol.35, pp.6797-6809, 1996.
8. L.G.Henyey, J.L. Greenstein, „Diffuse radiation in the galaxy", *Astrophys. J.*, Vol.93, pp.70-83, 1941.
9. S.Thomsen, S.Jacques, S.Flock, „Microscopic correlates of macroscopic optical property changes during thermal coagulation of myocardium", in *Laser-Tissue Interaction*, S.L.Jacques, eds., Proc.Soc.Photo-Opt. Instrum. Eng. Vol.1202, pp.2-10, 1990.
10. G.J.Derbyshire, D.K.Bogen, M.Unger, "Thermally induced optical property changes in myocardium at 1.06μm", *Las.Surg.Med.*, Vol.10, pp.28-34, 1990.

Pressure effects on soft tissues monitored by changes in tissue optical properties

HanQun Shangguan[a], Scott A. Prahl[a], Steven L. Jacques[a],
Lee W. Casperson[b], and Kenton W. Gregory [a]

[a]Oregon Medical Laser Center, 9205 SW Barnes Rd, Portland, OR 97225

[b]Department of Electrical Engineering, Portland State University, Portland, Oregon 97207

ABSTRACT

For pulsed laser tissue welding, an appropriate pressure needs to be applied to the tissues to achieve successful welds. In this study, we investigated the influences of pressure on *in vitro* optical properties of elastin biomaterial. The optical properties were measured as a function of pressure with a double integrating-sphere system. A He-Ne laser (633 nm) was used for all measurements. Each sample was sandwiched between microscope slides and then compressed with a spring-loaded apparatus. Transmittance and diffuse reflectance of each sample were measured under a pressure (0–1.5 kg/cm^2 and then released to 0). Absorption and reduced scattering coefficients were calculated using the inverse doubling method from the measured transmittance and reflectance values. Results from this study demonstrated: 1) The overall transmittance increased while the reflectance decreased as the tissue thicknesses were reduced up to 72% and the tissue weights were decreased about 40%, 2) The absorption and scattering coefficients increased with increasing the pressure, and 3) The pressure effects on the tissue optical properties were irreversible. Possible mechanisms responsible for the changes in the tissue optical properties were also investigated by changing tissue thicknesses or weights (through dehydration). This study implies that changes in tissue thickness and water content are important factors that affect tissue optical properties in different ways.

Keywords: Hydration, transmittance, diffuse reflectance, adding-doubling.

1. INTRODUCTION

Patch welding with a pulsed diode laser and indocyanine green (ICG) has been shown a promising method to successfully fuse two pieces of tissue with strong mechanical strength.[1] The advantages of the patch welding are: 1) The welding process can be simplified by welding patches to flat surfaces and 2) Collateral tissue damage is minimized by heating only the area stained with ICG. Firm contact between the two surfaces is necessary to create strong welds and consequently, during welding, the laser light must pass through the compressed tissue. However, previous studies have demonstrated that tissue optical properties are changed under compression.[2,3] The decrease in tissue thickness and the loss of water content might lead to the changes. Hence the deposition of the thermal energy at the site of welding is not only a function of laser irradiation parameters, but also the changes of optical properties in the surrounding tissue. An understanding of the pressure effects on tissue optical properties will enhance our ability to estimate the photothermal response of tissue to laser irradiation during patch welding procedure.

From preliminary work, it had been observed that dehydration could also cause both a decrease in tissue thickness and a loss of water content. A study by Çilesiz *et al.* demonstrated that the absorption coefficient increased by 20–50% in the visible range when 40% of total tissue weight was lost through dehydration.[4] Moreover, it was also noticed that the more dehydrated the biomaterial, the less pressure was needed to weld.[1] Unfortunately, there is not a comparative study to investigate the mechanisms possibly causing the changes in tissue optical properties due to the mechanical pressure or dehydration. It also remains unclear whether the changes are reversible or irreversible when the pressure is released. Thus, the objective of this study was to investigate the pressure effects on soft tissues, specifically elastin biomaterial, and possible mechanisms responsible for these changes.

SPIE Vol. 3254 • 0277-786X/98/$10.00

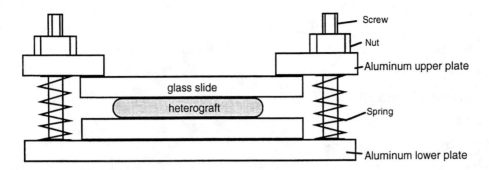

Figure 1. Cross section of the spring-loaded apparatus used for creating a constant pressure at the tissue sample. The apparatus consists of four posts with springs located at the corners of a 90×160 cm plate.

2. MATERIALS AND METHODS

2.1. Elastin Biomaterial

Porcine aorta were obtained at Carlton Packing Co., Carlton, OR. They were freshly cut and then were digested at 60°C for 1–1.5 hours in 0.5M sodium hydroxide (NaOH) to dissolve all tissue constituents but the elastin lamina. These modified vessels are termed elastin biomaterial. The biomaterial was placed in a room temperature deionized waterbath for 30 minutes, then boiled in deionized water for 30 minutes to remove the NaOH and to disinfect the vessels. The biomaterial was then kept in saline and autoclaved, and then stored at 4°C before use. Each sample was trimmed into about a 2×2 cm square using a sharp double-edged razor blade.

2.2. Experiments

Two experimental protocols were performed to investigate: 1) How does pressure affect tissue optical properties? and 2) What caused the changes? To address the first question, we measured tissue optical properties *in vitro* as a function of pressure with a double integrating-sphere system. A He-Ne laser (633 nm) was used for all measurements. Absorption and reduced scattering coefficients were calculated using the inverse doubling method[5] from the measured transmittance and reflectance values. The reflectance measurements were calibrated using a reflectance standard (Labsphere Inc.). Each sample was sandwiched between microscope slides. The glass slides were held together using a spring-loaded apparatus (Fig.1). This apparatus provided a constant force on the tissue sample. Four compression springs were calibrated using a universal material tester (V1000, LIVECO, Inc.), so that the applied pressure could be determined based on the tissue sample size (i.e., 2×2 cm square). The pressure was applied from 0, 0.5, 1, 1.5 kg/cm^2, and then released to 1, 0.5, 0 kg/cm^2 for each sample. For no pressure, each sample loosely adhered to the glass slides by tissue moisture. Tissue thickness was determined by averaging thicknesses measured at the center and near the edges of each sample using a micrometer. Five samples were used in this experiment.

To investigate the source of the changes, we measured tissue optical properties using the samples having either the same thickness or the same weight (through dehydration) as that of the compressed samples. To determine the weight loss, we weighed the samples before and after the dehydration. Each fresh sample was placed in a plastic container, and then slowly dehydrated at room temperature.

3. RESULTS

We observed that, in general, the overall transmittance increased and the diffuse reflectance decreased gradually as the pressure increased. The tissue thicknesses were reduced up to 72% and the tissue weights were decreased about 40%. Typical sample thicknesses and weights were 1.45 mm and 0.6 g respectively. A typical profile of the transmittance and the reflectance as a function of pressure is shown in Fig.2. Both the transmittance and the reflectance were irreversible; the transmittance increased up to 30% and the reflectance reduced by 12% from the initial values after the pressure was released. The corresponding absorption and scattering coefficients are shown in Fig.3. The absorption and scattering coefficients increased with increasing pressure, especially the absorption coefficient increased about twice as much as the initial value. The differences between the initial values and the final values (i.e., after compression) represent the irreversible optical properties due to the pressure effects.

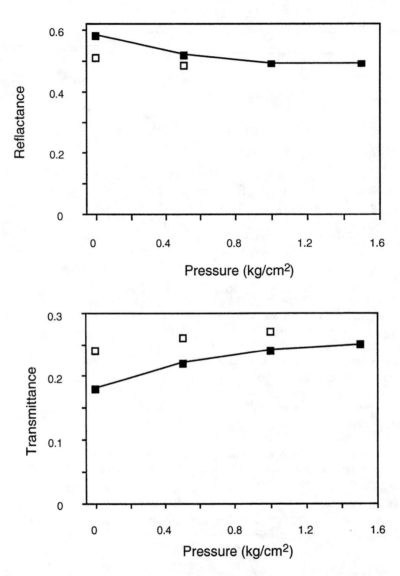

Figure 2. Elastin heterograft diffuse reflectance (top) and transmittance (bottom) as function of pressure. The filled marks represent the data measured with increasing pressure, while the open marks are the data measured as the pressure is released.

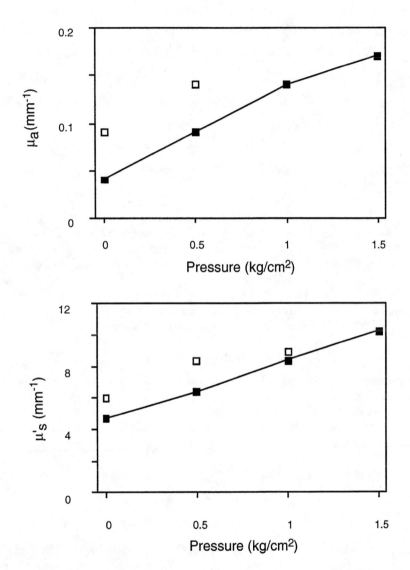

Figure 3. Elastin heterograft absorption coefficient (top) and reduced scattering coefficient (bottom) as function of pressure. The filled marks represent the data measured with increasing pressure, while the open marks are the data measured as the pressure is released.

Table 1. Optical properties of the samples with similar thickness. The tabulated values are the average of three samples. The errors are the standard deviation.

	Thickness (mm) ±0.02	Trans. (%) ±0.02	Refl. (%) ±0.02	μ_a (mm^{-1}) ±0.02	μ_s' (mm^{-1}) ±0.80
No pressure	0.54	0.35	0.45	0.09	5.37
Compressed (1 kg/cm^2)	0.53	0.24	0.49	0.14	8.31

Table 2. Optical properties of the samples with similar weight. The tabulated values are the average of three samples. The errors are the standard deviation.

	Weight (g) ±0.02	Thickness (mm) ±0.02	Trans. (%) ±0.02	Refl. (%) ±0.02	μ_a (mm^{-1}) ±0.02	μ_s' (mm^{-1}) ±0.80
Dehydrated	0.32	0.72	0.29	0.57	0.04	6.46
Compressed (1.5 kg/cm^2)	0.36	0.42	0.25	0.49	0.17	10.20

The measurements for the samples with similar thickness are listed in Table 1 and those with similar weight are listed in Table 2. The samples with similar thicknesses did not have similar optical properties (see Table 1). More light was transmitted through the compressed sample than the normal one, although the absorption and scattering coefficients for the compressed sample were greater than those for the uncompressed sample. The dehydrated samples were thicker than the compressed samples with similar weight (see Table 2). The transmittance and reflectance for the dehydrated samples were slightly greater than those of the compressed sample, while differences in the absorption and reduced scattering coefficients between them were significantly different.

4. DISCUSSION

In this study the pressure effects on tissue optical properties and the possible mechanisms for these changes were investigated. We observed that, in general, under compression the transmittance, absorption, and reduced scattering increased while the diffuse reflectance decreased. Compression caused the reduction in sample thickness and leakage of fluids from the sample. The overall transmittance increased gradually with decreasing the sample thickness. These observations may be explained with the following two equations[6]:

$$\mu_a = \rho\sigma_a \tag{1}$$

$$\mu_s = \rho\sigma_s \tag{2}$$

where μ_a and μ_s are absorption and scattering coefficients of the biomaterial respectively, ρ is the density of the absorbing or scattering centers. σ_a and σ_s are the absorption cross section and the scattering cross section. If variation in tissue density and refractive index cause light scattering in soft tissue, then under compression ρ increased as a result of reduction in the spacing among the cellular components, while σ_a and σ_s remained roughly constant or were slowly decreased because a more index-matched environment might be created as the proteins refractive index became closer to that of the elastin fibrils. Thus, the absorption and scattering coefficients were increased. Chan et al. suggested that the increase of the volumetric water concentration because of the reduction in tissue thickness may also be an explanation for the increase of absorption coefficient with compression.[3]

Previous investigations have shown that the optical properties of aorta at 633 nm for different species (e.g., bovine and human) were different. For example, values of the optical properties of bovine aorta were 0.04 mm^{-1} for the absorption coefficient and 2.19 mm^{-1} for the reduced scattering coefficient at 633 nm,[7] while values from normal human aorta were $0.05\,\mathrm{mm}^{-1}$ and $4.1\,\mathrm{mm}^{-1}$ for the absorption coefficient and for the reduced scattering coefficient respectively.[8] The results of this study showed that the optical properties of elastin biomaterial were similar to those of normal human aorta (see Fig. 3 and Table 1), although there are several tissue constituents (e.g., collagen, fiber, elastin) in the normal human aorta, while only elastin in the elastin biomaterial used in this study.

The absorption coefficient for the compressed tissue sample was greater than that for the uncompressed one, although they had the similar thicknesses (see Table 1). However, the compressed samples were very dense and compact, while the physical structures of the uncompressed samples were loose under light microscopy. The changes in the physical structure under compression may give rise to the increase in absorption and scattering due to the reasons mentioned above. Furthermore, the results of this study showed that the pressure effects on the tissue optical properties were greater than the effects of dehydration for the samples with similar weights. Although both compression and dehydration cause a reduction in tissue thickness and a loss of water content, the processes were different. Under compression, tissue thickness was reduced because spacing of elastin layers was decreased after the water was squeezed out, and even the elastin layers were squeezed as sufficient pressure was applied. On the other hand, the process for dehydration was slow (e.g., it took at least 3 hours to obtain the sample with the similar weight through dehydration.). The loss of water content was due to the evaporation rather than using extra pressure. The elastin layers may remain loose even after dehydration, so that the sample did not become very dense. Moreover, the terms, σ_a and σ_s, in Eqs. 1 and 2 may also remain roughly constant, since the samples were not deeply dehydrated in this study. Thus, the absorption and scattering coefficients for the dehydrated samples were less than those for the compressed samples.

The changes in the physical structure of soft tissue are most likely responsible for the changes in soft tissue optical properties under compression. The changes will be irreversible if the structure cannot recover after compression. We observed that the tissue thickness did not return to its initial value after releasing the pressure. This may be an explanation for the irreversible changes in the optical properties after releasing the pressure.

In conclusion, this study demonstrated: 1) The overall transmittance increased while the reflectance decreased as the tissue thicknesses were reduced up to 72% and the tissue weights were decreased about 40%, 2) The absorption and scattering coefficients increased with increasing the pressure, and 3) The pressure effects on the tissue optical properties were irreversible. Possible mechanisms responsible for the changes in the tissue optical properties were also investigated by changing tissue thicknesses or weights (through dehydration). This study implies that changes in tissue thickness and water content are important factors alerting tissue optical properties, but the contributions they make are different.

ACKNOWLEDGEMENTS

The authors wish to thank Dr. R-Q. Qian for useful discussion. This work was supported primarily by the Department of the US Army, Combat Casualty Care Division (US AMRMC contract 95221N-02).

REFERENCES

1. E. N. La Joie, A. D. Barofsky, K. W. Gregory, and S. A. Prahl, "Patch welding with a pulsed diode laser and indocyanine green," *Laser Med. Sci.* **12**, pp. 49–54, 1997.
2. A. Vogel, C. Dlugos, R. Nuffer, and R. Birngruber, "Optical properties of human sclera, and their consequences for transscleral laser applications," *Lasers Surg. Med.* **11**, pp. 331–340, 1991.
3. E. K. Chan, B. Sorg, D. Protsenko, M. O'Neil, M. Motamedi, and A. J. Welch, "Effects of compression on soft tissue optical properties," *IEEE J. Selected Topics in Quantum Electronics* **2**, pp. 943–950, 1996.
4. I. F. Çilesiz and A. J. Welch, "Light dosimetry: Effects of dehydration and thermal damage on the optical properties of the human aorta," *Appl. Opt.* **32**, pp. 477–487, 1993.
5. S. A. Prahl, "A user's manual for the inverse adding-doubling program: a compendium of worries," 1993.
6. A. Ishimaru, *Wave Propagation and Scattering in Random Media*, vol. 1, Academic Press, New York, 1978.
7. E. K. Chan, T. Menovsky, and A. J. Welch, "Effects of cryogenic grinding on soft-tissue optical properties," *Appl. Opt.* **35**, pp. 4526–4532, 1996.
8. G. Yoon, *Absorption and Scattering of Laser Light in Biological Media — Mathematical Modeling and Methods for Determining Optical Properties.* PhD thesis, University of Texas at Austin, 1988.

Time-Resolved Detection of Small Objects in Turbid Media by Diffusive Light: Simulation versus Experiment

K. Michielsen and H. De Raedt

Institute for Theoretical Physics and Materials Science Centre
University of Groningen, Nijenborgh 4
NL-9747 AG Groningen, The Netherlands

and

J. Calsamiglia, N. García and J. Przeslawski

Laboratorio de Física de Sistemas Pequeños y Nanotecnología
Consejo Superior de Investigaciones Científicas,
Serrano 144, Madrid E-28006, Spain

ABSTRACT

A method is presented to simulate the light propagation in turbid media. Based on a numerical algorithm to solve the time-dependent diffusion equation, the method takes into account spatial variations of the reduced scattering and absorption factors of the medium due to the presence of objects as well as random fluctuations of these factors. The simulation results for tissuelike phantoms are compared to experimental data and excellent agreement is found. The technique is employed to explore the possibility of locating millimeter-sized objects, immersed in turbid media, from time-resolved measurements of the transmitted or reflected (near-infrared) light. A method is proposed to enhance the imaging power of the time-resolved technique. Using the data-processing technique we find that it is possible to detect 1 mm-diameter objects, independent of their location within the sample and under unfavorable conditions. Experimental data of a time-resolved reflection experiment on a 1 mm diameter tube filled with blood and embedded in an intralipid solution are presented. The results show that, using the data processing technique, it is possible to detect the tube to a depth of 15 mm from the illuminated surface in a 70 mm thick sample. Simulation data are in excellent agreement with these experimental results.

Keywords: Time-resolved imaging, optical transillumination and reflection, diaphanography, breast cancer, tissue optical properties

1. Introduction

Breast cancer is the most common cancer in women and one of the leading causes of death in women. A successful screening method should be able to distinguish small tumors from surrounding healthy tissue before metastasis occurs.[1] The most common imaging method at this moment,

SPIE Vol. 3254 • 0277-786X/98/$10.00

x-ray mammography, is not very sensitive to differences between normal fibrotic tissue and cancer, making it less suitable for imaging young dense breasts which usually are fibrotic.[2,3] Moreover the x-ray imaging technique exposes the body to potentially harmful, ionizing radiation and increases the risk of contracting cancer. Therefore one would like to avoid using this technique for extensive routine screening.

The need for diagnostic imaging equipment that is non-invasive, safe, compact and capable of monitoring tissue chemistry in vivo, together with the advent of picosecond pulse lasers in the near-infrared wavelength regime and fast optical detectors able to resolve such pulses, has increased the interest in optical techniques as a tool for early breast cancer detection. For diagnostic optical imaging the wavelengths of interest are in the range 650 – 1300 nm: Near-infrared light is not as strongly absorbed by human tissue than visible light[2,4] and so will have higher transmission and less likelihood of causing burns. Breast imaging with red and near-infrared light relies on the differences in the optical properties of breast tissue and cancerous tissue. In cancerous tissue the incident light is strongly absorbed due to the higher blood content in the neovascular zone surrounding most malignant tumors.[5,6]

The dilemma encountered with optical imaging of human breasts is that although the wavelength of the light can be chosen such as to minimize the absorption it is impossible to avoid the blurring of the images due to strong scattering by the tissue. Light entering a strongly scattering medium (e.g. the woman breast) that contains one or more small objects (with reduced scattering and/or absorption coefficients different from that of the surrounding medium, e.g. malignant tumors) can arrive at a detector by two different routes:

1) By ballistic transport, in which the light travels without scattering through the sample to yield a projection of the object(s). The unscattered light (ballistic component) can be selected by means of a very fast (ps) time gate. A systematic study of the time-gating technique has shown that it is highly sensitive with respect to spatial variations in the absorption or reduced scattering factors,[7] in particular under conditions that are similar to those of biological systems of interest.[7] However, any technique based on the detection of unscattered light only for image formation is subject to intrinsic physical limitations. As the signal at the detector contains only an exponentially small fraction of the number of photons in the light pulse emitted by the source, the signal-to-noise ratio is low. For applications to optical breast imaging, the intensity of these photons seems to be too low to be of practical use.[7]

2) By diffusion, in which the light is scattered many times before it reaches the detector. Amplitude modulated light injected into a scattering medium generates diffusive light-intensity waves.[8] These waves have been shown to behave, in many respects, like propagating waves.[8,9,10] Inverse scattering techniques in combination with perturbation schemes have been employed to compute spatial variations in the absorption factor and the diffusion coefficient from knowledge of the phase and amplitude of these waves at various source and detector positions.[11] The diffusive character of the light transport through turbid media usually prohibits the direct detection of weakly absorbing objects hidden in the medium by direct continuous-wave measurement of the transmitted or reflected light intensity. Only if the diffusion factors of the object and the medium differ considerably, direct detection is possible.[12]

2. Model

Most of the light entering a turbid medium is scattered many times before it reaches the detector. For weakly absorbing media the propagation of the light is, to a good approximation, described by the time-dependent diffusion equation[13,14] (TDDE)

$$\frac{\partial I(\mathbf{r},t)}{\partial t} = \nabla \cdot D(\mathbf{r})\nabla I(\mathbf{r},t) - v\mu_a(\mathbf{r})I(\mathbf{r},t) + S(\mathbf{r},t) \quad , \tag{1}$$

where $I(\mathbf{r},t)$ is the intensity of light at a point $\mathbf{r}$ and at time t, $D(\mathbf{r}) = v/3[\mu'_s(\mathbf{r}) + \mu_a(\mathbf{r})]$ is the diffusion coefficient, $\mu'_s(\mathbf{r})$ is the reduced scattering factor, $\mu_a(\mathbf{r})$ denotes the absorption factor, and v is the velocity of light in the medium in the absence of objects. The light source is represented by $S(\mathbf{r},t)$. The presence of objects in the medium is reflected by spatial variations in the absorption factor and/or the reduced scattering factor. In general, both the absorption and the reduced scattering factor of the medium will fluctuate randomly around their spatial averages, denoted $\bar{\mu}_a$ and $\bar{\mu}'_s$, respectively. For weakly absorbing media, $\bar{\mu}_a \ll \bar{\mu}'_s$.

For purposes of notation it is convenient to write the intensity distribution as a "vector" $|I(t)\rangle$, i.e. $I(\mathbf{r},t) = \langle \mathbf{r}|I(t)\rangle$ where $\langle.|.\rangle$ denotes the inner product of two vectors. The intensity at a point $\mathbf{r}$ and time t is given by $\langle \mathbf{r}|e^{-tH}|s\rangle$, where $|s\rangle$ is the intensity distribution at time $t = 0$. The time evolution of the light intensity is governed by the "Hamiltonian" $H = -\nabla \cdot D(\mathbf{r})\nabla + V(\mathbf{r})$. For later convenience, we have introduced the "potential" $V(\mathbf{r}) = v\mu_a(\mathbf{r})$.

2.1 Algorithm

According to Eq. (1) the time evolution of the light intensity at time $t + \tau$ is related to the light intensity at time t through

$$|I(t+\tau)\rangle = e^{-\tau H}\left[|I(t)\rangle + \int_0^\tau d\tau' \, e^{\tau' H}|S(t+\tau')\rangle\right] \quad , \tag{2}$$

where τ denotes the time step. From Eq. (2) it follows that all we need to solve the TDDE (1) is an algorithm to compute $\exp(-\tau H)A(\mathbf{r})$ for arbitrary $A(\mathbf{r})$. We have developed an algorithm to compute $\exp(-\tau H)A(\mathbf{r})$, based on the fractal decomposition of matrix exponentials proposed by Suzuki.[15] It is accurate to second order in the spatial mesh size δ and to fourth order in the temporal mesh size τ. Conceptually the algorithm is closely related to the one that we developed for the time-dependent Schrödinger equation.[16] The first step in setting up a numerical method to solve the TDDE (1) is to discretize the derivatives with respect to the spatial coordinates. The simplest approximation scheme having satisfactory properties is[17]

$$K_x I(\mathbf{r},t) \equiv -\left.\frac{\partial}{\partial x}\left(D(\mathbf{r})\frac{\partial}{\partial x}I(\mathbf{r},t)\right)\right|_{\mathbf{r}=(i\delta,j\delta,k\delta)} \approx -\frac{D_{i+1,j,k} + D_{i,j,k}}{2\delta^2}I_{i+1,j,k}$$

$$+ \frac{D_{i+1,j,k} + 2D_{i,j,k} + D_{i-1,j,k}}{2\delta^2}I_{i,j,k} - \frac{D_{i-1,j,k} + D_{i,j,k}}{2\delta^2}I_{i-1,j,k} \quad , \tag{3}$$

where $I_{i,j,k} = I(\mathbf{r} = (i\delta, j\delta, k\delta))$ and $D_{i,j,k} = D(\mathbf{r} = (i\delta, j\delta, k\delta))$. For the derivatives with respect to y and z we use expressions similar to (3).

Proceeding as in the case of the time-dependent Schrödinger equation, the time-step operator $e^{-\tau H}$ is approximated by a product of matrix exponentials. An approximation correct to second order in the time-step τ is given by[18,19]

$$e^{-\tau H} \approx e^{-\tau K_z/2} e^{-\tau K_y/2} e^{-\tau K_x/2} e^{-\tau V} e^{-\tau K_x/2} e^{-\tau K_y/2} e^{-\tau K_z/2} \quad . \tag{4}$$

Instead of using Fast-Fourier-Transform methods[20] to compute $e^{-\tau K_x/2} A(\mathbf{r})$, we replace $e^{-\tau K_x/2}$ by a first-order product-formula approximation and obtain[21]

$$e^{-\tau K_x/2} \approx X(\tau/2) = \prod_{j,k} \left[\prod_{i \in \mathcal{E}} \frac{1}{2} \begin{pmatrix} 1 + e^{-\tau a_{i,j,k}} & 1 - e^{-\tau a_{i,j,k}} \\ 1 - e^{-\tau a_{i,j,k}} & 1 + e^{-\tau a_{i,j,k}} \end{pmatrix}^{(i,i+1)} \right]$$
$$\times \left[\prod_{i \in \mathcal{O}} \frac{1}{2} \begin{pmatrix} 1 + e^{-\tau a_{i,j,k}} & 1 - e^{-\tau a_{i,j,k}} \\ 1 - e^{-\tau a_{i,j,k}} & 1 + e^{-\tau a_{i,j,k}} \end{pmatrix}^{(i,i+1)} \right] \quad , \tag{5}$$

where the triples (i, j, k) appearing in (5) represent a point on the lattice, $\mathcal{E}$ and $\mathcal{O}$ are the sets of even and odd numbers respectively and $a_{i,j,k} = \delta^{-2}(D_{i,j,k} + D_{i+1,j,k})/2$. The superscripts $(i, i+1)$ labeling the two-by-two matrices indicate that this matrix operates on the vector $(I_{i,j,k}, I_{i+1,j,k})$ only. In (4) we replace $e^{-\tau K_y/2}$ and $e^{-\tau K_z/2}$ by similar approximations, $Y(\tau/2)$ and $Z(\tau/2)$ respectively. The resulting product formula remains correct up to order τ^2. It is also of interest to note that all the matrix elements of both $e^{-\tau K_x/2}$ and $X(\tau/2)$ are positive so that approximation (5) has the desirable feature that it will never lead to negative light intensities. The accuracy of the second-order algorithm may be insufficient if we want to solve the TDDE for long times. In practice this is only a minor complication because the second-order algorithm can be re-used to build an algorithm that is correct to fourth order in the time step. According to Suzuki's fractal decomposition,[15]

$$S_4(\tau) = S_2(p\tau) S_2(p\tau) S_2((1 - 4p)\tau) S_2(p\tau) S_2(p\tau) \quad , \tag{6}$$

will be an approximation to the time-step operator that is correct to fourth order in τ provided $p = (4 - 4^{1/3})^{-1}$. In our simulations we have used both (4) and (6) and obtained quantitatively similar results.

The contribution from the source $S(\mathbf{r}, t)$ is computed using the standard Simpson rule[22]

$$e^{-\tau H} \int_0^\tau d\tau' \, e^{\tau' H} |S(t + \tau')\rangle \approx \frac{\tau}{6} \left(e^{-\tau H} |S(t)\rangle + 4 e^{-\tau H/2} |S(t + \tfrac{\tau}{2})\rangle + |S(t + \tau)\rangle \right) \quad , \tag{7}$$

which is correct to fourth order in τ.

From the structure of (3) and $S_2(\tau)$ it is clear that the propagation of light over a time-step τ has been reduced to elementary operations: Repeated multiplications of two elements of a vector by the corresponding two elements of another vector (in the case of $e^{-\tau V}$), or of matrix-vector multiplications involving two-by-two matrices only. The resulting algorithm is fast, stable and flexible. For practical applications to the tumor detection problem it is important that the software can deal with irregulary shaped samples. As the Suzuki-product-formula based algorithm presented above operates on numbers labeled by real-space indices only, it is as easy to solve the TDDE for a particular shape as it is to solve the TDDE for a rectangular box.

2.2 Simulation software

Our current version of the software solves Eq. (1) in two and three dimensions subject to perfectly reflecting and/or perfectly absorbing boundary conditions. The intensity of light transmitted by the sample is collected by detectors located at $\mathbf{r} = (L_x, y, z)$, where L_x denotes the size of the simulation box in the direction of the incident light. The reflected light intensity is recorded at $\mathbf{r} = (0, y, z)$. The light source is placed at $x = 0$ [i. e. $S(\mathbf{r}, t) = 0$ unless $\mathbf{r} = (0, y, z)$]. We have carried out simulations using sources of variable size, including the cases of a point source [$S(\mathbf{r}, t) = S_0(t)\delta(x)\delta(y - y_0)\delta(z - z_0)$] and uniform illumination [$S(\mathbf{r}, t) = S_0(t)\delta(x)$]. At $t = 0$ the source starts to illuminate the system, until $t = t_p$ when it is turned off. Detection of the light intensity starts at t_d ($t_d > t_p$). Our simulation software allows the detectors to record the instantaneous or the time-integrated light intensity.

For a representative sample of 71 mm × 71 mm, using a mesh size of $\delta = 1$ mm ($L_x = L_y = 71$), and a time step of 1 ps it takes about 1 minute on a Pentium Pro 200 Mhz system to carry out 1000 time steps. The CPU time required to solve the TDDE by the algorithm presented above scales linearly with the number of time steps and the total number of grid points. Calculation of the time-evolution of the light intensity for a grid of $63 \times 63 \times 63 = 250047$ points and 1480 time steps takes 6 minutes on a Cray C98 (single processor), 42 minutes on a SGI Power Challenger (single processor), and 65 minutes on an IBM RS/6000 model 43P workstation. For exploratory purposes it is advantageous to simulate two-dimensional (2D) systems. Then, for selected cases, we simulate the corresponding three-dimensional (3D) system. On a qualitative level there seems to be little difference between the results obtained from 2D or 3D simulations. In fact we never encountered a 3D simulation that forced us to change a conclusion drawn from 2D simulation data.

3. Comparison with experiments

We have tested our software and the validity of the TDDE model by comparing simulation data[23] with the experimental results of Ref. 7 for exactly the same systems as those studied in Ref. 7. We made simulations for systems of size 40 mm ×127 mm, with a spatial mesh-size $\delta = 1$ mm, a time step $\tau = 1$ ps, $t_p = 7$ ps, $t_d = 350$ ps and the speed of light in the medium $v = 0.222$ mm/ps. We verified (by reducing the mesh size and the time step) that the numerical results are, for all practical purposes, exact. The simulation itself is carried out in a manner identical to the procedure used in the time-gating technique.[7] The sample is illuminated uniformly by the pulsed light source. This corresponds to the experimental situation in which the phantom is located on an x-y stage and is moved in the horizontal plane under computer control.[7] The detector accumulates the light intensity over the interval $t_d < t < t + \Delta t$ where Δt denotes the time gate.

In Fig. 1 we depict our simulation results (dashed curves) and the experimental data (solid curves) which are taken from Fig. 12b of Ref. 7. The medium contains a plastic tube (8 mm

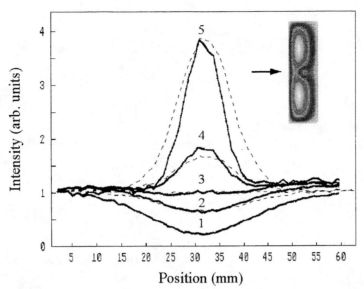

Fig. 1 Comparison of experimental[7] (solid curves) and computer simulation (dashed curves) results for the time-resolved transilluminated light intensity. In experiment and simulation the turbid medium has a reduced scattering factor $\mu'_s = 0.9\,\mathrm{mm}^{-1}$ and an absorption factor $\mu_a < 0.001\,\mathrm{mm}^{-1}$. The 8 mm-diameter tube, located in the centre of the sample, has $\mu_a = 0.13\,\mathrm{mm}^{-1}$ and $\mu'_s = 0$.[7] As in Fig. 12b of Ref. 7 : 1, continuous-wave case (experimental data only); 2, $\Delta t = 960\,\mathrm{ps}$; 3, $\Delta t = 480\,\mathrm{ps}$; 4, $\Delta t = 240\,\mathrm{ps}$; 5, $\Delta t = 30\,\mathrm{ps}$. The inset shows the light distribution inside the sample for $\Delta t = 960\,\mathrm{ps}$; the arrow indicates the direction of the incident light. See also Fig. 12b of Ref. 7.

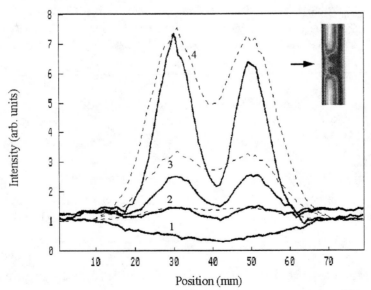

Fig. 2 Same as Fig. 1 except that instead of one there are two 10 mm-diameter objects, separated by 20 mm, with an absorption factor $\mu_a = 0.029\,\mathrm{mm}^{-1}$.[7] See also Fig. 13a of Ref. 7.

diameter) filled with diluted ink, positioned in the center of the sample. In the simulation both the absorption and the reduced scattering factors are allowed to fluctuate randomly within 10% of their values specified in Ref. 7. Our numerical results are in remarkably good agreement with the experimental data. The inset shows the distribution of light inside the sample at $\Delta t = 960$ ps. The object is clearly visible.

Simulation and experimental[7] data for a medium containing bead pairs are shown in Fig. 2. The agreement between experiment and theory is remarkable, when one takes into account that no attempt has been made to make a best fit. The above simulation results and others[23] (not shown) demonstrate that our simulation software reproduces all the features observed in the experiments on the tissuelike phantoms reported in Ref. 7.

4. Time-resolved reflection experiments on breast phantoms

Our simulation software reproduces, without fitting, the data obtained from time-resolved transillumination measurements on turbid media containing relatively large (± 8 mm diameter) objects. Hence it can be used to explore different techniques for improving the detection methods. We have used our simulation method to devise a data processing technique to enhance the quality of the images. An obvious approach is to compare the data with other data obtained from a reference, or model, system. In the case at hand we know that the immense scattering of light is responsible for the blurring of the images of the objects. The variations of both the reduced scattering and absorption factor due to the objects are relatively small. Therefore as a starting point, it is reasonable to take as a reference model a system with a constant diffusion coefficient. In practice the data processing method works as follows: We measure the integrated intensity I of the sample, calculate or measure the reference signal corresponding to a "test" model and compute $\ln(I/I_0)$ or $I - I_0$ for various source and detector positions. The resulting distribution should reveal whether there are hidden objects or not. The mathematical justification of the method is based on a generalization of inequalities of Symanzik[24] but is out of the scope of this paper and will therefore be presented elsewhere.

An illustration of the usefulness of this image processing method is given in Figs. 3-5. Unless explicitly mentioned otherwise, the spatial mesh size $\delta = 1$ mm, the time step $\tau = 1$ ps, the source pulse time $t_p = 10$ ps, the time at which the detectors start to record intensity $t_d = 500$ ps, and the speed of light in the medium $v = 0.222$ mm/ps. Guided by the experimemts on breast tissue[7,25−28] in our simulations we will assume that the turbid medium is characterized by an absorption and reduced scattering factor $\mu_a = 0.01$ mm^{-1} and $\mu'_s = 0.9$ mm^{-1}, respectively. For tumor tissue we will take $\mu_a = 0.1$ mm^{-1} and $\mu'_s = 0.9$ mm^{-1}, unless explicitly mentioned otherwise.

We will use the short-hand notation $\bar{I}_T$ and $\bar{I}_R$ for the transmitted and reflected intensity respectively, integrated over the corresponding detection area. All intensities given below are normalized with respect to the light intensity supplied by the source.

In Fig. 3 we show results of a simulation for a sample of size 71 mm $\times$ 71 mm, containing an object of 2.5 mm radius, positioned at $(36, 26)$ mm. The sample is illuminated by a source of diameter 1 mm centered around $(0, 36$ mm$)$. Figs. 3a,c show the integrated intensity while Figs. 3b,d show the corresponding processed signal. For $\Delta t = 612$ ps (Figs. 3a,b), it is clear that the object leaves no trace in the transmitted and reflected intensity whereas the processed data clearly

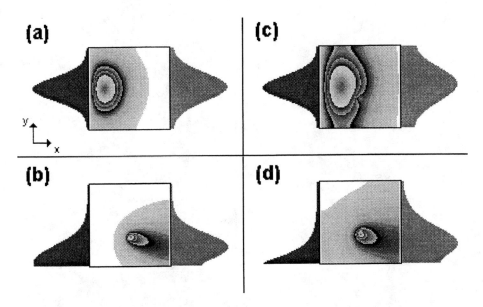

Fig. 3 Simulation of a time-resolved experiment on a turbid medium with a reduced scattering factor $\mu'_s = 0.9 \, \text{mm}^{-1}$ and an absorption factor $\mu_a = 0.01 \, \text{mm}^{-1}$ containing a 2.5 mm-radius object with absorption and reduced scattering factors $\mu_a = 0.1 \, \text{mm}^{-1}$ and $\mu'_s = 0.9 \, \text{mm}^{-1}$, respectively. The dimensions of the sample are 71 mm × 71 mm. The object is located at (36, 26) mm. The sample is illuminated by a source of diameter 1 mm centered around (0, 36 mm) during a time $t_p = 10$ ps. (a) Time-integrated transmitted (right) and reflected (left) intensity for $\Delta t = 612$ ps. $\bar{I}_T \approx 0.6 \times 10^{-8}$ and $\bar{I}_R \approx 0.2 \times 10^{-2}$; (b) processed signal corresponding to (a); (c) same as (a) except that $\Delta t = 1836$ ps. $\bar{I}_T \approx 0.5 \times 10^{-6}$ and $\bar{I}_R \approx 0.3 \times 10^{-2}$; (d) processed signal corresponding to (c); The (processed) light intensities inside the sample are also shown.

indicate that there is an object inside the sample. For $\Delta t = 1836$ ps (Figs. 3c,d) the transmitted intensity shows an asymmetry. Since the light source is positioned at (0, 36 mm) this asymmetry indicates that there is an object immersed in the sample. In the reflected intensity, however, the object leaves no trace. In the processed reflected intensity the object is clearly visible.

Fig. 4 depicts simulation results for uniform illumination of a three-dimensional sample of size 63 mm × 63 mm × 63 mm, on its whole left plane. In Figs. 4a,b the sample contains a 2.5 mm sphere, while in Figs. 4c,d the sample contains a 0.5 mm sphere. The sphere is positioned at (32, 30, 36) mm. Figs. 4a,b show the transmitted and reflected intensities and Figs. 4c,d show the corresponding processed signals. Only in the case of the 2.5 mm radius object there is a weak signal of the object in the transmitted intensity. In the processed signals, however, there is a clear signal of both the 2.5 mm radius object and the 0.5 mm object.

As shown above the data processing method is very useful in the simulation of object detection in turbid media. Hence it can be used to explore its usefulness in time-resolved reflection experiments on tissuelike phantoms. The experimental set-up we used for time-resolved diffused light reflectance is described in Ref. 29. In the experiment we used a vessel (70 mm × 70 mm × 70 mm) filled with a 10% of commercial intralipid solution ($\mu'_s = 1.1 \, \text{mm}^{-1}$ and $\mu_a = 0.01 \, \text{mm}^{-1}$). At ($x = d, y = 25$ mm) we placed a 1 mm diameter tube filled with blood. We varied d from 5 mm to 15 mm. To compare with the experimental results we performed simulations for exactly the same

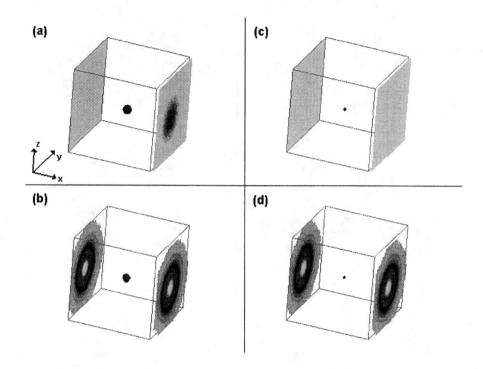

Fig. 4 Simulation of a time-resolved experiment on a turbid medium with a reduced scattering factor $\mu'_s = 0.9\,\mathrm{mm}^{-1}$ and an absorption factor $\mu_a = 0.01\,\mathrm{mm}^{-1}$ containing a sphere with absorption and reduced scattering factors $\mu_a = 0.1\,\mathrm{mm}^{-1}$ and $\mu'_s = 0.9\,\mathrm{mm}^{-1}$, respectively. The dimensions of the sample are $63\,\mathrm{mm} \times 63\,\mathrm{mm} \times 63\,\mathrm{mm}$. The sample is illuminated uniformly on its whole left plane. The object is located at $(32, 30, 36)\,\mathrm{mm}$. The sphere inside the sample denotes the position of the object. (a) Time-integrated transmitted (right) and reflected (left) signal for $\Delta t = 875\,\mathrm{ps}$. The sample contains a 2.5 mm object. (b) processed signal corresponding to (a); (c) same as (a) except that that the radius of the object is 0.5 mm; (d) processed signal corresponding to (c).

system. The simulation is carried out in a manner identical to the procedure used in the time-resolved reflection technique.[29] In Fig. 5 we show the experimental and simulation data which are taken from Figs. 3,5 of Ref. 29. Fig.5a depicts the experimental data and Fig.5b depicts the simulation data. The reflected intensities are shown on the left while the processed reflected intensities are shown on the right. In the processed intensities the tube is clearly distinguishable to depths of 15 mm from the illuminated surface. The simulation results are in excellent agreement with the experimental data.

5. Conclusions

We have developed software to simulate time-resolved near-infrared diffuse light imaging experiments in turbid media. Our simulation technique reproduces experimental data of time-resolved transillumination experiments on 8 mm tubes hidden in turbid media without the need of fitting parameters. Simulation results suggest that under conditions similar to those of human tissue

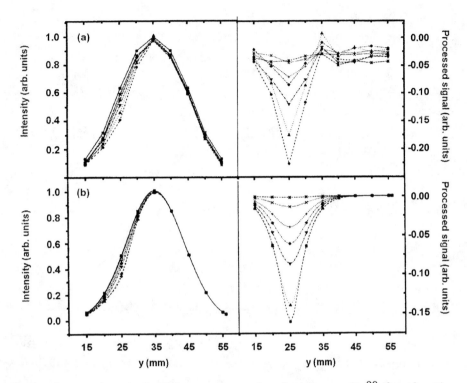

Fig. 5 Comparison of experimental and computer simulation results[29] for the time-resolved reflected light intensity. In the experiment and simulation the turbid medium has a reduced scattering factor $\mu'_s = 1\,\mathrm{mm}^{-1}$ and an absorption factor $\mu_a = 0.01\,\mathrm{mm}^{-1}$. The 1 mm-diameter tube, located at $(x = d, y = 25\,\mathrm{mm})$, is filled with blood. In the simulations the tube has $\mu_a = 0.1\,\mathrm{mm}^{-1}$ and $\mu'_s = 1$. The sample is illuminated uniformly on the $x = 0$ plane. Circle: $d = 5\,\mathrm{mm}$; up triangle: $d = 6\,\mathrm{mm}$; down triangle: $d = 8\,\mathrm{mm}$; diamond: $d = 9\,\mathrm{mm}$, cross (+): $d = 10\,\mathrm{mm}$; cross (x): $d = 12\,\mathrm{mm}$, star: $d = 15\,\mathrm{mm}$; square: No object. (a) Experimental results for the reflected intensity (left) and the processed signal (right) for $t_d = 395\,\mathrm{ps}$ and $\Delta t = 50\,\mathrm{ps}$; (b) same as (a) but for the simulation results. See also Figs. 3,5 of Ref.29.

with tumors, objects of 1 mm radius can be located in a 60 mm thick sample, independent of their location within the sample, if a data processing technique is used. We performed time-gated reflection experiments on 1 mm blood tubes hidden in an intralipid solution. The data show that, using the data processing technique, the tube can be detected to a depth of 15 mm from the illuminated surface in a 70 mm thick sample. Simulation results are also in excellent agreement with these experimental data. Hence, the numerical method can be applied to look for the best experimental conditions for detection and localization of various objects in turbid media with both time-resolved transillumination and reflection techniques.

ACKNOWLEDGEMENTS

This work is supported by EEC and Spanish research contracts and by a supercomputer grant of the "Stichting Nationale Computer Faciliteiten (NCF)".

References

1. J.C. Hebden, D.J. Hall, M. Firbank, and D.T. Delpy, "Time-resolved optical imaging of a solid tissue-equivalent phantom", Appl. Opt. **34**, 8038 – 8047, 1995.

2. E. Carlsen, "Transillumination light scanning, Diagnostic Imaging", 28 – 33 (+60), 1982.

3. S. Nioka, M. Miwa, S. Orel, M. Shnall, M. Haida, S. Zhao, and B. Chance, "Optical Imaging of Human Breast Cancer", Oxygen Transport to Tissue XVI, M.C. Hogan *et al.* eds., Plenum Press, New York, 1994, p. 171 – 179.

4. S. Ertefai, and A.E. Profio, "Spectral Transmittance and Contrast in Breast Diaphanography", Med. Phys. **12**, 393 – 400, 1985.

5. D.J. Watmough, "Diaphanography: Mechanism responsible for the imaging", Act. Radiol. Oncol. **21**, 11 – 15, 1982.

6. A.E. Profio, G.A. Navarro, O.W. Sartorius, "Scientific basis of breast diaphanography, Med. Phys. **16**, 60 – 65, 1989.

7. G. Mitic, J. Kölzer, J. Otto, E. Plies, G. Sölkner, and W. Zinth, "Time-gated transillumination of biological tissues and tissuelike phantoms", Appl. Opt. **33**, 6699 – 6710, 1994.

8. J.B. Fishkin, and E. Gratton, "Propagation of photon-density waves in strongly scattering media containing an absorbing semi-infinite plane bounded by a straight edge", J. Opt. Soc. Am. A **10**, 127 – 140, 1993.

9. B.J. Tromberg, L.O. Svaasand, T.T. Tsay, and R.C. Haskell, "Properties of photon density waves in multiple-scattering media", Appl. Opt. **32**, 607 – 616, 1993.

10. J.M. Schmitt, A. Knüttel, and J.R. Knutson, "Interference of diffusive light waves", J. Opt. Soc. Am. A **9**, 1832 – 1843, 1992.

11. M.A. O'Leary, D.A. Boas, B. Chance, and A.G. Yodh," Experimental images of heterogeneous turbid media by frequency-domain diffusing-photon tomography", Opt. Lett. **20**, 426 – 428, 1995.

12. P.N. den Outer, Th. M. Nieuwenhuizen, and A. Lagendijk, "Location of objects in multiple-scattering media", J. Opt. Soc. Am. A **10**, 1209 – 1218, 1993.

13. A. Ishimaru, *Wave Propagation and Scattering in Random Media*, (Academic, New York, 1978).

14. H.C. van de Hulst, *Multiple Light Scattering*, (Academic, New York, 1980).

15. M. Suzuki, "General theory of fractal path integrals with applications to many-body theories and statistical physics", J. Math. Phys. **32**, 400 – 407, 1991.

16. H. De Raedt, and K. Michielsen, "Algorithm to solve the time-dependent Schrödinger equation for a charged particle in an inhomogeneous magnetic field: Application to the Aharonov-Bohm effect", Computers in Physics **8**, 600 – 607, 1994.

17. G.D. Smith, *Numerical solution of partial differential equations*, (Clarendon, Oxford, 1985).

18. H. De Raedt, and B. De Raedt, "Applications of the Generalized Trotter Formula", Phys. Rev. A**28**, 3575 – 3580, 1983.

19. M. Suzuki, "Decomposition Formulas of Exponential Operators and Lie Exponentials with some Applications to Quantum Mechanics and Statistical Physics", J. Math. Phys. **26**, 601 – 612, 1985.

20. W.A. Press, B.P. Flannery, S.A. Teukolsky, W.T. Vetterling, *Numerical Recipes*, (Cambridge University Press, 1986).

21. H. De Raedt, "Product Formula Algorithms for Solving the Time-Dependent Schrödinger Equation", Comp. Phys. Rep. **7**, 1 – 72, 1987.

22. M. Abramowitz, and I.A. Stegun (eds.), *Handbook of Mathematical Functions*, (National Bureau of Standards, Washington DC, 1964).

23. K. Michielsen, H. De Raedt, and N. García, "Time-gated transillumination and reflection by biological tissues and tissuelike phantoms: Simulation versus experiment" J. Opt. Soc. Am. (in press).

24. K. Symanzik, "Proof and Refinements of an Inequality of Feynman", J. Math. Phys. **6**, 1155 – 1156, 1965.

25. V.G. Peters, D.R. Wyman, M.S. Patterson, and G.L. Frank, "Optical properties of normal and diseased human breast tissues in the visible and near infrared", Phys. Med. Biol. **9**, 1317 – 1334, 1990.

26. H. Key, E.R. Davies, P.C. Jackson, and P.N.T. Wells, "Optical attenuation characteristics of breast tissues at visible and near-infrared wavelengths", Phys. Med. Biol. **36**, 579 – 590, 1991.

27. R. Marchesini, A. Bertoni, S. Andreola, E. Melloni, and A.E. Sichirollo, "Extinction and absorption coefficients and scattering phase functions of human tissue *in vitro*", Appl. Opt. **28**, 2318 – 2324, 1989.

28. K. Suzuki, Y. Yamashita, K. Ohta, and B. Chance, "Quantitative measurement of optical parameters in the breast using time-resolved spectroscopy", Invest. Radiol. **29**, 410 – 414, 1994.

29. J. Przeslawski, J. Calsamiglia, N. García, H. De Raedt, K. Michielsen, and M. Nieto-Vesperinas, "Detection of 1 mm size hidden object in tissuelike phantoms by backscattered diffused light", submitted to Opt. Lett..

For further author information:

K.M.: e-mail: k.f.l.michielsen@phys.rug.nl, Phone: ++31-50-3634950, Fax: ++31-50-363947

H.D.R.: e-mail: h.a.de.raedt@phys.rug.nl, Phone: ++31-50-3634950, Fax: ++31-50-363947

J.C.: e-mail: jcalsamig@fsp.csic.es, Phone: ++34-1-5631854, Fax: ++34-1-5631560

N.G.: e-mail: nikolas.garcia@fsp.csic.es, Phone: ++34-1-5631854, Fax: ++34-1-5631560

J.P.: e-mail: janusz@fsp.csic.es, Phone: ++34-1-5631854, Fax: ++34-1-5631560

SESSION 13

Poster Session

System of measurement of the transmission spectrum of "in vitro" corneas for eye banks

Josemilson de M. Bispo, Liliane Ventura, Carlos Roberto de Carvalho Júnior, Sidney Júlio de Faria e Sousa and Caio Chiaradia

(JMB, LV, CRCJ, SJFS, CC - Laboratório de Física Oftálmica - FMRP-USP- Av. Bandeirantes 3900, 14049-900 Ribeirão Preto - SP - Brasil) (JMB, Departamento de Física e Matemática - FFCLRP-USP).

Keywords: Transmission Spectrum of "In Vitro" Cornea, Donated Corneas Evaluation, Corneal Transparency

ABSTRACT

The donated cornea transparency is one of the features to be analyzed previously to its indication for the transplant. Hence we have developed a system to evaluate the transmission spectrum of "In Vitro" corneas in its preservative medium, in the range of 400-700nm, to be implemented in an Eye Bank. The cornea in its preservative medium is illuminated by collimated white light beams which strike a diffraction grid, passes through an optical system and a selecting filter (400-800nm) and then is detected by a linear CCD detector (2048 photodiodes). The data is displayed in a PC monitor via a commercial interface device. A dedicated software has been developed to plot the transmission spectrum profile and provide an objective and standard information about the transparency of the donated cornea.

1. INTRODUCTION

The anterior transparent part of the human eye is known as the cornea[1]. The donated cornea transparency is one of the features to be analyzed previously to its indication for the transplant.

According to the statistics of the Hospital das Clínicas Eye Bank (in Ribeirão Preto - Brasil) 50% of the donated corneas are rejected to be used for transplants by presenting doubtful aspect regarding its transparency and the number of endothelium cells. Therefore, some of them are despised by excess of zeal. This is quite necessary in order to protect the patient who will receive the donated cornea, but on the other hand this is an undesirable loss of such a precious tissue. Hence, we have developed a system to evaluate the transmission spectrum of "in vitro" cornea in its preservative medium, in order to standardize the approval of the analyzed corneas.

2. MATERIALS AND METHODS

Figure 1 shows the schematic set up of the system.

The white light beams diverge from a slit and become parallel after leaving the convergent lens, L_1, whose focus is 120mm (see figures 1 and 2). These collimated beams pass through a pin-hole, in order to provide that just the cornea's central portion is illuminated. The cornea, in its preservative medium, is illuminated by white light beams which strike a diffraction grid (responsible for spreading the white light in its several wavelengths[2]), and passes through a selecting filter (400-700nm). Then, the light passes through another converging lens, L_2 (focal length = 90mm), that forms the image of the spectrum on the detector. When every ray of same wavelengths are parallel, they are focused and detected by a linear CCD detector (2048 photodiodes). Rays of different wavelengths, are not parallel and, therefore, are focused at different positions[3] on the CCD, placed on the focal plane of lens L_2, according to figure 1.

SPIE Vol. 3254 • 0277-786X/98/$10.00

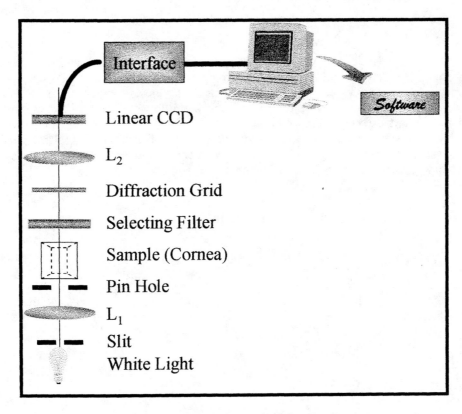

Figure 1: Schematic set up of the system.

The data is displayed in a PC monitor, where a dedicated software has been developed to plot the transmission spectrum profile.

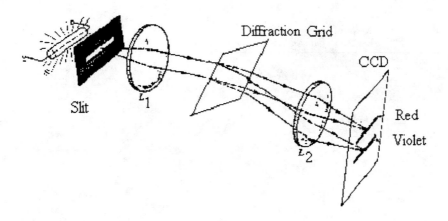

Figure 2: Ssytem for obtaining a defined spectrum of the white light.

3. RESULTS

The spectrum processing is done in a determined sequence of events. First the dedicated software records the signal of the scattered light by the diffraction grid and then is detected by a linear CCD detector, so the data is displayed in a PC monitor via a commercial interface device (ADC-10). Afterwards, all the process must be repeated for the light passing trough the sample. As this data is available, the software divides the signals, which provides the transmission spectrum of the sample. Figures 3a shows a spectrum obtained in our system of a well known optical filter and 3b shows the spectrum of the same filter obtained in a commercial spectrophotometer. Although they just have large bandwidth, they are illustrative to show thar our system is precise enough for the donated corneas measurements. Figure 4 shows the transmission spectrum of a human donated cornea 4 days after the death.

4. CONCLUSIONS

The system has been presenting good results and the processing time is fast enough for the Eyes Bank routine (15s for a PC-386, 4MB-RAM). Also the precision of the system is 2nm for the cornea spectra, which is sufficient for this kind of measurement. The system should be implemented in an Eye Bank in the next months providing objective measurements in order to standardize the approval of the analyzed corneas. Figure 3 shows a spectrum of an optical filter obtained by our system and by a commercial spectrophotometer in order to compare the spectra.

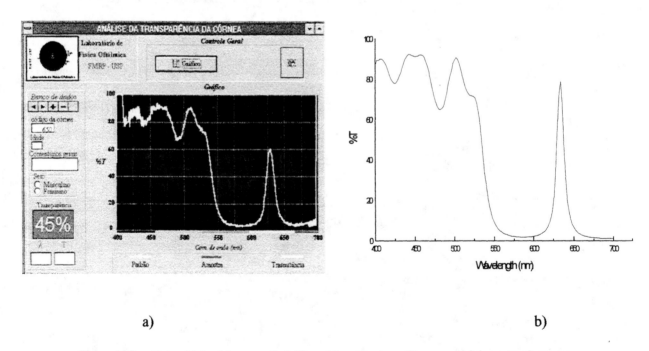

a)   b)

Figure 3: Spectrum obtained for an optical filter: (a) our system; (b) commercial spectrophotometer.

Figure 4 presents the spectrum of a donated cornea. Figure 4a is the spectrum of the cornea plus its preservative medium. Figure 4b is the spectrum of the cornea itself. We should notice that the cornea has an almost continuum spectrum in the range of 400-700nm.

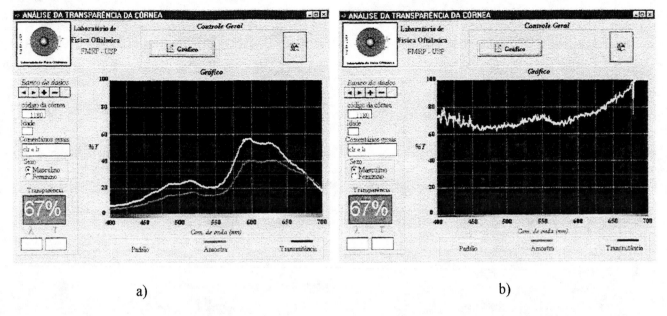

a)   b)

Figure 4: Spectrum obtained for an "in vitro" cornea: (a) cornea + the preservative medium; (b) cornea itself.

Several measurements were done and the spectra are in good agreement with the data obtained from commercial spectrophotometer, BECKMAN DU-70.

5. ACKNOWLEDGMENTS

The authors would like to thank FAPESP (proc. n°: 95/9702-8) for all financial support for this research, CNPq, CAPES and Hospital das Cínicas de Ribeirão Preto, particularly Banco de Olhos do Hospital das Clínicas de Ribeirão Preto.

6. REFERENCES

1. Vaughan, D.; Asbury, T., Oftalmologia Geral, 2° Ed., Chapter 8.
2. Sears, F. W., Física Óptica, vol III, 1964, Ao livro técnico Ltda, ch. 7.
3. James, J. F.; Sterberg, R.S., The design of optical spectrometers, ch. 9.

In situ observation of IR and UV - solid state laser modifications of lens and cornea

V. Kamensky[1*], R.Kuranov[*], G.Gelikonov[*], S.Muraviov[*], A.Malyshev[*], A.Yurkin[**], F.Feldchtein[*], and N.Bityurin[*]

[*]Institute of Applied Physics of Russian Academy of Sciences, Uljanov , st. 46, 603600, Nizhny Novgorod, Russia

[**]Design and Technology Institute of Single Crystals, Siberian Branch of RAS, 43, Russkaja str., 630058, Novosibirsk, Russia

ABSTRACT

Pulse - to - pulse kinetics of laser ablation of porcine cornea *in vitro* by a YAG:Er laser ($\lambda = 2.94$ μm) and by fifth harmonic of a YAP:Nd laser ($\lambda = 216$ nm) as well as preablation transformations of cataracted human lens *in vitro* irradiated by Glass:Er laser ($\lambda = 1.54$ μm) are followed by Optical Coherence Tomography (OCT).
In the latter case kinetics of tissue swelling is studied.
Observation of tissue surface with temporal resolution better than pulse train duration by means of cw probe laser reveals evidences of outburst of "dynamic" hump.

Keywords: Ablation, swelling, thermally damaged area, Optical Coherence Tomography, time resolved experiments.

1. INTRODUCTION

The real time investigation of laser ablation and tissue modifications kinetics provide information which can be of significant interest to maintain the real model of laser-matter interactions.

In our previous publications [1–4] we demonstrated the possibility to employ the Optical Coherence Tomography (OCT) for *in situ* monitoring of the pulse-to-pulse kinetics of laser ablation and modification of turbid biological tissue. As an example of tissue we used the cataract - suffered human lens *in vitro*. As radiation sources we used different kinds of IR lasers with wavelengths corresponding to different initial absorption coefficients of water, α. We employed a YAG:Er laser with $\lambda = 2.94$ μm (α ~17700 cm^{-1}), a Glass:Er laser with $\lambda = 1.54$ μm (α ~10 cm^{-1}) and a YAG:Nd laser with $\lambda = 1.32$ μm (α ~1 cm^{-1}). These lasers operate in the free-running regime with pulse train duration of 300 μs.

OCT makes use of a low coherence light source and Michelson interferometer to isolate photons undergoing a single backscattering event in tissue, at a given depth. It has allowed studying irradiation of biotissues *in situ* optically, while an observation of biotissue modification by means of conventional optical techniques is difficult because of the high light scattering.

The recent advances in OCT technique specially intended for contrasting images in highly scattering media enable controlling of the ablation process in biotissues as well as monitoring of the area of thermal laser induced damage in tissues adjacent to the ablation crater. On the other hand, the nondestructive control of laser-treated tissue permits to elucidate the hidden features of laser-matter interactions.

In the present publication we demonstrate the possibility to monitor the pulse-to-pulse kinetics of laser ablation of porcine cornea by IR and UV lasers. As a source of UV laser radiation we use the fifth harmonic of a YAP:Nd laser with wavelength 216 nm and pulse duration of 10 ns. The OCT image of ablation crater produced by this laser is compared to the effect of YAG:Er laser.

Afterwards we review the main features of pulse-to-pulse kinetics of hump growth. This hump appears when tissue

---

[1] Further author information -

V.K. (correspondence): E-mail: vlad@ufp.appl.sci-nnov.ru, phone +7 8312 384503, telefax +7 8312 363792

SPIE Vol. 3254 • 0277-786X/98/$10.00

is irradiated with fluences below ablation threshold. In our previous publications we followed the hump growth phenomena by means of OCT facilities. In the present paper we report the results of time resolved experiments on hump evolution with temporal resolution better than pulse duration.

2. OCT IMAGING OF PULSE-TO-PULSE KINETICS OF LASER ABLATION OF PORCINE CORNEA.

The schematic of OCT monitoring of ablation process was described in [1-4]. In those publications we investigated the ablation of human cataract lens *in vitro* by different kind of mid IR lasers.

Here we demonstrate *in situ* monitoring of pulse-to-pulse kinetics of laser ablation of porcine cornea *in vitro*.

OCT records X-Z cross-sectional image (Z being in-depth direction). The image consists of 200×200 pixels. The images are obtained with the frequency of 0.5 Hz.

We irradiated cornea by a YAG:Er laser operating in free-running mode (Fig.1), and by the fifth harmonic of a Q-switched YAP:Nd laser at the wavelength 216 nm (Fig.2.).

Because of the high values of absorption coefficient the digging of the crater in both cases is a layer-by-layer process. Using OCT technique we can, in principle, follow not only the depth of crater but also the formation and development of adjacent to crater surface thermally damaged layer. It has been demonstrated in [1-4]. As can be seen in Figures 1,2 in both cases of ablation of cornea the thickness of discussed above thermally damaged layer is comparable with the OCT resolution limit, which, under these experimental conditions, may be estimated to be 15 μm.

It should be noted that the same technique could be used for *in vivo* imaging of laser ablation kinetics of human cornea. It could be used for controlling the processes of laser microsurgery eye treatment during e.g. photorefractive *keratectomy*.

3. THE PULSE-TO-PULSE KINETICS OF HUMP GROWTH

The swelling of cornea due to heating is well known and widely used in photothermal *keratoplasty* treatment [5,6]. Here YAG:Ho laser radiation is commonly used. This effect is usually associated with denaturation of collagens.

On the other hand, the swelling of material, hump formation, irradiated at laser fluences below ablation threshold was observed in artificial polymers (see e.g. [7]).

In [4] we performed the investigation of main features of hump formation in cataracted human lens *in vitro* when irradiated by Glass:Er (λ = 1.54 μm). The radiation of this laser has greater depth of light penetration into the material than radiation of YAG:Er laser.

The main features of hump formation can be formulated as follows:

There exists a single shot threshold fluence of hump formation. This threshold fluence is smaller than ablation threshold.

When irradiation of tissue is performed with fluences smaller than single pulse threshold, incubation occurs. In this case a hump appears after several pulses. The needed number of pulses increases with decreasing fluence.

Figures 3 a,b show the formation of a hump with the height up to 0.2 mm over the irradiated surface as a single shot response of tissue. Pictures are made by means of OCT. The radiation is focused onto the surface of the extracted cataracted human lens by lens with F=2.7 cm. Pulse train energy was 80 mJ. The initial divergence of the beam was 3 mrad. Figures 3 c,d show the effect of following pulses of the same fluence. It is seen than the subsequent pulses make hump broader rather than higher.

In order to investigate the incubation (see Fig. 4), we employed the laser pulses with fluences less than threshold one but several shots were used to irradiate the same part of tissue. The repetition rate was one pulse per 25 seconds and was slow enough to avoid the heat accumulation in treated zone from pulse to pulse. It is seen that the effect of successive subthreshold pulses manifests itself by the creation and developing of the cloudy zone beneath the surface with subsequent formation of a hump. The incubation may be connected with the gradual changing in mechanical and thermophysical properties of subsurface layers of irradiated material accounted for the partial dehydration of tissue and collagen denaturation. These changes cause the decrease of thermal diffusivity due to creation of pores and the loss of elasticity due to modification of material.

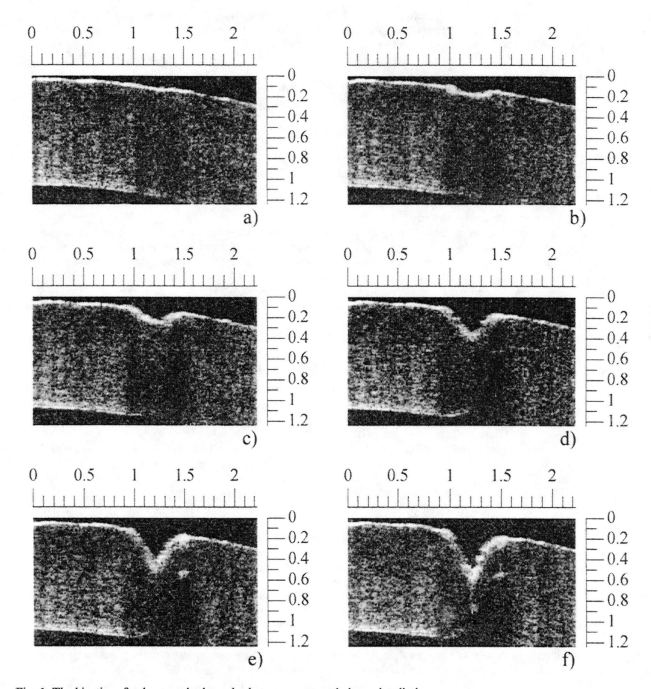

Fig. 1. The kinetics of pulse-to-pulse layer-by-layer crater growth due to irradiation of porcine cornea by YAG:Er laser (repetition rate 3 Hz, pulse train energy -15 mJ) a) initial, b) 20 s.,c) 50 s., d) 100 s., e) 150 s., f) 200s

Scale unit corresponds to 1 mm

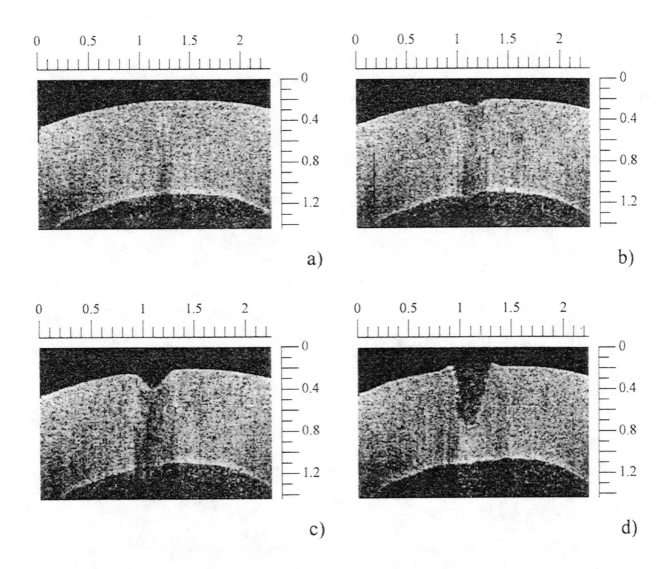

Fig. 2. The kinetics of pulse-to-pulse crater growth due to irradiation of porcine cornea by the fifth harmonic of Nd:YAP laser (λ=216 nm, repetition rate 10 Hz, fluence=270 mJ/cm^2) a) initial, b) 9 s.,c) 40 s., d) 180 s.,

Scale unit corresponds to 1 mm

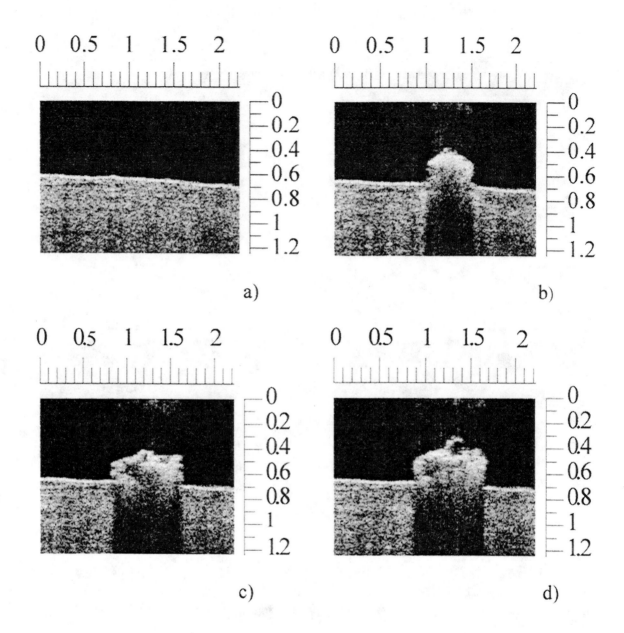

Fig. 3. Pulse-to-pulse kinetics of hump growth (Glass:Er; $\lambda = 1.54$ μm).
Fluence is 120 % of the threshold.
a) - initial, b) -1 pulse, c) -2 pulses, d) -3 pulses.

Scale unit corresponds to 1 mm

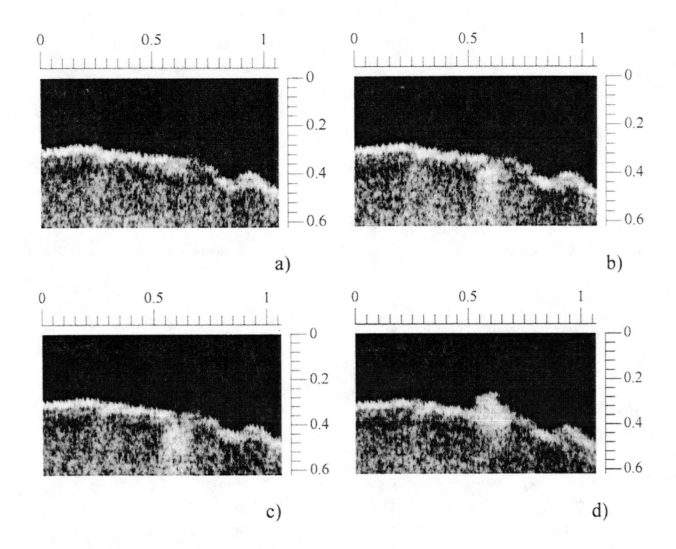

Fig. 4. Pulse-to-pulse kinetics of hump growth (Glass:Er; $\lambda = 1.54$ μm).
Fluence is 60 % of the threshold
 a)- initial, b) -1 pulse, c) -3 pulses, d) -4 pulses.

Scale unit corresponds to 1 mm

4. TIME-RESOLVED DYNAMICS OF HUMP FORMATION

In order to observe the laser modification dynamics with temporal resolution which is comparable to the pulse train duration we measured the changes in transmission through the hump of the probe radiation from the single transverse mode (TEM_{00}) stabilized CW 0.83 μm diode laser (see Fig. 5).

Probe CW laser radiation was transported perpendicular to the beam of a high-power Glass:Er laser and close to the tissue surface.

The oscillograms (see Fig. 6) show the effect of blocking of a CW beam by a cataractous lens material, which is swelled out due to interaction of high-power radiation with lens.

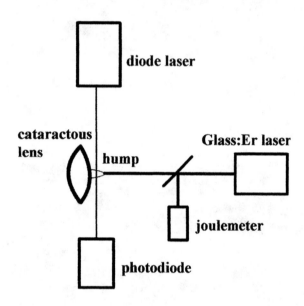

Fig. 5. The schematic of time-resolved study of hump formation.

When laser fluence is smaller than the threshold one, we observe the emergence of a "dynamic hump" which disappeared after several milliseconds. (Curves 1,2, Fig. 6) When fluence is higher than threshold, the probe radiation is blocked off according to the oscillogram 3 (Fig. 6). After irradiation the remaining hump can be visually observed. To prove that this effect does not occur as a response of the whole object to the blowing up of decomposition products, we take the probe radiation 1 mm aside from the treated zone along the lens surface. The probe radiation is not blocked in this case.

In our opinion, the temporal swelling, which we call "dynamic hump" cannot be connected only with the thermal denaturation which is practically irreversible. We suggest that mechanical stresses are essential here and attribute the irreversible hump growth phenomena to the nonelastic viscous flow driven by the pressure of water heated due to irradiation and boiling at temperatures somewhat higher than 100°C.

5. CONCLUSIONS

The possibility of *in situ* OCT monitoring of pulse-to-pulse kinetics of laser ablation of cornea is demonstrated. As radiation sources we used a YAG:Er laser ($\lambda = 2.94$ μm), and fifth harmonic of a YAP:Nd laser ($\lambda = 216$ nm). In both cases the thickness of thermally damaged layer adjacent to the ablation crater appeared to be less than or comparable to the OCT resolution limit.

The swelling of cataractous human lens irradiated by a Glass:Er laser at preablation fluences is followed by OCT technique. It permits to monitor the pulse-to-pulse kinetics. The incubation is demonstrated.

Time-resolved investigation of near threshold swelling was performed by means of cw probe laser technique. It reveals the existence of temporal swelling, which we call "dynamic hump".

The features of time-resolved dynamics of hump formation suggest that tissue swelling in this case cannot be attributed solely to pure thermal collagen denaturation. The movement of the outer part of tissue caused by pressure originated from the heating of water is also significant.

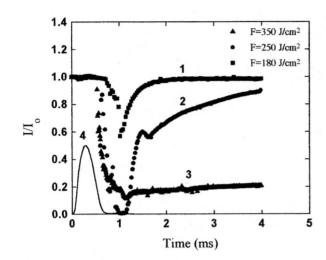

Fig. 6. Oscillograms of shielding of probe CW laser radiation by hump.
I_0 - initial intensity of aiming cw laser,
1-fluence of powerful laser radiation is 180 J/cm^2,
2-fluence is 250 J/cm^2,
3-fluence is 350 J/cm^2,
4- pulse train envelope.

6. REFERENCES

1. V.Kamensky, V.Gelikonov, G.Gelikonov, K.Pravdenko, N.Bityurin, A.Sergeev, F.Feldchtein, A.Pushkin, I.Skripatshev, M.Tshurbanov, "YAG:Er laser system for eye microsurgery with OCT monitoring", *CLEO'96 Technical Digest Series*, v.9, p. 60.

2. V.Kamensky, V.Gelikonov, G.Gelikonov, F.Feldchtein , A.Sergeev, K.Pravdenko, N.Artemiev, N.Bityurin, I.Skripachev, A.Pushkin, G.Snopatin, "In *situ* monitoring of the middle IR laser ablation of cataract-suffered human lens by optical coherent tomography". in *Lasers in Ophthalmology IV*, Reginald Birngruber; Adolf F. Fercher; Philippe Sourdille; Eds. *Proc. SPIE*, v.2930, pp. 222-229, 1996.

3. V.Kamensky, V.Gelikonov, G.Gelikonov, F.Feldchtein , A.Sergeev, K.Pravdenko, N.Artemiev, N.Bityurin, I.Skripachev, G. Snopatin, "YAG:Er laser system for microsurgery treatment of cataract-suffered human lens ", in *Laser Applications Engineering (LAE-96)*, Vadim P. Veiko; Ed. *Proc.SPIE*, v.3091, pp. 129-134, 1997.

4. V.Kamensky, F.Feldchtein, K.Pravdenko, V.Gelikonov, G.Gelikonov, A.Sergeev, and N.Bityurin, "Monitoring and animation of laser ablation process in catatacted eye lens using coherence tomography", in *Coherence Domain Optical Methods in Biomedical Science and Clinical Applications*, Valery V. Tuchin; Halina Podbielska; Ben Ovryn; Eds. *Proc. SPIE*, v.2981, pp.94-102, 1997.

5. K.P. Thompson, Q.S. Ren, J.-M. Parel, "Therapeutic and diagnostic application of lasers in ophthalmology", Proc. *IEEE*, v.80, N.6, pp. 838-859, 1992.

6. Q. Ren, R.H. Keates, R.A. Hill, M.W. Berns, "Laser refractive surgery: a review and current status", *Optical Engineering*, v.34, N.3, pp. 642-659, 1995.

7. M. Himmelbauer, N.Arnold, N.Bityurin, E. Arenholz, D.Baeuerle, "UV-laser -induced periodic surface structures in Polyimide", *Appl.Phys.A*, v.64, N.5, pp.451-456, 1997.

Optical properties of nasal septum cartilage.

Nodar V. Bagratashvili, Alexander P. Sviridov, Emil N. Sobol, Michael S. Kitai.

Research Center for Technological Lasers, Russian Academy of Sciences,

142092, Troitsk, Moscow Region, Pionerskaya st. 2, Russia.

ABSTRACT

Optical parameters (scattering coefficient s, absorption coefficient k and scattering anisotropy coefficient g) of hyaline cartilage were studied for the first time. Optical properties of human and pig nasal septum cartilage, and of bovine ear cartilage were examined using a spectrophotometer with an integrating sphere, and an Optical Multi-Channel Analyser. We measured total transmission T_t, total reflection R_t and on-axis transmission T_a for light propagating through cartilage sample, over the visible spectral range (14000-28000 cm^{-1}). It is shown that transmission and reflection spectra of human, pig and bovine cartilage are rather similar. It allows us to conclude that the pig cartilage can be used for *in-vivo* studies instead of human cartilage. The data obtained were treated by means of the one-dimensional diffusion approximation solution of the optical transport equation. We have found scattering coefficient s, absorption coefficient k and scattering anisotropy coefficient g by the iterative comparison of measured and calculated T_t, R_t and T_a values for human and pig cartilage. We found, in particular, that for 500 nm irradiation $s=37,6\pm3.5 cm^{-1}$, $g=0,56 \pm0.05$, $k\cong0,5\pm0.3$ cm^{-1}. The above data were used in Monte Carlo simulation for spatial intensity profile of light scattered by a cartilage sample. The computed profile was very similar to the profile measured using an Optical Multi-Channel Analyzer (OMA).

Keywords: cartilage, optical properties, Monte Carlo simulation.

1. INTRODUCTION

Optical properties of various biological tissues are data of importance for laser applications in medicine and biology. In particular, we have to know the optical properties of human nasal septum cartilage when developing or applying a technique of laser reshaping of cartilage[1]. It is known that cartilage of various types have different composition and structure[2]. However, there is a very limited information in the literature about optical properties of cartilage[3]. The aim of this paper is experimental and theoretical study of optical coefficients for human and pig nasal cartilage and also for bovine ear cartilage..

Two different theoretical approaches are usually applied to model the light propagation in biological tissues: diffusion model[4] and the Monte Carlo simulation[5]. Each approach has its own limitation, and it is not obvious that results obtained with above approaches will be in agreement with experimental data obtained for cartilage of different types.

We measured the total transmission T_t , the total reflection R_t and on-axis (collimated) transmission T_a. of cartilage samples using spectrophotometer with integrating sphere. Diffusion approximation does not allow to obtain exact expressions to calculate the optical coefficients from experimentally measured data, but we can obtain values of this coefficients by the iterative comparison of experimentally measured and computed values of T_t, R_t and T_a.

The Monte Carlo simulation is a very effective method to study the propagation of light in biological tissues[5], but it requires some preliminary information about the optical properties of a tissue and the character of light photon-material interaction. We computed spatial intensity profile of light, scattered by the cartilage upon Monte Carlo simulation, using the data of optical coefficients, obtained by the spectrophotometric measurements. The computed profile was compared with the real profile, measured using an Optical Multi-Channel Analyser (OMA). From this comparison we derived an additional information about the optical properties of cartilage.

2.MATERIALS AND METHODS

2.1.Sample preparation

A health adult human nasal cartilage, pig nasal cartilage, and bovine ear cartilage were excised in 1 x 1 cm rectangular samples of 300-900 micrometers in thickness. Samples of different thickness were prepared using a microtom. Human cartilage was removed after routine surgery on bent nasal septum of patients. Removed cartilage were immediately placed into the 0,9 % NaCl solution. All the measurements were made on the day when cartilage was extracted. We used a special system, which humidified the sample during experiment to avoid the drying of cartilage, which may disturb the measured values of transmission and reflection of cartilage .

2.2. Spectrophotometric studies

A standard integrating sphere spectrophotometer SPECORD M-40 measured the total transmission, T_t , total reflection R_t , and on-axis transmission (transmission in incident light axis direction), T_a (Fig.1) for collimated light that propagated through the sample normally to the sample

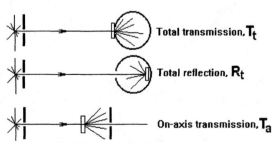

Fig.1 Scheme of optical measurements conducted on cartilage sample.

surface over the visible spectrum (14000-28000 cm^{-1}). T_a was measured with the replaced integrating sphere. We can not measure the T_a value for bovine ear cartilage sample, because it has an on-axis transmission value less then our spectrophotometer limit. The reflectivity of our spectrophotometer was calibrated with $BaSO_4$ powder (99,999%).

2.3. Optical Multi Channel Analyser

An Optical Multi-Channel Analyser (OMA) allows to obtain a spatial profile of light intensity. Our OMA represents set of 3000 light detectors of 8 micrometers in size each. Signal from every detector is processed by the computer, and we can save it and make further processing. Cartilage sample was

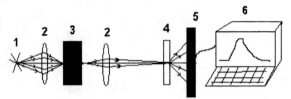

Fig.2. Scattered light spatial intensity measuring system. *1-light source, 2- lense, 3- monochromator, 4-sample, 5- Optical Multi-Channel Analyser, 6- computer.*

placed on the path of incident collimated monochromatic light beam. The signal, scattered by the cartilage was recorded by the OMA, and analyzed by the computer (Fig.2). Typical exposition time for OMA experiments was 10-100 milliseconds.

3. THEORETICAL TREATMENT

3.1. One-dimensional diffusion approximation

Diffusion approximation solution to the 1-D optical transport equation[6] usually applies as a theoretical model for light distribution in turbid media with more than 1% of scattering units. This solution was obtained in assumption, that scattering coefficient *s* is much more than absorption coefficient *k*. Diffusion approximation does not allow to obtain analytical expressions to calculate the optical coefficients from experimentally measured data, but we can obtain values of this coefficients by the iterative comparison of experimentally measured and computed T_t, R_t and T_a values.

The values of total transmission T_t, total reflection R_t and on-axis transmission T_a of flat sample, in the frameworks of one-dimensional approach to diffusion approximation are [6]:

$$T_t = (1 - R_{s1})[T_d + (1 - R_{s2})T_à]$$

$$R_t = R_{s1} + (1 - R_{s1})R_d \tag{1}$$

$$T_à = exp(-(s+k)d),$$

where R_{s1} and R_{s2} are coefficients of reflections from front and bottom sample surface, *k* is the absorption coefficient, d is the sample thickness, and T_d and R_d are diffuse transmission and reflection.

They are depends of coefficients *s, k, g* . This expressions are results of the one-dimensional diffusion approximation solution to the optical transport equation [6]:

$$a \nabla I(r,a) = -(s+k) I(r,a) + [(s+k)/4\pi] \int_{4\pi} p(a,a^*) I(r,a^*)dw^*, \tag{2}$$

where I(a,s) is total specific intensity at position r in the direction of unit vector **a** and dw* is differential solid angle in the direction **a***. The phase function p(a,a*) represents the fraction of light scattered from the direction **a** into the direction **a***. In diffusion approximation the Heney-Greenstein expression for phase function is usually applied:

$$P(\alpha)=(s/s+k)(1-g^2)/(1+g^2-2g \, cos \, (\alpha))^{-3/2} \tag{3}$$

where α is scattering angle (angle between **a** and **a***). The scattering anisotropy coefficient is defined as the average cosine of the phase function:

$$g = [(s + k) / 4\pi s] \int_{4\pi} p(cos \, (\alpha)) \, cos\alpha \, dw^*$$

We cannot obtain analytical expressions for the *s*, *k*, and *g* coefficients from the equations (1). The values of this coefficients are obtained as follows:

Firstly we measured total transmission, total reflection and on-axis transmission for some spectral range. Further processing of these data is an iterative comparison with a diffusion theory: initially we set the spatial grid of values of optical coefficients with a some step, then we calculated (in accordance with (1)) the appropriate values of total transmission T_t, total reflection R_t and on-axis transmission T_a for every unit of the grid. Values of R_{s1} and R_{s2} in (1) were accepted equal to water reflection coefficient (appr.4%). Then we find the unit of grid, whose calculated values are nearest to some real values corresponding to the point of experimental spectrum of T_t, R_t and T_a. The set of optical coefficients corresponding to the unit of grid with the minimal deviation from experimental values of T_t, R_t and T_a is considered as corresponding to this point of spectrum. Total deviation Δ is given as follows:

$$\Delta = (T_t- T_{texp})^2/ T_{texp}^2 + (R_t- R_{texp})^2/ R_{texp}^2 + (T_a- T_{aexp})^2/ T_{aexp}^2 \tag{4}$$

where T_{texp}, R_{texp}, and T_{aexp} are experimental values, and T_t, R_t, and T_a. are calculated values. Value of deviation may be reduced by reducing the grid step. We kept calculations to reach a deviation $\Delta < 1$.

3.2.Monte Carlo Simulation

We applied a standard method to calculate a propagation of photon in scattering media [5]. We consider
the path of photon consisting of steps of
varying length between interaction
(scattering) events (Fig.3). The length of
each path step is calculated from random
number RND as:

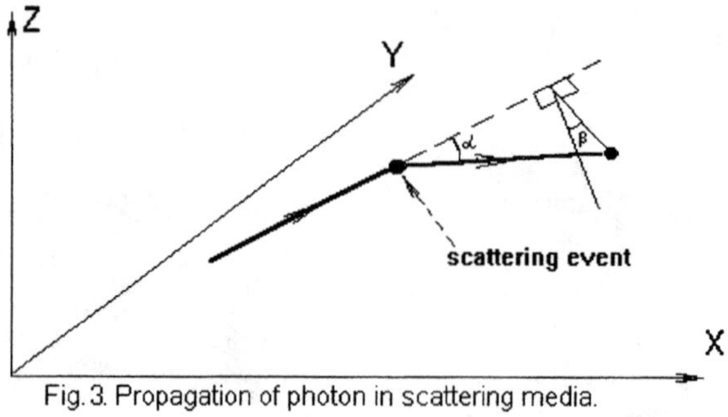

Fig. 3. Propagation of photon in scattering media.

$$L = -ln(RND)/s$$

where s is scattering coefficient, RND is the
random number between 0 and 1. Then we defined if photon had been absorbed in this step. If:

$$exp(-kL) > RND$$

$(k$ is absorption coefficient), than we assumed that photon was absorbed. If it was not, than we defined
angle α (Fig. 3) between old and new trajectories by Heney-Greenstein expression [6]:

$$\alpha = arccos[(1+g^2) - (1-g^2)^2/(1-g+2g\ RND)^2]/2g$$

Azimuthal angle β (Fig.3) is

$$\beta = 2\pi RND$$

Now we have all the values to
define the position of photon in
three-dimensional space. The
coordinates of n-th interaction
event are (Fig.4):

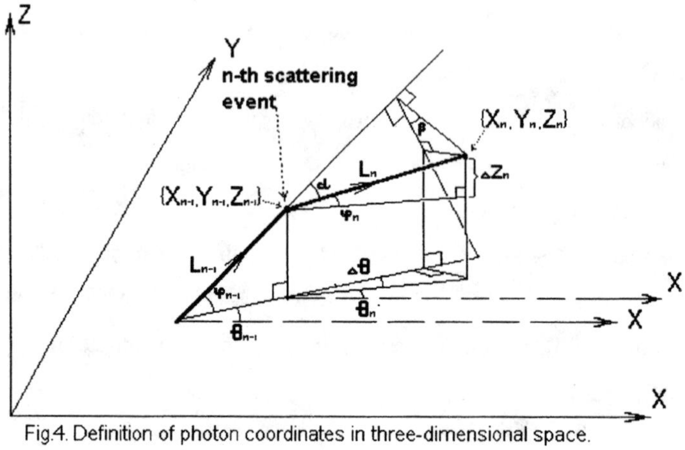

Fig.4. Definition of photon coordinates in three-dimensional space.

$$X_n = X_{n-1} + L\ cos(\varphi_n)sin(\theta_n)$$

$$Y_n = Y_{n-1} + L\ cos(\varphi_n)cos(\theta_n)$$

$$Z_n = Z_{n-1} + \Delta Z_n,$$

where X_{n-1}, Y_{n-1} and Z_{n-1} are coordinates of previous interaction event, ΔZ_n is change of Z coordinate
between n-1 and n interaction events, φ_n- angle between trajectory from n-1 to n interaction event and

XY plate, θ_n- angle between projection of this trajectory and X axis (azimuthal angle). ΔZ_n , φ_n and θ_n are defined by the iterative process:

$$\Delta Z_n = L[cos(\alpha)sin(\varphi_0)-sin(\alpha)cos(\beta)cos(\varphi_{n-1})],$$

where φ_{n-1} is the previous value of φ angle.

$$sin(\varphi_n)=\Delta Z_n/ L$$

$$cos(\theta_n)=sin(\theta_{n-1})cos(\Delta\theta) - cos(\theta_{n-1})sin(\Delta\theta),$$

where θ_{n-1} is the previous value of θ angle,

$$sin(\Delta\theta)=sin(\alpha)sin(\beta) / cos(\varphi_{n-1}),$$

Initial values of φ and θ are set proceeding from the initial spatial profile of real light source, whose interaction with media is needed for modeling., For point source, for example,

$$\varphi_0=\pi / 2,$$
$$\theta_0= 0$$

Anyway, the axis of symmetry of light beam is parallel to Z axis.

Thus, we can define the position of photon after n scattering events. When Z coordinate becomes more then sample thickness, we consider that photon left the sample. Thus, we can define the position of photon at any distance from the sample surface proceeding from values of X, Y, φ and θ at the moment of exit. We have developed the original computer program to calculate these data.

4. RESULTS AND DISCUSSION

The typical spectra of total transmission T_t, total reflection R_t for human and pig nasal cartilage samples of the same thickness and, also, bovine ear cartilage sample are shown at Figs.5 and 6. Spectra of on-axis transmission T_a for human and pig nasal cartilage samples are shown in Fig.7.

The calculated spectra of scattering coefficient s, absorption coefficient k, and scattering anisotropy coefficient g values for human and pig nasal cartilage are shown in Fig. 8-10. Every point of each curve is an average value over 10 samples of various thickness. The calculated values for s, k, and g of human nasal cartilage are also summarized in Table 1. Note, that the spectra of T_t, R_t and T_a , and also, the spectra of s, k and g are rather similar for all the samples of human and pig cartilage. This allows to use a pig nasal cartilage in preliminary *in-vivo* experiments instead of human cartilage. Also a

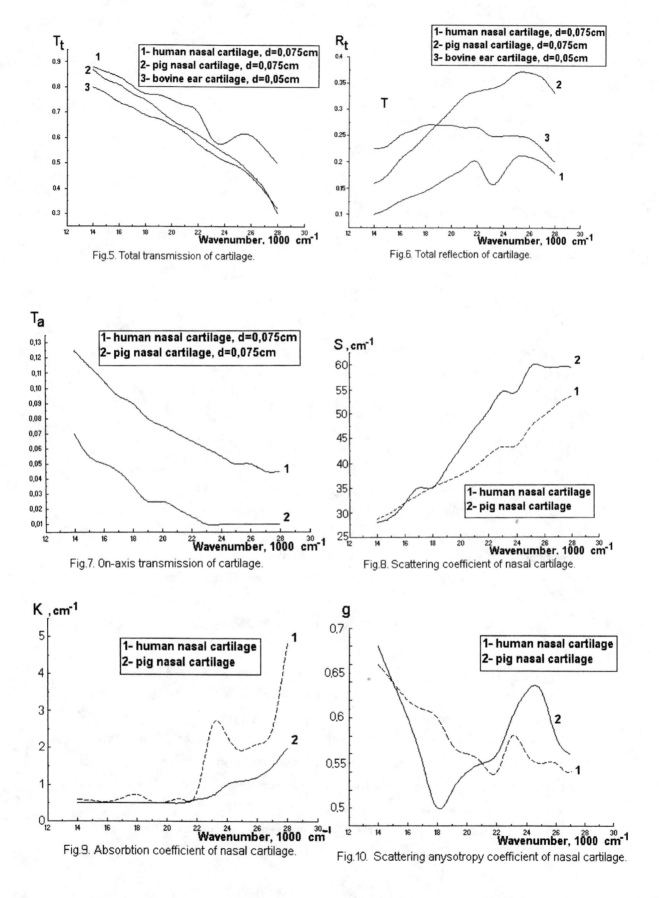

Fig.5. Total transmission of cartilage.

Fig.6. Total reflection of cartilage.

Fig.7. On-axis transmission of cartilage.

Fig.8. Scattering coefficient of nasal cartilage.

Fig.9. Absorbtion coefficient of nasal cartilage.

Fig.10. Scattering anysotropy coefficient of nasal cartilage.

pig cartilage can be selected as a representative material for measuring the dynamics of optical properties under laser treatment.

Table 1. Summary of calculated optical parameters for human nasal cartilage. Scattering coefficient **S**, absorbtion coefficient **K**, scattering anysotropy coefficient **g**.

wavenumber, cm⁻¹	S, cm⁻¹	K, cm⁻¹	g
14000	28,6±0.44	0,6 ±0,46	0,66 ±0,04
15000	30 ±0,66	0,56±0,48	0,64 ±0,05
16000	31,9±1,6	0,53±0,44	0,62 ±0,05
17000	33,6±1,6	0,63±0,44	0,61 ±0,05
18000	35,1±2,6	0,73±0,44	0,6 ±0,05
19000	36,3±2,44	0,53±0,37	0,57 ±0,05
20000	37,6±3.5	0,53±0,31	0,56 ±0,05
21000	39,3±4,4	0,6 ±0,2	0,55 ±0,04
22000	41,6±5,5	0,83±0,44	0,54 ±0,03
23000	43,3±6,4	2,6 ±0,13	0,58 ±0,03
24000	43,6±9,5	2,33±0,08	0,56 ±0,03
25000	47,3±9,7	1,93±0,31	0,55 ±0,03
26000	49,6±11,5	2,1 ±0,53	0,55 ±0,03
27000	52 ±16	2,53±0,31	0,54 ±0,03
28000	53,6±16	4,86±1,15	0,56 ±0,04

It should be noted that total accuracy of our calculations is rather low. Cartilage has a complicated internal structure[2], and the one-dimensional diffusion approximation can be considered as just a first, rather rough approximation. One of the disadvantages of this method is a low accuracy for absorption coefficient k. Any changes in k value in the range from 0.2 to 2.0 1/cm did not affect materially the computed spectra. The scattering coefficient s can be obtained much more precisely (when the relation $s \gg k$ is valid) from the following formula:

$$T_å = \exp\left(-(s+k)\, d\right).$$

We cannot also estimate an accuracy for calculations of the scattering anisotropy coefficient g. The g values obtained for cartilage are slightly lower than that for skin and for other soft biological tissues ($g \approx 0,74$ for skin[4], $g \approx 0,91$ for artery tissue[5], $g \approx 0,6$ for nasal cartilage at 500 nm wavelength)

Our calculations (for varied g value) shows that small change in g results in the significant changes of the computed transmission intensity profile. It allows us to assume that the accuracy of g value calculations is adequate to the accuracy of our experimental measurements.

The optical properties obtained from above experiments and calculations were used for the Monte Carlo calculations of a spatial profile of light intensity, scattered by a human cartilage

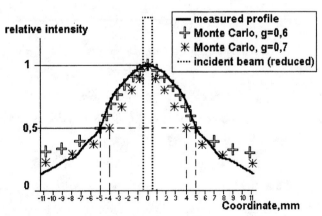

Fig.11. Spatial intensity profile of light, scattered by the carilage sample. Comparsion of measured and computed upon Monte Carlo simulation profiles. Sample thickness d=0.035cm.

sample of 350 micrometers in thickness. This calculations (for $s=37\,\text{cm}^{-1}$, $k=0.5\,\text{cm}^{-1}$, $g=0.6$) were compared with the results of our OMA measurements for 20000 cm⁻¹ irradiation (Fig.11). The incident light beam had a rectangular spatial profile with 5^0 divergence angle. The computed profile was obtained for 100,000 generated photons. The ratio of half-height widths of incident beam to that for the profile of the scattered light intensity, is about 10, for both computed and experimentally measured profiles.

Fig.11 also presents the spatial intensity profile computed for the other value of scattering anisotropy coefficient g =0.7. In this case a deviation on calculated and measured profile widths is significant (more then 20%). This means that the g value obtained from the diffusion approximation is quite reliable.

5. CONCLUSIONS

Optical properties of hyaline cartilage involving scattering coefficient s, absorption coefficient k and scattering anisotropy coefficient g were studied for the first time. The characters of transmission and reflection spectra behaviour for human and pig nasal septum cartilage are rather similar. This allows to use a pig nasal cartilage as a good model of human cartilage in the most of optical *in-vivo* experiments.

The combination of two theoretical approaches (diffusion approximation and Monte Carlo simulation) allows us to obtain for cartilage the quite reliable values of scattering and scattering anisotropy coefficients, when the absorption coefficient is small and do not affect significantly the light propagation through a tissue.

6.ACKNOWLEDGEMENTS

We would like to thank Prof. V.N.Bagratashvili and Dr.A.I.Omel'chenko for their support and stimulating discussions and, also, Russian foundation for Basic Research (Grant 97-02-17465).

7. REFERENCES

1. Sobol E.N., Bagratashvili V.N., Sviridov A.P., Omelchenko A.I. *"Cartilage Shaping Under Laser Irradiation."*, *Proc SPIE ,Vol.2128, pp.43-49, 1994.*

2. D.Comper. "Physicochemical aspects of cartilage extracellular matrix» in: «Cartilage: Molecular Aspects», *eds.B.Hall, S.Newman, CRC Press, Boca Raton, 1991.*

3. Juergen Raunest, Hans-Joachim Schwarzmaier "Optical Properties of Human Articular Cartilage as Implication for a Selective Laser Application in Arthroscopic Surgery.", *Lasers in Surgery and Medicine vol.16, pp.253-261, 1995.*

4. Steven L. Jacques, Scott A. Prahl "Modeling Optical and Thermal Distributions in Tissue During Laser Irradiation", *Lasers in Surgery and Medicine vol.6, pp.494-503, 1987.*

5. Marleen Keijzer, Steven L. Jacques, Scott A. Prahl, Ashley J. Welch "Light Distributions in Artery Tissue: Monte Carlo Simulations for Finite-Diameter Laser Beam", *Lasers in Surgery and Medicine vol.9, pp.148-154, 1989.*

6. Ishimaru A. "Wave Propagation and Scattering in Random Media", *New York, Academic Press, 1978.*

Investigation of the efficiency of laser action on hemoglobin and oxyhemoglobin in the skin blood vessels.

Mustafo M. Asimov, Rustam M. Asimov, Anatoly N. Rubinov.

Institute of Physics Academy of Sciences of Belarus. Skarina Pr.70,
Minsk. 220072. Belarus.

ABSTRACT

The efficiency of light absorption by oxyhemoglobin and deoxyhemoglobin in cutaneous blood vessels in dependence of the radiation wavelength and optical properties of the tissue is investigated. The main goal is to develop the practical application of long pulse flashlamp-pumped dye lasers in the treatment of different cutaneous lesions, based on the selective photothermolysis. The spectra of laser action both on oxyhemoglobin and deoxyhemoglobin of blood vessels at different depths of the tissue layer were calculated using the Kubelka-Munk optical model of the tissue. The obtained results allow to choose the proper wavelength of laser radiation for the selective and efficient influence on the blood chromophores. It is shown that for blood vessels located in tissue up to the depth of 2500 μ the action spectra of laser radiation follow the shape of the Q - absorption bands of oxyhemoglobin and deoxyhemoglobin. At deeper layers the action spectra become very narrow ($\Delta\lambda \sim$ 25-30 nm) and shift to the long wavelength with maximum at 585 nm and 570 nm for oxyhemoglobin and deoxyhemoglobin, accordingly. The action spectra in the near infrared region remain very broad and cover the range from 600 nm to 1200 nm. It is shown that these bands play the dominant role in the absorption of laser radiation in deeper layers of tissue.

Key Words: flashlamp - pumped dye laser, tissue, melanin, oxyhemoglobin, deoxyhemoglobin, action spectrum, photo-dissosiation, biostimulation

INTRODUCTION

In the last years medicine and biology has attract increasing attention the specialists in laser physics, laser spectroscopy and photochemistry. The formation of the new branch of science "Lasers in the Life Sciences" took place. The significant place in this field belongs to the medical application of lasers. It should be noted that the successes in application of lasers practically in all areas of modern medicine are caused by two factors: pioneering investigations by enthusiasts, which started practically from the time of discovery of laser, and by modern development of laser technique. One of the significant achievements in recent time is the application of the flashlamp-pumped dye lasers in dermatology for the treatment of cutaneous vascular lesions.[1-6] This achievement is based on theoretical conception of selective photothermolysis,[7] which consider two basic optical and thermal properties of pigmented tissue targets. It is required that the time of heat generation by chromophores due to selective absorption of high power laser radiation will be shorter then the thermal relaxation time of the target. In this case the major part of absorbed energy is concentrated within the target structure and undesirable thermal damage of surrounding tissue is minimized.[8-10] Thus, the flashlamp-pumped dye laser with pulse duration up to 450 μsec was developed and applied for the treatment of a variety of cutaneous vascular lesions. In particular, the significant success has been achieved in the treatment of Port-Wine-Stains.[4-6] In the clinical practice, the radiation at wavelength of 577 nm was primarily used, as it correlates with the one of the maximum of oxyhemoglobin absorption. Recently, it was demonstrated that the radiation at 585 nm is also very effective because of its deep penetration into tissue. It should be noted that most of the efforts to-day are concentrated on the developing high power laser systems to reach maximal absorption by oxyhemoglobin at λ = 577 nm and λ = 585 nm.

Future author information -
M.M.A. (correspondence): Email: mustafo@asimov.belpak.minsk.by; Telephone: 375(0172) 683-549; Fax: 375(0172) 393-131
R.M.A.: Email: roustam@asimov.belpak.minsk.by; Telephone: 375(0172) 683-549.
A.N.R.: Email: rubinov@ifanbel.bas-net.by; Telephone: 375(0172) 684-646.

Unfortunately, the absorption by deoxyhemoglobin, which is contained in significant amounts in venous blood, so far is practically ignored and needs investigation.[11] To consider the treatment of vascular lesions, located in deeper layers of dermas, it is important to investigate the efficiency of laser absorption at IR bands by both oxyhemoglobin and deoxyhemoglobin.

There is one more interesting aspect of laser-tissue interaction by means of low energy laser radiation as well as light effect on oxyhemoglobin of human skin blood vessels. It is connected with the photodissociation of oxyhemoglobin, which leads to local increase of the oxygen concentration. These phenomena probably may be considered as a possible primary mechanism of biostimulation effect of low energy laser radiation.

In this report the result of investigation of the laser interaction efficiency on oxyhemoglobin and deoxyhemoglobin of the skin blood vessels both in two aspects on selective photothermolysis and biostimulation effect are presented. The action spectra of laser radiation on oxyhemoglobin and deoxyhemoglobin of cutaneous blood vessels in dependence of wavelength and the depth of penetration on tissue are investigated. The future development of the practical application of long pulse flashlamp-pumped dye lasers in the treatment of vascular cutaneous lesions is discussed.

2. BASIC CONCEPTIONS

As is well known, the skin has complex structure with three basic layers: epidermis, derma and hypodermic fatty tissue. The thickens of skin without hypodermic fatty tissue layer can reach 4 mm. Architecture of tissue and wavelength of laser radiation determine the peculiarities of laser light interaction with tissue. At first, there is a partial reflection of light from the surface layer of epidermis. Deeper epidermis layer contains melanin pigment, which is one of the basic chromophores intensively absorbing light in a wide spectral range. Derma contains collagen, which causes strong scattering of light. Tissue has a rich net of cutaneous blood vessels containing oxyhemoglobin and deoxyhemoglobin chromophores with strong absorption bands in the visible region. It should be noted that cutaneous blood vessels are located basically in two layers: in a superficial layer close to epidermis and the deeper one on the border with hypodermic fatty tissue. These basic components of tissue determine the depth of penetration of incident light into skin in dependence on the light wavelength. Thus, the laser radiation incident on the skin is partially reflected by epidermis, partially scattered by collagen of derma, and partially absorbed by pigments of melanin, oxyhemoglobin and deoxyhemoglobin.

The typical absorption[12] spectra of Q - band and in IR-band of oxyhemoglobin and hemoglobin are presented in Fig. 1. The absorption of light by oxyhemoglobin and hemoglobin of cutaneous blood vessels allows to consider and discuss the following photophysical and photochemical processes.

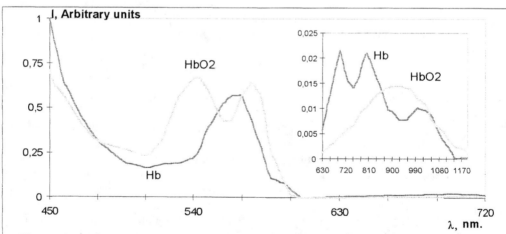

Fig. 1. Absorption Spectra of Q - band and in IR spectral range of oxyhemoglobin (HbO2) and hemoglobin (Hb) of cutaneous blood vessels .

The photophysical processes are connected with nonradiative dissipation of the electronic excitation energy by oxyhemoglobin and deoxyhemoglobin. The heat generated in this process is transferred to the blood capillaries, which has the characteristic time of thermal relaxation of 0,05-1,2 msec.[7] The mechanism of the laser light influence on the a human body is very much dependent on the output laser energy. The effect of high energy lasers is quite clear, it is based on the photothermal processes such as selective photothermolysis.

Contrary to that the mechanism of biostimulation by low energy laser radiation is still not established[15] in spite of the numerous publications in this field. As a result the correct interpretation of experimental data received in clinical practice remains to be difficult. The absence of quantitative interrelation between parameters of laser radiation and object of interaction complicates search for the optimal methods of treatment. From the first experiments till the present time the question of existence of the fundamental differences in the biological effect on human organism of low energy laser radiation and of conventional light is widely discussed.

It is clear that the effect of heating via absorption of low intensity laser radiation in a tissue is not very important. Estimate shows that in typical case the local increase of temperature only by $0,1 - 0,5$ ^{0}C may be expected[13]. Such a small raise of a local temperature may promote only some improvement in capillary microcirculation of blood and by this perhaps somewhat stimulate the metabolism processes. We suppose that in a case of low intensity lasers the most important process is the photodissociation of oxyhemoglobin, whose main biological function is the transport of molecular oxygen. The molecular oxygen is generated due to the light absorption by oxyhemoglobin in blood vessels which allows to control the local increase of oxygen concentration at irradiated region. Quantum yield of this process in a spectral range of 300 - 600 nm is close to 0,1 while it seems to drop by factor of 50 at the wavelength of excitation $\lambda \geq 1060$ nm[14].

It is worth to note that the above reasoning may be equally related to oxymioglobin, the function of which is to accept molecular oxygen from oxyhemoglobin. The spectral properties of oxyhemoglobin and oxymioglobin are similar as they are defined by identical structure of hem.

It follows from the above considerations that efficiency of therapeutic effect of low intensity lasers must be directly dependent on the efficiency of laser radiation absorption by oxyhemoglobin. From this point of view it is important to know a real spectra of action on oxyhemoglobin and deoxyhemoglobin of cutaneous blood vessels, taking into account both their absorption spectra and the change of spectrum of incident light at penetration of beam into the skin.

We have calculated the action spectra of laser radiation on oxyhemoglobin and deoxyhemoglobin in dependence on the location depth of cutaneous blood vessels in tissue. Calculations were carried out by the method of computer modeling using in Cubelka - Munk model[12] of tissue was used to describe its optical properties.

3. RESULTS AND DISCUSSIONS

The calculated action spectra of laser radiation on oxyhemoglobin and deoxyhemoglobin are presented in Fig. 2 and 3. These spectra are normalized to the maximum of correlated absorption bands in order to demonstrate their transformation at penetration of radiation into tissue.

As it is seen from Fig. 2 the action spectra of laser radiation on oxyhemoglobin and deoxyhemoglobin in deeper layers of tissue shift to the long wavelength with maximum at $\lambda= 585$ nm and $\lambda= 570$ nm, accordingly, and become very narrow ($\Delta\lambda\sim25$-30 nm). These results are consistent with experimental data on low efficiency of argon laser radiation at wavelengths 488 and 514 nm and predict the high efficiency of application of Rhodamine 6G dye laser.

The action spectra of laser radiation in near and IR range have rather broad bands and cover spectral region from 600 nm up to 1200 nm. The obtained results show that these bands must play a dominant role in absorption of laser radiation by oxyhemoglobin and deoxyhemoglobin in deep layers of tissue.

Thus, there are two preferable wavelengths in the Infrared for irradiation of deoxyhemoglobin ($\lambda \sim 800$ nm and $\lambda \sim 1000$ nm) and one at $\lambda \sim 960$ nm for oxyhemoglobin. The efficiency of laser radiation absorption by oxyhemoglobin at widely used in clinical practice wavelength 585 nm as compared to the absorption at $\lambda = 960$ nm at different depths of tissue is shown in Fig. 4.

As it seen the efficiency of absorption at $\lambda = 585$ nm remains higher than at $\lambda = 960$ nm up to 2 mm of the tissue depth and at the depth of about 2,5 mm they become equal. In the deeper layers of tissue IR band of oxyhemoglobin play the dominant role in the absorption of laser radiation. So the wavelength 585 nm may be recommended as the most efficient one for the treatment of vascular lesion located at the depth of tissue down to 2.5 mm while for the deeper layers of tissue the most suitable wavelength is 960 nm.

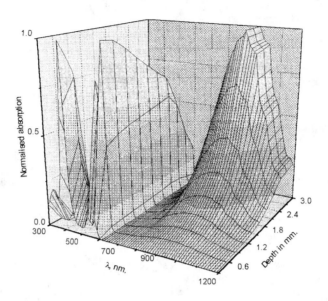

Fig. 2. Action spectrum of laser radiation normalized to the maximum of oxyhemoglobin bands in dependence of the penetration depth into tissue.

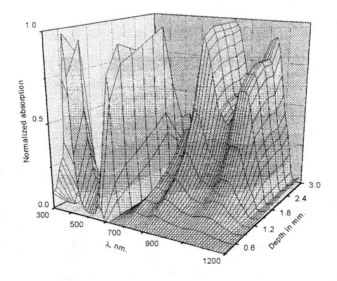

Fig. 3. Normalized spectrum of laser action on deoxyhemoglobin in dependence on the penetration depth into tissue.

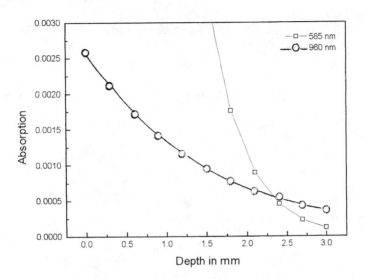

Fig. 4. The efficiency of laser radiation absorption by oxyhemoglobin at maximum of Q-band (585 nm) and of IR band (960 nm) in dependence on the tissue depth.

In practice different semi-conductor lasers (820 nm, 870 nm, 880 nm, 904 nm) are widely used for wound healing and treatment of various diseases. As is seen from the Fig. 2, all these wavelength are well correlated with the IR band of oxyhemoglobin action spectrum. As to the He-Ne laser the role of oxyhemoglobin photodissociation under irradiation at 632, 8 nm demands additional investigation because of absence of exact data on a quantum yield of oxyhemoglobin photo-dissociation in this spectral range. He-Ne laser was evidently chosen because of its simplicity, reliability and low cost. At the same time it must be stressed once again that the wavelength 585 nm is expected to be the most effective in the action on the blood. It should be noted in this respect that the improvement of efficiency and photostability of flashlamp pumped dye lasers, producing radiation at 585 nm, still remains to be an important practical problem to solve. We hope that application of new watersoluble laser dyes on the basis of inclusion complexes of organic molecules with cyclodextrins [16] may significantly improve the above mentioned parameters.

4. CONCLUSION

The obtained results demonstrate the necessity of binding of parameters of the laser to effect on cutaneous blood vessels in consideration of laser therapeutic effect. High spectral selectivity of laser action on oxyhemoglobin and deoxyhemoglo-bin of cutaneous blood vessels is determined mainly by absorption of melanin in epidermis. Thus, the efficiency of laser-tissue interaction is depended on the degree of skin pigmentation.

Some important conclusions may be drawn from the analysis of the spectra of laser action on oxyhemoglobin. For the first, one may expect the increase of therapeutic effect under irradiation directly at the maximum ($\lambda = 585$ nm) of oxyhe-moglobin action spectrum. For the second, considerable therapeutic effect is expected under laser irradiation directly at maximum of oxyhemoglobin and deoxyhemoglobin action spectra in IR spectral region.

More definite conclusion on the role of oxyhemoglobin photodissociation in mechanism of biostimulation could be drawn only after comparative experimental investigations of the effect of low intensity laser radiation at various wave-lengths.

REFERENCES

1. E. Gonzalez, R.W. Gange, Kh. T. Momtaz. «Treatment of telagiectases and other benign vascular lesions with the 577 nm pulsed dye laser», J. Am. Acad. Dermatol. **27**, pp. 220 - 226, 1992.

2. T.A. Abd-el-Raheem, U. Hohenleuter, M. Landthaler. «Granuloma pyogenicum as a complication of flashlamp - pumped dye laser», Dermatol. **189**, pp. 283 - 285, 1994.

3. T.S. Alster, A.K. Kurban, G.L. Grove at all. «Alteration of argon laser-induced scars by the pulsed dye laser», Lasers Surg. Med. **13**, pp. 368 - 373, 1993.

4. T.S. Alster, F. Wilson. Ann. «Treatment of Port-Wine-Stain with the flashlamp - pumped pulsed dye laser: extended clinical experience in children and adults», Plast. Surg. **32**, pp. 478 - 484, 1994.

5. R. Ashinoff, R.G. Geronemus. «Flashlamp - pumped dye laser for Port-Wine-stains in infancy: Early versus later treatment», J. Am. Acad. Dermatol. **24**, pp. 467 - 472, 1990.

6. C. Raulin, S. Helwig. «Efficiency and limitations of the pulsed dye laser», H + G. **71**, pp. 96 - 102, 1996.

7. R.R. Anderson, J.A. Perrish. «Selective photothermolysis: Precise microsurgery by selective absorption of pulsed radiation», Science. **220**, pp. 524 - 527, 1985.

8. E. Glasberg, GP, Lask, EML. Tan, J. Uitto. «Cellular effects of the pulsed tunable dy laser at 577 nm on human endothelial cells, fibroplasts and erythrocytes. An in vivo study». Lasers Surg. Med. **8**, pp. 567 - 572, 1988.

9. E. Glasberg, GP, Lask, EML. Tan, J. Uitto. «The flashlamp pumped 577 nm tunable dye laser: Clinical efficacy and in vitro studies». J. Dermatol Surg Oncol **14**, pp. 1200 - 1208, 1988.

10. LM. Garden, LL. PolLa, OT. Tan. «The treatment of portwine stains by the pulsed dye laser: Analysis of pulse duration and long-term therapy». Arch Dermatol **124**, pp. 889 - 896, 1988.

11. J.L. Ratz. «Laser physics». Clinics Dermatol **13**, pp. 11 - 20, 1995.

12. R.R. Anderson, J.A. Parrish. «The optics of human skin», J. Invest. Dermatol. **77**, pp. 13 - 19, 1981.

13. J.R. Basford. «Low - energy laser therapy: Controversies and new research findings», Lasers Surg. Med. **9**, pp.1 - 5, 1989.

14. B.M. Jagarov, V.S. Chirvoniy, G.P. Gurinovich. «Electronic excited states and photodissosiation of oxyhemoglobin», Laser picosecond spectroscopy and photochemistry of biomolecules. P.203 -212, M. "Nauka". 1987.

15. R. Babapour, E. Glassberg, G. P. Lask. «Low - Energy Laser Systems», Clinics in Dermatol. **13,** pp. 87 - 90, 1995.

16. M.M. Asimov, V.P. Chuev, S.N. Kovalenko, V.M. Nikitchenko, A.N. Rubinov. «Effect of cyclodextrins and water-soluble polymers on spectral and laser properties of rodamine 6G» Optica and Spektr. (Russ.) **70**, pp. 544 - 546, 1991.

Part B

SOFT-TISSUE MODELING

SESSION 14

Soft-Tissue Modeling

Dynamic Simulation of the Mastication Muscles

T. Weingärtner[a] and J. Albrecht[b]

[a]Institute for Real-Time Computer Control Systems & Robotics, University of Karlsruhe
76128 Karlsruhe, Germany, weinga@ira.uka.de
[b]Surgical Robotics Lab, Maxillofacial Surgery (MKG), Virchow-Hospital
13353 Berlin, Germany, jochen@ukrv.de

ABSTRACT

The purpose of a simulated operation system in craniofacial surgery is to evaluate and visualize the results of operations on the overall facial shape of the patient and on the functionality of his jaw. This paper presents the analyzation of muscle movements in the mastication system by applying real jaw movements to the simulation. With this method an accurate modeling of the mastication muscles can be performed which is a prerequisite for a realistic simulation and precise intra-operative registration. According to this results a large-scale musculoskeletal model of the mastication system is generated including kinematic and dynamic parameters.

By integrating distance sensors in the simulation of a segmented CT (computer tomograph) image of the maxilla and mandible the motions of the masticatory muscles during different kinds of jaw movements have been analyzed. The data for this motions have been recorded by a commercial system (CONDYLOCOMP LR3) on a test person and transformed to the graphical simulation system. This method for the first time allows to observe the dynamics of the mastication muscles and their different parameters like muscle length ratio and velocity. The integration of a kinematic model for the jaw movement makes it possible to analyze non traced movements.

Keywords: - Mastication simulation, craniofacial surgery, deformable models, muscle analyzation, tracking human movements

1. INTRODUCTION

Today, computer based simulation in craniofacial surgery is performed statically. This means incisions in the jaw are simulated and the static pieces are repositioned. Some systems like[1] include the simulation of soft tissue displacements but in these cases only the static changes are calculated. There exists no dynamic simulation of the jaw movement including soft tissue. Our system is an approach towards such a dynamic mastication simulation.

The clinical relevance is given, since the anatomical conditions in the region of the head are very complex and the surgeon has to consider all of them during the planning of the operation. Up to now the planning of an operation in cases of reconstructive surgery or corrections of malformations in the area of the mandible and the mid-face was done with the help of two-dimensional teleradiography and an orthopantomogramm. The adjustment of the occlusional contacts between the rows of teeth was performed with the help of plaster models. These models are fitted into so-called articulators for the mechanical simulation of the movement of the mandible. However, this method only replicates the pathway. The functional dynamics of the muscular system are not taken into account at all. Also, planning the operation by shifting these plaster models is only a static process. Modeling the dynamics of the movement of the mandible in the articulator is severely limited.

Our research approach includes a three-dimensional collection of image data using computerized tomography, magnet resonance tomography and surface scan-methods as opposed to the two-dimensional based analysis used up to now. Afterwards the muscles and bone structures are segmented. These three-dimensional diagnostics allow a detailed analysis of the asymmetry and the deviation from the normal values. The kinematic model which has been described in[2,3] is adapted to the data set and defines the constraints for the movement of the mandible. This model rebuilds the complex sliding and gliding movements of the lower jaw by several axes. Using the developed inverse kinematic model, the position and orientation of the mandible for a given point can be calculated and allows the simulation of mastication movements by a given path of one point on the mandible.

SPIE Vol. 3254 • 0277-786X/98/$10.00

The simulation of the mouth aperture and muscle function shows a dynamic masticatory-functional view of the surgical procedure as opposed to the static three-dimensional planning. This should enable us to further optimize the surgical procedures as described above and to improve the stability of the operational result. It also appears to be possible to reduce the period of intermaxillary fixation of several weeks customary till now or even to avoid it altogether. (This period of time is quite stressful for the patient since he can not open his mouth.)

The software developments should contribute to the individual patient-specific planning. The planning will also be used within the scope of surgeries in order to realize the planning precisely with the help of methods of the computer-aided surgery (navigation of instruments, robotics). These techniques can also be used for the training of surgeons in simulators.

This paper deals with the application of tracked, real jaw movements to the simulation and the analyzation of the muscle movements performed during the mastication. The goal of our research is to get a deeper knowledge of the jaw muscles and their movements during the mastication process. Section 2 describes the state of the art in jaw simulation and tracking human movements. In section 3 the data acquisition process is described starting with a short description of the registration device and the conversion into transformation commands for the simulation. An overview of the simulation system is given in section 4. Here, also the methods for simulating the mastication muscles are shown. Section 5 demonstrates the results of the analyzation and a conclusion is given in section 6.

2. STATE OF THE ART

Due to its importance, the temporomandibular joint (TMJ) has been an area of active research in dentistry for many years. The main reason for this is the strong influence of this joint on the occlusion.[4] An optimal occlusion is the goal of any dental therapy. Dysfunctions in the area of the TMJ entail a disorder of the occlusion like the supernatural wear or loosening of the teeth and severe pain disorders. The state of the art for our system can be divided into three parts: medical analysis of the jaw movement, computer simulations of the jaw movement and tracking human movements.

2.1. Medical analysis of the jaw movement

To get a better view on the occlusion, physicians use articulators. In these mechanical devices plaster-casts of the teeth are fixed. By adjusting the hinge axis position, the inclination of the trajectory of the condylus, and the Bennett angle the individual geometric parameters of the patient are identified. Articulators are used to show a view of the occlusion and the initial opening and closing movement. But these devices have significant disadvantages: they do not allow a simulation of a whole chewing cycle, the muscular functions can not be integrated in any way and as these are mechanical devices, they have to be operated by hand.

2.2. Computer simulations of the jaw movement

There exist some computer animations of the mandible movement, like for computer-aided production of ceramic dental restorations and diagnosis for occlusal therapy as the Intelligent Dental Care System (IDCS).[5] This system provides a playback of the recorded jaw movement and can be used as a "software articulator". Since those systems do not build a kinematic model of the jaw movement which can be changed, there exists no simulation of jaw replacements. They can only give a better view on measured data.

A research group at the Waseda University in Japan has been working for several years on a chewing robot.[6-8] The third version of this robot (WJ-3) consists of a skull model which is moved by motors and wires. Its kinematics is fixed and given through the mechanical assembly and the muscle functions are modeled by artificial muscle actuators (AMA). This is the first and only simulation known to the authors, which enables a reproduction of a whole three-dimensional chewing cycle including muscular functions. Due to the fact that an adaption to the patients individual parameters is not possible, a robot like this can only be used for research in the field of the TMJ and the mastication muscles. In addition, it is not possible to track trajectories of the patients mandible and repeat them with such a device.

A graphical simulation of the mandible movements including the muscle functions is not known to the authors. The tool presented in this paper is useful in simulation, analysis, and planning of operations. It is especially valuable since it enables a simple adaption to the patients parameters and the possibility of reproducing mastication movements of the patient. The simulation enables a better view to the pre-operative situation, facilitates precise pre-operative planning, and makes predictions of post-operative results more reliable.

2.3. Tracking human movements

The tracking of human movements has many practical applications and is done in medicine, biomechanics and robotics. There are different devices which allow the recoding of momentary positions of body parts. Four different techniques can be distinguished: magnetic devices, acoustic devices, optical devices, and mechanical devices. All of them have their limitations. Magnetic devices like the Polhemus system[9] allow the recording of positions and orientations in a large working area but their susceptibility to electro-magnetic distortions like from computer monitors or ferro magnetic objects is very large.[10] Their resolution is not very high. Devices based on ultrasound have a higher resolution but can be disturbed by other acoustical waves. Optical devices are very robust and have a high resolution but tracked objects have to be visible during the whole process. Mechanical devices can not be used for recording the jaw movements, since their weight and mechanics affect the trackes.

There exist some special devices for the motion recording of the mandible, since dentists need this information for the diagnostics. In this project the CONDYLOCOMP LR3 from Dentron[11] was used, which records the 3D movement of the lower jaw in the area of the condyls with 10 IR-diodes. The accuracy of this device is $\pm 0.3mm$ and $0.3°$.[12] Dentists use this device to diagnose of different diseases of the temporomandibular joint, but they only use the 2D representations of the motion in different directions which are supported by the software. For the simulation of mandible and mastication muscle movements a 3D representation is needed. Therefore a special reconstruction which is not included in the analyzation software had to be implemented and integrated.

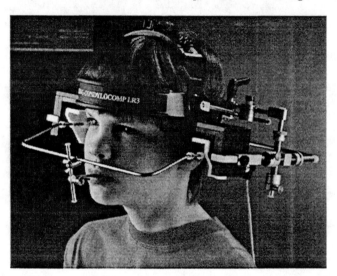

Figure 1. The registration apparatus can be mounted on the patient within minutes. Thereby the maxilla remains untouched. The lower measuring bow is extremely light-weighted. The contact-less measurement is made by a light reflexion method. (Picture from[11])

3. DATA ACQUISITION

3.1. Recording device for jaw motion

The CONDYLOCOMP LR3 is an opto-electronic measuring device for the registration of all mandibular movements (translations and rotations) using personal computers, which tracks all 6 degrees of freedom that are necessary for the recording of the jaw motions. It is normally used for the diagnostics of TMJ derangement and functional disorders of the stomatognatic system, for high quality prosthetics and orthodontics and in the splint therapy.

The CONDYLOCOMP LR3 is significantly different to normal registration systems. The contact-less measurement is carried out by a light reflecting method. The maxilla is not touched. Occlusal surfaces and tongue area are completely free because of the paraocclusal fixation of the very light lower measuring bow (see figure 1). By means of a patented procedure essential advantages like easy usage and high precision are the results for mounting, recording and analysis. A microprocessor controlled device is the bridge between the registration apparatus on the patient and the computer.

But there are also some disadvantages of this system. The registration procedure is not trivial and has to be performed by a physician since some anatomical parameters have to be measured. Furthermore the device is designed only for recording the jaw movement. Other movements can not be tracked.

3.2. Measurement principles

The movements of the lower measuring bow (see figure 1) are registered with a contact-less light reflecting method measuring near to the TMJ by 5 sensors on each side with a resolution of 1/100 mm. Thereby all possible degrees of freedom (translation and rotation) are tracked by the registration device and the obtained data can be used for the analysis and simulation of the jaw muscle motions.

Figure 2 shows the reflector fixed with the mandible and the measurement sensors of the registration apparatus mounted on the head of the patient. Three sensors marked with **H** in the figure – one is behind the reflector – are used for the translation, the other two sensors marked with **N** are used for the rotation. These data are registered with the CONDYLOCOMP and transmitted to the computer.

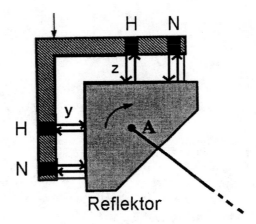

Figure 2. Light reflecting method of the CONDYLOCOMP LR3[13]

3.3. Conversion into transformation commands

The registered data of the device contain the spatial coordinates of both condyls and the angle of the jaw opening. They have to be converted in a special way to be suitable for the graphical simulation system. Homogeneous coordinate matrices are used to describe the transformation between two measurements. First the translations of the left and right condyls are calculated. Afterwards the rotation around the hinge axis, which is located through both condyls, is identified. These calculations have to be performed for each mandible position provided by the CONDYLOCOMP with a rate of $100Hz$. The moving coordinate frame of the mandible has been defined in the left condylus.

Since the sensors are mounted on the head of the patient the relation between fixed maxilla and moving mandible the simulation is correct even if the patient moves his head during the recording.

4. SIMULATION SYSTEM

For this project the visualization system KaVis[14] developed at the Institute for Real-Time Computer Control Systems & Robotics at the University of Karlsruhe is used. With this tool geometric objects can be visualized on a workstation using Open Inventor^{TM} (SGI) files. Originally, this visualization tool was developed for the simulation and animation of robot movements. Our kinematic model of the jaw has been rebuild in the simulation and can be adapted to the patients values.

An extension of KaVis made it possible to either visualize the muscles by passive flexible objects, which act like elastic bands, to show movements of the muscles force vectors (see figure 3 left), or to visualize them by flexible surfaces to show a realistic image of the muscles (see figure 3 right). For the purpose of tracking the muscle movements the first method is used. These flexible objects have a starting point and an ending point and adapt themself to movements by keeping these points. The muscle tissue in this simulation is fixed to a segmented computer tomograph image of the skull.

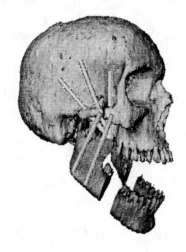 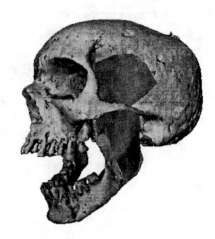

Figure 3. Flexible objects (left) and flexible surfaces (right) in the simulation.

When visualizing the real jaw movements the change of the muscle lengths is recorded and can be used for the analysis and evaluation of the contraction of the jaw muscles during motion. For the first time, it is possible to visualize real jaw muscle movements in a graphical simulation and to evaluate their alteration of length in diagrams. This analysis and the result of our project can be used for further studies like generating a model of the human mastication system or in the diagnosis and therapy of malfunctions.

The system developed in this project provides a planning tool for the user or physician and is easy to understand and to handle. For the routine course an application-oriented graphical user interface was designed which satisfies the mentioned requirements. After the CT-scanning of the patient and registering the jaw movements the user can choose the segmented skull from the menu. Alternatively a reference skull can be matched to the dimensions of the patient by using the Least Square method. The recorded jaw motion has to be transformed in 4×4 homogeneous matrices which is done by a special computer program. Finally, the registered jaw motion can be visualized in real time and the muscle length can be saved for the further analysis.

5. RESULTS

After the visualization and animation of the jaw motion the contraction of the jaw muscles can be analyzed and evaluated using the recorded motion of the flexible objects representing the muscle length. So far, the opening and closing of the mouth as well as protrusions, retrusions, laterotrusions and mediotrusions movements have been analyzed. The analysis diagrams show the muscle lengths and velocities with respect to the time.

As an example of the result of our study a comparison of the muscle lengths of the musculus pterygoideus lateralis and the musculus temporalis during an opening and closing of the mouth is presented. The m. pterygoideus lateralis initiates the motion (see figure 4 (1)), then the other muscles follow. The curve of the m. temporalis rises rapidly (see figure 5), the opening is done by a rotation of the temporomandibular joint. At point (2) in figure 5 the opening continues with a constant velocity. Before closing the mouth by a continuous contracting of the muscle the test person relaxed for a short moment (point 3 to 4).

In contrast to the other muscles the m. pterygoideus lateralis shows a different curve (see figure 4). At first, the muscle contract during the opening (point 1 to 2) and then relax to their initial length (point 3 to 4). This behavior is based anatomically.

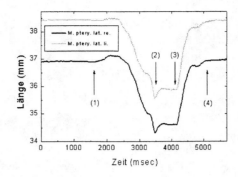

Figure 4. M. pterygoideus lateralis left and right during the opening and closing of the mouth

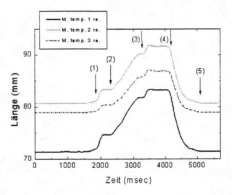

Figure 5. M. temporalis right during the opening and closing of the mouth

6. CONCLUSION

A new approach of recording the dynamic changes of the mastication muscles has been presented. Using the CONDY-LOCOMP recording device and increasing its functionality three dimensional jaw movements are recorded and converted into iterative transformation commands for the mandible. By applying these transformations to the jaw in the simulation system an animation of the records is possible. The developed flexible objects act as length sensors during this movement and make it possible for the first time to analyze the lengths and velocities of the muscles.

This analyzation can be used in diagnostics of jaw malfunctions and prediction of the results of craniofacial surgeries. Furthermore, it can be used in craniofacial research to retrieve more information about jaw and mastication muscle movements.

ACKNOWLEDGMENTS

This work has been supported by the German Research Foundation by the SFB 414 "Informationstechnik in der Medizin – Rechner- und sensorgestützte Chirurgie", Project Q4. It has been performed at the Institute for Real-Time Computer Control Systems & Robotics, Prof. Dr.-Ing. H. Wörn, Prof. Dr.-Ing. U. Rembold and Prof. Dr.-Ing. R. Dillmann, Department of Computer Science, University of Karlsruhe and the Clinic for Oral and Maxillofacial Surgery, Prof. Dr. Dr. J. Mühling, University of Heidelberg, Medical Department, Heidelberg, Germany.

REFERENCES

1. E. Keeve, S. Girod, and B. Girod, "Computer-aided craniofacial surgery," in *Computer Assisted Radiology (CAR) 96*, H. L. et.al., ed., pp. 757–763, Elsevier, (Amsterdam), June 1996.

2. T. Weingärtner and R. Dillmann, "Simulation of jaw-movements for the musculoskeletal diagnoses." Accepted at the MMVR '97, San Diego, Jan. 1997.

3. T. Weingärtner, S. Haßfeld, and R. Dillmann, "Dynamic simulation of the jaw and chewing muscles for maxilofacial s urgery," in *Proceedings of the IEEE Nonrigid and Articulated Motion Workshop (NRAMW '97)*, (Puerto Rico), June 1997.

4. B. Koeck, ed., *Funktionsstörungen des Kauorgans*, vol. 8 of *Praxis der Zahnheilkunde*, pp. 116–149. Urban & Schwarzenberg, München, 3 ed., 1995.

5. J. Herder, K. Myszkowski, T. Kunii, and M. Ibuski, "A virtual reality interface to an intelligent dental care system," in *Proceedings of the Medicine Meets Virtual Reality 4, Health Care in the Information Age*, H. Sieburg, S. Weghorst, and K. Morgan, eds., IOS Press and Ohmsha, 1996.

6. A. Takanishi, T. Tanase, M. Kumei, and I. Kato, "Development of 3 DOF jaw robot WJ-2 as a human's mastication simulator," in *Proceedings of the International Conference on Advanced Robotics ICAR*, pp. 277–282, (Pisa (Italy)), 1991.

7. H. Takanobu, A. Takanishi, and I. Kato, "Control of a mastication robot for reduction of jaw joint force focusing on musculus temporalis," in *IROS*, (München), 1994.

8. H. Takanobu, T. Yajima, and A. Takanishi, "Development of a mastication robot using nonlinear viscoelastic mechanism," in *Proceedings of the IEEE/RSJ International Conference on Intelligent Robots and Systems (IROS)*, vol. 3, pp. 1527–1532, (Grenoble, France), Sept. 1997.

9. Polhemus, *3 Space User's Manual*. Vermont, USA, revision f ed., 1993.

10. M. Stasch, "Entwicklung und Aufbau eines magnetfeldbasierten Positionssensors," Master's thesis, University of Karlsruhe, Institute for Real-Time Computer Control Systems & Robotics, June 1997.

11. Dentron, *String CONDYLOCOMP LR3 Manual*, DENTRON GmbH, 1996.

12. A. Hugger, B. Kordaß, E. Edinger, and U. Stüttgen, "Simultane Bewegungsaufzeichnungen mit zwei berührungslos messenden Registriersystemen," *Deutsche Zahnärztliche Zeitschrift* **52**, pp. 536–539, Aug. 1997.

13. J. Albrecht, "Übertragung von Bewegungsaufnahmen des Kiefers auf eine Simu lation und Analyse von Muskelbewegungen," Master's thesis, University of Karlsruhe, Institute for Real-Time Computer Control Systems & Robotics, Aug. 1997.

14. H. Schaude et al., "Documentation for KaVis," tech. rep., University of Karlsruhe, Institute for Real-Time Computer Control Systems & Robotics, 1997.

Shape reconstruction and subsequent deformation of soleus muscle models using B-spline solid primitives.

Victor Ng-Thow-Hing[a], Anne Agur[b], Kevin Ball[c], Eugene Fiume[a], and Nancy McKee[d]

[a]Department of Computer Science, University of Toronto, Toronto, Canada

[b]Department of Anatomy and Cell Biology, University of Toronto,

[c]School of Physical and Health Education, University of Toronto,

[d]Department of Surgery, University of Toronto

ABSTRACT

We introduce a mathematical primitive called the B-spline solid that can be used to create deformable models of muscle shape. B-spline solids can be used to model skeletal muscle for the purpose of building a data library of reusable, deformable muscles that are reconstructed from actual muscle data. Algorithms are provided for minimizing shape distortions that may be caused when fitting discrete sampled data to a continuous B-spline solid model. Visible Human image data provides a good indication of the perimeter of a muscle, but is not suitable for providing internal muscle fiber bundle arrangements which are important for physical simulation of muscle function. To obtain these fiber bundle orientations, we obtain 3-D muscle fiber bundle coordinates by triangulating optical images taken from three different camera views of serially dissected human soleus specimens. B-spline solids are represented as mathematical three-dimensional vector functions which can parameterize an enclosed volume as well as its boundary surface. They are based on B-spline basis functions, allowing local deformations via adjustable control points and smooth continuity of shape. After the B-spline solid muscle model is fitted with its external surface and internal volume arrangements, we can subsequently deform its shape to allow simulation of animated muscle tissue.

Keywords: deformable models, B-spline solids, soleus, muscle modeling

1. INTRODUCTION

The emergence of imaging techniques such as computer tomography (CT) and magnetic resonance imaging (MRI) combined with the use of computer graphics has provided researchers and practitioners with the ability to study and view anatomy in novel ways. Using images from the Visible Human data set,[1] it is possible to perform volume reconstructions of anatomic structures throughout the human body. Although we can navigate around the models of reconstructed anatomy, they are often static and cannot be deformed. To simulate living tissue, researchers have started using Visible Human data to transform static images into dynamic structures to perform virtual tasks such as facial surgery.[2]

However, there are cases where the inherent representation of the human body into a set of axial (transverse) slices of fixed orientation makes it difficult or impossible to extract structural information that is required for functional studies of various tissue. For example, it is difficult to identify and track individual muscle fiber bundles to determine their orientations due to the lack of continuity cues between adjacent image slices. In addition, the image resolution of the Visible Human data set is not high enough to retrieve finer structural details of individual muscle fiber bundles. Muscle fiber orientation is important for calculating force generation, visualizing shape changes, and understanding the role of skeletal muscles in the creation of human movement.

The architecture of a muscle consists of its external configuration and dimensions, and the internal arrangement and morphology of its contractile elements. Grossly, skeletal muscle has been described as being parallel, circular or

---

Other author information:

V.N.: E-mail: victorng@dgp.toronto.edu

A.A.: E-mail: anne.agur@utoronto.ca

K.B.: E-mail: ball@phe.utoronto.ca

E.F.: E-mail: elf@dgp.toronto.edu

N.M.: E-mail: n.mckee@utoronto.ca

pennate in fiber arrangement. Historically muscle architecture studies have been purely descriptive in nature, but a quantitative analysis of muscle architecture is important because the structural parameters have a profound effect on muscle function.[3] Previous work has focused on the muscle as a whole with little attention being paid to different regions within a muscle. Commonly, structural parameters have been recorded as single values for the whole muscle, regardless of the complexity of pennation. Parameters measured have included muscle length, fiber length, angle of pennation etc.[4–6] What is of great interest and has not been documented is the specific architecture of multi-pennate muscle. Knowledge of structural properties of each part of the muscle would help to establish the overall function, where function may include more sophisticated factors than simply the amount of shortening between the origin and insertion. The detailed measurement and modeling of the architectural characteristics of the soleus muscle (Figure 1) was chosen as the focus of this study, since these muscles are major contributors to human ambulatory power.

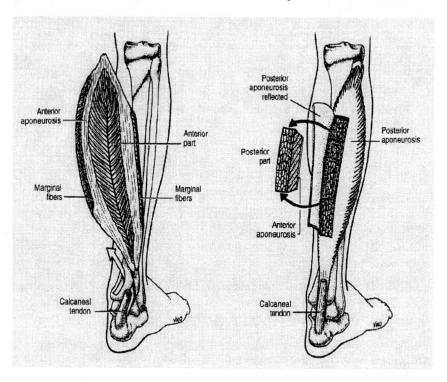

Figure 1. Marginal (M), posterior (P) and anterior (A) fibers in the soleus muscle (*illustrator Valerie Oxorn*[7])

In creating a detailed model of muscle, there is a need to represent its smooth shape properties while simultaneously being able to specify its internal architecture. Such a model must also be capable of deformations to reproduce the shape changes that occur when active muscle contracts. We introduce B-spline solids as useful modeling primitives for skeletal muscle as well as for potentially other anatomic structures. The properties of B-spline basis functions allow local deformations in shape. A continuous solid domain can be defined with inherent smoothness properties as well as an internal coordinate system that allows parameterization of vector and scalar properties within the entire solid as well as on its boundary surface. The inherent smoothness and compactness of representation in B-spline solids make them an interesting alternative to the more faceted polygon representations that are often created using the *Marching Cubes algorithm*.[8] Quantities like surface normals and volume can be computed directly from B-spline solids without the need for approximation.

This form of three-dimensional parameterization can also be used to nest or restrict the deformations of solids within the volume of another solid that contains it. By using B-spline solids, animation and modification of shape at interactive rates is possible. Solids can be created from a relatively sparse amount of data through the use of 3-D sampling function techniques. The mathematical formulation of B-spline solids allows them to be applicable to optimization methods that can constrain the nature of shape changes, similar to finite element techniques.[9] We will show how B-spline solids can be used to create deformable models of soleus muscle from both the Visible Human dataset and from dissected soleus specimens. From this, we will compare the quality of the reconstructed shapes in each case. Before describing the procedure for constructing deformable models of soleus muscle, the mathematical formulation of B-spline solids will be reviewed.

2. INTRODUCTION TO B-SPLINE SOLIDS

B-spline solids are straightforward extensions of B-spline curves and surfaces into the volumetric domain. A third parameter is added to the function to allow enumeration of points throughout a volume in addition to an iso-surface (one parameter constant) or a streamline curve (two parameters constant). Mathematically, a B-spline solid is represented by the following equation:

$$\mathbf{V}(u, v, w) = \sum_{i=0}^{l} \sum_{j=0}^{m} \sum_{k=0}^{n} B_i^u(u) B_j^v(v) B_k^w(w) \mathbf{C}_{ijk} \tag{1}$$

where each $\mathbf{C}_{ijk} \in \mathcal{R}^3$. The set $\mathbf{C} = \{\mathbf{C}_{ijk}\}$ of points form a control point lattice which will influence the shape of the B-spline solid (Figure 2A). $\mathbf{V}$ describes a parametric solid given by the tritensor product of these B-spline basis functions (in this case, the polynomials $B_i^u(u), B_j^v(v), B_k^w(w)$) with the control points in $\mathbf{C}$. We can substitute the control points $\mathbf{C}$ with other vector or scalar values to define other continuous fields or functions within the solid such as continuous internal forces. The basis functions for each parameter need not all have the same order and each basis function family is indexed depending on the size of its associated knot vector, U, V or W. The knot vectors form a sequence of points that partitions the parameter domain space, determining the local region of influence for each basis function. As each control point is weighted with B-spline basis functions, moving a point will deform a region of the solid as dictated by the shape of the B-spline basis functions which are in turn determined by the knot vectors (see Figure 2). For a more detailed description of the properties and evaluation of B-spline basis functions, please refer to Hoschek and Lasser.[9]

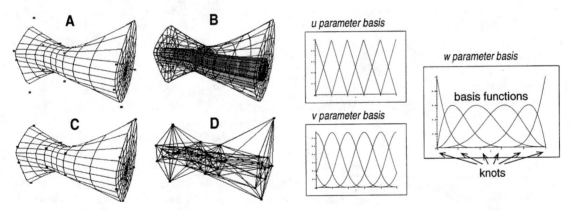

Figure 2. Features of B-spline solids. (A) B-spline solid with control points. (B) Iso-parameteric surfaces of a B-spline solid. (C) B-spline solid with sample points. (D) Sample points are connected with a viscoelastic network. On the right, the uniform basis functions for the u, v, and w parameters of a B-spline solid are displayed.

2.1. Control point lattice design

The control point lattice determines the shape of the B-spline object. The coordinate system used to represent and position control points will determine the space in which the object will be displayed. Although any three-dimensional coordinate system can be used for solids, we chose the cartesian coordinate system to represent geometry for 3-D graphics.

The topology of the lattice defines the topology and the control point indexing of its associated B-spline solid. Therefore, the design of the control point lattice is influential in creating the user interface handles that can be used to modify the object's shape.[10] The indexing of control points will affect the interpretation of the solid's iso-parametric surfaces or curves when one or more parameters is held constant (see Figure 2B).

The choice of a control point lattice depends on the type of object that is being modeled. We chose a natural cylindrical indexing that allowed us to retain the basic cylindrical topology of muscle-like bundles after shape deformation. The topology of a cylindrical lattice is actually the same as that of a tube since it includes outer and inner surfaces, with the main axis corresponding to the inner surface where all the surface points are coincident on the axis curve (see Figure 3).

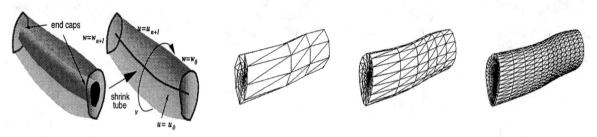

Figure 3. Left: The parameterization of the cylindrical B-spline solid. The topology of the solid is actually the same as a tube. Right: B-spline solids can be retessellated to any desired level of detail.

2.2. Interactive display of B-spline solids

For the purposes of animation, we need to quickly display and update the changing shape of B-spline solids. A key advantage of using a solid formulation instead of a surface parameterization is that the solid produces a unified model that allows us the flexibility of displaying arbitrary iso-surfaces within the solid. It is possible to display subvolumes within the solid (Figure 2B) by displaying different iso-parametric surfaces. To visualize the closed outer surface of the solid, we simply draw iso-parametric surfaces (holding one parameter constant while varying the other two over their respective domains) that correspond to the boundary of the parameter domains. Although it is possible to create a closed cylindrical surface with a single B-spline surface, duplicate control points or additional knots must be inserted to create discontinuities at the edges between the caps and the outer shell of the cylindrical shape.

Due to the use of multiple knots in the u and w parameter domains, the external control points are solely responsible for the shape of the solid's boundary since the internal basis functions evaluate to zero at the boundaries. Consequently, the outer surface of a B-spline solid is equivalent to a standard B-spline surface,[9] making it possible to apply standard acceleration techniques to interactively update and display B-spline solids. To take advantage of graphics hardware, it is necessary to tessellate the B-spline solid surfaces. By pre-evaluating the B-spline basis functions at tessellation points and storing these basis function values in a table, we can quickly update a pre-existing tessellation whenever a control point is changed. A given control point will affect only a finite set of tessellation points which correspond to the parameter values of u,v, and w where $B_i^u(u)B_j^v(v)B_k^w(w) \neq 0$ for a control point $\mathbf{C}_{ijk}$. By storing the non-zero $B_i^u(u)B_j^v(v)B_k^w(w)$ for each control point, we can achieve fast incremental updates of the solid deformations at interactive rates. Choosing the density of tessellation points allows us to produce different levels of detail of each model (Figure 3), which will be needed to display very complex scenes with hundreds of these solids in them.

3. METHODS AND MATERIALS

The process of producing deformable models of soleus muscle from various sources of data can be divided into several stages:

1. 3-D data is obtained from the Visible Human data set and from serially dissected human soleus specimens.

2. From the sampled data, a *continuous volume sampling function* (CVSF) is built which has a domain consisting of three parameters $(\tilde{u}, \tilde{v}, \tilde{w}) \in [0,1]^3$. The parameter space maps to a continuous volume that approximates the volume of the anatomic structure with the characteristic that the volume intersects the original data that was used to build the function . During the construction of this function, steps can be taken to produce evenly distributed samples.

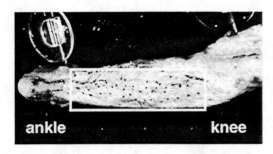 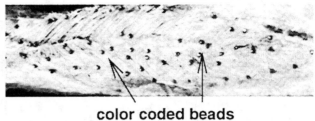

color coded beads

Figure 4. Dissection of anterior soleus (inside the rectangle). The fiber bundles are pinned with color-coded beads and the specimen with marker clusters is placed on the base plate.

3. Once the CVSF is available, samples can be freely selected and used in a data-fitting process with a B-spline solid that guarantees intersection of the sample points. Samples are chosen both on the surface and in the interior of the solid.

4. Having obtained a B-spline solid approximation of the muscle, we can perform volume visualizations of muscle fiber orientations, or subsequently deform the shape for simulation or user adjustment purposes.

We will now discuss each of these stages in more detail.

3.1. Obtaining 3-D data from anatomical specimens

3.1.1. Visible Human data

We obtained a subset of images of soleus muscle from the Visible Human Male data set. To avoid managing the large amount of data, we used lower resolution 24 bit images at 800x500 (MRI data is 256x256 and CT is 512x512)[1] resolution instead of the original axial images of 2048x1216. Every tenth slice (intervals of 1cm) was used in a sequence of images bounding the posterior and anterior soleus of the right leg.

As we could not reliably segment the individual posterior and anterior regions of the soleus by automatic means, an anatomist examined each of the data images and delineated the different regions, outlining the boundaries using a dark thick line with an image paint program. This facilitated the use of active contours ("snakes")[11] to quickly guide a deformable contour curve to the marked boundaries. From the active contour software, we were able to obtain two sets of contour curves, made up of a sequence of 3-D coordinates, for each of the posterior and anterior soleus. The contour curves for each set had the same number of points, allowing one-to-one mappings between the points on the adjacent contours.

3.1.2. Dissected soleus specimens

The human soleus muscle has three parts: *posterior, marginal and anterior*[12] (Figure 1). To develop the model, the soleus muscle, located in situ, was serially dissected from posterior to anterior. At each level the beginning and end of 50-100 representative fiber bundles distributed throughout the muscle volume were identified and pinned with color coded beads. The specimen was placed on a calibrated base plate and photographs were taken at each level of the serial dissection using three 35mm cameras that were calibrated using the *direct linear transformation* (DLT)[13] (Figure 4). These images were transferred to CD-ROM and the locations of the beads digitized. Visible in each image were two rigid objects of known dimensions. These objects were attached directly to the bones of the specimen. Reference points on these objects were digitized and rigid body procedures were used,[14,15] on a level by level basis, to achieve a consistent alignment of all of the 3-D coordinates that were viewed across the muscle's dissected surface. These muscle-related coordinates were ordered to generate line segments that represented the fiber orientations. This entire procedure will be referred to as *anatomical photogrammetry*. Plots of the muscle in whole and in part were created to observe and verify the architecture seen in the cadaveric specimen.

3.2. Constructing the continuous volume sampling function

We needed to develop two different approaches to create *continuous volume sampling functions* (CVSFs) for the Visible Human and dissected soleus data sets. The form of the CVSF is:

$$CVSF(\tilde{u}, \tilde{v}, \tilde{w}) = \mathbf{s}_{\tilde{u}\tilde{v}\tilde{w}} \tag{2}$$

where the three parameters $(\tilde{u}, \tilde{v}, \tilde{w}) \in [0,1]^3$. This allows a relatively sparse amount of data to be used to specify the shape of a B-spline solid as the $CVSF$ will interpolate between the given data. A sample point, $\mathbf{s}_{\tilde{u}\tilde{v}\tilde{w}}$, is a 3-D point that can be chosen anywhere within the continuous volume defined by the $CVSF$ using the parameters $(\tilde{u}, \tilde{v}, \tilde{w})$. Sample points are used for defining the B-spline solid's shape during the data-fitting process.

3.2.1. Visible Human

The Visible Human data produced a set of contour curves for an individual muscle where each contour curve is an ordered set of points that make up a closed polygon. This data was obtained directly from the active contour image processing program we used. The contours belonging to a common set were re-indexed by offsetting the ordering to minimize the least squared distance between adjacent points sharing the same index. This helped to reduce twisting distortions in shape along the muscle axis. We chose the parameter $\tilde{u}$ to correspond roughly to the radial distance formed by the centroid axis of the contours, $\tilde{v}$ to span a distance around the circumference of the axis and $\tilde{w}$ to represent the fractional length along the longitudinal axis of the muscle (Figure 5). To retrieve a given sample point, we first create an interpolating spline, $\mathbf{c}_i(v), i = 0, 1, \ldots, n$, for each of the $n+1$ contour curves making up a muscle. Arc length parameterization is used to obtain a point at the fractional distance $\tilde{v}$ around the circumference of each of the contours. Another interpolating B-spline, $\mathbf{l}$, is used that consists of the sequence of points $\mathbf{c}_i(\tilde{v})$ that are chosen from each of the $n+1$ contours. A point $\mathbf{l}(\tilde{w})$ is evaluated that corresponds to the fractional length $\tilde{w}$ along the spline curve $\mathbf{l}$. A second point $\mathbf{a}(\tilde{w})$ was taken that coincided with the fractional length $\tilde{w}$ along an interpolating spline made up of the centroids of each axis.

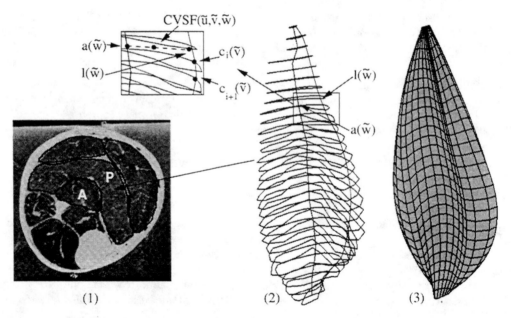

Figure 5. Stages of data fitting for Visible Human data. (1) Contours of the posterior (P) and anterior (A) soleus are extracted from images. (2) CVSF is built to generate sample points (only posterior contours are shown). (3) B-spline solid is generated to intersect the sample points.

Second degree interpolating curves were used to create a C^1 continuous volume shape. Higher degree splines introduced unwanted oscillations in shape and were more expensive to compute. The final desired sample points $\mathbf{s}_{\tilde{u}\tilde{v}\tilde{w}}$ were obtained by linear interpolation between $\mathbf{l}(\tilde{w})$ and $\mathbf{a}(\tilde{w})$ (Figure 5). Higher-order interpolation schemes could be applied by using more sample points in the interior of the solid, but we found that linear interpolation produces an even distribution of fibers in the solid.

3.2.2. Dissected soleus

We developed a method of constructing the CVSF from a series of profile curves that follow the edges formed by the ends of the line segments that were retrieved using anatomic photogrammetry. By parameterizing profile curves so that the same parameter in two curves produces the end points of the same line segment, we guarantee that muscle fiber bundle orientations are preserved. The CVSF volume is formed by interpolating or sweeping between the profile curves. For example, if we are given two end cap curves and an axis curve that outline a cylindrical shape (Figure 3), the swept volume creating the CVSF is computed as:

$$\mathbf{CVSF}(\tilde{u}, \tilde{v}, \tilde{w}) = (1 - \tilde{u})\mathbf{axis}(\tilde{w}) + \tilde{u}[(1 - \tilde{w})\mathbf{cap}_1(\tilde{v}) + \tilde{w}\mathbf{cap}_2(\tilde{v})]. \tag{3}$$

We illustrate the method by showing the CVSFs developed for marginal (M), posterior (P) and anterior (A) soleus regions in Figure 6.

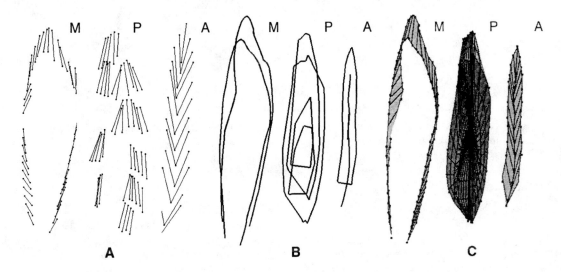

Figure 6. Creating the CVSF with profile curves. (A) 3-D points and line-segments are retrieved from soleus using anatomical photogrammetry. (B) Profile curves are created to define the CVSF. (C) The resulting B-spline solids with the sample points used to define its shape.

3.3. Fitting the data to the B-spline solid shape

With the creation of the continuous function **CVSF**, we are free to sample any number of points anywhere within the domain of **CVSF**. However, we restrict the number of samples we wish to take to be equal to the number of degrees of freedom (control points) in our B-spline solid. This allows us to create a set of linear systems through which we can solve for the control points efficiently. In contrast to Hsu *et al.*,[16] who developed a general direct manipulation interface for any point within a free form deformation lattice, we restrict manipulation to the original sample points used for data fitting.

The control points cannot all be solved for in a single large linear system containing the sample points. This is because linear dependencies arise due to multiple knot vectors occurring at the boundaries of the B-spline solid's knot vectors. For example, the control points around the outer ring of an end cap of a cylindrical B-spline solid is sufficient to completely specify the shape of the cap's boundary. Including these control points in a larger linear system would over-constrain the problem and create a singular matrix. The solution is to solve a sequence of linear systems that partition the unknown control points into solvable sets. The boundary conditions of the solid are solved first. These boundary control points can then be used to solve for the internal control points within the solid. Figure 7 illustrates the sequence that the various sets of control points must be solved in. The general form of these linear systems is:

$$\mathbf{Bc} = \mathbf{s} - \mathbf{b} \tag{4}$$

where **c** are the control point components to solve, **s** are the sample points to fit, and **B** is a matrix where each row is made up of the evaluated basis functions at the parameter values assigned to the sample point stored in the same row

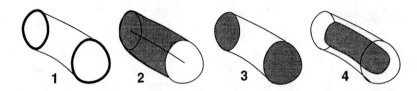

Figure 7. Proper sequence for solving all the control points for a B-spline solid. 1. Cap rings. 2. Outer shell and inner axis. 3. Inner caps. 4. Remaining region between the outer shell, axis and caps.

of **s**. In cases where the boundary control points have been solved, **b** will store the product of these solved control points and their corresponding evaluated basis functions which will be subtracted from **s** to maintain an independent set of equations. In some cases, the data fitting matrices, **B**, for two systems are identical due to symmetries in the boundary conditions of the solid. This allows us to solve two simultaneous systems in one pass. In all cases, we perform an LU factorization of the matrix **B** and use the factors to solve two simpler linear systems with triangular matrices to significantly accelerate the solution of the linear systems.[17] Since we must repetitively solve the system each time the sample points are moved, the acceleration technique is very important. These factors can be stored and reused to recompute the new control points for an animated set of sample points very quickly without the need to expensively compute inverse matrices.

The choice of sample points and their corresponding parameters within the B-spline solid determines how the shape will change as sample points are moved. We choose sample point parameters that locate the maximum of each basis function of the B-spline basis for each parameter dimension. This adjusts the weighting of control points that must be moved to interpolate the sample point so that the corresponding control point of the basis function has the greatest influence on the sample point. Forsey and Bartels[18] use a similar formulation for direct manipulation of hierarchical B-spline surfaces. They avoid solving linear systems by restricting the manipulation of sample points to only one at a time.

Sample points are an effective alternative to control points because they allow the user to specify the exact placement of the solid in space. The use of sample points becomes very useful when fitting a viscoelastic system over these points instead of the control points. Spatial constraints between sample points create direct correlations between actual points in the solid. In contrast, constraints acting between control points can create undesirable deformations in the underlying solid shape.

4. RESULTS

4.1. Obtaining muscle fiber orientations

Once the B-spline model is obtained, we can visualize the iso-surfaces or streamlines within the solid. Figure 8 illustrates streamlines for B-spline solids, representing parts of the posterior and anterior soleus, extracted from both the Visible Human and dissected soleus specimens with various streamlines and iso-surfaces displayed. The Visible Human data provides a nicer overall shape definition due to the higher density of original sample points. However, the internal fiber orientations are incorrect due to the lack of internal markers within the contours to construct an accurate CVSF. In contrast, using the profile curves to create the CVSF allowed close matching of fiber end points in the dissected soleus specimens than in the Visible Human data set derived models. With the dissected soleus specimens, we were able to resolve the soleus into marginal, posterior and anterior fiber groups. This level of detail was not apparent from the Visible Human images.

4.2. Deforming B-spline solids

Control points on the original sample points of the B-spline solids can be directly manipulated to locally deform the solid shape at interactive rates. Notice that the control points may not necessarily lie on the solid's surface or within its volume (except in degree 1 B-spline solids). For direct manipulation of solids, we used the set of sample points $\mathbf{s}_{\bar{u}\bar{v}\bar{w}}$ that were used to fit the B-spline solid's shape and solved for a new configuration of control points to define the resulting shape change. For simulation, it is necessary to coordinate the movement of many control or sample points simultaneously. We are currently experimenting with two techniques: (1) a network of viscoelastic units connecting the sample points and (2) nonlinear constrained optimization techniques[19] that seek to minimize energy functionals of the control points while conserving volume. It is possible for a modeler to define different

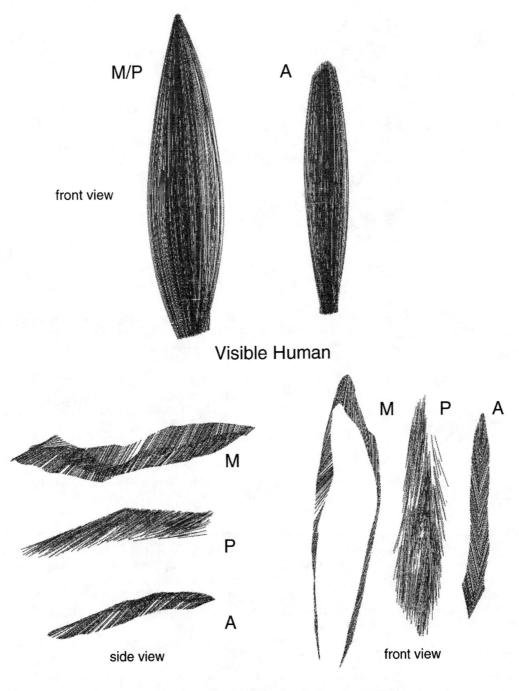

Figure 8. Fiber orientations derived from Visible Human data and serially dissected soleus. Multiple views of the fibers obtained from photogrammetry of dissected soleus show that orientations are accurately reconstructed (M=marginal fibers, P=posterior fibers, A=anterior fibers). In the Visible Human data, it is impossible to distinguish between posterior and marginal fibers. Note that the aspect ratio of the Visible Human image has been adjusted to correct for the 3:1 height to width ratio in the data set.

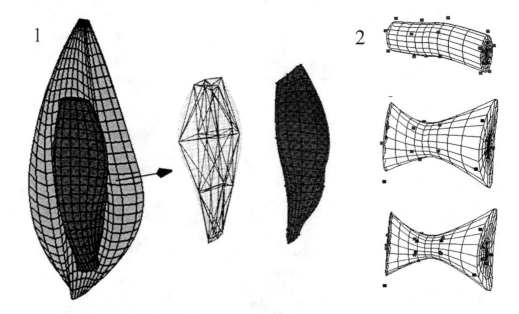

Figure 9. (1) The anterior soleus has a viscoelastic network applied to its sample points that deforms its shape. (2) The B-spline solid optimizes its least squares change in control points while conserving volume. The top shape is deformed to create the middle shape. After optimization, the bottom shape has the same volume as the top one.

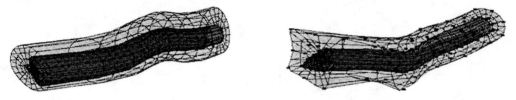

Figure 10. B-spline solids can be nested within each other to allow modeling of components within an anatomic structure. As the outer solid changes shape, the nested solid deforms with it.

stiffness or damping coefficients for the viscoelastic units, allowing nonhomogenous physical properties throughout the solid. The speed of the simulation depends on the number of sample points, the number of springs and the degree of the basis functions of the B-spline solid. For optimization, we experimented with a simple case using only control point values to minimize the least-squares distance between the control point configurations of an initial B-spline solid shape and the deformed solid while conserving volume (Figure 9). In addition, the mathematical formulation of B-spline solids can potentially be applied to finite element analysis by defining energy functionals that can be minimized to find the optimal control point configuration.

4.3. Nesting solids

The three-dimensional parameter space of a B-spline solid can be used to nest other solids within each other, similar to a technique in computer graphics called *free-form deformations*.[20] We used nonlinear least squares numerical techniques[21] to solve the inverse problem of finding the parameters u, v, w for a given point that lies within a solid. If every control or sample point in a B-spline solid lies entirely within another solid, we can deform the outer solid while simultaneously deforming the solids that reside within it (Figure 10). This can be used to model substructures within anatomy. For example, fiber bundles can be modeled as individual solids residing within a larger solid that represents the envelope of outer deep fascia tissue. This technique can also be used to link solids together at common points.

5. CONCLUSIONS AND DISCUSSION

We have shown that B-spline solids can be a useful primitive for developing deformable models of skeletal muscle. Techniques have been introduced to construct continuous representations of volume from discrete data. Since B-spline solids can be defined completely with its control points and knot vectors, they can require significantly less storage than a dense set of polygons.

The three dimensional parameterization allows true volume analysis of the shapes, providing arbitrary streamline or iso-surface visualizations. In the case of streamline construction, careful design of the CVSF can provide accurate depictions of muscle fiber orientations in soleus for subsequent use in functional simulation of muscle. This was aided with the use of dissection and optical recording techniques designed solely for capturing muscle fiber orientations (anatomical photogrammetry). Although the Visible Human data is helpful for delineating gross sections of anatomy by segmenting the regions using axial boundary information, internal muscle architecture cannot be determined. The correct fiber arrangements provided from the serially dissected soleus will allow future studies to examine muscle contraction and subsequent force generation with accurate muscle pennation effects.

We hope to refine the B-spline solid model to set the stage for further research on applying B-spline solids for non-invasive surgical simulation using functional, deformable models of tissue, especially with skeletal muscles. B-spline solids can have other topologies such as tubular and ellipsoidal shapes to allow modeling of a wider variety of shapes. Nonuniform knot vectors can potentially lead to better data-fitting of solids with less sample points required or the knot vectors can be adjusted to allow greater shape control in selected regions of the solid.

We intend to continue exploring the use of viscoelastic networks in combination with volume-preserving constraints. This promises the development of faster interactive visualizations that can be used for functional studies of muscle and their role in creating movement in animals. For example, B-spline solids could be incorporated as muscle primitives in a system where they can be attached to an underlying skeleton and create active motion. Such a tool would be useful for the exploration of biological systems without the need to perform invasive procedures.

We found it exciting that this work arose out of the common interests from three different disciplines: computer animation, clinical anatomy and biomechanics. Anatomy provided the methods to perform serial dissections to categorize the different orientations of muscle fibers in the soleus. Optical triangulation techniques used in biomechanics made it possible to convert markers on muscle fibers to three dimensional points. Computer animation research drove the development of B-spline solid primitives to create deformable shapes for the muscles. Each discipline has gained from the synergies that have resulted from this co-disciplinary work.

6. ACKNOWLEDGEMENTS

This work was partially funded by NSERC, ITRC of Ontario, AO/ASIF - Foundation of Switzerland and the Department of Surgery, Faculty of Medicine, University of Toronto.

REFERENCES

1. U. N. L. of Medicine, "The visible human project." MRI, CT, and axial anatomical images of human body, October 1996.
2. R. Koch, M. Gross, F. Carls, D. von Buren, and Y. Parish, "Simulating facial surgery using finite element models," in *Computer Graphics (SIGGRAPH '96 Proceedings)*, pp. 421–428, 1996.
3. R. Woittiez, P. Huijing, and R. Rozendal, "Influence of muscle architecture on the length-force diagram: a model and its verification.," *Pflugers Arch.* **397**, pp. 73–74, 1983.
4. T. Wickiewicz, R. Roy, P. Powell, and V. Edgerton, "Muscle architecture of the human lower limb.," *Clinical Orthopaedics and Related Research* **179**, pp. 275–283, 1983.
5. J. Friederich and R. Brand, "Muscle fibre architecture in the human lower limb.," *Journal of Biomechanics* **23**, pp. 91–95, 1990.
6. G. Yamaguchi, A. Sawa, D. Moran, M. Fessler, and J. Winters, "A survey of human musculotendon actuator parameters.," in *Multiple muscle systems: Biomechanics and movement organization*, J. Winters and S. Woo, eds., pp. 717–773, New York: Springer-Verlag, 1990.
7. V. Oxorn, A. Agur, and N. McKee, "Resolving discrepancies in image research: The importance of direct observation in the illustration of the human soleus muscle.," *Journal of Biocommunication* **25**(1), 1998.

8. W. E. Lorensen and H. E. Cline, "Marching cubes: A high resolution 3D surface construction algorithm," in *Computer Graphics (SIGGRAPH '87 Proceedings)*, M. C. Stone, ed., vol. 21, pp. 163–169, July 1987.

9. J. Hoschek and D. Lasser, *Fundamentals of Computer Aided Geometric Design*, A K Peters, 1989.

10. S. Coquillart, "Extended free-form deformation: A sculpturing tool for 3D geometric modeling," in *Computer Graphics (SIGGRAPH '90 Proceedings)*, F. Baskett, ed., vol. 24, pp. 187–196, Aug. 1990.

11. M. Kass, A. Witkin, and D. Terzopoulos, "Snakes: Active contour models," *International Journal of Computer Vision* **1**(4), pp. 321–331, 1987.

12. A. Agur and N. McKee, "Soleus muscle: Fiber orientation.," *Clinical Anatomy* **10**, p. 130, 1997. Abstract.

13. Y. Abdel-Aziz and H. Karara, "Direct linear transformation into object space coordinates in close-range photogrammetry," in *Symposium on Close-Range Photogrammetry*, pp. 1–19, 1971.

14. K. Ball and M. Pierrynowski, "Estimation of six degree of freedom rigid body segment motion from two dimensional data.," *Human Movement Science* **14**, pp. 139–154, 1995.

15. K. Ball and M. Pierrynowski, "Classification of errors in locating a rigid body.," *Journal of Biomechanics* **29**, pp. 1213–1217, 1996.

16. W. M. Hsu, J. F. Hughes, and H. Kaufman, "Direct manipulation of free-form deformations," in *Computer Graphics (SIGGRAPH '92 Proceedings)*, vol. 26, pp. 177–184, 1992.

17. W. H. Press, S. A. Teukolsky, W. T. Vetterling, and B. P. Flannery, *Numerical Recipes in C*, Cambridge University Press, second ed., 1992.

18. D. R. Forsey and R. H. Bartels, "Hierarchical B-spline refinement," in *Computer Graphics (SIGGRAPH '88 Proceedings)*, J. Dill, ed., vol. 22, pp. 205–212, Aug. 1988.

19. P. E. Gill, W. Murray, and M. H. Wright, *Practical Optimization*, Academic Press, 1981.

20. T. W. Sederberg and S. R. Parry, "Free-form deformation of solid geometric models," in *Computer Graphics (SIGGRAPH '86 Proceedings)*, D. C. Evans and R. J. Athay, eds., vol. 20, pp. 151–160, August 1986.

21. V. Ng-Thow-Hing and E. Fiume, "Interactive display and animation of b-spline solids as muscle shape primitives," in *Computer Animation and Simulation '97*, pp. 81–97, Springer-Verlag/Wien, 1997.

Modeling of the pliant surfaces of the thigh and leg during gait

Kevin A. Ball[a] and Michael R. Pierrynowski[b]

[a]Community Health (Exercise Sciences), University of Toronto, Toronto, ON M5S 3J7
[b]Rehabilitation Sciences, McMaster University, Hamilton, ON L8N 3Z5

ABSTRACT

Rigid Body Modeling, a 6 degree of freedom (DOF) method, provides state of the art human movement analysis, but with one critical limitation; it assumes segment rigidity. A non-rigid 12 DOF method, Pliant Surface Modeling (PSM) was developed to model the simultaneous pliant characteristics (scaling and shearing) of the human body's soft tissues. For validation, bone pins were surgically inserted into the tibia and femur of three volunteers. Infrared markers (44) were placed upon the thigh, leg and bone pin surfaces. Two synchronized OPTOTRAK/3020™ cameras (Northern Digital Inc., Waterloo, ON) were used to record 120 seconds of treadmill gait per subject. In comparison to the "gold standard" bone pin rotational results, PSM located the tibia, femur and tibiofemoral joint with root mean square (RMS) errors of 2.4°, 4.0° and 4.6°, respectively. These performances met or exceeded (P<.01) the current state of the art for surface data, Rigid Surface Modeling. The thigh's measured surface experienced uniform repeatable changes in scale: 40% mediolateral, 5% anterioposterior, 5% superioinferior, and planar shears of: 25° transverse, 15° sagittal, 5° frontal. With the brief exception of push-off, the lower leg demonstrated much greater rigidity: <5% scaling and <5° shearing. Thus, PSM offers superior "rigid" estimates of knee motion with the ability to quantify "pliant" surface changes.

Keywords: human movement, rigid body modeling, deformable models, pliant modeling

1. INTRODUCTION

Qualitative assessments of human movement typically involve visual inspections of the rotational and translational movements that occur within the bodys' joints and body segments. In a less obvious way, such assessments also include recognition that the segments of the body have the ability to undergo modest shape changes. Within the human movement literature, numerous quantitative techniques exist for the measurement of Rigid Body motion,[1-6] yet virtually none exists to describe the concomitant motion of the body's soft-tissues. This paper introduces Pliant Surface modeling, a non-rigid approach for the measurement of human movement. Use of this method provides simultaneous quantification of a body segment's "rigid" (rotations and translations) and "pliant" (scales and shears) motion characteristics. Assessments of body segment shape change should prove useful in several ways. They may allow designers to enhance the fit of objects that function in dynamic contact with the body's external surfaces: orthoses, sports equipment and clothing are examples of this. Moreover, since human movement analysis, itself, typically involves the use of surface observations, it will be shown that the Pliant Surface model actually enhances the accuracy of skeletal motion estimates.

1.1. Techniques of Rigid modeling

If the spatial positions of at least three non-collinear points are known on an object, in both, their static control point locations, $\mathbf{P}_C$, as well as in their dynamic observed locations, $\mathbf{P}_T$, then the 6 Degree of Freedom (DOF) movement of that object can be completely described. These measures are related as follows:

$$\mathbf{P}_T = \mathbf{R}_T \, \mathbf{P}_C + \mathbf{T}_T, \tag{1}$$

where $\mathbf{P}_T$ and $\mathbf{P}_C$, are $3 \times N$ matrices with $N \geq 3$, $\mathbf{T}_T$ is a 3×1 vector that represents 3 DOF translation between the origins of the control and observed objects, and $\mathbf{R}_T$ is a 3×3 rotation matrix that contains 3 rotational DOF.

K.A.B. (correspondence): Email: ball@phe.utoronto.ca; Telephone: 416-978-3196; Fax: 416-978-4384
M.R.P. (correspondence): Email: pierryn@fhs.mcmaster.ca; Telephone: 905-525-9140 x22910; Fax: 905-522-6095

Note also that rotation matrices, denoted generically as $\mathbf{R}$, possess the properties: $\det(\mathbf{R}) = +1$ and $\mathbf{R}^T\mathbf{R} = \mathbf{I}$, where $\mathbf{I}$ is the 3×3 identity matrix.

In (1), if the points measured in $\mathbf{P_T}$ and $\mathbf{P_C}$ are error-free, and the object is indeed rigid, then the solutions for $\mathbf{R_T}$ and $\mathbf{T_T}$ can be easily determined, but as is more often the case,

$$\mathbf{P}_O = \mathbf{R}_M\,\mathbf{P_C} + \mathbf{T}_M + \varepsilon, \tag{2}$$

where ε is a $3 \times N$ error matrix, $\mathbf{R_M}$ (3×3) and $\mathbf{T_T}$ (3×1) are modeled estimates of $\mathbf{R_T}$ and $\mathbf{T_T}$, and the $3 \times N$ observations in $\mathbf{P_O}$ are thought to contain error since $\mathbf{P_C}$ is usually assumed to be error free[4]. A random and Gaussian distribution is often assumed for the error[7] in ε, as such, several researchers have developed numerical methods[2,3,4,6] for the purpose of finding the best rigid fit to $\mathbf{P_O}$. In this sense, $|\varepsilon|$ is minimized (least-squares), hence,

$$\mathbf{P}_M = \mathbf{R}_M\,\mathbf{P_C} + \mathbf{T}_M, \tag{3}$$

where the $3 \times N$ matrix, $\mathbf{P_M}$, represents the best rigidly modeled alias of $\mathbf{P_O}$. From these calculations, the expression,

$$\mathbf{E}_{OM} = \mathbf{P}_O - \mathbf{P}_M, \tag{4}$$

may be readily derived. Here, the $3 \times N$ matrix, $\mathbf{E_{OM}}$, contains the overall Measured Error[8] of Rigid Body modeling. Note that $\mathbf{E_{OM}}$ is identical to ε, however, specific characterization of this quantity is useful.

For human movement analysis, the techniques of Rigid Body modeling have been applied in two ways: marker laden rigid objects have been attached to the bodys' segments,[9-11] or markers have been affixed directly to the bodys' surface;[12-15] this latter technique can be called Rigid Surface modeling. Regardless of the approach taken to marker placement, it has been recognized that the skin and soft-tissue shifts that accompany human movement represent the greatest impediment towards determining skeletal motion accuracy[15]. Nevertheless, it has also been observed that Rigid modeling techniques currently represent the state of the art in human movement analysis[16].

1.2. Towards a Pliant Surface model

Since methods for routinely quantifying the non-rigid characteristics of body segments were not available in the human movement literature, a cross-discipline search was conducted. Fortunately, the computer graphics literature contained numerous descriptions of numerical methods that had been used to modify the shape of virtual objects[17]. Such techniques included affine[18] and freeform deformation[19] models. The direct suitability of these techniques, however, presented certain challenges. Whereas, it is common for animators to create deformations through a trial and error process, human movement analysts must uniquely quantify what has already happened. In this manner, the two tasks appeared to be the virtual opposites of each other.

Another factor also guided the development of Pliant Surface modeling. Since the current procedures for collecting human movement data are typically easy to perform, an emphasis was placed upon developing procedures that would differ little from those that are already in use in human movement laboratories. To this end, solutions that were judged expensive in either hardware, or time, were avoided. From these efforts, a compromise was reached. The details are described below.

Within the Computer Graphics literature, the term, affine deformation, is used to describe the set of numerical matrices that can be linearly combined to produce changes in object shape and position[17]. Affine matrices include those for rotation, scaling, shearing and translation; the latter, however, requires homogeneous coordinates. Given these definitions, Rigid Body modeling can be said to consist of affine transformations, yet only those of rotation and translation are employed. Thus, to enable the measurement of pliant surfaces, the following model was constructed:

$$\mathbf{P}_O = \mathbf{R}_M \, \mathbf{H}_M \, \mathbf{S}_M \, \mathbf{P}_C + \mathbf{T}_M + \varepsilon, \tag{5}$$

where, like $\mathbf{R}_M$, the new entries, $\mathbf{H}_M$ and $\mathbf{S}_M$ possessed a 3×3 matrix form. These two matrices specifically incorporate the use of the other types of affine matrices, scaling and shearing.

The general 3×3 scaling matrix $\mathbf{S}$ has the form,

$$\mathbf{S} = \begin{bmatrix} sx & 0 & 0 \\ 0 & sy & 0 \\ 0 & 0 & sz \end{bmatrix}, \tag{6}$$

where sx, sy and sz represent respective scaling multipliers for the x, y and z coordinates. The complete 3×3 shearing matrix is defined as,

$$\mathbf{H} = \begin{bmatrix} 1 & hxy & hxz \\ hyx & 1 & hyz \\ hzx & hzy & 1 \end{bmatrix}. \tag{7}$$

Here, the off-diagonal elements represent shearing in the first coordinate direction with respect to the second, i.e. hxy creates x coordinate changes in an object that are proportional to it's y values. Defined in this manner, $\mathbf{H}$ and $\mathbf{S}$ can be combined to create,

$$\mathbf{D} = \mathbf{H} \, \mathbf{S}, \tag{8}$$

where the matrix elements of $\mathbf{D}$ are,

$$\mathbf{D} = \begin{bmatrix} sx & sy \, hxy & sz \, hxz \\ sx \, hyx & sy & sz \, hyz \\ sx \, hzx & sy \, hzy & sz \end{bmatrix}. \tag{9}$$

In constructing (14) it was recognized that $\mathbf{S}$ and $\mathbf{H}$ could be combined in a different order ($\mathbf{H}$ would have to be transposed), but this choice was made since it was felt that $\mathbf{S}$ should be placed rightmost (see 8). This was done in preparation for concatenation of the deformation matrix with the target matrix, $\mathbf{P}_C$. In this way, a given object will be scaled, then sheared, rather than the other way around.

The symbolic matrix $\mathbf{D}$ contains 9 different variables, but in practice this expression presents certain difficulties. The version of $\mathbf{D}$ used for Pliant Surface modeling must contain only 6 DOF. This restriction is explained as follows. If one examines the pairs of off-diagonal terms in $\mathbf{H}$: (hxy, hyx), (hxz, hzx) and (hyz, hzy), one will note that each pair indicates the total amount of shear that can be specified within a given plane. While the elements in these pairs may seem to be independent, in essence they are not. Both will produce the rotation of a specific axis within the same given plane, albeit they move in opposite directions. Thus, with respect to the z axis (and the xy plane), an hxy shear represents a rotation of the y axis towards x, while an hyx shear represents a rotation of x towards y. In light of these relationships, it can be concluded that interdependencies exists between shearing and rotation.

Fortunately, this uncertainty can be easily avoided. In (7), and hence in (9), specific choices can be made as to the elements in each $\mathbf{H}$ pair that one wishes to keep. These choices should not be made on an arbitrary basis, but instead should reflect the qualitative characteristics of the shape changes that one would expect to see for a given body segment. This process is demonstrated as follows.

Assume that we have chosen our specific shearing model to include hxy, hxz and hzy. From (7), $\mathbf{H_M}$ will be derived with hyx, hzx and hyz set to zero. Additionally, in specifying $\mathbf{S_M}$, it can be shown that it is necessary to restrict $\mathbf{S} > 0$. Having constructed these matrices, the specific version of $\mathbf{D_M}$ can be created as follows:

$$\mathbf{D}_M = \begin{bmatrix} sx & sy\ hxy & sz\ hxz \\ 0 & sy & 0 \\ 0 & sy\ hzy & sz \end{bmatrix}, \tag{10}$$

from whence, the relationships in (5) may be re-expressed as:

$$\mathbf{P}_O = \mathbf{R}_M\ \mathbf{D}_M\ \mathbf{P_C} + \mathbf{T}_M + \varepsilon, \tag{11}$$

and hence, the Pliant Model's expression for $\mathbf{P_M}$ is,

$$\mathbf{P}_M = \mathbf{R}_M\ \mathbf{D}_M\ \mathbf{P_C} + \mathbf{T}_M. \tag{12}$$

Inspection reveals that (11) contains 12 DOF, however, care must be taken in deriving these individual solutions. As was stated, coupling exists between the rotational DOF and the various entries that were chosen for the shearing matrix. As such, if one desires to find a best-fitting solution for $\mathbf{R_M}$, then care must be taken in defining the characteristics of $\mathbf{D_M}$. A similar interdependency can also be shown for translation and scaling, $\mathbf{T_M}$ and $\mathbf{S_M}$, respectively. This problem is presently dealt with by assuming that $\mathbf{T_M}$ quantifies the linear distance between the numerical centroids of $\mathbf{P_C}$ and $\mathbf{P_O}$. Performed in this way, the translational DOF may be derived *a priori*.

Cursory comparisons of the models expressed in (2) and (11) yields one obvious observation; that the Pliant Surface model differs only by the inclusion of $\mathbf{D_M}$. Introduction of this matrix, however, produces several interesting effects. First, since the Pliant Model includes scaling and shearing, this model should be expected to produce better estimates of $\mathbf{P_M}$, hence this will reduce the magnitude of $\mathbf{E_{OM}}$ (see 4). This ability to more faithfully match the observations of markers on a body segment also provides human movement researchers with the ability to model shape changes. Second, since one can actually specify the contents of $\mathbf{D_M}$ (and hence, its characterization of pliant motion), this process offers the prospect that more accurate estimates of $\mathbf{R_M}$ can be derived. This process, however, also offers the opposite potential, that inappropriate selections can be made for $\mathbf{D_M}$. Third, while Rigid modeling procedures require the use of matched data from 3 or more non-collinear markers, the procedures for Pliant Surface modeling actually demand that 4 or more, non-coplanar, markers be viewed upon each body segment. This adaptation is required since the solution for (11) involves the calculation of 12, not 6, kinematic DOF.

1.3. Experimental validation of Pliant Surface modeling

For the purposes of conducting definitive experimental comparisons it was necessary to obtain "Gold Standard" human movement data. Fortunately, the simultaneous use of Rigid Body modeling, along with invasive methods of data collection had been shown to provide such results[14,20,21]. In their studies, researchers had surgically inserted bone pin(s) into the tibia and femur of their subjects. Most, had also used these procedures (called Rigid Invasive modeling) to examine gait. Thus, measurements of the knee's gait patterns were selected as the test-bed for examining the relative performances of the Pliant and Rigid Surface models.

2. METHODS

2.1. Subject selection

All subjects (N=3) volunteered to participate in the experiments. Prior to the data collection sessions, each subject completed a signed consent form. The subject group had the following characteristics: 37 ± 3 yrs., 1.81 ± 0.07m, 82.7 ± 4.5 kg. Each subject possessed a typical walking pattern, but one of the subjects had undergone a partial medial menisectomy, non-arthroscopically, 15 years earlier.

2.2. Surgical insertion of bone pins

Two pin sites were used: one on the tibia, the other on the femur. Both sites were selected such that bone pins (Howmedica self-tapping, self-screwing 150 mm in length, 4 mm diameter) could be inserted without having to pass through large amounts of muscle or soft tissue. Gerdy's tubercle was chosen as the pin site for the tibia, while the greater trochanter was selected for the femur. This latter site featured much greater proximity to the hip than it did to the knee but it was preferred for three reasons. First, the femur is a relatively rigid structure. Second, the greater trochanter site avoided possible complications with movements of the iliotibial band over the lateral border of the knee. Third, the lateral placement of both pin sites avoided possible collisions between the opposite knee and the pins.

2.3. Measurement of 3D coordinates

2.3.1. Camera systems

Two OptoTrak Model 3020 camera systems (Northern Digital, Waterloo, Ontario, Canada) working in parallel were used to record the 3D point data. Each camera system consisted of 3 one-dimensional sensors housed within a single enclosure. Each sensor digitized infrared light with 16-bit precision. The two units were synchronized and calibrated such that both systems contributed to the measurement of 3D coordinates within the experimental volume. Each OptoTrak camera exclusively records infrared light, as such, the system uses active (light-emitting) infrared markers called IREDS. This design offers great advantages in terms of both processing time and ease of use. The system unit sequentially fires the IREDS, while at the same time the sensors on the camera(s) are notified. In this way, positional time-series data can be determined for each IRED by each sensor automatically. These data can also be combined, without significant user intervention, to generate lists of individual 3D coordinates. The manufacturer stated that each system alone has a 3D reconstruction accuracy of 0.15 mm at a distance of 2.5 m, but used together the total system accuracy should have been better still. The software used for the tasks of 3D calibration and data collection was provided by the system manufacturer.

2.3.2. Experimental volume

The experimental volume approximated 2 m in length, 2 m in width, and 2 m in height. All physical activities were conducted such that the subjects performed centrally within this volume. The cameras were located such that the entire lateral surface and much of the anterior surface of each subject's leg could be kept constantly in view. With respect to each subject's control position (described below), both cameras were placed approximately 3 m away. One camera viewed the subject's anteriolateral surface from a position that was approximately 30° removed in a horizontal direction from the plane of progression. The second camera recorded the lateral surface of the subject from a position that was approximately 10° posteriorly removed along the horizontal plane from an imaginary line drawn perpendicular to the sagittal plane.

2.3.3. Placement of markers

While the definition of only two body segments, the upper and lower leg, would normally be required for the measurement of knee motion, four representative body segments were actually defined since these experiments sought to evaluate the abilities of three different kinematic models: Rigid Invasive, Rigid Surface and Pliant Surface modeling. Two of the segments were associated with motions of the lower leg, while the other two were used to measure the thigh's activities. Table 1 describes the characteristics of these marker placements.

Body Segment	# IREDS	Cluster Shape	Cluster Rigidity	Approximate Dimensions (cm)	Placement Characteristics	Place of Attachment
Tibial Object	4	disk	rigid	spaced at 3.5 cm radius	planar: circular	bone pin into Gerdy's tubercle
Leg Surface	16	hemi-cylindrical	non-rigid	height * width: 20 * 15 cm	non-planar: random, distributed	approximately 1/2 of the leg's surface
Femoral Object	4	disk	rigid	spaced at 3.5 cm radius	planar: circular	bone pin into the greater trochanter
Thigh Surface	20	hemi-cylindrical	non-rigid	height * width: 30 * 20 cm	non-planar: random, distributed,	approximately 1/2 of the thigh's surface

Table 1. Characteristics of the 4 body segments. The Tibial Object and Leg Surface were associated with the lower leg, while the Femoral Object and Thigh Surface were used for the upper leg.

2.4. Experimental protocol

2.4.1. Static data - control position

The subjects stood upright with their feet shoulder width apart, toes pointing forward in their own comfortable stance position. None of the subjects showed a typical predisposition towards knee hyperextension. Data were collected for 3 seconds at 50 Hz in this static position. These data served to define the body segment Control Points, P_C, for each of the subjects.

2.4.2. Dynamic data - treadmill trials

A small treadmill (Quinton Instruments, Seattle, WA., Model 4-44B) was used. Each subject was acclimatized to the treadmill by having them walk at their own self-selected speed and pace. Kinematic data were collected for three velocities of treadmill gait, Slow (0.66 ms^{-1}), Medium (1.10 ms^{-1}) and Fast (1.54 ms^{-1}). These data served to define the observed points, P_O. In each trial, the subjects were asked to walk at a specified velocity using their own self-selected pace. Once their gait pattern had become stable, they indicated this, then kinematic data were collected at 50 Hz for a period of 20 seconds. Each data collection captured from 12 to 20 strides of gait. The actual number of strides depended upon the preset treadmill velocity and the subject's own self-selected cadence.

2.5. Data analysis

As described in section 1.1, the methods of Rigid modeling were used to analyze the motion of the surface and bone pin markers. This resulted in the production of 6 DOF Rigid Surface and Rigid Invasive modeled data. Similarly, the methods of Pliant Surface modeling, described in section 1.2, were used to analyze the surface marker data. Selected *a priori*, the Pliant Model featured greater rigidity in its superior/inferior direction, and greater pliancy in its anterior/posterior dimension. These analyses resulted in 12 DOF descriptions of segment motion: 6 rigid and 6 pliant motion characteristics. Since the input data were collected simultaneously for all three models, a number of interesting comparisons could be performed. First, the segmental data were geometrically compared for the purposes of deriving joint data. Second, since the Rigid Invasive model produced sets of Gold Standard results, the 6 DOF differences (geometric) between these data and those from the Rigid Surface and Pliant Surface models were calculated at both the joint and segmental levels. Third, these segmental and joint differences were summarized by determining their overall root mean squares (RMS). Fourth, the RMS data were statistically compared by performing chi-square tests (p<.01) of the comparisons between variances. Fifth, the Pliant Surface model's scaling and shearing results were converted into a meaningful form: scaling was expressed as a % change from the object's original size, and shearing was described in angular form as the amount by which the object's shape differed from its original orthogonality. Sixth, based only on the abilities of the Rigid and Pliant Surface technique's to model the thigh and leg's 3D surface data, simple comparisons (ratios) were performed. Finally, it should be noted that the results for the joint translation data will not be presented here.

3. RESULTS

Although three different velocities of gait were investigated, the RMS data associated with these estimates of rotation were ultimately pooled across the velocity condition since no significant difference were noted between the two models (N = 8142 frames, N = 276 strides). However, within the models, the velocity condition did produce slightly higher measurement errors, and a moderate increase in pliant activity.

3.1. Estimates of skeletal motion

Presented in Figure 1 is a representative trial of the 3 rotational DOF tibiofemoral motion that was measured from one of the subjects. This data was obtained through the use of bone pins and Rigid Invasive modeling. Table 2 presents an overall summary of the RMS errors that were produced by the Pliant and Rigid Surface models in estimating this rotation. In general, these data indicate that the motions of the tibia could be estimated with nearly twice the accuracy of the femur. The overall errors associated with the estimates of tibiofemoral motion were only slightly higher than those for the femur alone. Nevertheless, the performances of the Pliant Surface were found to be statistically superior to those of the Rigid Surface model (p<.01) in estimating both femoral and tibiofemoral motion; no significant differences were noted for tibial motion.

3.2. Pliant motion characteristics

Figures 2 and 3 provide representative samples of the pliant motions that were measured for the gait cycle. These data were actually determined from the same gait trial (for the same subject) as was presented in Figure 1. The largest scale changes (Figure 2) were found to occur across the lateral dimensions of both the Leg and Thigh Surfaces. Sizable shearing effects (Figure 3) were seen to occur in all three anatomical planes for both segments. With respect to the two body segments: the pliant changes in the Leg Surface (left plots) appeared to be more specifically related to the activities of push-off (at approximately 60% of the gait stride), while the thigh's pliant effects were both, larger in magnitude, and more evenly distributed throughout, than those for the lower leg.

3.3. Modeling of the 3D surface points

With respect to the abilities of the two Surface models to follow the approximate motions of the observed 3D coordinates, the Pliant Surface model produced lower RMS errors in every trial. In fact, where the Rigid Surface results for the Leg and Thigh Surface (3.8 and 4.8 mm, respectively) were used as a baseline, the Pliant Surface technique used its non-rigid capabilities to reduce these errors by 56% and 45%, respectively.

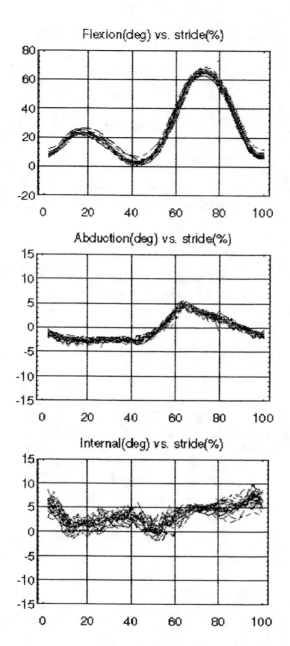

Figure 1. A representative sample of one subject's tibiofemoral rotation as measured during the gait cycle. These results were obtained through the use of Rigid Invasive modeling. The stance phase occurred for approximately the first 60% of each stride. The subject walked at a rate of 1.54 ms^{-1}. A total of 19 gait strides, collected over 20 seconds, are presented. No techniques of temporal data smoothing were applied to these data.

Model	Tibia		Femur		Tibiofemoral Joint	
	Pliant Surface	Rigid Surface	Pliant Surface	Rigid Surface	Pliant Surface	Rigid Surface
High CI	2.50°	2.43°	4.00°	4.35°	4.75°	5.24°
Low CI	2.41°	2.35°	3.86°	4.20°	4.58°	5.05°

Table 2. Comparison of the abilities of the Pliant Surface and Rigid Surface models to estimate tibial, femoral and tibiofemoral motion. Overall root mean square differences between the modeled surface, and gold standard bone pin data are presented. High and low 99% confidence intervals (CI) are stated for each condition. Where CI overlap exists, the performances of the models were not significantly different. Conversely, the Pliant Surface model provided significantly more accurate estimates of Femoral and Tibiofemoral motion.

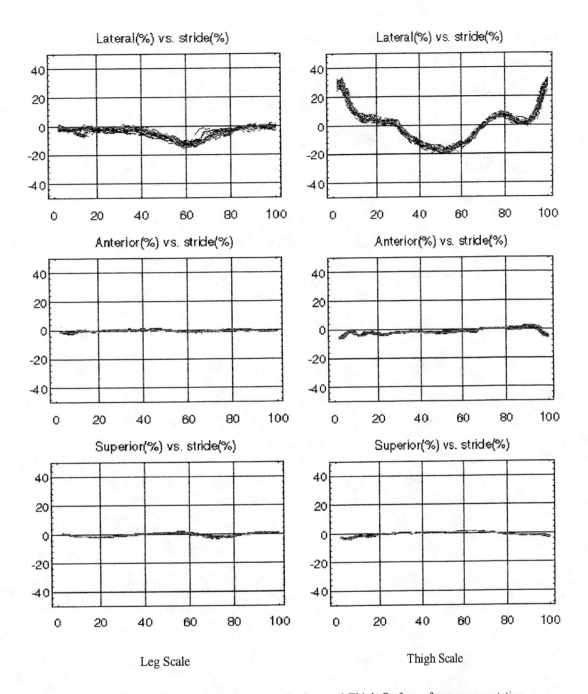

Leg Scale   Thigh Scale

Figure 2. Scale changes (%) in the Leg Surface and Thigh Surface of one representative subject as measured during the gait cycle. Pliant Surface modeling was used to obtained these results. The subject walked at a rate of 1.54 ms⁻¹. A total of 19 gait strides, collected over 20 seconds, are presented. No techniques of temporal data smoothing were applied to these data.

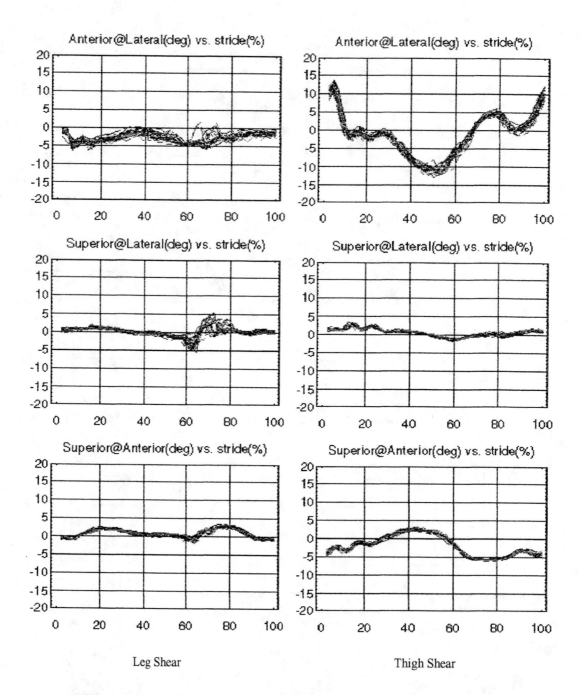

Leg Shear

Thigh Shear

Figure 3. Shear changes (°) in the Leg Surface and Thigh Surface of one representative subject as measured during the gait cycle. Viewed from top to bottom, these plots demonstrate shearing in the transverse, frontal and sagittal planes. Pliant Surface modeling was used to obtained these data. The subject walked at a rate of 1.54 ms⁻¹. A total of 19 gait strides, collected over 20 seconds, are presented. No techniques of temporal data smoothing were applied.

4. DISCUSSION

Kinematic methods, such as Rigid Surface modeling, have typically regarded the body's natural soft-tissue motions as if they were the result of experimental error. In this context, researchers have used the methods of Rigid Body modeling to identify physical locations on the human body that have the lowest potential for tissue shift[14,22,23]. It is these locations that have been suggested for marker placement. Despite these efforts, only limited success will ever be achieved. Human movement, by its very nature, depends upon soft-tissue movement.

The skeleton provides the body with an internal rigid framework. The muscles act as its shape transducers. Given neural stimulation, the muscles rearrange their own specific volumes. In doing so, they create movements within the joints of the human body. The skin and its underlying fascia, quite naturally, must provide adequate distensability for these activities. However, it is at this external interface that the problems of human movement research have typically occurred.

At present, the procedures of Pliant Surface modeling have been limited to the measurement of affine deformations. It is clearly recognized, however, that the soft tissues of the body may exhibit many specific local patterns of movement. Identification of these phenomena may prove quite useful (i.e. patellar tracking). To quantify these motions, future models may be able to borrow upon the more advanced techniques of deformable solid modeling[18] and freeform deformation[19]. Additionally, recent developments in the use of B-spline solid primitives[24] show considerable promise. Such efforts will require the registration of even greater numbers of DOF. These efforts are strongly encouraged.

5. CONCLUSIONS

Pliant Surface modeling offers exciting new opportunities for the assessment of human motion. Where typical methods of movement analysis have only offered the ability to model a body segment's rigid characteristics (3 rotations and 3 translations), Pliant Surface modeling is designed to quantify 6 additional DOF (3 scales and 3 shears). Validation experiments have shown that this added complexity can be quite advantageous: 1) the Pliant Surface model produced more accurate estimates of femoral and tibiofemoral motion, 2) the Pliant model produced unique repeatable patterns of scaling and shearing, 3) the non-rigidity within the Leg and Thigh Surfaces was made evident; where the 3D results for the Rigid Surface model were used as a baseline, the Pliant Surface model reduced these measurement errors by 56% and 45%, respectively. Despite these clear advantages, the Pliant Surface model also offers considerable ease of use. In comparison with Rigid Surface modeling, only one additional marker is required per body segment (non-coplanar). Future efforts on Pliant Surface modeling will investigate: marker placement sensitivities, the automatic configuration of Pliant Models, and the ability to quantify other forms of pliant motion, i.e. bends, twists. In closing, it is hoped that Pliant Surface modeling will gain future acceptance, in both basic and applied research settings, as a useful tool for the evaluation of human movement.

6. REFERENCES

1. K.A. Ball and M.R. Pierrynowski, "Estimation of six degree of freedom rigid body segment motion from two dimensional data", *Human Movement Science* **14**, pp. 139-154, 1995.
2. B.K.P. Horn, "Closed-form solution of absolute orientation using quaternions", *J. Opt. Soc. Am. A.* **4**, pp. 629-641, 1987.
3. I. Söderkvist and P.-A. Wedin, "Determining the movement of the skeleton using well-configured markers", *Journal of Biomechanics* **26**, pp. 1473-1477, 1993.
4. C.W. Spoor and F.E. Veldpaus, "Rigid body motion calculated from spatial coordinates of markers", *Journal of Biomechanics* **13**, pp. 391-393, 1980.
5. S.J. Tupling and M.R. Pierrynowski, "Use of Cardan angles to locate rigid bodies in three-dimensional space", *Med. Biol. Engng. Comput.* **25**, pp. 527-532, 1987.
6. F.E. Veldpaus, H.J. Woltring and L.J.M.G. Dortmans, "A least squares algorithm for the equiform transformation from spatial marker coordinates", *Journal of Biomechanics* **21**, pp. 45-54 ,1988.

7. H.J. Woltring, R. Huiskes and A. de Lange, "Finite centroid and helical axis estimation from noisy landmark measurements in the study of human joint kinematics", *Journal of Biomechanics* **18**, pp. 379-389, 1985.

8. K.A. Ball and M.R. Pierrynowski, "Classification of errors in locating a rigid body", *Journal of Biomechanics* **29**(9), pp. 1213-1217 ,1996.

9. J.L. Ronsky and B.M. Nigg, "Error in kinematic data due to marker attachment methods", In *Proceedings of the XIIIth Congress of Biomechanics.* (pp. 390-392). Perth, Australia: The University of Western Australia, 1991.

10. C. Angeloni, A. Cappozzo, F. Catani, and A. Leardini, "Quantification of relative displacement of skin- and plate- mounted markers with respect to the bones" (Abstract), *Journal of Biomechanics*, **26**, pp. 864, 1993.

11. F.L. Buczek, T.M., Kepple, K. Lohmann Siegel and S. Stanhope, "Translational and rotational joint power terms in a six degree-of-freedom model of the normal ankle complex", *Journal of Biomechanics* **27**(12), pp. 1447-1457, 1994.

12. J.M. Laviolette and M.R. Pierrynowski, "Optimal marker placement for kinematic studies of the human lower extremity", In *Proceedings of the Canadian Society for Biomechanics, Locomotion Conference*, Ottawa, Ontario, pp. 38-39 ,1988.

13. A. Cappozzo, F. Catani, U. Della Croce and A. Leardini, "Position and orientation in space of bones during movement: Anatomical frame definition and determination", *Clinical Biomechanics* **10**, pp. 171-178, 1995.

14. C. Reinschmidt, "Three-Dimensional Tibiocalcaneal and Tibiofemoral Kinematics during Human Locomotion - Measured with External and Bone Markers", Doctor of Philosophy dissertation, University of Calgary, Calgary, Alberta, 1996.

15. A. Cappozzo, "Three-dimensional analysis of human walking: Experimental methods and associated artifacts", *Human Movement Science 10, pp.* 589-602, 1991.

16. H.J. Woltring, "One Hundred Years of Photogrammetry in Biolocomotion". In A. Cappozzo, M. Marchetti, & V. Tosi (Eds.), *Biolocomotion: A Century of Research using Moving Pictures,* pp. 199-225, Rome: Promograph, 1992.

17. D.F. Rogers and J.A. Adams, *Mathematical Elements for Computer Graphics, second edition*, New York: McGraw-Hill Publishing Company, 1990.

18. A.H. Barr, "Global and local deformations of solid primitives", *Computer Graphics* **18**(3), pp. 21-30, 1984.

19. T.W. Sederberg and S.R. Parry, "Freeform deformation of solid geometric models", *Computer Graphics* **20**(4), pp. 18-22, 1986.

20. M.A. Lafortune, "The Use of Intra-corticol Pins to Measure the Motion of the Knee Joint during Walking", Doctor of Philosophy dissertation, The Pennsylvania State University, 1984.

21. M.C. Murphy, "Geometry and the kinematics of the normal human knee", Doctor of Philosophy dissertation, Massachusetts Institute of Technology, 1990.

22. M.A. Lafortune and M.J. Lake, "Errors in 3D analysis of human movement", In *Proceedings of the International Conference on 3-D Analysis of Human Movement*, Quebec City, pp. 55-56, 1991.

23. A. Cappozzo, F. Catani, A. Leardini, M.G. Benedetti and U. Della Croce, "Position and orientation in space of bones during movement: experimental artifacts", *Clinical Biomechanics* **11***, pp.* 90-100 ,1996.

24. V. Ng-Thow-Hing, A. Agur, K.A. Ball, E. Fiume and N. McKee, "Shape reconstruction and subsequent deformation of soleus muscle models using B-spline solid primitives". In *Proceedings of SPIE - The International Society for Optical Engineering, BiOS ' 98 - International Biomedical Optics Symposium*, 24-30 January, 1998, San Jose, CA, 1998.

The Subcutaneous Adipose Tissue Topography (SAT-Top) by means of the optical device Lipometer is highly correlated to plasma leptin levels in obese boys.

Karl Sudi[1], Reinhard Möller[2], Erwin Tafeit[2], Elke Reiterer[3], Martin Borkenstein[3], Karoline Vrecko[2], Renate Horejsi[2], Gilbert Reibnegger[2] and Peter Hofmann[1]

[1] Institute for Sport Sciences, Karl-Franzens University Graz; 8010 Graz - Austria
[2] Institute for Medical Chemistry and Pregl-Laboratory, Karl-Franzens University Graz; 8010 Graz - Austria; [3] Department for Diabetology and Endocrinology, Pediatric Hospital Graz; 8044 Graz - Austria

ABSTRACT

The product of the ob-gene named *leptin* is correlated with body fat mass in humans. Little evidence exists if the same holds true for body fat distribution. In this study we therefore investigated plasma leptin levels and the subcutaneous adipose tissue topography (SAT-Top) by means of the newly developed optical device Lipometer before and after a 3 week weight reduction camp. 34 obese boys (mean age 12a) took part in this study. Body fat distribution were assessed by means of Lipometer to measure the thickness of a subcutaneous fat layer at 15 standardised body sites (SAT-Top). Plasma leptin levels (*LL*) were measured by radioimmunoassay. All measurements were taken at the beginning and at the end of the camp. By dividing all boys according chronological age (group A: age <12a, n=17/ group B: >12a, n=17) we found correlations with the combination of measured body sites (*MBS*) before (A: *MBS* vs. *LL*, R^2=0.79; p<0.01 / B: *MBS* vs. *LL*, R^2=0.35; n.s.) and after (A: *MBS* vs. *LL*, R^2=0.83; p<0.01 / B: *MBS* vs. *LL*, R^2=0.70; p<0.01) the intervention. Our study confirms that the subcutaneous adipose tissue topography (SAT-Top) by means of the optical device Lipometer serves as a marker of plasma leptin levels in obese boys and highlights the use of this optical device in a predictive manner.

Keywords: Subcutaneous Adipose Tissue Topography (SAT-Top), Optical device, Lipometer, Obesity, Leptin, Boys

1. INTRODUCTION

In 1994 the positional cloning of the mouse *ob* gene and its human homologue by Zhang et al.[1] and the identification and expression cloning of a leptin receptor by Tartaglia et al.[2] was an outstanding success in research concerning body weight regulation mechanisms. The product of the *ob* gene named leptin is a 16-kDa plasma protein hormone which is expressed in white adipocytes and also synthesized in human placentae at delivery[3]. Although the mechanisms by which leptin acts are not clearly understood it is possible that due to the presence of leptin receptors the brain is one of the target organs of leptin`s action[4].

During the last years it has been established that weight loss in humans can reduce plasma leptin concentrations [5-7]. If obese people were set on hypocaloric diet the reduction in leptin levels uncouples from changes in body fat mass[7].

Studies concerning obesity research have shown that leptin is direct related to nearly all parameters of body composition. A very simple model like the Body Mass Index (*BMI*) provides evidence that height and body weight may be determinants of circulating leptin levels. More sophisticated methods to determine body composition e.g. bioelectrical impedance analysis (*BIA*), underwater weighing (*UWW*), near infrared interactance (*NIR*) or imaging techniques (Computed Tomography *CT*, Magnetic Resonance Imaging *MRI*) are limited for several reasons[8]. All studies investigating leptin levels under different aims found strong positive correlations with total body fat mass as measured by several methods of body composition assessment. Additionally it was shown that leptin might be related to specific fat depots measured by magnetic resonance[9]. It is therefore possible that leptin concentrations are more closely linked to the subcutaneous than the visceral fat mass especially in children and young adults.

This field of leptin and adiposity research underlines the necessity to use more appropriate methods to measure body fat distribution. The aim of this study was therefore to investigate the relationship between subcutaneous adipose tissue distribution (subcutaneous adipose tissue topography; *SAT-Top*) measured by the optical device *Lipometer* and leptin levels in obese boys before and after a 3 week diet intervention including intense physical activity for a reduction in body weight and body fat mass.

2. SUBJECTS AND METHODS

34 obese boys were investigated before and after a weight reduction camp. Metabolic and anthropometric characteristics are given in Table 1. Boys were assigned to a low-caloric diet depending on the degree of overweight and age. Physical activity was performed thrice daily and consisted of activities like biking, swimming and playing soccer. Body fat distribution were assessed by means of the newly developed optical device *Lipometer* to measure the thickness of a subcutaneous fat layer at 15 standardised body sites (SAT-Top). The technical characteristics have already been published[10]. Briefly, the Lipometer uses light emitting diodes which illuminate the interesting subcutaneous fatty layer. A photodiode measures the corresponding light intensities backscattered. These light signals are amplified, digitised and stored in a computer.

The 15 body sites for the measurement of SAT-Top are distributed over the whole body from neck to calf at the right body site (Fig. 1). For these measurements boys were in standing position. Plasma leptin levels were measured by radioimmunoassay (Linco, Res. Inc., standard available kit) (Table 1). Measurements for leptin and SAT-Top were performed at the beginning and at the end of the camp after an overnight fast.

Standard statistical analysis was performed. For normally distributed data Student`s t-test and Pearson correlation coefficient were used for analysis. For data not normally distributed non-parametric statistics were employed. P values less than 0.05 were considered significant. All values are Means ± SD.

3. RESULTS

Body mass (-5.1kg ± 1.5kg) and leptin levels (-6.6 ng/ml ± 4.6 ng/ml) decreased in the boys over the 3 week period (all p<0.0001). The best correlations between leptin levels (*LL*) and the thickness of the different body sites (SAT-layers) were found for the following body sites before (pre) the intervention: *LL*/neck; R^2= 0.41, *LL*/upper back; R^2= 0.33 and *LL*/lateral chest; R^2= 0.25. For all the other body sites correlations (R^2) are ranged between 0.02 and 0.23. After the intervention (post) the correlation between *LL* and the thickness of the measured body sites increased in all cases. Some of the highest correlations (and corresponding increases) for the above mentioned association were noticed for *LL*/biceps; post: R^2= 0.61 vs. pre: R^2= 0.07 (Fig. 2), *LL*/upper back; post: R^2= 0.69 vs. pre: R^2= 0.33 (Fig. 3). All coefficients (R^2) for leptin levels and the measured body sites are given in the *Leptinogram* (Table 2). The best overall indicator of any association between SAT-topography and leptin levels was found for the mean value of the sum of 3 measured body sites (biceps, upper back and rear thigh) after the intervention (R^2= 0.69; Fig. 4). No significant correlation was found between leptin levels and body weight before and after the diet intervention whereas the absolute amount of body fat mass calculated by means of Lipometer showed a significant correlation with leptin levels before (r= 0.59; p=0.0002) and after (r= 0.71; p<0.0001) the 3 weeks (data not shown in this work).

By dividing all boys according their Tanner stages (pubic hair and testes volume) to identify biological development (*group A*: prepubertal-, *group B*: pubertal stage) there was no clear distinction between these stages regarding the related SAT-Top of the boys. After splitting in a younger group of boys (Y: age <12a, n=17) and an older one (O: >12a, n=17) we identified strong correlations with the combination of measured body sites (*MBS*) before (pre: Y: *MBS* vs. *LL*, R^2=0.79; p<0.01 / O: *MBS* vs. *LL*, R^2=0.35; n.s.) and after (post: Y: *MBS* vs. *LL*, R^2=0.83; p<0.01 / O: *MBS* vs. *LL*, R^2=0.70; p<0.01) the intervention.

4. DISCUSSION

Our study investigated the subcutaneous adipose tissue topography (SAT-Top) by means of the optical device Lipometer and their association with leptin levels in obese boys. We found strong correlation between the combination of measured body sites and leptin levels. These associations between leptin and different body sites were pronounced after the intervention which suggests a common basis of an energy related factor, leptin, and physiological pathways connecting body fat and physical activity.

There is however a possible sex related difference to be mentioned. The allways reported sexual dimorphism in leptin levels, women showing elevated leptin levels even after correction for the higher body fat mass, but couldn't be explained until the work of Wabitsch et al. 1997 investigated the effects of testosterone and dihydrotestosterone on human adipocytes in primary culture[11]. Wabitsch and co-workers showed that androgens are able to reduce leptin secretion into the culture medium which might be the reason for the observed differences in leptin concentrations between boys and girls. Leptin therefore might be involved in growth and development related factors. It is not astonishing that leptin levels are correlated with those of GH-binding protein in prepubertal children[12]. Furthermore it was shown that growth hormone secretion is regulated by leptin[13]. We, on the other hand, did neither controll for levels of androgens nor levels of other growth related factors in the obese boys.

Additionally, our results might be limited for an extended interpretation because we did not compare leptin levels of the obese boys with that of age and sex matched normal weight controls.

How might the findings of our investigation be linked to subcutaneous adipose tissue ?

A possible explanation was suggested by a putative hypothalamic-pituitary-adrenal-adipose axis which in turn could be up- or downregulated by leptin (Heiman et al. 1997)[14].

The observation that leptin fits better to body fat distribution (or vice versa) after a diet and sport intervention programe in obese boys could be a sign for an improved sensitivity of leptin and (or) the endocrine system in general. This restoration of a relative leptin resistance could therefore be the main benefit of such an intervention programe. On the other hand there exists no study which examined the effects of diet and physical activity on the long-term outcome in respect of leptin levels. If low leptin levels are associated with decreased energy expenditure and higher food intake one would ask where is the ratio behind the results of our study. Low leptin levels as measured in the obese boys after the intervention could therefore be a sign of further weight gain. In contrast to this assumption it is possible to speculate about a higher degree of leptin sensitivity after a diet and sport intervention programe. This could be a necessary condition for a subsequent restoration of blunted metabolic pathways in obese boys.

Future studies will have to rely on the impact of weight reduction programes on different body fat tissue compartments in boys and girls. This will include the investigations of hormones, e.g. testosterone, insulin, and growth-hormone-related factors, and their association with body fat distribution. In addition to, these studies will consider the effects of different modes of exercise training on body weight regulation mechanisms in the long-term outcome.

We might conclude that the optical device Lipometer is an accurate and valid method to measure the thickness of the subcutaneous adipose tissue layer. Moreover we emphasize the Subcutaneous Adipose Tissue Topography (SAT-Top) as a non-invasive, rapid and safe approach to describe the link of metabolic related biochemical variables with body fat distribution.

5. REFERENCES

1. Y. Zhang, R. Proenca, M. Maffei, M. Barone, I. Leopold, and J.M. Friedman, „Positional cloning of the mouse *ob*-gene and its human homologue", *Nature* 372; pp. 425-432, 1994.

2. L. Tartaglia, M. Dembski, X. Weng, N. Deng, J. Culpepper, R. Devos, et al., „Identification and expression cloning of a leptin receptor, *OB*-R", *Cell* 83; pp. 1263-1271, 1995.

3. R. Senaris, T. Garcia-Caballero, X. Casabiell, R. Gallego, R. Castro, et al., „Synthesis of Leptin in human placenta", *Endocrinology* 138 (10); pp. 4501-4504, 1997.

4. F. Rohner-Jeanrenaud and B. Jeanrenaud, „Obesity, Leptin, And The Brain",
The New England Journal of Medicine 334 (5); pp. 324-325, 1996.

5. M. Maffei, J. Halaas, E. Ravussin, R.E. Pratley, G.H. Lee, et al., „Leptin levels in human and rodent: measurement of plasma leptin and ob RNA in obese and weight-reduced subjects",
Nature Medicine 1; pp. 1155-1161, 1995.

6. R.V. Considine, M.K. Sinha, M.L. Heiman, A. Kriauciunas, T.W. Stephens, et al.,
„Serum immunoreactive-leptin concentration in normal-weight and obese humans",
The New England Journal of Medicine 334; pp. 292-295, 1996.

7. G.H. Scholz, P. Englaro, I. Thiele, M. Scholz, T. Klusmann, et al., „Dissociation of serum leptin concentration and body fat content during long-term dietary intervention in obese individuals",
Hormone and Metabolic Research 28 (12); pp. 718-723, 1996.

8. H.C. Lukaski, „Methods for the assessment of human body composition: traditional and new", American Journal of Clinical Nutrition 46; pp. 537-556, 1987.

9. S. Caprio, W.V. Tamberlane, D. Silver, C. Robinson, R. Leibel, et al., „Hyperleptinemia: an early sign of juvenile obesity. Relations to body fat depots and insulin concentrations",
American Journal of Physiology 271 (3); pp. E626-E630, 1996.

10. R. Möller, E. Tafeit, K.H. Smolle, P. Kullnig, „Lipometer: determining the thickness of an subcutaneous fatty layer", *Biosensorics and Bioelectronics* 9; pp. xiii-xvi, 1994.

11. M. Wabitsch, W.F. Blume, R. Muche, M. Braun, F. Hube, et al., „Contribution of androgens to the gender differences in leptin production in obese children and adolescents", *Journal of Clinical Investigation* 100 (4); pp. 808-813, 1997.

12. R. Bjarnason, M. Boguszewski, J. Dahlgren, J. Gelander, B. Kriström, et al.,
„Leptin levels are strongly correlated with those of GH-binding protein in prepubertal children",
European Journal of Endocrinology 137; pp. 68-73, 1997.

13. E. Carro, R. Senaris, R.V. Considine, F.F. Casanueva, C. Dieguez, „Regulation of in vivo growth hormone secretion by leptin", *Endocrinology* 138 (5); pp. 2203-2206, 1997.

14. M.L. Heiman, R.S. Ahima, L.S. Craft, B. Schoner, T.W. Stephens, and J.S. Flier,
„Leptin inhibition of the hypothalamic-pituitary-adrenal axis in response to stress",
Endocrinology 138 (9); pp. 3859-3863, 1997.

Table 1. Anthropometric characteristics and leptin values of obese boys before and after the weight reduction programme. Values are mean, standard deviations are in parentheses

Boys (n=36)	Before	Post	Difference	P
Age (y)	12 (1.7)			
Height (cm)	155.5 (10.2)			
Body Mass (kg)	65.3 (14.6)	60.2 (13.4)	5.1 (1.5)	a
Leptin (ng/ml)	12.7 (6.2)	5.9 (2.4)	6.6 (4.6)	a

Note. n= Numbers. P Significance between before and post intervention; a: p< 0.0001

Body site	R^2 pre	R^2 post
1-neck	0,42	0,54
2-triceps	0,24	0,56
3-biceps	0,09	0,69
4-up.back	0,33	0,75
5-fr.chest	0,21	0,69
6-lat.chest	0,26	0,58
7-up.abd.	0,12	0,42
8-lo.abd.	0,12	0,19
9-lo.back	0,19	0,58
10-hip	0,08	0,60
11-fr.thigh	0,15	0,46
12-lat.thigh	0,05	0,39
13-r.thigh	0,26	0,31
14-in.thigh	0,10	0,32
15-calf	0,14	0,20

Table 2. *Leptinogram*: Correlation between serum leptin levels and all body sites measured show the varying interrelations before and after the diet and sport intervention programe.

LIPOMETER Standardised body sites

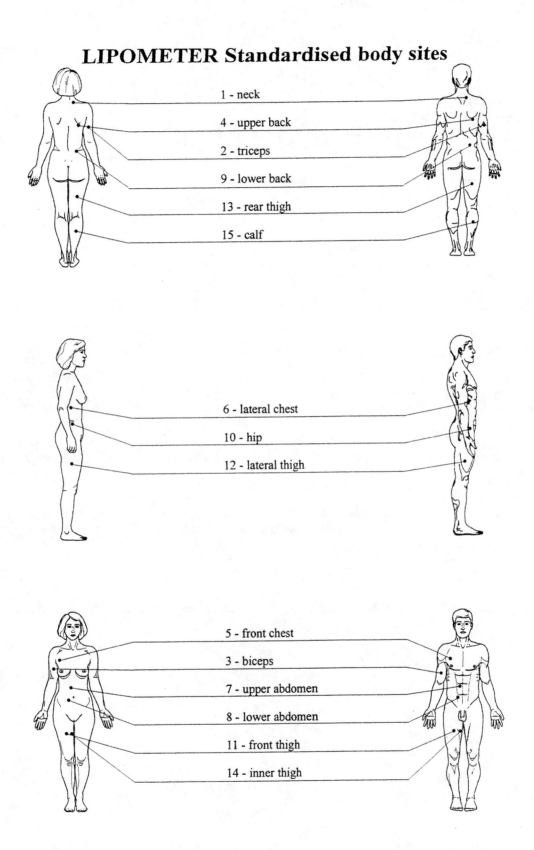

1 - neck

4 - upper back

2 - triceps

9 - lower back

13 - rear thigh

15 - calf

6 - lateral chest

10 - hip

12 - lateral thigh

5 - front chest

3 - biceps

7 - upper abdomen

8 - lower abdomen

11 - front thigh

14 - inner thigh

Figure 1. Standardised body sites (n=15) for the measurement of subcutaneous adipose tissue topography (SAT-Top) by means of *Lipometer*

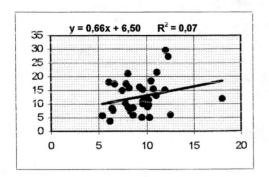
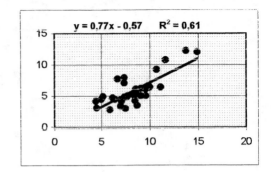

Figure 2. Linear regression between *leptin levels* (ng/ml; y-axis) and the thickness of the body site *biceps* (mm; x-axis) in obese boys before (left fig.) and after (right fig.) the diet and sport intervention programe

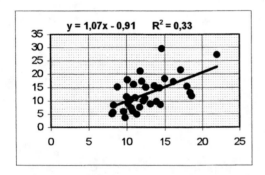
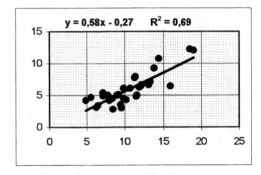

Figure 3. Linear regression between *leptin levels* (ng/ml; y-axis) and the thickness of the body site *upper back* (mm; x-axis) in obese boys before (left fig.) and after (right fig.) the diet and sport intervention programe

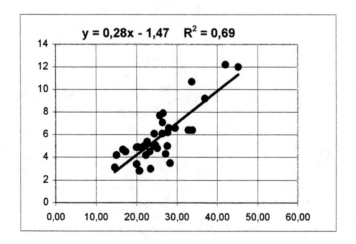

Figure 4. Linear regression between *leptin levels* (ng/ml; y-axis) and the sum of 3 body sites measured: *biceps, upper back,* and *rear thigh* (mm; x-axis) in obese boys after the diet and sport intervention programe

Lipometer-Subcutaneous Adipose Tissue Topography (SAT-Top) reflects serum leptin levels both varying in circadian rhythms

Reinhard Möller[1], Erwin Tafeit[1], Karl Sudi[2], Karoline Vrecko[1], Renate Horejsi[1], Helmut Hinghofer-Szalkay[3] and Gilbert Reibnegger[1]

[1]Institute for Medical Chemistry and Pregl-Laboratory, Karl-Franzens University Graz; 8010 Graz - Austria, [2]Institute for Sport Sciences, Karl-Franzens University Graz; 8010 Graz - Austria, [3]ASM Institute for Adaptive and Spaceflight Physiology; 8010 Graz-Austria

ABSTRACT

Recent advances in obesity research have shown that the product of the ob-gene named leptin is related to to total body fat mass in humans. There is, however, a debate if leptin levels are pulsatile and linked to body fat distribution. In this study we therefore investigated the subcutaneous adipose tissue topography (SAT-Top) measured by means of the newly developed device Lipometer and leptin levels during a 24 hours beginning at 0715am ending the same time in the next day. Blood samples for measurement of leptin were taken every 3 hours in a male subject. Measurements of SAT-Top were performed at 15 body sites from neck to calf at the left and right body site at the same time intervall. We observed an almost symmetrically reaction of the left and right body site with a maximum of the mean value of all body sites in the evening at 0715pm. There was a negative correlation between serum leptin levels and SAT-Top using the set of certain body sites (R^2=0.80, p=0.01). If these combination of body sites is inversed and set against serum leptin levels, both curves show almost identical sahpe and time dependence. We conclude that SAT-Top by means of Lipometer is changed in a short time and related to leptin levels in the investigated male subject.

Keywords: Subcutaneous Adipose Tissue Topography (SAT-Top), Optical Device, Lipometer, Leptin

1. INTRODUCTION

Advances in obesity research have shown that the product of the ob-gene, named leptin, is direct related to nearly all parameters of body composition. Leptin is primarily secreted in white adipocytes and in human placenta at delivery. There is evidence that leptin plays a physiological role in regulating energy expenditure and food intake[1-4].

A very simple model like the Body Mass Index (*BMI*) provides evidence that height and body weight may be determinants of circulating leptin levels. More sophisticated methods to determine body composition i.e Bioelectrical Impedance Analysis (*BIA*), underwater weighing (*UWW*), near infrared interactance (*NIR*) or imaging techniques (Computed Tomography *CT*, Magnetic Resonance Imaging *MRI*) are limited for several reasons[5].

All studies investigating leptin levels under different aims found strong positive correlations with total body fat mass as measured by different methods. These observations lead to the conclusion that leptin is a metabolic signal of the total amount of body fat stored [6-7].

It is interestingly to notice that some authors found different results, suggesting that not body fat mass alone but body fat distribution as well might be related with leptin levels[8-10].

If this would suggest a possible role for leptin in the controll of adipose tissue distribution is questionable but it highlights the role of body fat distribution as a marker of leptin and perhaps of the endocrine system.

In an outstanding paper Licinio et al. 1997 published the observation that total circulating leptin levels exhibited a pattern indicative of pulsatile release[11]. They showed a mean of 32 pulses every 24 hours with the highest leptin values in all subjects studied in the night (20-24h) and early morning (0-4h). This raises the hypothetical assumption that changes in leptin levels could be related with changes in body fat distribution. This field of leptin and adiposity research therefore underlines the necessity to use adequate methods to measure body fat distribution and moreover subcutaneous adipose tissue distribution.

The aim of the study was therefore to investigate serum leptin levels in a male subject during a 24 hours period. Additionally we measured subcutaneous adipose tissue topography (SAT-Top) by means of the newly developed optical device Lipometer to investigate if and to what extent body fat distribution can serve as a marker of leptin levels.

2. SUBJECT AND METHODS

A healthy, trained male subject (33 years of age) was set on a 11700 kJ of energy per day diet for 3 months. Diet consisted of approximately 65% carbohydrate, 15% proteins and 20% fat. Carbohydrate intake consisted primarily of rice, potatoes, pasta and oats. Sources of protein were lean red meat, chicken breast, low-fat milk products and fish. No fatty products e.g. chocolate, nuts, butter were ingested throughout this diet regimen. Body weight (70.5 kg) was stable the last 8 weeks before the investigation. Bllood samples were taken from the antecubital vein every 3 hours starting at 0715am ending at the same time the next day. Leptin levels were estimated by a radioimmunological assay (Linco Res. Inc.; standard available kit). Body fat distribution were assessed by means of the newly developed optical device *LIPOMETER* to measure the thickness of a subcutaneous fat layer at 15 standardised body sites (SAT-Top). The technical characteristics have already been published[12]. Briefly, the Lipometer uses light emitting diodes which illuminate the interesting subcutaneous fatty layer. A photodiode measures the corresponding light intensities backscattered. These light signals are amplified, digitised and stored in a computer. The 15 body sites for the measurement of SAT-Top are distributed over the whole body from neck to calf at the right body site (Fig. 1). Measurements of SAT-Top were performed at the right and the left body site thereby resulting in a total of 30 body sites measured. All measurements were done in standing position. Standard statistical analysis was performed using software package *SPSS*. Pearson correlation coefficient were used for analysis. P values less than 0.05 were considered significant.

3. RESULTS

Most of the SAT-Top body sites showed rhythmic decrease and increase. The same was observed for the mean value of all body sites with a maximum in the evening at 0715pm. The right and the left body sites reacted almost symmetrically (Fig. 2). We found strong negative correlation between a combination of measured body sites from the left body site (biceps, lateral chest, hip, front thigh) and the right body site (biceps, hip and rear thigh) and serum leptin levels ($R^2 = 0.80$; $p<0.01$). This indicates that serum leptin levels reaches their nadir when the thickness of the measured body sites showe a peak value during the 24 hours period. If these aforementioned body sites are inversed and set against serum leptin levels both curves show an almost identical shape (Fig. 3).

4. DISCUSSION

The aim of our study was to investigate subcutaneous adipose tissue topography (SAT-Top) and its possible link with leptin levels during a 24 hours period. We found strong correlation between the combination of measured body sites and leptin levels. Moreover the curves of leptin and different body sites show a similar pattern when the mean value of all body sites is inversed and set against leptin levels.

The study of Licinio et al. suggests that leptin levels are highly pulsatile with a diurnal variation during a 24 hours period[11]. This rhythmicity could be a physiological sign of a time dependence of an energy related factor. The results of our study support this assumption but are limited because we collected blood samples only 9 time througout the entire period. It is interesting to notice that serum leptin reaches a first peak before lunch although high leptin levels are said to be a sign of increased energy expenditure and a relative state of satiety. There is however a surprisingly accordance of leptin levels with measured SAT-Top which is difficult to explain. The changes in SAT-Top observed during one day can be attributable to differences in energy intake by the size of meals and energy turnover. This study however was performed during a normal day of living with no substantial differences in environmental factors e.g. quantity and quality of food intake and modes of physical activities than the weeks before. So it is quite possible that changes in SAT-Top reflect normal fluctuations of subcutaneous fat tissues in one day. It is not clear from our results if the increase or decrease in the mean value of SAT-Top consists primarily of subcutaneous body fat and (or) fluids. The existence of an error in the measurement of 30 body is conceivable. It is not easy to provide an accurate and reproducable measurement at the surface of a biological tissue. All body sites were therefore marked to minimize an error of measurement but it is possible that the geometric pattern of underlying tissues of the subcutaneous fat pads vary with time.

In conclusion the results of our study suggest a common basis of endocrine pathways connecting the regulation of leptin with that of subcutaneous adipose tissue distribution. This seems to be in accordance with the suggestion of putative hypothalamic-pituitary-adrenal-adipose axis which in turn could be up- or downregulated by leptin (Heiman et al. 1997)[13].

We might conclude that the optical device Lipometer is an accurate and valid method to measure the thickness of the subcutaneous adipose tissue layer. Moreover we emphasize the Subcutaneous Adipose Tissue Topography (SAT-Top) as a non-invasive, rapid and safe approach to describe the link of leptin with body fat distribution both varying in circadian rhythm.

5. REFERENCES

1. Y. Zhang, R. Proenca, M. Maffei, M. Barone, I. Leopold, and J.M. Friedman, „Positional cloning of the mouse *ob*-gene and its human homologue", *Nature* 372; pp. 425-432, 1994.

2. L. Tartaglia, M. Dembski, X. Weng, N. Deng, J. Culpepper, R. Devos, et al., „Identification and expression cloning of a leptin receptor, *OB*-R", *Cell* 83; pp. 1263-1271, 1995.

3. R. Senaris, T. Garcia-Caballero, X. Casabiell, R. Gallego, R. Castro, et al., „Synthesis of Leptin in human placenta", *Endocrinology* 138 (10); pp. 4501-4504, 1997.

4. F. Rohner-Jeanrenaud and B. Jeanrenaud, „Obesity, Leptin, And The Brain", *The New England Journal of Medicine* 334 (5); pp. 324-325, 1996.

5. H.C. Lukaski, „Methods for the assessment of human body composition: traditional and new", *American Journal of Clinical Nutrition* 46; pp. 537-556, 1987.

6. M. Maffei, J. Halaas, E. Ravussin, R.E. Pratley, G.H. Lee, et al., „Leptin levels in human and rodent: measurement of plasma leptin and ob RNA in obese and weight-reduced subjects", *Nature Medicine* 1; pp. 1155-1161, 1995.

7. R.V. Considine, M.K. Sinha, M.L. Heiman, A. Kriauciunas, T.W. Stephens, et al., „Serum immunoreactive-leptin concentration in normal-weight and obese humans", *The New England Journal of Medicine* 334; pp. 292-295, 1996.

8. S. Caprio, W.V. Tamberlane, D. Silver, C. Robinson, R. Leibel, et al., „Hyperleptinemia: an early sign of juvenile obesity. Relations to body fat depots and insulin concentrations", *American Journal of Physiology* 271 (3); pp. E626-E630, 1996.

9. C.T. Montague, J.B. Prins, L. Sanders, J.E. Digby, S. O`Rahilly, „Depot- and sex-specific differences in human leptin mRNA expression. Implications for the control of regional fat distribution", *Diabetes* 46 (3); pp. 342-347, 1997.

10. M. Takahashi, T. Funahashi, I. Shimomura, K. Miyaoka, Y. Matsuzawa, „Plasma leptin levels and body fat distribution", *Hormone and Metabolic Research* 28 (12); pp. 751-752, 1996.

11. J. Licinio, C. Mantzoros, A.B. Negrao, G. Cizza, M-L. Wong, „Human leptin levels are pulsatile and inversely related to pituitary-adrenal function", *Nature Medicine* 3 (5); pp. 575-579, 1997.

12. R. Möller, E. Tafeit, K.H. Smolle, P. Kullnig, „Lipometer: determining the thickness of an subcutaneous fatty layer", *Biosensorics and Bioelectronics* 9; pp. xiii-xvi, 1994.

13. M.L. Heiman, R.S. Ahima, L.S. Craft, B. Schoner, T.W. Stephens, and J.S. Flier, „Leptin inhibition of the hypothalamic-pituitary-adrenal axis in response to stress", *Endocrinology* 138 (9); pp. 3859-3863, 1997.

LIPOMETER Standardised body sites

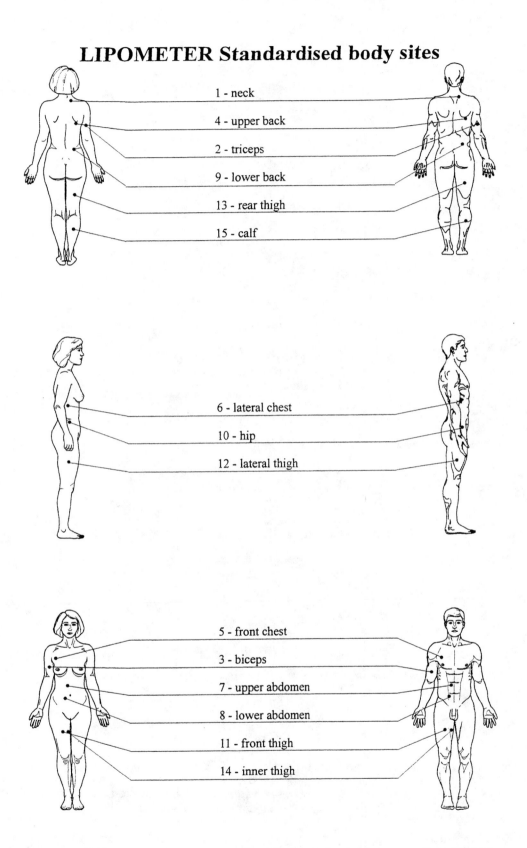

1 - neck

4 - upper back

2 - triceps

9 - lower back

13 - rear thigh

15 - calf

6 - lateral chest

10 - hip

12 - lateral thigh

5 - front chest

3 - biceps

7 - upper abdomen

8 - lower abdomen

11 - front thigh

14 - inner thigh

Figure 1. Standardised body sites (n=15) for the measurement of subcutaneous adipose tissue topography (SAT-Top) by means of *Lipometer*

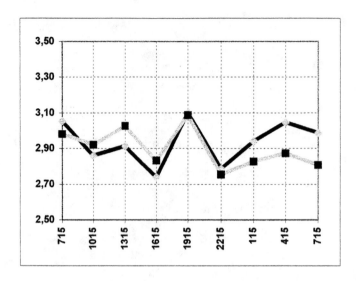

Figure 2. Changes in the mean value of 15 measured body sites (y-axis) during the 24h
period (x-axis). Left body site: black coloured dashed line; right body site: light
grey coloured dashed line

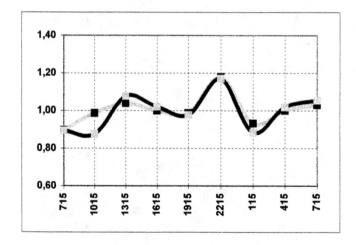

Figure 3. Inversed sum of different body sites (*SAT-Top*)from the left body site (biceps, lateral chest,
hip and front thigh) and the right body site (biceps, hip and rear thigh) versus relative leptin
levels during the 24h period. *Leptin levels*: light grey coloured dashed line; *SAT-Top*: black
coloured dashed line. Note the almost identical shape of both curves.

The comparative study of oxygen consumption during photodynamic reactions in human blood

A. Y. Douplik[1], V. B. Loshchenov[1], V. S. Lebedeva[2], V. M. Derkacheva[3], V. D. Rumyanceva[2], L.V. Chasovnikova[4], S. G. Kusmin[3], A. F. Mironov[2], E. A. Luk'Yanets[3], V. I. Sergienko[4]

[1]General Physics Institute of Russian Academy of Sciences,
Laser Biospectroscopy Lab., Vavilova St. 38, 117942, Moscow, Russia
[2]Institute of Fine Chemical Technology
[3]NIOPIK Institute of Organic Intermediates and Dyes
[4]Physicochemical Medicine Research Institute

Abstract

Comparative studies of oxygen consumption, surface activity, photodestruction of erythrocytes and hemoglobin were carried out during photodynamic reaction in human blood with Phthalocyanines, Chlorines, Porphyrins and Methylene blue photosensitizers in vitro.

Keywords: oxygenation, photodynamic therapy, blood.

1. Introduction

It is well known that the efficiency of the major part of modern photosensitizers used in photodynamic therapy (PDT) is related with the presence of the dissolved oxygen in the irradiated tissues. The interaction of the photosensitizer, photons, and oxygen molecules results in the formation of the active forms of oxygen such as singlet oxygen, oxygen radicals, etc. These forms can destroy different biomolecules, subcellular, and cellular structures [1]. In accordance with that, the level of oxygen consumption (the decrease of oxygen concentration in time) in course of PDT must correspond to the level of the photodynamic processes. Thus, one can estimate the rate of the photodynamic reaction by means of measuring of the oxygen consumption rate within the irradiated volume of the biological tissue.

There is a correlation between the concentration of the dissolved oxygen in blood and oxygenation of hemoglobin (Oxygen Saturation, %) inside erythrocytes [2]. Therefore, it is possible to monitor the photodynamic reaction in the whole blood by measuring the level of Oxygen Saturation.

Developing new methods of monitoring of photodynamic reactions with oxygen dependent photosensitizers we should interest what is the relationship between the studies in vitro and the real processes in vivo with the application of the given photosensitizer?

The photodynamic reaction in vivo can be also accompanied by disoxygenation of blood due to oxygen consumption. This process consists of two components: 1) photodynamic reaction in blood itself provided the concentration of photosensitizer in it is high enough at the moment of irradiation; 2) photodynamic reaction in the tissue surrounding the blood vessel that results in the local decrease of pO_2, formation of the gradient of oxygen concentration, and its diffusion from blood to the surrounding tissue. The latter process is possible in case of the sufficient level of blood microcirculation [3].

The evaluation of the hematoxicity of the photosensitizer, especially in case of its systematic application, is normally a part of the cytotoxicity tests performed during the pharmacological analyses of the given type of PDT. Note two parameters important for the physiological functions of blood: the level of photodestruction of erythrocytes (photohemolysis) and the level of photodestruction of hemoglobin. The cytotoxicity of the photosensitizer is in accordance with its ability to build into cellular or intracellular membrane. In turn the interaction between the photosensitizer molecule and cell membrane should depend on hydrophilic and hydrophobic properties of photosensitizer [4,5].

We believe that the studies of such photodynamic reactions as disoxygenation and photodestruction of erythrocytes and hemoglobin in human blood are not only quite urgent as model studies but are helpful for the development of the real clinical methods of monitoring of the photodynamic therapy.

2. Materials and methods

2.1 Preparation of blood.

We used heparinized and fully oxygenated whole blood from the healthy donors and patients of the Moscow Medical Academy. The value of hematocrit was from 41 to 43. Before preparation of the sample the blood was incubated with or without photosensitizer 30 minutes at 37 °C.

The control sample did not contain photosensitizer. The concentration of some of the photosensitizers in the test sample K (mg/ml) was close to its maximal level in the blood of a patient possibly being prepared for PDT. It was calculated as:

$$K(mg/ml) = K_w W/U$$

where: K_w - is the recommended concentration of a photosensitizer per kilogram of the body weight (mg/kg),

W - is the body weight (kg), and U is the total volume of blood (normally about 5000 ml) [2].

2.2 Photosensitizers

We studied four groups of the water-soluble photosensitizers (Table 1). PBS buffer was used as a solvent.

Table 1. Photosensitizers under study

Photosensitizers	Composition	Absorption maximum in red, nm. Ratio of the peaks heights Solution in PBS-buffer	Molecular weight
Phthalocyanines a)Aluminum phthalocyanine (Photosense®) b) Zinc phthalocyanine I c) Zinc phthalocyanine II d) Zinc phthalocyanine III e) Zinc phthalocyanine IV	percentage of groups with various degree of sulfonation a) tetra - 30, tri - 50, di - 20 b) tetra - 76, tri - 23, di - 1.5 c) tetra - 7, tri - 12, di - 75 d) tetra - 28, tri - 50, di - 22 e) tetra - 46, tri - 44, di - 10	a) 675 b) 665 c) 670 d) 675 e) 675	[6] a) 862 b-e) app. 870
Chlorines a) chlorine p6 I b) chlorine p6 II	a) trisodium salt Clp6 b) trisodium salt 3-divinyl- -3 formyl Clp6	a) 660 b) 692	[4] a) 648 b) 650
Porphyrins a) Hematoporphyrin derivate (Photogem®) b) Uroporphyrin III	a) 80% - oligomers, 20% monomers b) the mixture of isomers I and III	a) 630 b) 603 : 665 (9:1)	a) 598-2920 [5] b) 818 [7]
Methylene blue		600 : 655 (9:10)	373,9

2.3 The methods of the studies of the kinetics of photodynamic disoxygenation, photohemolysis, and photodestruction of hemoglobin

Blood oxygenation (Oxygen Saturation, %) was calculated from the relationship between the total transmission spectra of hemoglobin and oxyhemoglobin in the blood sample under study. Besides it, we irradiated separately the samples of the whole blood in the standard capillaries with the diameter of 1 mm for the subsequent analysis of the gas composition in blood gas analyzer CIBA-CORNING 238 (England).

To check up the erythrocytes ability to pass oxygen after uniform irradiation in standard capillaries we took blood with the help of a microsyringe and tried to restore the full oxygenation of the sample by means of mechanical manipulations.

Photohemolysis of the irradiated whole blood was determined as the change of the transmission spectrum integral within the range 500-700 nm. This method allows one to detect rather pronounced hemolysis (more than 5%).

We studied hemoglobin photodestruction in case the photodynamic reaction with the given photosensitizer resulted in photohemolysis. The photodynamic reaction was studied at the hemolyzed blood and the photodestruction of the hemoglobin was determined from the change of the integral of the absorption spectrum within the range 500-600 nm.

The standard methods of sample preparation for photometric studies were not good for the comparative studies of photodynamic reactions in blood. Blood in the cuvette undergoes the processes of sedimentation and its optical properties can not be treated as stationary within several hours after sample preparation. To overcome these difficulties we had to develop the methods enabling one to work with thin layers of the native whole blood fixing cells in space [8].

2.3.1 The method of the glass sandwich

0.08 ml of the whole blood, erythrocytes or hemolyzed blood was deposited on the standard sample glass. After that the blood droplet was covered by another sample glass to achieve homogeneous distribution between the glasses. Such a "sandwich" is cemented by the capillary forces. The thickness of the blood layer is from 10 to 25 microns. After 40 minutes of erythrocyte aggregation in such a blood layer the optical parameters of the sample become stationary in additional two hours. The reproducibility of the measurements of the optical parameters is 2-3%. The ability of entering the photodynamic reaction is retained in such a sample for one day.

For each sample with intact blood or the blood with the photosensitizer we measured the transmission and diffuse reflection of light within the range 500-600 nm with the help of the two-beam spectrophotometer with the integrating sphere HITACHI U-3400 (Japan) before and after the irradiation. The sample was irradiated outside the spectrophotometer.

Being simple and accessible the method has a substantial disadvantage. As it is impossible to set exactly the thickness of the blood layer, it is rather difficult to compare accurately, e.g., the dynamics of disoxygenation of different photosensitizers because the samples are different. Another method was developed for precise comparative studies of photodynamic reactions in blood.

2.3.2 The method of photodynamic prints

Erythrocytes or hemolysate with or without the photosensitizer are added to 1.8% solution of the ultra-low-temperature agarose in PBS buffer. The ability of such a sample with fixed thickness to enter the photodynamic reaction and the stability of its optical parameters are retained after polymerization for 2-3 days.

Placing a semitransparent item (e.g., a slide) between such a sample and the source of light one can obtain through Photodynamic disoxygenation a print of the item directly on blood in the scale of red with the resolution of 2-5 microns for the erythrocyte gel and about 10 nm for the hemoglobin gel.

Note that phthalocyanines block the polymerization process if one attempts to receive the photodynamic print on the polyacrylamide gel.

2.4 Irradiation of the samples

The absorbed power density was calculated in a way as follows:

$$P_v(mW/cm^2) = P_s(mW/cm^2)(1-Tt-Rd)$$

where P_s is the power density of the incident radiation, Tt is the total transmittance of blood layer, Rd is the diffuse reflection of the blood layer.

We used three light sources for irradiation of the blood samples: He-Ne laser (633 nm) coupled with the lightguide (diameter is 200 microns) with the output power at the end of the lightguide up to 20 mWt; confocal LED matrix (665-675 nm) with the output power density of 10 mWt/cm^2; and the diode laser (675 nm) with the output power up to 2.5 Wt (JSC «Biospec», Moscow).

2.5 Model estimation of the interaction between the photosensitizer molecule and cell membrane.

Taking into account that hydrophilic and hydrophobic properties of photosensitizer define its ability to connect with cellular membrane we evaluated surface activity of various photosensitizers in water and water-lipid solutions through measurement of surface tension depending on photosensitizer concentration. Photosense®, Photogem® and Chlorin I were investigated from this point of view.

The surface tension σ was measured by the Wilgelmi method, precision of measurement ± 0.1 mN/m. Determination of σ of the photosensitizer solution was as follows. A cleaned wet Wilgelmi glass plate was suspended above a round 20 ml cuvette until contact with the plate. If the depth of drawing in of the plate corresponded to the tabulated value for σ of water (72.2±0.2 mN/m) then a certain volume (5-200 μl) of the photosensitizer solution was introduced into the solution via a syringe and the kinetics of fall in σ monitored with constant weak agitation of the solution. The experiment was stopped if in 20-30 min the value σ remained unchanged. This equilibrium σ value ($σ_{eq}$) was taken as the surface tension of the photosensitizer solution of given concentration.

The surface activity of the photosensitizer is necessary condition of ability of the photosensitizer molecule to built in cellular membrane [4,5]. To confirm this chance we studied changes of the surface tension Δσ of cell membrane model (monolayer of soy lecithin (Natterman, Germany) on water surface) after injection of the photosensitizer under lipid monolayer. The quantity of the added photosensitizer has to be enough to create its dense monolayer on water surface. Such concentration for Photosense®, Photogem® and Chlorin I was 20 mg/ml, 10 mg/ml, 25 mg/ml correspondingly. Δσ was calculated as follows:

$$Δσ = σ_0 - σ_{phs}$$

where $σ_0$ - equilibrium value of the surface tension of water solution covered by lipid monolayer before addition of the photosensitizer,

$σ_{phs}$ - equilibrium value of the surface tension of water solution covered by lipid monolayer after creation of the above-mentioned content of the photosensitizer.

3. Results

The analysis of the spectra showed that there are no pronounced changes of the optical properties of blood samples without photosensitizers after laser irradiation.

The dynamics of the photodynamic disoxygenation in vitro are presented in Figs. 1-3.

We observed the decrease of pO$_2$ in the samples after irradiation from 100-170 mmHg down to 0-2 mmHg with the help of the blood gas analyzer. Both pH and pCO$_2$ were virtually stable. The attempt of the repeated oxygenation of the irradiated blood sample was successful. Gas analysis showed that the oxygenation level was restored to almost 97%.

The fastest photodynamic disoxygenation is observed for the whole blood photosensitized by zinc phthalocyanine IV (Fig. 1). There was no measurable disoxygenation for uroporphyrin III even for the power density of 300 mW/cm^2 (λ = 675 nm). There was also no disoxygenation effect for hematoporphyrin derivate (Photogem®) at λ=633 nm and P_v = 100 mW/cm^2.

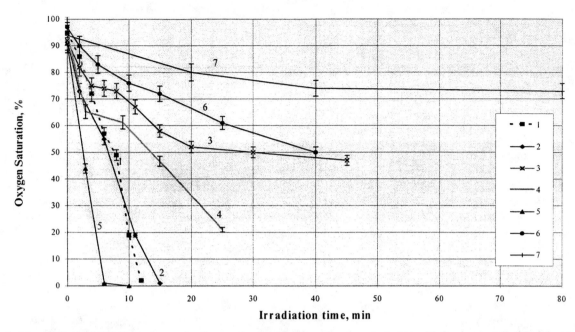

Fig. 1. Monitoring of the photodynamic disoxygenation in vitro for the whole blood by means of the glass sandwich method; λ = 665-675 nm, P_v = 10 mW/cm². (1) Aluminum phthalocyanine (Photosense®) - 0.01 mg/ml; (2) Zinc phthalocyanine I - 0.013 mg/ml; (3) Zinc phthalocyanine II - 0.013 mg/ml; (4) Zinc phthalocyanine III - 0.012 mg/ml; (5) Zinc phthalocyanine IV - 0.013 mg/ml; (6) Chlorine p6 I - 0.01 mg/ml; (7) chlorine p6 II - 0.01 mg/ml.

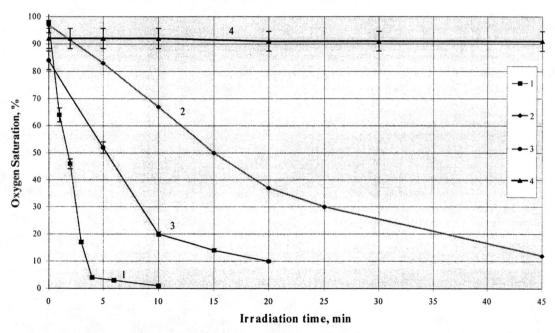

Fig. 2. Monitoring of the photodynamic disoxygenation in vitro for the whole blood by means of the glass sandwich method; λ = 675 nm, P_v = 35 mW/cm². (1) Chlorine p6 I - 0.025 mg/ml; (2) chlorine p6 II - 0.025 mg/ml; (3) Methylene blue - 0.01 mg/ml; (4) uroporphyrin III - 0.023 mg/ml.

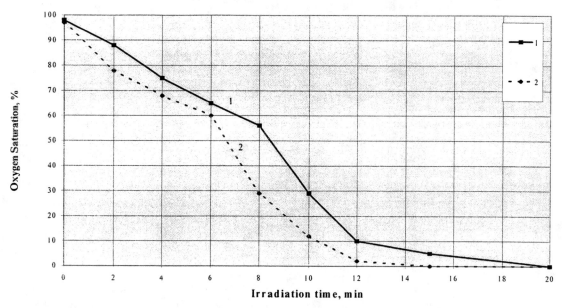

Fig. 3. Monitoring of the photodynamic disoxygenation in vitro for the erythrocyte suspension by means of the photodynamic prints method; λ=665-675 nm, P_v = 10 mW/cm². (1) Aluminum phthalocyanine (Photosense®) - 0.01 mg/ml; (2) Zinc phthalocyanine I - 0.013 mg/ml.

Photohemolysis was observed for chlorines (Fig. 4) and was not observed for phthalocyanines and methylene blue. Photohemolysis was detected for porphyrins at rather high power density of 500 mW/cm² (λ = 633 nm).

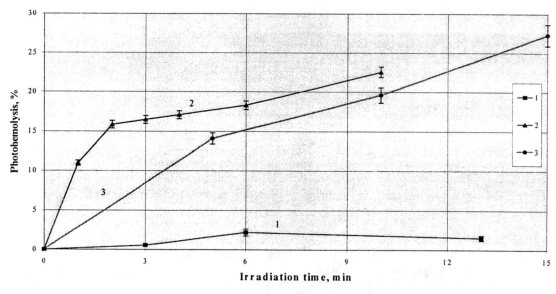

Fig. 4. Kinetics of the photohemolysis in vitro for the whole blood by means of the glass sandwich method. Photohemolysis is measured in percents of the control (nonirradiated) sample (0%); λ = 675 nm, P_v = 35 mW/cm². (1) - zinc phthalocyanine IV - 0.013 mg/ml; (2) chlorine p6 I - 0.025 mg/ml; (3) chlorine p6 II - 0.025 mg/ml.

As was shown above the most pronounced photohemolysis is observed for both chlorines p6. Moreover, we observed very high growth of viscosity in whole blood with chlorine p6 I in the cuvette after laser irradiation (λ = 675 nm, P_v = 150 mW/cm²). This effect was not observed for the samples with the other photosensitizers.

The results of the studies of hemoglobin photodestruction are presented in Fig. 5.

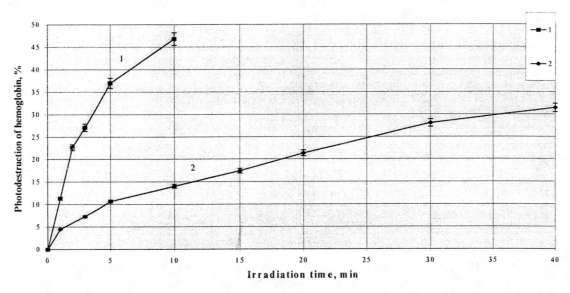

Fig. 5. Monitoring of hemoglobin destruction during irradiation in vitro for hemolyzed blood by means of the glass sandwich method. Photodestruction of hemoglobin is measured in percents of the control (nonirradiated) sample (0%); λ = 675 nm, P_v = 35 mW/cm². (1) chlorine p6 I - 0.025 mg/ml; (2) chlorine p6 II - 0.025 mg/ml.

Figure 6 presents a series of kinetic curves characterizing change in σ_{eq} of photosensitizers water solutions of various photosensitizers concentration. . The magnitude σ_{eq} characterizes the surface activity of the photosensitizer. As it is shown below, the addition of any photosensitizer causes decrease of surface tension, particularly for Trisodium salt Clp6 (Chlorin I).

Results obtained for water solution model correlates with results received for water- lipid model. $\Delta\sigma$ for Photosense®, Photogem® and Chlorin I was 3 mN/m, 15,5 mN/m, 22 mN/m accordingly. These results allow us to say that Photogem® and Trisodium salt Clp6 (Chlorin I) have the property of high ability to interact with lipid component of cell membrane comparing with Photosense®.

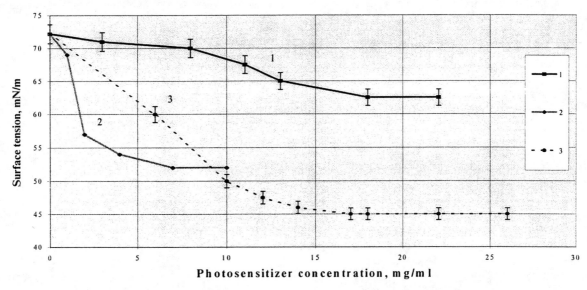

Fig. 6. Kinetics of surface tension of photosensitizers water solutions depending on photosensitizers concentration by means of Wilgelmi method. (1) - Photosense®; (2) -Photogem®; (3) - chlorine p6 I

Results showed on Fig.6 are in a good agreement with results presented on Fig. 4 and 5. Photosensitizers showing a high level of surface activity demonstrate a high level ability to destroy cell membrane. This feature is defined by ratio of hydrophilic and hydrophobic properties of the photosensitizer.

4. Conclusions

1. Photodynamic disoxygenation of blood is demonstrated in vitro.

2. Zinc phthalocyanine IV was determined to provide the maximal rate of the photodynamic disoxygenation of blood. This photosensitizer is a mixture of approximately equal parts of tetrasulfonated (46%) and trisulfonated (44%) forms with a minor content (10%) of the disulfonated form.

3. Maximal photohemolysis was achieved in the whole blood with the trisodium salt of chlorine p6 and trisodium salt 3-divinyl--3 formyl Chlorine p6. Maximal level of hemoglobin photodestruction was founded out under irradiation $\lambda = 675$ nm with the trisodium salt of chlorine p6. Trisodium salt Clp6 (Chlorin I) has the property of relatively high surface activity and ability to interact with lipid component of cell membrane.

5. Acknowledgments

We wish to thank Dr. Alexandre Guschin and Prof. Abram Sirkin for their assistance in experiments.

6. References

1. Vladimirov Y. A., Potapenko A. Y., «Mechanism of photosensitizing reactions in biological systems», Chap. 6 in «Physical-chemical basis of photobiology processes», pp. 116-129, Visshaya shkola, Moscow (1989).

2. G.I. Kosiskiy, «The physiology of blood system», Chap. 9 in «Human physiology», Ed. by G.I. Kosiskiy, pp. 211-216, Medicine, Moscow (1985).

3. A. Krug, M. Kessler, J. Hopper, S. Zellner, V. Sourdoulaud, «Analysis of downregulation of cellular energy demand by 2-D measurements of intracapillary HbO_2, Hb, pO_2 and redox state of cytochromes», SPIE-Proc., V. 2387, 257-268.

4. A. F. Mironov «Second generation photosensitizers based on natural chlorins and bacteriochlorins (Review)», SPIE-Proc., V. 2728, 150-164.

5. Chissov V. I., Scobelkin O. K., Mironov A.F. et al., «Photodynamic therapy and fluorescent diagnostics of cancer by drug «Photogem», Russian Oncology J., V. 12, 3-6 (1994).

6. Kasachkina N., Zharkova N., Fomina G., Yakbovskaya R., Sokolov V., Luk'Yanets E., «Pharmacokinetical study of Al- and Zn-sulphonated phtalocyanines», SPIE-Proc., V. 2924, 233-242.

7. A. Mironov «Methods of extraction of native porphirins and its analogs», Chap. 4 in «Porphirins: structure, properties, synthesis», pp. 282-332, Nauka, Moscow (1985).

8. A. Yu. Douplik «Investigation of influence of physiological parameters of human blood upon optical properties of the blood in visible and nearinfrared range», Ph. D. Dissertation, Dept. of Biophysics, Institute of Physical-Chemical Medicine, Moscow (1996).

Anatomical Registration and Segmentation by Warping Template Finite Element Models

Anton E. Bowden[1], Richard D. Rabbitt[1], and Jeffrey A. Weiss[1,2]

[1]Department of Bioengineering, University of Utah Salt Lake City, UT   84112-9202
[2]Orthopedic Biomechanics Institute, The Orthopedic Specialty Hospital, SLC, UT   84107

ABSTRACT

Image segmentation and anatomical registration play an important role in subject-specific computational modeling and image analysis. Often a three-dimensional (3D) segmentation is available for a canonical *template* image dataset of a single subject. The goal of the present work is to apply this *apriori* knowledge to facilitate segmentation of anatomical structures in other subjects. A "Warping" method was developed to deform the template anatomy and register it with specific *target* anatomies. This was achieved by direct incorporation of image data into a nonlinear finite element (FE) analysis program. The algorithm searches all admissible material configurations for the one which minimizes the difference between the target and the deformed template. FE models of specific anatomical structures were generated from the anatomy of one specific template subject. The FE model deforms under the laws of nonlinear continuum mechanics such that one-to-one correspondence of differential lines, areas, and volumes is guaranteed. The method has been successfully applied to 2D and 3D segmentation, registration, and geometrical model construction. Example results are provided for segmentation of the distal femur using X-ray computed tomography (CT) data, and registration of neuroanatomical structures using optical cryosection image data.

Keywords: nonlinear kinematics, tissue and organ segmentation, inter-subject registration, geometrical model generation, anatomical warping, global shape models

1. INTRODUCTION

Semi-automatic and automatic template-based registration techniques have been applied to a broad spectrum of uses in fields such as handwriting recognition,[1,2] vehicle classification,[3] facial feature recognition,[4] military target identification, manufacturing,[5] and nonlinear strain computation.[6] The principal use of such techniques to date is medical image segmentation and registration. The motivation for the use of deformable templates to automatically register and segment medical image data lies in the considerable human effort required to achieve these tasks manually. Manual segmentation is a painstaking process of selecting points within an image data set which lie on the boundaries of a region of interest (ROI). For many applications, the ROI must be identified on each slice of a 3D data set. Similar procedures are used in manual comparison of functional image data with a reference or atlas. Landmarks within a data set must be manually identified so that information from a specific patient data set can be transformed to a reference or template space. An example of this is the transformation of cortical information into the Talairach-Tournoux[7] space.

Recent attempts to automate the segmentation procedure using deformable templates have followed three distinct lines. Landmark or marker based identification techniques attempt to automatically align key points from a template image set with those in a target data set.[8] Principal Axis registration methods are based on low-dimensional translation, rotation, and scaling operations.[9,10] The third area of research is the more diverse field of deformable shape models. When these methods are rigorously applied, the template transformation is governed by principles of nonlinear differential geometry or continuum mechanics. Some methods focus on border information, such as the deformable contour models of Cohen.[11] Others have used full volumetric approaches using linear solid mechanics,[12] fluid mechanics,[13] or nonlinear continuum mechanics.[14]

Further author information:
A.E.B.(correspondence): Email: Anton.Bowden@m.cc.utah.edu; Telephone: 801-581-4549
R.D.R.: Email: R.Rabbitt@m.cc.utah.edu; Telephone: 801-581-6968
J.A.W.: Email: jeff@usi.utah.edu; Telephone: 801-269-4035

The present work applied the techniques described by Rabbitt, et. al.[14,6] to deform a discretized geometric representation of a 3D template data set subject to the laws of nonlinear continuum mechanics. This method required the solution of a nonlinear optimization problem to minimize the difference between target images collected from the subject of interest and images formed by mathematical interrogation of a deformed finite element (FE) model.

Two examples are presented. The first illustrates the ability to segment regions of the Macaque monkey brain using inter-subject registration of optical cryosection data. In the second example, CT data was used to register a 3D template model of the distal femur with a second subject. Results provide subject-specific tissue segmentation and FE mesh generation.

2. METHODS

2.1. Mathematical Basis

Only a descriptive outline of the mathematical basis of the method is presented here. For a more thorough treatment of the derivation, please refer to Rabbitt.[14,6] Briefly, using standard techniques from continuum mechanics, a deformation map φ was defined which related a reference configuration with material coordinates $\mathbf{X}$ to a target configuration with mapped material coordinates $\mathbf{x}$. A hyperelastic material model was used such that a strain energy density function $W(\mathbf{X}, \mathbf{C}(\varphi))$ was defined, where $\mathbf{C}(\varphi)$ is the right Cauchy strain tensor.[15] In addition to the strain energy density function, a Gaussian image-based energy density function $U(\mathbf{X}, \varphi)$ was used to relate the mathematically interrogated spatial information from the template to the target data.[13] Both energy terms were incorporated into a combined energy density functional:

$$E(\varphi) = \int_\beta W(\mathbf{X}, \mathbf{C}(\varphi(\mathbf{X})))dV + \int_\beta U(\mathbf{X}, \varphi(\mathbf{X}))dV \tag{1}$$

which was used to derive the weak form of the Euler-Lagrange equations. The domain of the template space was discretized and the FE method was used to survey all possible template configurations and select the one which minimized the combined energy functional. When solved using the penalty method,[16] this is equivalent to a Bayesian approach, where W defines the Gibbs form of the prior probability and U defines the likelihood.

2.2. Implementation

Solution of the problem is divided into three steps: preprocessing, processing, and postprocessing. In the preprocessing step, a geometric model is constructed, boundary conditions are specified, and material properties are assigned. The geometric model must span the ROI of the template image. In some cases it is necessary to histogram equalize the template and target images to correct for differences between scanners and data collection techniques. Figure 1 shows histograms from two image data sets. Differences such as these were accommodated by simply averaging the mean and amplitude of the histogram according to:

$$x^* = x\frac{\overline{x_1}}{\overline{x_2}}; \quad x \leq \overline{x_2} \tag{2}$$

$$x^* = (x - \overline{x_2})\frac{x_{max} - \overline{x_1}}{x_{max} - \overline{x_2}} + \overline{x1}; \quad x > \overline{x_2} \tag{3}$$

$$I_2^* = I_2\frac{\overline{I_1}}{\overline{I_2}} \tag{4}$$

$$I_2^{**}(x) = I_2^*(x^*) \tag{5}$$

where I is an index along the histogram (e.g. 0 to 255), and x is the frequency of occurrence of a particular intensity within the image.

The combined energy functional was minimized during the processing step by implementing equation 1 into the nonlinear finite element code NIKE3D.[17,6] Use of such a well-developed finite element package allowed for broad variation in both applied boundary conditions and material constitutive parameters which can be used to guide the registration process. It also allowed independence of the computational mesh from the spatial discretization of the

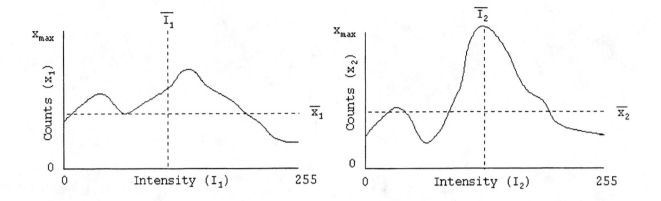

Figure 1. Description of a histogram equalization process. The equations governing the histogram transformation are given in (2)-(5)

image data. This independence can be important in reducing the computational size of the geometrical model and in cases where the ROI does not include an entire image data set. Template and target images are interpolated from voxel coordinates to the FE model to define a continuous mathematical representations of the data. These representations are updated as the material deforms through the spatially fixed image coordinates. Differences between intensity of the target and template images, as well as their gradients, contribute a spatially dependent body force which drives the registration process. These differences also contribute to the tangent stiffness in the FE implementation.

Field variables, including displacement, relative volume, and strain, were viewed using the postprocessor GRIZ.[18] Additional postprocessing software was written to output the deformed template as an image data set. This required interpolation of Lagrangian displacements to generate pixel locations and intensities within the Eulerian image-based coordinate frame. If the registration were perfect, subtraction of the deformed template from the target image would result in a zero difference image. Thus, visual inspection of the difference image provides a qualitative means to assess the registration.

3. RESULTS

3.1. 2D neuroanatomical slices

Results appearing previously in the literature for neuroanatomical registration often use rectangular computational grids associated with image voxels.[12,13] The present FE method allows for both rectangular and irregular mesh structure. This technique was applied to segment grey matter, white matter, and sulci of macaque monkey brains using optical images of stained cryosection slices. Results are provided for three different computation meshes: a simple regular mesh, a mesh conforming to a lobe of grey and white matter, and a mesh conforming to a layer of grey matter. In all cases, the material was modeled as an elastic-plastic solid with a low Poisson's ratio.[17] Deformation of the template brain slice was constrained to the plane of the image data.

3.1.1. Rectangular Mesh

Figure 2 provides results for a simple rectangular mesh constructed to span the domain of the image data. The outside edges of the mesh were aligned with the borders of the images and constrained from both vertical and horizontal motion. The template image is shown in panel A and the target image is shown in panel E. The goal is to find the deformation of the FE mesh (B) that aligns the deformed template with the target (E). Prior to deformation the difference image (Template-Target,C), contains regions of large magnitude intensities. After minimizing the functional (equation 1), the difference image is reduced from (C) to (D). The displacement magnitude (F), maximum shear strain (G), and relative volume (H) associated with the deformation are also shown. The final deformed

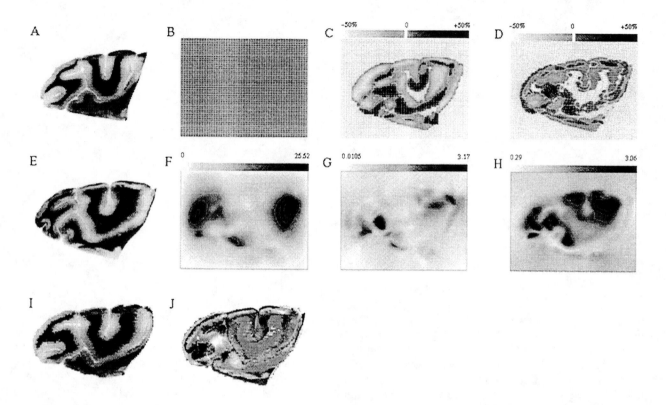

Figure 2. Regular mesh results. A) Template image. B) Computational mesh. C) Intensity difference before registration. D) Intensity difference after registration. E) Target image. F) Computed displacement magnitude. G) Computed principle shear strain. H) Computed relative volume. I) Deformed template image. J) Relative error. In F-H, the greyscale legend is given above each panel. Percent values in C-D correspond to the percentage of maximum initial difference in image intensity.

template, mapped to the image voxels, is shown in the lower left panel (I). Accuracy of spatial location in the segmentation is shown in the final difference image (E-I) in panel J. Note the large differences in location of sulci between the target (E) and the deformed template (I). These results represent a local minima in the energy function and are not considered acceptable.

3.1.2. Lobe Mesh

Better results were obtained using geometrical FE models that align with specific anatomical structures. Figure 3 provides results for an irregular mesh (B) constructed to span the white and grey matter between the central and rightmost sulci. No external boundary conditions were applied, so the edges of the mesh were free to move. Panels A-J correspond directly with those in figure 2. In both cases, results are computed on the geometrical model and thus are not available outside the spatial domain of the mesh. The registration results are much more acceptable with reference to both the difference in image intensity following registration (D) and the global positioning of the deformed template (I-J). The undeformed FE mesh is a segment of the template anatomy. The deformed mesh aligns well with the same region of the brain in the target anatomy, illustrating automatic segmentation.

3.1.3. Grey Matter Mesh

Figure 4 provides results for a FE mesh corresponding to a section of grey matter. Again the panels correspond to those shown in figure 2. Note the large volume changes associated with this registration (H). The difference in image intensity following the registration (D) has almost been reduced to zero. Automatic segmentation is demonstrated by the difference image (J) where the deformed FE mesh overlays the grey matter of the target.

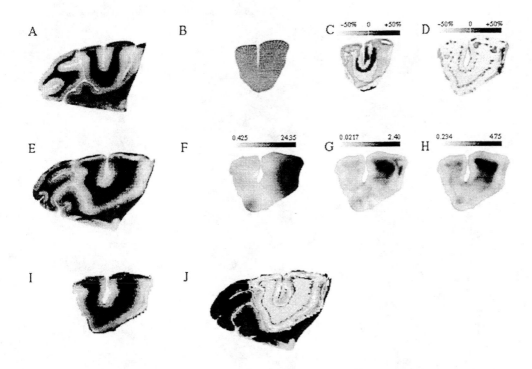

Figure 3. Center section results. Same notation as in figure 2.

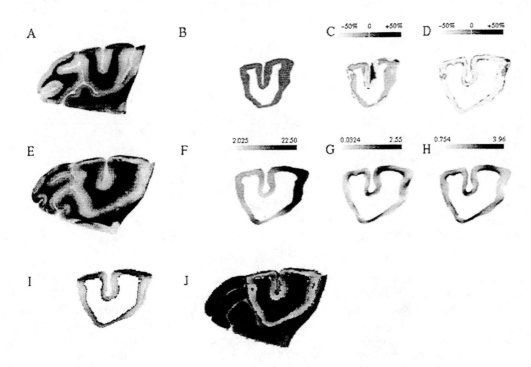

Figure 4. Grey matter results. Same notation as in figure 2.

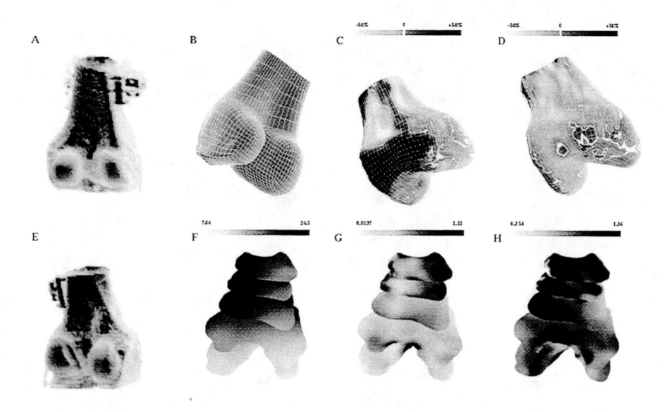

Figure 5. 3D femur results. A) Template data set. B) Template mesh. C) Intensity difference before registration. D) Intensity difference after registration. E) Target data set. F) Computed displacement magnitude. G) Computed principle shear strain. H) Computed relative volume.

3.2. 3D human femur

The method can also be applied to generate subject specific geometric models – a problem equivalent to tissue segmentation. This is illustrated in figure 5 where a FE model, generated from the CT data of one subject (template), is mapped to a second subject (target). Panels A and E show rendered views of the 3D CT data corresponding to the template and target respectively. The template FE mesh used for the registration is shown in panel B. Subtraction of the target CT image data from the deformed template generates a difference image. Values of the difference image are shown on the surface of the femur model before (C) and after (D) registration. Deformation results are presented on parallel slices through the long axis of the femur (F-H): displacement magnitude (F), maximum shear strain (G), and relative volume (H). The difference between the reference geometry (C) and the deformed configuration (D) is the result of rigid body translation and rotation, as well as fine scale deformation. Note the elongation and torsion induced on the mesh configuration (*cf.* C,D).

4. DISCUSSION

During image segmentation and registration, template and target images are typically taken from different subjects and hence the mapping is not a physical deformation. Rather, the mapping represents the optimal configuration that aligns the template and target data. Use of nonlinear continuum mechanics in the process guarantees a one-to-one mapping of differential lines, areas, and volumes between the template and its deformed configuration. This is required to insure that anatomical structures in the template remain continuous after the deformation. Paradoxically, this strength is sometimes a weakness in that strict adherence to the laws of mechanics can overpenalize some deformation fields. The severity depends upon the material properties used. In the registration problems we have run to date, acceptable results were obtained by *ad hoc* manual selection of material properties. Optimization of material parameters for anatomical registration remains a topic of future work.

The neuroanatomical registration results illustrate the difference in segmentation results achieved by a rectangular mesh versus a mesh corresponding to the tissue geometry. The rectangular mesh achieved unacceptable results because of the presence of a local minimum in the combined energy functional (equation 1). Experience has shown that local minima are more likely to occur during 2D segmentations on rectangular grids due to competing regions in the image data. Meshing only the ROI using an irregular mesh not only avoided such phenomena, but also reduced the computational size of the problem. An additional advantage to the irregular FE mesh was the direct segmentation afforded by the deformed template image (Panel I in figures 3 and 4). Although segmentation information could be extracted from the displacement field of a rectangular mesh, the transformation is not as obvious.

The 3D capabilities of the present method are demonstrated in the distal femur registration. In 3D segmentations, the independence of the computational mesh from the voxel space of the image data is especially relevant. A small ROI in a data set can be extracted without the computational burden of the bringing the whole image space into registration. This example further illustrates an important aspect of the present FE method. Considerable effort is required to construct structured computational meshes that accurately reflect the tissue geometry. The distal femur registration demonstrates a convenient way to automatically generate complex computational meshes by mapping a canonical template model to conform with the anatomy of an individual subject.

ACKNOWLEDGEMENTS

The finite element mesh and the computed tomography data used in the 3D femur registration were provided by John C. Gardiner of the Orthopedic Biomechanics Institute, Salt Lake City, UT. Cryosection data was provided by D. C. Van Essen of Washington University, St. Louis, MO. Partial support for this project was provided by the University of Utah Research Foundation, the University of Utah Center for High Performance Computing and the Human Brain Project (NIMH, NSF and NASA RO1 MH/DA52158).

REFERENCES

1. E. Lecolinet and L. Likforman-Sulem, "Handwriting analysis: Segmentation and recognition," *IEE Colloq Proc Eur Wkshp Handwriting Anal Recog: A European Perspective* **123**, pp. 17/1–17/8, 1994.

2. A. del Bimbo, S. Santini, and J. Sanz, "OCR from poor quality images by deformation of elastic templates," in *Proc Int Conf Pattern Recognit*, vol. 2, pp. 433–435, Oct 1994.

3. M. P. Dubuisson, S. Lakshmanan, and A. K. Jain, "Vehicle segmentation using deformable templates," in *Int Symp Comp Vision*, International Symposium – Coral Gables, FL, pp. 581–586, IEEE; Computer Society; Technical Committee for Pattern Analysis and Machine Intelligence, IEEE, Nov 1995.

4. K. Lam and H. Yan, "Facial feature location and extraction for computerized human face recognition," *Natl Conf Pub Inst Eng Aust* **1(94/9)**, pp. 167–171, 1994.

5. C. Gueudre, J. Moysan, and G. Corneloup, "Geometric characterization of a circumferential seam by automatic segmentation of digitized radioscopic images," *NDT & E International* **30**(5), pp. 279–285, 1997.

6. J. Weiss, R. Rabbitt, and A. Bowden, "Incorporation of medical image data in finite element models to track strain in soft tissues," *SPIE Biomed Optics Symp BiOS98* **3254**, 1998.

7. J. Talairach and P. Tournoux, "Co-planar stereotaxic atlas of the human brain," *Stuttgart, Germany:* **Thieme**, 1988.

8. Y. Amit, "Graphical shape templates for automatic anatomy detection with applications to MRI brain scans," *IEEE Trans Med Imaging* **16**, pp. 28–40, Feb 1997.

9. L. K. Arata, D. A. P., J. P. Broderick, M. F. Gaskil-Shipley, A. V. Levy, and N. D. Volkow, "Three-dimensional anatomical model-based segmentation of MR brain images through principal axis registration," *IEEE Trans Biomed Engineering* **42**, pp. 1069–1077, Nov 1995.

10. A. P. Dhawan, L. K. Arata, A. V. Levy, and J. Mantil, "Iterative principal axis registration method for analysis of MR-PET brain images," *IEEE Trans Biomed Engineering* **42**, pp. 1069–1077, Nov 1995.

11. L. Cohen and R. Kimmel, "Global minimum for active contour models: A minimal path approach," *Int J Comp Vision* **24**(1), pp. 57–78, 1997.

12. R. Bajcsy, R. Lieberson, and M. Reivich, "A computerized system for the elastic matching of deformed radiographic images to idealized atlas images," *J Comp Assist Tomography* **7**(4), pp. 618–625, 1983.

13. G. E. Christensen, R. D. Rabbitt, and M. Miller, "Deformable templates using large deformation kinematics," *IEEE Trans Image Process* **5**(10), pp. 1435–1447, 1996.

14. R. Rabbitt, J. Weiss, G. Christensen, and M. Miller, "Mapping of hyperelastic deformable templates," in *Proc Int Soc Optical Engineering*, vol. 252, pp. 252–265, SPIE, 1995.

15. A. Spencer, *Continuum Mechanics*, Longman Scientific & Technical, Essex, England, 1980.

16. K.-J. Bathe, *Finite Element Procedures*, Prentice-Hall, Englewood Cliffs, New Jersey, 1996.

17. B. Maker, R. Ferencz, and J. Hallquist, "NIKE3D a nonlinear, implicit, three-dimensional finite element code for solid and structural mechanics," *UC - Lawrence Livermore National Laboratory Report* **UCRL-MA-105268 rev 1**, 1995.

18. D. Dovey and T. Spelce, "GRIZ finite element analysis results visualization for unstructured grids," *UC - Lawrence Livermore National Laboratory Report* **UCRL-MA-115696**, 1993.

Incorporation of medical image data in finite element models to track strain in soft tissues

Jeffrey A. Weiss[1,2], Richard D. Rabbitt[2], Anton E. Bowden[2] and Bradley N. Maker[3]

([1]Orthopedic Biomechanics Institute, The Orthopedic Specialty Hospital, SLC, UT 84107)

([2]Department of Bioengineering, University of Utah Salt Lake City, UT 84112-9202)

([3]Livermore Software Technology Corporation, Livermore, CA 94550)

ABSTRACT

A new method has been developed to extract tissue strain from a sequence of two or more medical images. This was achieved by deforming a finite element (FE) model of the tissue under loads derived from the spatial differences between two sets of image data. One image data set deforms with the tissue, while the other remains stationary. The final configuration aligns the two sets of image data. The method accounts for convection of material points, modification of the Lagrangian material properties, and probabilistic features of the sensor. A FE model of the tissue must be constructed and assigned material properties. Image data are assigned to the model tissue such that the reference configuration of the FE model corresponds to one image. The image data is subject to change during the deformation. A nonlinear solution method determines the material configuration that minimizes the difference between the deformed image (deformed template) and the experimentally observed image (target image). In many cases the image data provide powerful constraints which allow estimation of material deformation even in the absence of known loads and/or boundary conditions. The method has been applied to estimate the motion and distribution of strain using MR and CT data.

Keywords: strain measurement, finite element, nonlinear kinematics, anatomical warping

1. INTRODUCTION

The accurate determination of strain in deforming biological tissues is a necessary and important part of many experimental investigations in biomechanics. Previous attempts to estimate nonlinear strains in biological tissues and cells usually employed fiducial markers.[1,3-9] In some cases, the 3D strain can be estimated directly from changes in the distances between groups of markers making up tetrahedral sets. Inhomogeneous strain fields and physical dimensions of the markers, however, can limit applicability of the method.[3,10,1] The ability to use textural inhomogeneities present in medical images rather than fiduciary markers considerably easier to implement and also would allow for the measurement of soft tissue deformation *in vivo*.

This paper describes a method to estimate stress and strain fields in biological soft tissues that may be applied in the absence of information regarding the tissue constitutive properties or discrete markers to track the deformation. The method makes use of medical image data to provide information about the deforming tissue and thus the strain and stress fields. Accurate stress determinations require a good approximation for the material properties of the tissues under consideration, but even in the absence of stress data, the kinematic data alone provide useful information in both applied and fundamental biomechanical studies ranging from joint mechanics to cell motility.[1,2]

Further author information:
J.A.W.(correspondence): Email: jeff@usi.utah.edu; Telephone: 801-269-4035
R.D.R.: Email: R.Rabbitt@m.cc.utah.edu; Telephone: 801-581-6968
A.E.B.: Email: Anton.Bowden@m.cc.utah.edu; Telephone: 801-581-4549
B.N.M: Email: maker@lstc.com; Telephone: 510-449-2500

2. METHODS

We have developed a method to combine medical image data with a standard solid mechanics analysis approach to allow the estimation of tissue strain fields in the absence of detailed information about boundary conditions and in some cases constitutive information. For the description to follow, it is assumed that a single imaging modality was used to interrogate a fixed 3D volume of space while the material was in a reference configuration (template image) and, at a later time, in a deformed configuration (target image). Standard segmentation and mesh generation methods were used to define a geometrical model of the tissue(s) in the reference configuration. The reference image data were interpolated to the FE model nodes to define a continuous template image intensity field. If CT image data are used, the template image data reflect the initial distribution of material density in the FE model. When the material is deformed, mathematical interrogation of the model generates image data representing a transformed version of the template image field. The mathematical problem is to search through all admissible configurations of the model for the one which minimizes the difference between the transformed template and actual data collected experimentally from the deformed material. There are two formulations of the problem. The first is to assume that the image data provide a hard constraint which must be satisfied exactly. The second is to combine a stochastic model of the imaging sensor (likelihood of the data) with the mechanical model (prior probability), yielding a soft constraint.[14–16] The first case uses Lagrange multipliers[17] or an augmented Lagrangian method[20] and the second uses Bayes theorem or the penalty method.[18] The most effective approach is application-dependent and hence we have used both approaches in the solution of test problems.

2.1. Variational Formulation

The nonlinear solid mechanics problem, subject to the soft (Bayesian) or hard (Lagrange multiplier) constraint imposed by the image data, can be cast in the form of a potential functional. This highly nonlinear functional can be linearized around a known configuration to form the basis for an incremental-iterative solution procedure using a Newton-type method. For an arbitrary domain and boundary conditions, the finite element method is used to discretize the geometry and describe the variations in the unknown field variables over the domain.

Following the standard convention in nonlinear continuum mechanics,[19] material coordinates in the reference configuration are denoted by vector $\mathbf{X}$ while coordinates in the current configuration are $\mathbf{x} = \varphi(\mathbf{X})$. Here φ is the deformation mapp. The deformation gradient is defined as $\mathbf{F} := \frac{\partial \varphi}{\partial \mathbf{X}}$. We provide here a brief derivation for the special case of a hyperelastic material, although the method is easily generalized for other material behaviors. In this case the standard mechanical strain-energy density $W(\mathbf{X}, \mathbf{C})$ is augmented with the Gibb's image-energy density $U(\mathbf{X}, \varphi(\mathbf{X}), \mathbf{F}(\mathbf{X}))$. The argument $\mathbf{X}$ denotes dependence of the image data on the initial material configuration and distribution of properties while $\varphi(\mathbf{X})$ and $\mathbf{F}(\mathbf{X})$ denote changes in the image data resulting from convection of the material as well as local deformation. The form of U depends, in part, upon the point-spread function and properties of the imaging hardware. In preliminary results U is taken as a simple Gaussian form, but can be modified to account for other sensor models (empirical or theoretical). The combined optimization problem is to minimize the functional E:

$$E(\varphi) = \int_{\mathcal{B}} W(\mathbf{X}, \mathbf{C}(\varphi(\mathbf{X}))) dV + \int_{\mathcal{B}} U(\mathbf{X}, \varphi(\mathbf{X}), \mathbf{F}(\mathbf{X})) dV, \qquad (2.1)$$

where $\mathcal{B}$ denotes integration over the reference configuration. The minimization of the energy functional E will simultaneously minimize internal forces derived from material stresses (W) and deformation-dependent body forces arising from differences between the transformed template image field and the target image data (U, see below). The linearized weak form (Euler-Lagrange equations) is obtained by taking the first and second variations of the energy functional $E(\varphi)$ with respect to the deformation to obtain:

$$\int_{\varphi(\mathcal{B})} \nabla \mathbf{u} \boldsymbol{\sigma} : \nabla \boldsymbol{\eta} \, dv + \int_{\varphi(\mathcal{B})} \nabla^s \mathbf{u} : \mathbf{C} : \nabla^s \boldsymbol{\eta} \, dv - \int_{\varphi(\mathcal{B})} \mathbf{u} \cdot \frac{\partial^2 U}{\partial \varphi \partial \varphi} \cdot \boldsymbol{\eta} \frac{dv}{J}$$
$$= \int_{\varphi(\mathcal{B})} \frac{\partial U}{\partial \varphi} \cdot \boldsymbol{\eta} \frac{dv}{J} - \int_{\varphi(\mathcal{B})} \boldsymbol{\sigma} : \nabla^s \boldsymbol{\eta} \, dv, \qquad (2.2)$$

Here, $\varphi(\mathcal{B})$ is the deformed configuration, $\mathbf{u}$ and $\boldsymbol{\eta}$ are 1st and 2nd spatial variations, dv denotes integration over the deformed body, $\mathbf{C}$ is the spatial version of the 2nd elasticity tensor (see Marsden and Hughes[19]) and J is the Jacobian. The 4th order elasticity tensor $\mathbf{C}$ provides the constitutive model contribution to the tangent stiffness.[21]

In addition to the standard mechanical terms, the image-based energy density contributes a new term to the tangent stiffness as well as a spatially distributed nonlinear body force. The term $\frac{\partial U}{\partial \varphi}$ provides a deformation-dependent body force, while the term $\frac{\partial^2 U}{\partial \varphi \partial \varphi}$ contributes to the tangent. The body force term provides the force which drives the deformation process. For the case of a single imaging modality with a Gaussian likelihood[16]:

$$U(\mathbf{X}, \varphi(\mathbf{X})) \;=\; \frac{\lambda}{2} \left(T(\mathbf{X}, \varphi) - S(\mathbf{X}, \varphi)\right)^2. \tag{2.3}$$

Here, T and S are the template and target image data fields, respectively.[11] The body force vector is derived from the first derivative of U with respect to the deformation map:

$$\frac{\partial U}{\partial \varphi} \;=\; \lambda \left(T(\mathbf{X}, \varphi(\mathbf{X})) - S(\mathbf{X}, \varphi(\mathbf{X}))\right) \left(\frac{\partial T}{\partial \varphi} - \frac{\partial S}{\partial \varphi}\right). \tag{2.4}$$

In the Bayesian approach, λ is related to the variance in the Gaussian imager model normalized for U to match the same energy density units used for the mechanics W. The Bayesian approach is directly analogous to the penalty method used in mechanics to enforce a constraint in an approximate sense.[18]

2.2. Solution Strategy using the FE Method

We have implemented the image driven algorithm in the nonlinear FE code NIKE3D.[11-13] The unknown variations in shape and displacement over the domain are discretized using the FE shape functions in the standard manner.[21] An iterative Newton procedure is used to obtain the nonlinear solution. Assuming that the solution at a configuration φ^* is known, we seek to determine a new configuration $\varphi^* + \mathbf{u}$ that results in a minimization of the energy functional $E(\varphi)$. Here $\mathbf{u}$ is a vector of incremental nodal displacements, and the configuration $\varphi^* + \mathbf{u}$ is such that the applied loads/displacements (including image-derived forces) are equilibrated with the internal stresses. The following linearized matrix equations result from the FE discretization:

$$\sum_{i=1}^{N_{\text{nodes}}} \sum_{j=1}^{N_{\text{nodes}}} \left({}^{M}\mathbf{K}(\varphi^*) + {}^{G}\mathbf{K}(\varphi^*) + {}^{I}\mathbf{K}(\varphi^*)\right)_{ij} \mathbf{u} \;=\; \sum_{i=1}^{N_{\text{nodes}}} \left({}^{ext}\mathbf{F}(\varphi^*) - {}^{int}\mathbf{F}(\varphi^*)\right)_{i}. \tag{2.5}$$

The term ${}^{M}\mathbf{K}$ is the material stiffness matrix, while the term ${}^{G}\mathbf{K}$ is the geometric (initial stress) stiffness matrix. These terms both arise in a traditional displacement-based nonlinear analysis. The image-based stiffness, ${}^{I}\mathbf{K}$, is a direct result of the fact that the image-based force changes with configuration. The image-based body forces are applied with other external forces via the vector ${}^{ext}\mathbf{F}$. By solving for $\mathbf{u}$, the configuration at $n+1$ is approximated as $\varphi_{n+1} = \varphi^* + s\mathbf{u}$. Here s is a scalar parameter between 0 and 1 determined by a line search. The determination of an accurate value for φ_{n+1} follows by iterative solution of (2.5) using a quasi-Newton strategy.[22]

Equation (2.4) shows that U and the associated driving force both vanish when transformed template image data $T(\mathbf{X}, \varphi)$ are equal to target image data $S(\mathbf{X}, \varphi)$. The driving body force is also zero if the gradients vanish. The gradient terms determine the direction of the force. Since the appropriate direction can not be determined on a local level without gradient information it is natural that this term vanishes in the absence of a spatial gradient. As a result, inhomogeneous images containing intensity variations and boundaries are most effective in driving the process. The image energy density U also contributes to the tangent stiffness in this implicit formulation.[12]

2.3. Test Problems

The following test problems illustrate the application of the method for strain and stress determination using both simulated and real image data. The first problem simulates the the deformation of a soft rubberlike material by compression between two plates. First, the problem is solved in the "forward" sense using applied displacements to drive the top plate towards the bottom plate. Next, all displacement and contact boundary conditions are removed and the analysis is driven using image data generated from the density distributions that the forward simulation predicted. Excellent agreement between the forward solution and the warping solution was achieved. The second problem utilizes MR image data of the intervertebral disc. In this case the correct strain field in the tissue is unknown and the image data before and after deformation provide a means to estimate it.

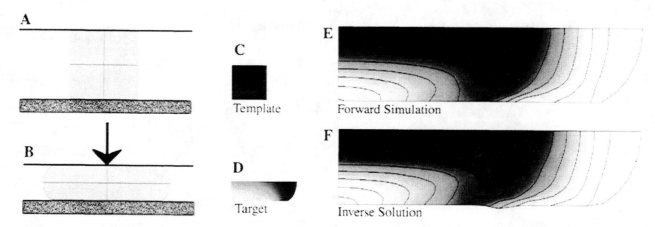

Figure 1. Deformation of a rectangular billet under compression. Panel A is the intial geometry of the billet compressed between two plates. Panel B is the deformed geometry obtained from the forward FE simulation. Panels C and D show the template and target images of the density distribution, used to drive the Warping analysis. Panel E shows the von Mises stress distribution obtained from the forward simulation. Panel F shows the results from the Warping analysis, obtained by removing all applied displacements and contact boundary conditions and using only the pointwise image intensity differences between Panels C and D to drive the analysis.

3. RESULTS

3.1. Stress/Strain Estimation using Simulated CT Data

To test the ability of the warping method to determine stress/strain distributions using "exact" representations for the image data, a traditional FE simulation was performed of a hyperelastic material compressed between two plates (Figure 1A). The material was assumed to be bonded to the plates, and the objective of the analysis was to deform the mesh to 50% axial compression. The sides of the mesh bulge out and eventually contact the plates on the top and bottom (Figure 1B). Contact was modeled with a standard penalty method. This problem is a challenging forward simulation because of the extreme deformation and the contact. The material was assumed to be hyperelastic (compressible Mooney-Rivlin Material model, A=10 MPa, B=5 MPa, bulk modulus=750 MPa) with initially homogeneous density.

Both the forward and inverse solutions were obtained. The forward problem was posed as a standard solid mechanics problem with applied displacements pushing the plates together and contact constraints so that no material would penetrate the infinite plates. For the inverse problem, the applied displacements and contact constraints were removed and the deformation was driven by forces derived from the image-based energy terms in equation (2.1). Images of the density in the reference and deformed configurations obtained from the forward simulation were used as the template and target image data, respectively (Figures 1C and 1D).

The deformed shape of a 1/4 symmetry model and the von Mises stress distribution obtained from the forward simulation are shown in Figure 1E with isocontours indicating lines of constant equivalent stress. To test the warping algorithm, we removed the boundary conditions and the applied loads but added the image-terms to the functional. The problem was then re-run with the two images (1C,D) driving the process. Fig. 1F shows the resulting configuration and isocontours of constant stress for this inverse problem. Notice the excellent correspondence with the forward solution (compare 1E & F). The small error (kink, 1F) at the bottom of the billet could not be eliminated with the image-driven analysis. This is due to the use of the penalty method where the parameter λ was increased during the simulation using a load curve. The maximum value of λ that can be used in the computation is controlled by numerical precision. Since the simulated CT data was perfect in this test case, λ should be allowed to approach infinity, in theory. This is not computationally feasible. An augmented Lagrangian or Lagrange multiplier method, in combination with a more refined mesh along the bottom edge of the domain, should alleviate this shortcoming.

Figure 2 illustrates a sequence of the deforming mesh for both the forward and inverse problems. The forward problem (top panels) proceeds by compression of the material as specified by the applied displacements and contact conditions. During the compression, the side of the original mesh eventually contacts the compressing plate and the material continues to bulge out between the plates. In the case of the inverse image-driven problem (bottom panels), the deformation proceeds along a very different path as specified by the pointwise difference in template and study intensities and their gradients. However, the end state is almost identical to that obtained from the forward solution. The actual path of deformation taken by the forward problem can only be reproduced in the inverse problem if a sufficient number of intermediate images are employed in the deformation process.

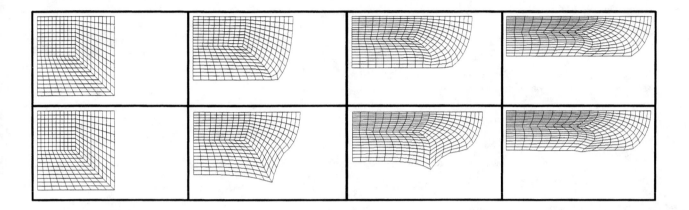

Figure 2. Sequence of images from the forward (top panels) and inverse (bottom panels) solution of the compression of a beam between two plates. Only the bottom right portion of the beam was modeled because of symmetry. The mesh of the forward solution is gradually compressed and eventually the side of the mesh contacts the plate as the deformation progresses to 50% axial compression. The inverse solution follows an entirely different path as dictated by the image data and its gradients, but eventually reaches the same final configuration.

3.2. Intervertebral disc strain extracted using MR images

We also have tested the FE implementation by using MR data to track strain in a spinal disc.[23] The human intervertebral disc is a complex combination of materials, including collagen, water, and a proteoglycan matrix. Material characterization and strain measurement are extremely difficult for the disc. Using a nonmagnetic compression frame and a MRI scanner, MR images of a L2-L3 motion segment were obtained before and after application of a 250 lb compressive load (data supplied by Chiu et al.,[24] Figs. 3A, B). The image in the reference configuration was used to generate geometrical models of the disc and bone. Pixel intensities from the reference image were assigned to the model to define the template image field. Image data were filtered at the spatial Nyquist frequency of the FE mesh to avoid aliasing. Representative hypoelastic material properties were estimated from the literature[25] as described by Bowden et al. (1997).[23] Differences between the template and target images defined the only input "force" driving the deformation of the disc and bone. As the Warping code registered the two images, strains developed in the spinal disc. The difference images before and after deformation illustrate the excellent registration that was achieved (Figs. 3C, D). Results show changes in volume of up to 15% and compressive strains as high as 20% within the disc[23] (Figs. 3E, F). The computed deformation was insensitive to changes in the elastic moduli due to the path independent nature of the elastic response. This insensitivity does not hold for Poisson's ratio owing to the interplay between the volume ratio and strain. Due to lack of volumetric information in two-dimensional problems the computed strain field is sensitive to the compressibility of the material. The best results for 2D data are therefore obtained when the model material properties match the actual tissue.[23]

4. DISCUSSION

The paper presented a finite-element based method that combines 2D or 3D image-based data with nonlinear continuum mechanics to track the motion and deformation of materials. This was achieved using a nonlinear variational approach which simultaneously minimizes energy functional associated with the image data and with the mechanical

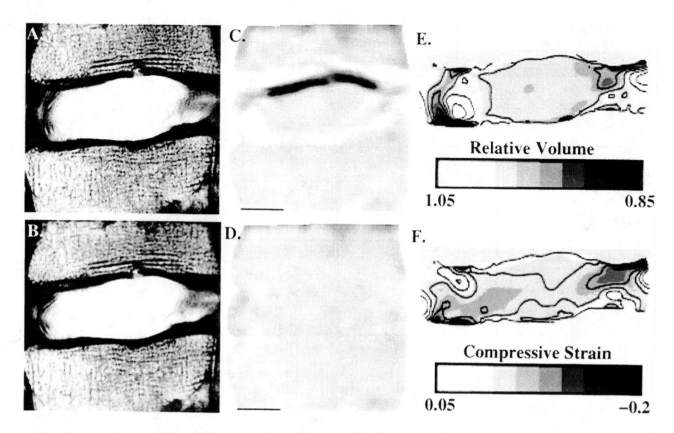

Figure 3. Intervertebral disc strain. Images on the left show the template (A) and target (B) images. Center panels show the difference images prior to deformation (C) and after deformation (D). The resulting volume ratio (E) and and compressive strain (F) are shown on the right with isocontours.

model. The derivation was presented for hyperelastic materials, but the approach is not in any way limited to this material type. When used with medical image data, it provides a means to estimate tissue strains *in vivo*.

The implementation must be modified to accommodate nonconservative systems which exhibit path dependent behavior. The time sequence of images shown in figure 2 clearly illustrate that the path determined by the image-driven deformation is distinct from the actual path, even though the final configuration is approximately the same. The difference in path is due to the fact that the deformation is driven only by the initial and final images. Intermediate images are not used in this example and hence the algorithm has no information concerning the path other than that built into the a priori mechanical model. Since the applied boundary conditions were neglected in the image-based result, the resulting path is different. For hyperelastic materials this difference does not influence the final stress state and therefore is not a concern. For general materials the path is crucial and must be accurately reproduced. One way to achieve this is to use a time sequence of images that are spaced so that the path is resolved sufficiently.

The specific content of the images can affect the ability of the method to reproduce a defined deformation field. Sharp boundaries, such as present in Example 1, provide strong gradient information that controls the direction of the image-derived body forces as defined in equation (2.4). This can result in better end-registration, but also causes severe nonlinearities for the incremental-iterative solution process. We have used image blurring to circumvent this problem. By starting with blurred versions of the template and target images and gradually sharpening them as the analysis proceeds, excellent results are often obtained. The opposite problem can occur when the image consists of diffuse gradient information. In this case local minima can complicate the solution process. Again image blurring or other ad-hoc processing techniques can be used in this case.

In summary, a method for combining medical image data with nonlinear continuum mechanics has been developed and used to determine strain distributions in the absence of detailed information about applied loads or boundary conditions. The method appears to hold promise for in vivo strain determination using image data obtained from noninvasive imaging modalities such as MR. Future work will assess the sensitivity and accuracy of the method for materials undergoing well-defined deformations.

ACKNOWLEDGEMENTS

Partial support for this work was provided by the Whitaker Foundation; The NIMH, NSF and NASA under the Human Brain Project, # RO1 MH/DA52158; The University of Utah Research Foundation; The University of Utah Center for High Performance Computing. MRI images of the intervertebral disc were provided by Elaine J. Chiu, Sharmila Majumdar, Neil A. Duncan and Jeffrey C. Lotz.

REFERENCES

1. S. I. Simon and G. W. Schmid-Schonbein, "Cytoplasmic strains and strain rates in motile polymorphonuclear leukocytes," *Biophysical J.* **58**, pp. 319–332, 1990.

2. R. Skalak, C. Dong, and C. Zhu, "Passive deformations and active motions of leukocytes," *J. Biomech. Eng.* **112**, pp. 295–302, 1990.

3. A. D. McCulloch, B. H. Smaill, and P. J. Hunter, "Regional left ventricular epicardial deformation in the passive dog heart," *Circ Res* **64**, pp. 721–733, 1989.

4. J. W. Holmes, Y. Takayama, I. LeGrice, and J. W. Covell, "Depressed regional deformation near anterior papillary muscle," *Am J Physiol* **269**(**1 Pt 2**), pp. H262–70, 1995.

5. Z. Jia and S. P. Shah, "Two-dimensional electronic-speckle-pattern interferometry and concrete-fracture processes," *Exp Mech* **34**(**3**), pp. 262–70, 1994.

6. E. H. Jordan, S. C. U. Ochi, D. Pease, and J. I. Budnick, "Microradiographic strain measurement using markers," *Exp Mech* **34**(**2**), pp. 155–165, 1994.

7. J. O. Hjortdal and P. K. Jensen, "In vitro measurement of corneal strain, thickness, and curvature using digital image processing," *Acta Ophthalmol Scand* **73**(**1**), pp. 5–11, 1995.

8. D. J. Wissuchek, T. J. Mackin, M. DeGraef, G. E. Lucas, and A. G. Evans, "Simple method for measuring surface strains around cracks," *Exp Mech* **36**(**2**), pp. 173–9, 1996.

9. H. van Bavel, M. R. Drost, J. D. L. Wielders, J. M. Huyghe, A. Huson, and J. D. Janssen, "Strain distribution on rat medial gastrocnemius (mg) during passive stretch)," *J Biomech* **29**(**8**), pp. 1069–74, 1996.

10. L. K. Waldman, Y. C. Fung, and J. W. Covell, "Transmural myocardial deformation in the canine left ventricle: Normal in vivo three-dimensional finite strains," *Circ Res* **57**, pp. 152–163, 1985.

11. R. D. Rabbitt, J. A. Weiss, G. E. Christensen, and M. I. Miller, "Mapping of hyperelastic deformable templates," in *Proceedings of the International Soc. for Optical Engineering*, vol. 252, pp. 252–265, SPIE, 1995.

12. J. Weiss, R. D. Rabbitt, and B. N. Maker, "Use of image data to regularize ill-posed problems in solid mechancis," *In Review, Int. J. Numer. Methods Engng.* , 1996.

13. B. N. Maker, R. M. Ferencz, and J. Hallquist, "Nike3d: A nonlinear, implicit, three-dimensional finite element code for solid and structural mechanics," *Lawrence Livermore National Laboratory Technical Report* **UCRL-MA**(105268 Rev. 1), 1995.

14. M. I. Miller, G. E. Christensen, Y. Amit, and U. Grenander, "Mathematical textbook of deformable neuroanatomies," *Proceedings of the National Academy of Science* **90**, pp. 144–48, dec 1993.

15. U. Grenander, *Lectures in Pattern Theory I, II, and III: Pattern Analysis, Pattern Synthesis and Regular Structures*, Springer-Verlag, 1976.

16. G. E. Christensen, R. D. Rabbitt, and M. I. Miller, "Deformable templates using large deformation kinematics," *IEEE Trans on Image Processing* **5**(10), pp. 1435–1447, 1996.

17. J. N. Reddy, *Energy and variational methods in applied mechanics*, John Wiley, 1984.

18. A. M. Maniatty and N. J. Zabaras, "Investigation of regularization parameters and error estimating in inverse elasticity problems," *Int J. for Numerical Meth. in Eng.* **37**, pp. 1039–1052, 1994.

19. J. E. Marsden and T. J. R. Hughes, *Mathematical Foundations of Elasticity*, Dover, Minneola, New York, 1994.

20. J. C. Simo and R. L. Taylor, "Quasi-incompressible finite elasticity in principal stretches: Continuum basis and numerical algorithms," *Comp Meth Appl Mech Engng* **85**, pp. 273–310, 1991.

21. K.-J. Bathe, *Finite Element Procedures*, Prentice-Hall, Englewood Cliffs, New Jersey, 1996.

22. H. Matthies and G. Strang, "The solution of nonlinear finite element equations," *Int J Numer Methods Eng* **14**, pp. 1613–1626, 1979.

23. A. Bowden, R. Rabbitt, J. Weiss, and B. Maker, "Use of medical image data to compute strain fields in biological tissue," *Proc ASME Bioengineering Conference* **BED-35**, pp. 191–192, 1997.

24. E. Chiu, J. Lotz, and S. Majumdar, "High resolution magnetic resonance imaging of the human intervertebral disc with compression," *Trans. 41st Orthopaedic Research Society* **20(2)**, p. 292, 1995.

25. Y. Liu, G. Ray, and C. Hirsch, "The resistance of the lumbar spine to direct shear," *Orthopadic Clinics of North America* **16(1)**, pp. 33–47, 1975.

In Vivo Facial Soft Tissue Thickness Measurement

Haidong Liang[1] Abdul Daya Steve Hughes

BioMedical Engineering Group School of Mechanical and Material Engineering

University of Surrey Guildford Surrey GU2 5XH UK

ABSTRACT

The purpose of this study is to determine the soft tissue thickness around the face using A-scan ultrasound, for incorporation into a 3D head model as a design tool for safety equipment and facial prostheses for patients following maxillofacial reconstruction.

Using very high frequency A-scan ultrasound allows the superficial tissue to be measured on volunteers without risk. The investigation covers 112 points on half of the face, linked to 11 defined morphological zones. The zonal boundaries are based on previous research and are initially identified by palpation of the face. The thickness of the facial soft tissue varies greatly between individuals but the calculations of average and standard deviation coefficients reveal that the distribution of the features in the same zone of an individual fits within a normal range of variation. The measurements presented for the thickness of soft tissues at different parts of the face can also be recommended for specialists in craniofacial identification. The results of this study will be presented and indications of its application to FEA modelling outlined.

Keywords: facial soft tissue; thickness measurement.

1. INTRODUCTION

A need for new equipment has arisen because of developments in modern aircraft. The high acceleration capabilities of the new aircraft results in the crew experiencing forces sufficient to deform their soft tissues. When this deformation occurs around the face, it can cause slipping of the helmet and mask. Consequently, the helmet may no longer be providing the protection it was designed to give. Leakage of the air supply between the mask and the maxillofacial area may also occur.

A soft tissue model is needed to assist designers in the development of helmets and oxygen masks. Data on the shape of the face together with the thickness of the tissues and their mechanical properties will be incorporated into a soft tissue model around which a new generation of helmets and masks for military aircraft crew will be designed using a CAD system..

High frequency ultrasound (13 MHz) was chosen in A-scan mode for this study. This offers a relatively low cost method with the potential for exploring the different layer within the soft tissues overlying the cranial and maxillofacial skeleton. It also allowed subjects to be measured in the upright seated position appropriate to the end objective of the work.

Anatomical landmarks are palpated to define regions of interest and ultrasound determination carried out to give thickness normal to the bone surface. Careful mapping of thickness not only provides the required data, but also enables validation testing of "iso-thickness zones" which has been proposed by previous researchers [1].

---

[1] Further author information-

H.L. (correspondence): H.Liang@surrey.ac.uk; http://www.surrey.ac.uk/MechEng/BioMed/; Telephone: +44 1483 259683; Fax: +44 1483 306039

The immediate aim of this study is to explore the iso-thickness zones and the inter zone boundaries.

Information concerning the internal structure of the human body can be obtained through the use of an ultrasound beam which is reflected from tissue and bone interface and subsequently displayed. Systems based on this method have been available for some time and are used in a variety of clinical and research situations. A block diagram of the system is shown in Fig. 1.

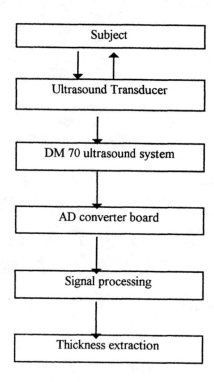

Fig. 1. Block diagram of system

2. Methods and Equipment

A-scan ultrasound was selected as the technique to be used in acquiring soft tissue thickness data around the head. Computer Tomography (CT) and Magnetic Resonance Imaging (MRI) are imaging tools that provide sequential two dimensional tomographic information, but require more processing time to extract tissue thickness and operate at a considerably higher cost

The transducer acts as both transmitter and receiver, operates in the pulsed ultrasound mode. A pulse is transmitted through a medium with an acoustic impedance $Z(kg/m^2 sec)$, which is defined as the product of the acoustic velocity (m/s) and mass density (kg/m^3) of the medium. At the interface between two mediums with different acoustic impedance, some of the incident pulse is transmitted through the second medium and some of the pulse is reflected back to the receiver. The proportion of wave transmitted and reflected is dependent upon the ratio of the impedance, i.e. a material with the higher density will act as a stronger reflector. [2,3,]

High-frequency pulse-echo ultrasound in the 10-50 MHz range offers the potential for non-invasive, *in vivo* visualisation of the microscopic anatomy of soft tissue. In order to examine internal tissue structures of interest, a spatial resolution on the order of 0.2 mm is desirable. We used an ultrasound transducer with a central frequency of 13 MHz, which gives a resolution of about 0.12 mm at the typical sound velocity in soft tissue of 1540 m/s [4].

While the wavelength provides a limit to the ultimate resolution attainable, the resolution of a pulse-echo ultrasound imaging system depends to a large degree upon the bandwidth of the overall system. Increasing the frequency further results in the system penetration being severely compromised, due to the exponentially increasing ultrasonic attenuation coefficient of tissue with frequency. In facial soft tissue, penetration can be substantially sacrificed for increased resolution. The maximum penetration that can be achieved is approximately 30 mm for a 13 MHz ultrasonic probe, which is ideal for measuring the thickness of maxillofacial soft tissues.

2.1 Hardware

The A-Scan ultrasound instrument used was the Dermal Monitor DM 70 (Cutech, (UK) limited.). This system was designed for the measurement of skin and scar tissue thickness. The Dermal Monitor is capable of measuring depths of 0.05-50 mm. The piezoelectric transducer transmits and receives that pulse after interaction with the tissue. Strong reflectors are air and bone. The incident pulse is transmitted through the various interfaces of soft tissue until it reaches an air canal or bone structure, at which point, most of the remaining pulse is reflected back to the transducer (the pulse echo). By measuring the time between the transmitted and received pulse, the distance travelled is derived using the average velocity of sound through soft tissue as 1540m/s. The received electric signal is directed toward either a radio frequency (RF) or video amplifier. The video amplifier will rectify the signal to unipolar. Outputs from either one of the amplifiers are possible for examination of the return echoes, but the original signal (RF) rather than partially processed (video) data are used. The amplifier has a bandwidth of 70 MHz with a variable gain control for optimisation of signal to noise ratio and selection of greatest dynamic range. The analogue signal was digitised with a resolution of 8 bits at a sampling rate of up to 250 Mega samples per second by the Gage CompuScope CS2125 AD converter board (Gage Applied Sciences Inc.). All data acquisition and processing was done using a PII-266 personal computer.

2.2 Signal processing

Three basic processing techniques (Fig. 2) have been used to increase resolution and enhance coherent energy echoes. The first of these is simply averaging echoes over several cycles in order to decrease random noise. The signal to noise ratio is increased by a factor equal to the square root of the number of cycles used for averaging provided the following conditions are met:

- the original (RF) rather than partially processed (video) data are used;

- the structures producing the echoes do not move significantly during the period of averaging.

Clearly this method is most useful in areas of small movement, such as the head, and is most limited with rapidly moving structures such as heart valves. It was found that averaging with more than 32 cycles produced little improvement in the visible noise on the display.

The moving average is used to remove the unwanted high frequency noise prior to band pass filtering. The use of digital filters enable selective matching of the frequency region with the greatest signal-to-noise ratio. Following the filtering process, the signal is differentiated and envelope-detected to extract the thickness data.

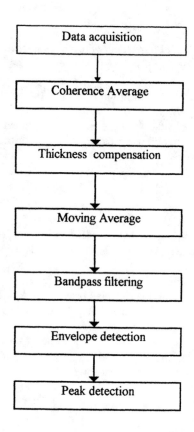

Fig. 2 Data acquisition and processing software diagram

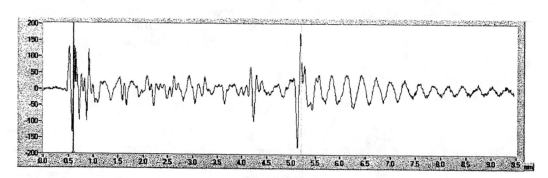

Fig. 3 The original signal on forehead

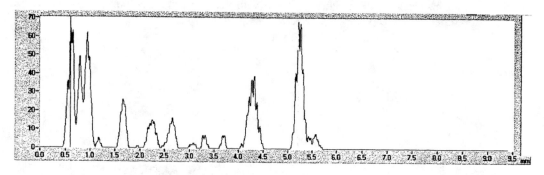

Fig. 4 Processed signal from which thickness data is extracted between the first and last peak.

2.3 Measurement protocol

Jelier and Hughes [1] proposed the hypothesis, based on sample tissue thickness data and the anatomic skeletal and muscular structure, that zones could be designated so that there is a large thickness variation between the zones, but there is not great variation within the zones. One thickness measurement could be taken to represent each zone for using the design model.

This proposal simplifies the creation of the head soft tissue model.

In preparation for this study, a series of tests were conducted to:

- calibrate the ultrasound scanner
- determine the accuracy and repeatability of the operator in locating landmarks using repeated laser scans.

The sites chosen as landmarks for ultrasonic measurement conformed to a set of requirements. These were that the sites should:

- include locations similar to those used by other workers to enable comparability,
- be the same landmarks for all subjects,
- be positioned over flat bone where possible,
- lie at the prominence like glabella, angle of jaw, or in depressions and folds such as the soft nasion or nasolabial fold.

Some landmarks were located by relating them to a surface feature of the face. Others could only be determined by first palpating the underlying bone and then marking the skin.

The technique used to obtain thickness must be done with care. The central beam should be directed at right angles to the under lying bone and the probe must maintain contact with skin without depressing it. Different pressure is applied at each measuring point. For example, the cheek is easily displaced inwards even though the skin itself may not be compacted and a very light pressure must be employed in this region. It is quite permissible to circumduct the probe whist maintaining the landmark as centre, until an echo is picked up. However caution is advised not to wander off target in order to find a more 'suitable' point.

The amplitude of the echo peak at bone/tissue interface is used to determine if the underlying bone is perpendicular to the transmitting pulse. This is done by moving the probe around fixed point so that maximum peak is achieved. The probe is then moved axially to off-load any pressure.

Only half of the face is measured so as to complete the test within an acceptable test time period. The relative symmetry of thickness has been previous established [5]. Eleven zonal boundaries were identified by palpation on each half of the face (Fig. 5): Frontal bone, brow, temporal, zygomatic arch, zygomatic bone, cheek, masseter muscle, ramus, lip, chin and bottom mandible. 112 points were measured to determine the thickness variation between zones. The zone were determined by palpation. The exact location of the 112 points was determined by the requirement for a reliable ultrasound echo approximately normal to the underlying bone or reflecting tissue interface to get the greatest ultrasound echoes. The frontal bone provided the most reliable and easily obtainable echoes. Obtaining reliable echoes from the cheek was often time consuming, sometimes reflection from an air interface lateral from the mouth was achieved but more usually from a tooth or gum.

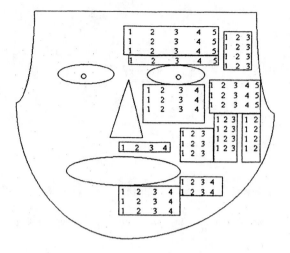

Fig. 5 pre-defined 11 zones

3. RESULT AND DISCUSSION

The present study has produced a set of average facial soft tissue depth measurements for the healthy 11 European male , 10 female and 10 Chinese male aged from 18 to 39.

These data (Table 1) were compared with the work of Rhine and Campbell [5] who measured soft tissue thickness at 21 sites (Fig. 6) using American white cadavers and Phillips and Smuts [6] who used CT to measure the facial soft tissue thickness of mixed race groups in Cape Town in South Africa. It can be seen that at most points, there is no significant difference between our findings and that of Rhine and Campbell except around the supra orbital, lateral orbit, occlusal line, Sub M2 (mandible) and supra M2 (maxilla). For these sites, we compared our data with the that measured by Phillips and Smuts, our data had no significant variation to theirs, the only difference was observed in the occlusal site

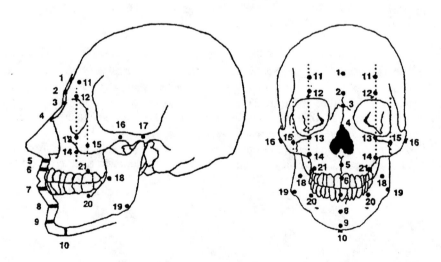

Fig. 6 landmarks determined by other forensic scientists [6].

Table 1: The thickness data comparison with Rhine and Campbell, Phillips and Smuts

| Position | Rhine and Campbell | | | | Phillips and Smuts | | Surrey | | | | |
	Blk/M	Blk/F	Whi/M	Whi/F	Mix/M (S.D.)	Mix/F (S.D.)	Whi/M (S.D.)	Whi/F	STD V	Chinese/M	STD V
Supraglabella 1	4.75	4.5	4.25	3.5	5.36 (1.44)	4.88 (1.02)	4.68 (0.47)	4.34(0.31)	0.31	4.94	0.62
Glabella 2	6.25	6.25	5.25	4.75	5.47 (0.68)	5.64 (1.42)	5.22 (0.45)	4.81	0.52	5.07	0.48
Mid-philtrum 5	12.25	11.25	10	8.5	12.25 (2.97)	10.13 (2.48)	9.95 (1.29)	8.88	0.91	9.94	0.78
chin-lip fold 8	12	12	10.75	9.5	12.02 (2.07)	11.70 (1.66)	11.3 (2.04)	9.29	0.73	10.84	2.23
Mental eminence 9	12.25	12.25	11.25	10	8.94 (2.42)	9.57 (2.36)	10.68 (1.62)	9.06	1.3	10.61	1.62
Frontal eminence 11	8.75	8	4.25	3.5	4.51 (1.40)	4.78 (1.74)	4.96 (0.36)	4.36	0.48	4.88	0.61
Supra orbital 12	4.75	4.5	8.25	7	5.46 (1.31)	5.79 (1.89)	5.23 (0.78)	5.36	0.69	5.47	0.46
Infra orbital 13	7.75	8.25	5.75	6	5.97 (2.87)	6.42 (3.83)	6.67 (1.19)	6.48	1.45	6.3	0.44
Inferior malar 14	17	17.75	13.25	12.75			12.68 (1.45)	13.26	2.1	15.62	2.61
Lateral orbit 15	13.25	12.75	10	10.75	7.54 (1.49)	8.25 (2.52)	8.5 (1.09)	7.64	0.8	8.3	1.28
Zygomatic arch 16	8.5	9	7.25	7.5	6.49 (2.50)	9.30 (3.21)	8.45 (1.53)	7.61	0.91	7.83	1.75
Supra glenoid 17	11.75	12.25	8.5	8	9.10 (4.04)	8.44 (3.84)	8.72 (1.67)	9.1	2.48	8.33	1.81
Occlusal line 18	19	19.25	18.25	17	19.06 (9.08)	21.26 (8.37)	14.7 (2.03)	15.14	1.84	16.46	2.24
Gonion 19	14.75	14.25	11.5	12	14.20 (6.08)	13.50 (6.60)	12.21 (3.2)	10.5	1.5	12.34	2.05
Sub M2 (mandible) 20	16.5	17.25	16	15.5	13.13 (5.31)	11.88 (5.95)	10.69 (1.77)	10.35	1.37	11.34	2.05
Supra M2 (maxilla) 21	22	21.25	19.5	19.25	12.68 (2.10)	12.99 (4.45)	13.74 (1.9)	14.84	2.58	15.55	1.83

Fig. 7 represents the facial tissue thickness distribution in and between the 11 pre-defined zones. Areas of high tissue thickness can be identified with increasing grey scale. It was observed there was a large variation in thickness between the defined zones with little or no significant variation within the zones. Table 2 is the range of thickness distribution within zones. The mean thickness for each zone was calculated for all the subjects to identify the maximum and minimum value over the subjects range. The average thickness of frontal bone was calculated for each subject. Then the minimum and maximum value of the means for the 21 males was obtained, which was 4.24 and 5.26 mm respectively.

Table 2 Range of thickness distribution in zones (Surrey)

| Zones | Male (21) | | | | Female (10) | | | |
| | Means within zones (mm) | | Std Dev respectively (mm) | | Means within zones(mm) | | Std Dev respectively (mm) | |
	min	max.	min	max.	min	max.	min	max.
frontal bone	4.24	5.26	0.17	0.61	4.09	4.83	0.22	0.38
brow	4.24	5.72	0.15	0.78	4.17	5.45	0.13	0.76
temporal	8.76	12.05	0.5	2.89	8.4	12	1.27	2.45
zygomatic arch	6.43	9.64	0.52	1.75	7.24	7.95	0.63	1.37
zygomatic bone	5.48	7.97	0.56	1.41	5.99	9.1	0.5	1.35
cheek	11.7	19.94	1.07	2.36	12.4	16.11	1.04	2.05
masseter muscle	12.75	20.13	0.73	2.5	15.1	16.53	1.16	2.29
ramus	6.61	9.72	0.38	1.79	7.15	9.65	0.63	1.62
lip	8.32	11.4	0.32	1.33	7.45	9.39	0.7	1.96
chin	8.14	12.63	0.51	2.74	7.64	9.94	0.57	1.29
bottom mandible	9.05	13.4	1.14	3.63	8.67	11.82	0.33	1.64

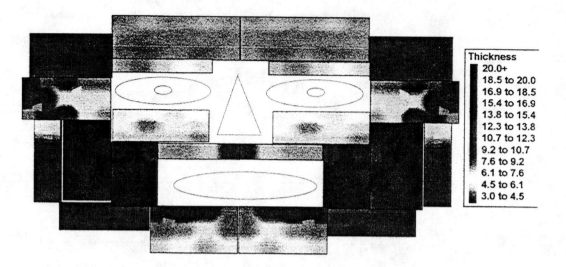

Fig. 7 spectral plot of thickness within zones.

The preliminary work of the FEA analysis (ABAQUS) on the facial soft tissue mode was also done [7]. A vertical downward acceleration of 10g was analysed. It emulated the forces experienced by a fighter pilot during flight.

A side view of the deformation plot of the 10g loaded head is shown in Fig. 8. The deflected model is shown as light, the original as dark. It can be seen that the areas of greatest deflection occur around the fleshiest regions of the face, namely the throat, chin, lips and nose tip areas. Currently, the tissue is assumed to have linear material properties and the values of density, Young's modules and Poisson's Ratio are only approximate

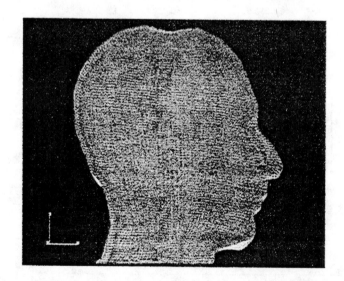

Fig. 8. Side view of the deformation plot of the 10g loaded head.

4. CONCLUSION

The use of A-scan in determining facial tissue thickness distribution was found to be valuable for this purpose and the software was demonstrated to be both robust and reliable. Zonal hypothesis was also found to be valid for the application intended. The results of this study have shown that our facial tissue thickness data compares well to previous finding and adds to the range of measurement of races.

5. REFERENCE

1. Jelier, P. and S. C. Hughes, "Laser scanning as a source of 3D head anthropometric data". New developments in mechanics -- Biomechanics and design aspects of military helmets, Defence Research Agency Farnborough, Hampshire, England (1993).

2. Daly, C. H. and J. B. Wheeler, "The use of ultrasonic thickness measurement in the clinical evaluation of the oral soft tissues." International Dental Journal 21: 418-429. 1971.

3. Alexander, H. and D. L. Miller (1979). "Determining Skin Thickness with Pulsed Ultrasound." Journal of Investigative Dermatology. 72: 17-19. 1979.

4. McDicken, W. N., Diagnostic Ultrasonics. Principles and Use of Instruments. John Wiley and Sons Inc. New York., 1981.

5. Rhine, J. S. and H. R. Campbell "Thickness in Facial Tissue in American Blacks." Journal of Forensic Sciences, 25(4): 847-858. 1980.

6. Phillips, V. M. and N. A. Smuts. "Facial reconstruction - utilisation of computerised-tomography to measure facial tissue thickness in a mixed racial population." Forensic Science International, 83:51-59. 1996.

7. Humphries, W, A and A. Crocombe "Finite Element Modelling of human Head". Report to DERA, Farnborough, UK. 1995

3D Maxillofacial Soft Tissue Model in Laser Scanned Head

Haidong Liang[1] Steve Hughes

BioMedical Engineering Group School of Mechanical and Material Engineering
University of Surrey Guildford Surrey GU2 5XH UK

ABSTRACT

The purpose of this study is to incorporate thickness data into a soft tissue model in a laser scanned head data base, for use in FEA modelling of the behaviour of the soft tissue layer under mechanical loads.

Using a magnetic-based, spatial acquisition system (Polhemus) into which is incorporated an ultrasound sensor the position and orientation of tissue thickness vectors are obtained. By combining this with 3D high resolution head shape data from our laser scanner, a model of the head complete with soft tissue thickness is to be developed.

We have implemented an initial version of software for the integration of laser scanning and facial soft tissue thickness measurement. The package displays facial images and performs basic image processing. The co-ordinate systems of the two methods are matched with the help of markers fixed on known head landmarks and a 3D digitiser (Polhemus). The computed source locations can be instantly superimposed on the facial images during the analysis.

Key words: head model; space registration.

1. INTRODUCTION

In the past, anthropometric data bases have consisted of standard linear measurements taken with fundamental equipment such as callipers and anthropometric rigs [1] While the sample sizes of the databases have been reasonably large, it has involved much effort and time. Advance laser scanning technology has enabled vast quantities of data to be acquired in relatively small time scales [2]. The 40,000 to 100,000 data points that are common to these acquisition systems, in combination with surface interpolation over this data, provides us with further surface and curvature information that is necessary to have in present day design e.g. of headworn protective equipment.

The overall objective of this work is to measure the soft tissue thickness of face and measure the surface shape of the face, then incorporate the thickness data and shape together to create a soft tissue shell model. The investigation and measurement of soft tissue geometry is a major and parallel part of the study to obtain data suitable for incorporation of a soft tissue layer in the model.

---

[1] Further author information-

H.L. (correspondence): H.Liang@surrey.ac.uk; http://www.surrey.ac.uk/MechEng/BioMed/; Telephone: +44 1483 259683; Fax: +44 1483 306039

2. EQUIPMENT AND METHODS

2.1 Laser scanner

The equipment used is a scanner system selected to serve the BioMedical Engineering Group's interest in the medical needs of maxillofacial prosthesis development and fabrication. The scanner was developed initially by staff in University College, London and is subsequently being marketed by 3D Scanners ltd., UK [3].

The laser scanner provides detailed high resolution images of the head and face, where high resolution is taken here to mean an ability to discriminate objects (or surface features) down to ±0.5 mm. Each scan amounts to a data set of over 75,000 data points. It is very compact in its operation, consisting of one laser, scanning a rotating subject, viewed by one camera. The complete set-up (Fig. 1) occupies a floor space of approximately 2 metres × 3 metres.

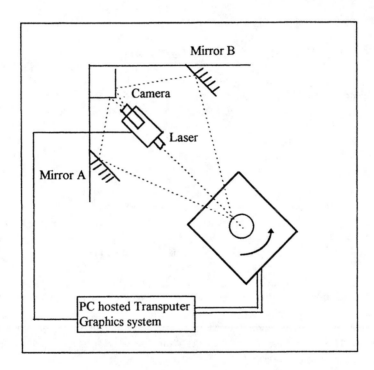

Fig. 1 The outlay of laser scanning system

As a subject is rotated 360° in the darkness, the laser illuminates a profile line which is reflected on to the mirrors and in turn, reflected on to the camera. The software mirrors the two profiles together and uses the calibration data to derive the "best fit" profile. The scan resolultion is 1.46° throuth-out the full 360° giving a total of 245 profiles.. The entire scanning process takes approximately 10-15 seconds. The raw data format is in terms of a shaft encoder value and parameters of the CCD camera in cylindrical co-ordinates. The data can be reformatted to Cartesian co-ordinates and modelled in commercial 3D software as required.

2.2 Ultrasound scanning

This element of the project was directed at acquiring tissue thickness data for an unstructured sample population of healthy young volunteers for incorporating it directly into the 3D Modeller database.

A-scan ultrasound was selected as the technique to be used in acquiring soft tissue thickness data around the head. B-scan ultrasound, its related grey scale and real time scanning, and Computer Tomography (CT) and Magnetic Resonance Imaging (MRI) are imaging tools that provide two dimensional tomographic information, but require more processing time to extract tissue thickness and operate at a considerably higher cost. A-scan signals are more suitable for providing better contrast and axial resolution.

The A-Scan ultrasound instrument used is the Dermal Monitor DM 70 (Cutech, Stiefel laboratories (UK) limited.). This system was designed for measurement of skin and scar tissue thickness. The Dermal Monitor is capable of measuring depths of 0.05-50 mm. The piezoelectric transducer transmits and receives that pulse after interaction with the tissue. The incident pulse is transmitted through the various interfaces of soft tissue until it reaches an air canal or bone structure, at which time, most of the remaining pulse is reflected back to the transducer (the pulse echo). By measuring the time between the transmitted and received pulse, the distance travelled is derived using the average velocity of sound through soft tissue as 1540m/s. The amplifier has a bandwidth of 70 MHz and a variable gain, use of which allowed optimisation of signal to noise ratio. There is also a trigger pulse output to synchronise the data acquisition unit to the DM70. The Gain and Delay of the signal and trigger are controllable to alter the magnitude and view particular parts of the signal. The ultrasound signal was digitised the Gage CompuScope CS2125 AD converter board met (Gage Applied Science Inc., Canada) with a resolution of 8 bits at a sampling rate of up to 250 Mega samples per second.

2.3 Space registration

The acquisition of surface anthropometric data and soft tissue thickness of a human head is described above. This information is valuable in itself. However, the combination of these data sets into one comprehensive data set, resulting in a solid soft tissue model, is more informative as a design tool. Space registration refers to the techniques used to identify in each data set in a "world" reference frame, enabling aggregation of the data, resulting in soft tissue detail related to anatomical location.

The underlying rationale for building a soft tissue shell is that for every surface point, a known vector can be subtracted, in 3D space, to define the position of the inner surface of the soft tissue shell. The magnitude of the vector corresponds to the thickness measurement of the ultrasound. The orientation of the vector is dependent on the orientation of the ultrasound signal when propagated through tissue and reflected off the underlying bone surface or air pocket. Therefore to get an accurate inner shell shape (a shape broadly similar to the skull), the orientation of the ultrasound probe against the outer surface as a critical piece of information needs to be incorporated into the model.

A type of "spacing system" was needed to record location and orientation data of the ultrasound probe tip at the surface of the skin, relative to the reference frame of the laser scanned data at a resolution of 1 mm and ±0.50°. A facility to acquire space data upon command by a PC was a requirement to be able to record the position of the ultrasound probe tip nearly simultaneous to the acquisition of the ultrasound signal.

Magnetic-based, spatial acquisition system was chosen because it met the requirements mentioned above and was sensitive to most positions and orientations within a defined volume. Magnetic spacing systems in general consist of either one or two magnetic field transmitters and one to four sensors. The transmitter is secured to a stationary surface while the sensors are attached to the object whose position and orientation is desired. Inside the transmitter are three orthogonal coils which when sequentially electronically excited in each of the axis directions, produce a magnetic field in the respective axis plane. Each sensor also contains three orthogonal coils which all detect the transmitted magnetic field from each of the x, y and z coils in the transmitter. The magnitude of the sensed voltage is determined by magnitude and direction of the magnetic field, and thus, the position along each reference axis. The ratios of the voltages determine the orientation in space of the sensor. Thus six degrees of freedom: x, y, z, α, β, γ are an output from the system's calculations. The 3D registration device used was a six degree-of-freedom magnetic field sensor (Polhemus Fastrack, Colchester, VT, USA). This device, shown schematically in Fig. 2, consists of a transmitter placed close to the subject and a receiver mounted on the probe. The transmitter produces a spatially varying magnetic field, and the receiver 2 measures the field strength and receiver 1 monitors the movement of the head. By measuring the local magnetic field, the position and angulation of the receiver relative to the transmitter can be determined. Typically, field measurements are made at 100 Hz, thus allowing continuous monitoring the movement of the ultrasound transducer. The receiver size is about $15 \times 15 \times 23$ mm^3, allowing for easy mounting on the ultrasound transducer without interference with its usual use.

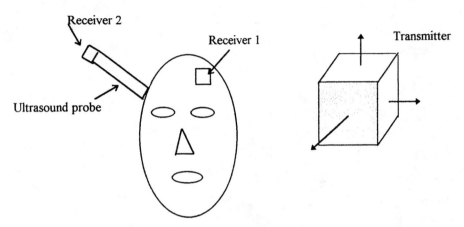

Fig. 2 The space registration system

Although this approach is very flexible, accurate 3-D reconstruction requires that electromagnetic interference be minimised, the transmitter be close to the receiver to allow field measurements with sufficient signal-to-noise ratio (SNR), and that ferrous or highly conductive metals be absent from the vicinity, since they can distort the magnetic field. These limitations can be overcome with special precautions, yielding high quality images.

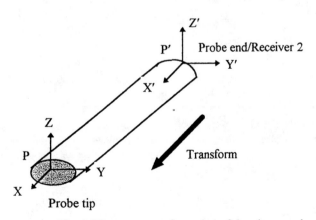

Fig. 3 The space transformation of the ultrasound probe

Fig. 3 is the configuration of the ultrasound probe. The receptacles at the end of the ultrasound probe are made of nylon with a groove cut to the shape of the sensor, enabling it to lie firmly within. After the laser scanning, the sensor was placed in the receptacle for the duration of the ultrasound measurement. At the tip of the probe is the ultrasound transducer. At the end of the probe is the Polhemus receiver 2. Receiver 2 was mounted so that its central axis coincided with that of the probe, thus the orientation of the sensor was also the orientation of the probe.

The co-ordinate of point P were calculated from the position and orientation of the end of the ultrasound probe end P'when the ultrasound was taken,

$$P = M * P'$$ (1)

M is the space translation matrix to transform the P' to P.

$$M = \begin{vmatrix} & & & 0 \\ & Mr & & 0 \\ & & & lp \\ \hline 0 & 0 & 0 & 1 \end{vmatrix}$$ (2)

lp is the length from the probe tip to the Polhemus receiver 2.

$$Mr = \begin{bmatrix} C\alpha C\beta & C\alpha S\beta S\gamma - S\alpha C\gamma & C\alpha S\beta C\gamma + S\alpha S\gamma \\ S\alpha C\beta & S\alpha S\beta S\gamma + C\alpha C\gamma & S\alpha S\beta C\gamma - C\alpha S\gamma \\ -S\beta & C\beta S\gamma & C\beta C\gamma \end{bmatrix}$$ (3)

Mr is the rotation matrix. C stands for cos function and S for sin. α is the angle rotating about OX axis (pitch), β is the angle rotating about OY axis (row) and γ is the angle rotating about OZ axis (yaw).

The receiver 1 (R1) that monitor the head movement was directly adhered to the forehead using double-sided sticky tape so that the change in orientation and position of the head from the reference position was monitored (Fig. 4). Next, the spatial data was taken around the head using the second sensor (R2) which was positioned at the end of the ultrasound probe. An arbitrary position of R1 was registered to which all of the subsequent data was later transferred so that even when subjects moves his head, the relative position between P2, R1 and P2' and R1' will remain constant.

2.4 Integration of shell thickness into the laser surface data.

To be able to reference the Polhemus data set to the laser scanning data, a common datum, identifiable in both data sets, had to be designated so that the two sets of surface data could be merged together.

During the laser scanning, four green light-absorbing dots, 8 mm in diameter and with adhesive backing were positioned on the subject's forehead. Due to the light absorption when the subject was scanned, these four dots appeared as marked "bad" points in the file on the otherwise good data of the forehead. The centre of the dots was detected with an accuracy of ±0.25 mm.

The dots were left on the subject's forehead during the ultrasound and corresponding spatial acquisition. Before the facial soft tissue thickness measurement started, the position of the four green dots was recorded. During the thickness measurement, the space co-ordinates of probe end was recorded, and the position of the probe tip was found by calculation. When the thickness was extracted, the position of the facial bone surface or the air pocket was also determined. For every position measured, there are three features to be recorded: the thickness, the position of outer surface (skin) and inner surface (tissue/bone or tissue/air).

Following the ultrasound measurement, the space data was incorporated into laser scanned data using the space translation method. As the four dots measured by the laser scanner and Polhemus should correspond to each other, the space translation matrix was found from (4) and (5).

498

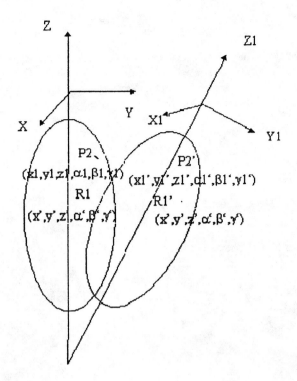

Fig. 4 Detection of the head movement

$$S_{laser} = M * S_{polhemus} \qquad (4)$$

$$M = S_{laser} * S_{polhemus}^{-1} \qquad (5)$$

S_{laser} are the four reference points measured by laser scanning.

S_{laser} are the four reference points measured by Polhemus.

M is the 4×4 space translation matrix with the follow format:

$$M = \begin{vmatrix} & & & Xt \\ & Mr & & Yt \\ & & & Zt \\ \hline 0 & 0 & 0 & 1 \end{vmatrix} \qquad (6)$$

Mr is same as (3) and Xt,Yt, Zt are the homogenous translation. 4 dots (3 co-ordinates × 4 =12) are needed to determine the 12 unknown parameters of M.

After the M was determined, all the data measured by the Polhemus can be translated into the laser data by equation (4) if we replace the $S_{polhemus}$ with data set from every point. Because the facial soft tissue thickness does not vary greatly within a small area on the face [4], the thickness measurement was simplified by measuring the zonal position and the thickness of one point to represent the whole thickness in that zone. The zone position was determined by four points on the boundary of that zone. The thickness between the zones was interpolated.

3. RESULTS

A shell model is shown in Fig. 5. The same tissue thickness in each zone was removed from the laser scanner data from all points with the thickness being subtracted normal to both the vertical and radial tangents at the particular surface points. Fig. 5a is the outside surface of soft tissue, and 5b is the inner surface of the soft tissue or the interface of the bone/tissue or air/tissue. Areas of high tissue thickness can be identified with increasing grey scale.

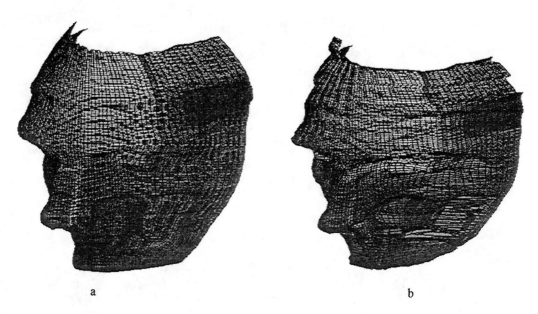

a   b

Fig. 5 a) outside surface   b) inside surface of a shell model.

4. CONCLUSION

This paper has presented a way to create accurate 3D facial reconstruction from laser scanned images and measure facial soft tissue thickness, and incorporating the thickness data into the face model to create a shell model. This form of model offers a direct route to both FEA modelling or to a range of commercially available 3D CAD modelling.

5. REFERENCE

1. Bolton, C., M. Kenward, et al. "An Anthropometric Survey of 2000 Royal Air Force Aircrew", 1970/1971. Royal Aircraft Establishment, 1973

2. Jelier, P. and S. C. Hughes. "Laser scanning as a source of 3D head athropometric data". New developents in mechanics - - Biomechanics and design aspects of military helmets, Defence Research Agency Fanborough, Hampshire, England, 1993

3. Moss, J. P., A. D. Linney, et al. "A laser scanning system for the measurement of facial surface morphology." Optics and Lasers in Engineering. **10**: 179-190, 1989.

4. Liang, H, A.Daya, S. C. Hughes, "In vivo facial soft tissue thickness measurement" SPIE Proc *Vol. 3254.*San. Jose, 1998.

Modeling Surgical Loads to Account for Subsurface Tissue Deformation During Stereotactic Neurosurgery

Michael I. Miga[*], Keith D. Paulsen[*+#0], Francis E. Kennedy[*],
P. Jack Hoopes[*+#], Alex Hartov[*+], David W. Roberts[+#]

[*]Thayer School of Engineering, Dartmouth College, Hanover, N.H., 03755
[+]Dartmouth Hitchcock Medical Center, Lebanon, N.H., 03756
[#]Norris Cotton Cancer Center, Lebanon, N.H., 03756

ABSTRACT

For more than a decade, surgical procedures have benefited significantly from the advent of OR (operating room) coregistered preoperative CT (computed tomographic) and MR (magnetic resonance) imaging. Despite advances in imaging and image registration, one of the most challenging problems is accounting for intraoperative tissue motion resulting from surgical loading conditions. Due to the considerable expense and cumbersome nature of intraoperative MR/CT scanners and the lack of high spatial definition of intracranial anatomy with ultrasound, we have elected to pursue a physics-based computational approach to account for tissue deformation in the context of frameless stereotactic neurosurgery. We have developed a computational model of the brain based on porous media physics and have begun to quantify subsurface deformation due to comparable surgical loads using an *in vivo* porcine model. Templates of CT-observable markers are implanted in a grid-like fashion in the pig brain to quantify tissue motion. Preliminary results based on the simplest of model assumptions are encouraging and have predicted displacement within 15% of measured values. In this paper, a series of computations is compared to experimental data to further understand the impact of material properties and pressure gradients within a homogenous model of brain deformation. The results show that the best fits are obtained with Young's moduli and Poisson's ratio which are smaller than those values typically reported in the literature. As the Poisson ratio decreases towards 0.4 the corresponding Young's modulus increases towards the low end of the values contained in the literature. The optimal pressure gradient is found to be within physiological limits but generally higher than literature values would suggest for a given level of imparted loading, although differences between our experiments and those in the literature with respect to tissue loading conditions are noted.

Key Words: stereotactic neurosurgery, subsurface brain deformation model, brain material properties

1. INTRODUCTION

In recent years, imaging technology has allowed the coregistration of surgical instrument spatial location with preoperative images obtained from modalities such as CT and MR. In the context of neurosurgery, the capability of registering OR and image spaces has provided the possibility of performing stereotactic tasks without the need for a frame attached to the cranium[1-6]. Further, the ability to track instrument location relative to patient-specific anatomical landmarks visible through volumetric image information offers navigational assistance to the neurosurgeon that leads to procedures which are safer, more precise and less invasive. However, because the coregistration is based on preoperative data, brain shift which occurs intraoperatively is not considered but has the

---

[0]For further information contact: keith.paulsen@dartmouth.edu, 8000 Cummings Hall, Hanover, N.H. 03755, Office: 603-646-2695 , Fax: 603-646-3856.

potential to produce inaccuracies that could invalidate the frameless stereotactic approach. In previous studies, we have shown that the average shift of the cortical surface of the brain during various neurosurgical procedures is 1 cm with a definite predisposition of the brain surface to move in the direction of gravity[7]. Dickhaus et al. quantified brain shift specifically for tumor resections by tracking brain structures using MR pre- and intraoperatively. They found that surface motion was on the order of 2 cm, and subsurface shift was 6 to 7 mm for positions located at the interhemisphere fissure and the lateral ventricles[8]. These studies highlight the fact that centimeter-scale motion routinely occurs during neurosurgery suggesting that intraoperative brain shift cannot be ignored during frameless stereotactic procedures.

To address this problem, we have adopted a physics-based modeling approach to predict deformation from surgical loads in order to update the neurosurgeon's navigational perspective intraoperatively. Our initial modeling efforts have been based on a biphasic porous media representation of brain tissue in which case we have been able to predict *in vivo* displacements in the porcine brain within an average error of 15% under the simplest of model assumptions[9,10]. Ultimately, we envision that a computational model of brain tissue deformation would be used in conjunction with a limited amount of concurrently obtained operative data (e.g. video-tracked surface movement and subsurface ultrasound) in order to estimate subsurface tissue motion and thereby provide updated anatomical information for improved navigational assistance during frameless stereotaxy procedures.

In previous work[9,10], we have used a homogenous representation of the brain with displacement and pressure boundary conditions to represent comparable surgical loads. Unfortunately, only a modest amount of data on brain tissue mechanical properties has been reported in the literature. Early studies used mechanical devices to measure properties *in vivo* but were semi-quantitative at best[11-15]. A new and exciting area of research has emerged using MR and ultrasound to image transverse strain waves thereby allowing the calculation of regional mechanical properties based on strain measurements[16,17]. While more quantitative tissue property information can be anticipated in the future based on these newer techniques, the current uncertainty in brain tissue mechanical properties has led us to investigate the effect of varying Young's modulus and Poisson's ratio in our simplified homogenous model as well as the pressure gradient which acts as a distributed body force with respect to elastic deformation. The goal is to shed some light on the range of mechanical properties of brain tissue by comparing a series of computations with experimental data. The results show that an optimal Young's modulus exists which varies with Poisson's ratio. The calculations indicate that an optimal pressure gradient for a given Young's modulus and Poisson's ratio also exists.

2. THE COMPUTATIONAL MODEL

Previous literature reflects the existence of two major subcategories of brain tissue modeling. The first results from a substantial effort which appeared in the 1970's and centered around brain injury effects. These models were concerned with brain trauma resulting from impacts during automobile crashes [18-20]. Loading conditions for these studies were large accelerations of the cranium followed by sharp decelerations or impact. An example of a recent study in this area was performed by Ruan et al. and consisted of a 2D axisymmetric plane strain finite element computation incorporating a modest number of elements, an idealized skull and a layered structure of cranial contents[21].

The second major subcategory of brain tissue modeling has resulted in simulations of the brain in the context of pathophysiologies such as hydrocephalus and hemorrhage[22-27]. This work involved a more complex representation of the brain as a multi-phasic porous medium. Prior to our recent developments, these computations were performed only in 2D and demonstrated qualitative promise. We have recently extended this approach contributing the first 3D calculations in the context of modeling brain motion under surgically-induced loading conditions and have provided the first *in vivo* attempts to quantify its 3D predictive potential[10].

The theory underpinning this type of brain tissue model originates from the soil mechanics literature and describes the process of consolidation[28]. Consolidation theory is biphasic in nature where the medium consists of a solid matrix/tissue that is saturated with an incompressible fluid throughout the interstitial spaces. Subject to a deformation source, tissue consolidation results in an instantaneous deformation at the area of contact followed by additional deformation caused from exiting interstitial fluid driven by a pressure gradient. Others have recognized the utility of applying consolidation theory to soft tissue mechanics, including Taylor[29,30] who created an interstitial transport model taking into account plasma protein movement and interstitial swelling. Basser[31] has also used a consolidation approach to model infusion-induced swelling in the brain. Computationally, at least in terms of brain tissue mechanics, the work of Nagashima et al. represents the first and most extensive experience with consolidation in the neuroanatomy context[22-24].

The governing equations we have considered for consolidation in soft-tissue can be written as

$$\nabla \cdot G\nabla \mathbf{u} + \nabla \frac{G}{1-2\nu}(\nabla \cdot \mathbf{u}) - \alpha\nabla p = 0 \tag{1a}$$

$$\alpha\frac{\partial}{\partial t}(\nabla \cdot \mathbf{u}) + \frac{1}{S}\frac{\partial p}{\partial t} - \nabla \cdot k\nabla p = 0 \tag{1b}$$

where,

G is shear modulus,
ν is Poisson's ratio,
$\mathbf{u}$ is the displacement vector,
p is the pore fluid pressure,
α is the ratio of fluid volume extracted to volume change of the tissue under compression,
k is the hydraulic conductivity, and
$1\backslash S$ is the amount of water which can be forced into the tissue under constant volume.

These equations assume that the tissue is linearly elastic and that the interstitial fluid is incompressible. Equation (1a) represents classic static mechanical equilibrium subject to a body force represented by an interstitial fluid pressure gradient across the medium. Equation (1b) provides the constitutive relationship between volumetric strain and fluid pressure. Generally, the brain can be considered as a saturated medium which eliminates the time rate of change in pressure from equation (1b) (i.e. $\alpha = 1$, $1\backslash S = 0$), and we have made this assumption in the results reported herein. Although more complex theories exist for soft tissue modeling[32-35], consolidation seems to be a natural starting point in the development of a brain tissue model. It has an advantage over simple linear elasticity due to the added fluid component; this allows access to more realistic boundary conditions related to intracranial pressure and cerebrospinal fluid (CSF) drainage while still maintaining the computational advantages of a linear theory.

3. METHODS

The equations described in (1a-b) have been solved in three dimensions using the Galerkin finite element method (FEM) and were compared to analytical and numerical benchmarks in the literature which has shown that our computational approach is highly accurate (errors less than 2% of applied load on modest levels of finite element mesh resolution). In addition, we have also performed a stability analysis of the equations to better understand the propagation of numerical errors[36]. We have quantified our preliminary experiences with an *in vivo* porcine model

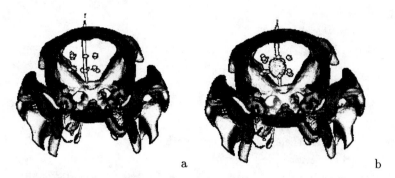

a   b

Figure 1. Experimental porcine model with centrally placed balloon catheter, tissue thresholded out, and surrounding grid of 1mm ss markers: (a) baseline volume with uninflated catheter; (b) 1cc inflation with subsequent bead movement.

and have found we can predict the total average displacement to within 15% of the maximum imparted measured displacement[10].

The experimental surgical procedure involved implanting a pig brain with small 1mm beads in a grid-like fashion in the parenchyma which serve as tissue displacement markers. Following implantation and evaluation of the marker fixation, a balloon catheter filled with contrast agent was inserted in the cranium. All objects were easily seen in a CT scanner and were monitored during subsequent balloon inflations thus creating deformation maps which can be compared to model calculations. Figure 1 shows an example of a pig cranium during a 1cc inflation of the balloon with the tissue thresholded out and the markers/balloon easily observable. Prior to the surgical procedure, a complete set of MR images were taken of the pig cranium. These scans serve as the basis of the FEM discretization process. Using **ANALYZE Version 7.5 - Biomedical Imaging Resource** (Mayo Foundation, Rochester, M.N.), we segmented the 3D volume of interest and used **MATLAB** (Math Works Inc., Natick Mass.) to render the surface boundary description of the brain and any surgical implants. We then produced a tetrahedral grid on the interior using mesh generation software[37] which completed the discretization process. Figure 2 displays a typical mesh in the 1cc deformed state (i.e. after computation) where volume elements are approximately 1 mm^3 inside the tissue (prior to calculation) and 0.025 mm^3 near the implanted catheter (prior to calculation). The mesh contained 11,923 nodes and 62,439 tetrahedral elements.

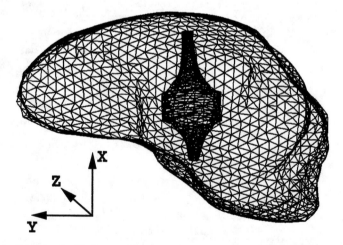

Figure 2. Deformed boundary at the 1cc inflation level.

4. RESULTS

In previous work[10], we have shown that we are capable of predicting the total average displacement level to within 14% and 19% of the maximum bead displacement over 1cc and 2cc inflation levels, respectively. Figure 2 represents the typical geometries resulting from our calculations. This example was computed using the following properties,

Material Properties: $E = 2100\ Pa$, $\nu = 0.45$, $k = 1e - 7\ \frac{m^3 s}{kg}$
Running Properties: $dt = 1e4\ s$, $\theta = 1$, # steps=5.

In terms of boundary conditions, the balloon catheter was divided into two sections which included deformed (cylindrical portion of catheter with 5.45 mm outward expansion) and free surface components (necked portion of catheter). The interstitial pressure at the balloon/tissue interface was taken to be constant at 6000 Pa (or 45 mmHg) which is within the range of values recorded by Wolfla et al.[38,39] under conditions of acute balloon inflation within a closed cranial cavity of the pig. The outer cortical brain surface was prescribed as a fixed (no displacement) boundary with zero fluid pressure.

Starting with the above boundary conditions and varying Young's modulus and Poisson's ratio, we have been able to produce a description of how the average total displacement error varies over the solution domain. Figure 3 represents the average match between the data and calculations for the total displacement of the 15 beads that were tracked in the CT for the 1cc inflation level. It demonstrates that as the solid matrix becomes more incompressible ($\nu \rightarrow 0.5$) the minimum error occurs at lower moduli for the homogenous case. Another interesting phenomena is that the convexity of the minimum becomes more pronounced with decreasing Poisson's ratio. From Figure 3, an average total displacement error of 13.8% occurs at a Young's Modulus of 1800 Pa and Poisson's ratio of 0.45. Figure 4 displays the complete comparison between experiment and calculation for each bead displacement directional component as well as the total displacement for these values of Young's modulus and Poisson's ratio.

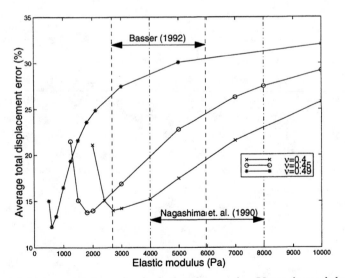

Figure 3. Average match between data and calculation for varying Young's modulus and Poisson's ratio.

In addition to total displacement, the average error in each bead's directional component can be analyzed in a similar fashion to that of Figure 3. These results are shown in Figure 5 and demonstrate that a similar shift in minimum error values is accompanied with increasing Poisson's ratio. Figures 3 and 5 also indicate some brain

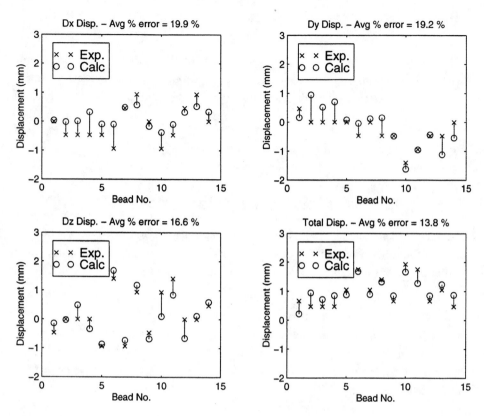

Figure 4. Comparison between measured and calculated data for displacement error at the 1cc inflation level of the balloon catheter.

moduli ranges from the literature where the lower values represent white matter and the upper values correspond to gray matter. The Nagashima et al. and Basser papers used Poisson's ratios used of 0.47 and 0.49 respectively.

We have also quantified how the solution is influenced by the pressure gradient across the tissue which is another important model variable beyond the solid matrix material properties. Figure 6 represents the effect of pressure on each average directional error component as well as the total displacement error. Interestingly, the pressure gradients which correspond to the minimum error in the directional components occur at quite different values. Based on this results, it follows that the minimum total displacement error exists at a gradient value which is a weighting of the different minima that appear in Figure 5. In addition to our calculations, pressure ranges are shown from the Wolfla et al. data which was obtained in a porcine model[38,39]. The 1996 data represents the approximate maximum/minimum interstitial pressure ranges for 1cc-3cc inflation levels of an acute expanding frontal epidural mass (balloon catheter)[38]. The 1997 data represents the pressures associated with the same inflation level range for an acute expanding extradural temporal mass[39].

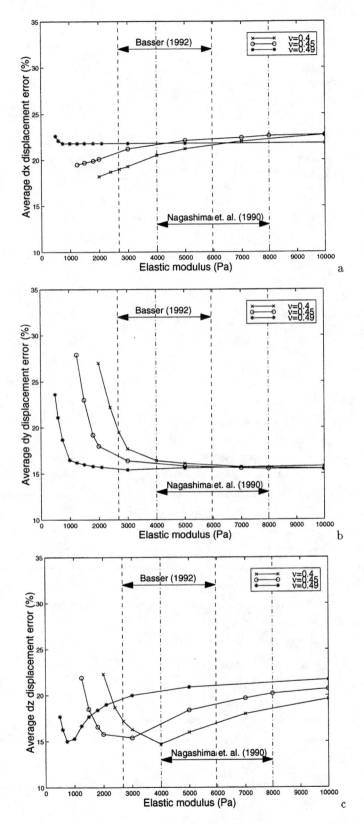

Figure 5. Comparison between measured and calculated data for average directional displacement error for 1cc inflation level of balloon catheter for varying Young's modulus and Poisson's ratio.

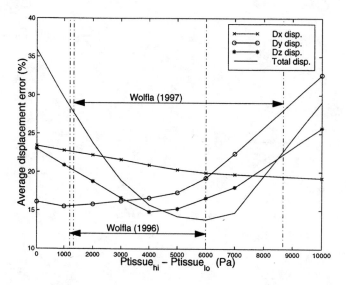

Figure 6. Comparison between measured and calculated data for average displacement error for 1cc inflation level of balloon catheter while varying pressure across the tissue.

5. CONCLUSIONS

We have shown in the case of a homogenous model of brain deformation based on consolidation theory subject to displacement and pressure boundary conditions that minimum average displacement error varies with Young's modulus, Poisson's ratio, and pressure gradient. We have also found that as the solid matrix becomes more incompressible (i.e. $\nu \rightarrow 0.5$), the error minimum shifts downward towards a smaller Young's modulus. Typically the literature has considered brain tissue as nearly incompressible. Interestingly, we observe that the ranges of accepted moduli values for brain do not correlate with the typical Poisson's ratio cited (assuming that brain moduli ranges are close in value across species). This is not to say that the incompressible assumptions made in previous studies are incorrect but the results do suggest that further study is required. With respect to the effect of tissue pressure gradients, we find that our optimal gradient falls inside the range of physiological limits. Although the lower values of the Wolfla range (1cc inflation level) are significantly lower than our optimum, it is important to recognize that our balloon placement was intraparenchymal and its effects are not yet quantified. The variation in the upper range for the two different placements in the Wolfla studies suggests that placement could indeed have a substantial effect on the pressure gradients that occur in tissue under acute expansion.

Clearly, one of the major assumptions in these calculations is tissue homogeneity. Effort is currently underway to employ a heterogeneous model to further investigation of the effects of varying moduli and Poisson's ratio in our *in vivo* model. We are also developing more refined techniques for imparting tissue displacement in a more controlled and quantifiable manner. It is the hope that these studies will lay the ground work for a real-time, model-based updating of surgeon's navigational fields in the context of frameless stereotactic neurosurgery.

Acknowledgement: This work was supported by National Institutes of Health grant R01-NS33900 awarded by the National Institute of Neurological Disorders and Stroke. ANALYZE software was provided in collaboration with the Mayo Foundation.

6. REFERENCES

1. T. Peters, B. Davey, P. Munger, R. Comeau, A. Evans, and A. Olivier, 'Three-dimensional multimodal image-guidance for neurosurgery',*IEEE Trans. Med. Imaging*, vol. 15, pp. 121-128, 1996.

2. W. E. L. Grimson, G. J. Ettlinger, S. J. White, T. Lozano-Perez, W. M. Wells 3rd, and R. Kikinis, 'An automated registration method for frameless stereotaxy, image guided surgery and enhanced reality visualization', it IEEE Trans. Med. Imaging, vol. 15, pp. 129-140, 1996.

3. D. W. Roberts, J. W. Strohbehn, J. F. Hatch, W. Murray, and H. Kettenberger, ' A frameless stereotactic integration of computerized tomographic imaging and the operating microscope', *J. Neurosurg.*, vol. 65, pp. 545-549, 1986.

4. R. L. Galloway, R. J. Maciunas, and C. A. Edwards, 'Interactive image-guided neurosurgery', *IEEE Trans. Biomed. Eng.*, vol. 39, pp. 1226-1231, 1992.

5. G. H. Barnette, D. W. Kormos, and C. P. Steiner, 'Use of a frameless, armless stereotactic wand for brain tumor localization with 2D and 3D neuroimaging', *Neurosurgery*, vol. 33, pp. 674-678, 1993.

6. D. R. Sanderman, and S. S. Gill, 'The impact of interactive image guided surgery: the Bristol experience with the ISF/Elekta viewing wand', *Acta Neurochirurgica, Suppl.*, vol. 64, pp. 54-58, 1995.

7. D. W. Roberts, A. Hartov, F.E. Kennedy, M. I. Miga, K. D. Paulsen, 'Intraoperative brain shift and deformation: a quantitative clinical analysis of cortical displacements in 28 cases', *Neurosurgery*, (submitted), 1997.

8. H. Dickhaus, K. Ganser, A. Staubert, M. M. Bonsanto, C. R. Wirtz, V. M. Tronnier, and S. Kunze, 'Quantification of brain shift effects by mr-imaging', *Proc. An. Int. Conf. IEEE Eng. Med. Biology Soc.*, 1997.

9. M. I. Miga, K. D. Paulsen, F. E. Kennedy, P. J. Hoopes, A. Hartov, and D. W. Roberts, 'A 3D brain deformation model experiencing comparable surgical loads', *Proc. 19th An. Int. Conf. IEEE Eng. Med. Biology Soc.*, 773-776, 1997.

10. K. D. Paulsen, M. I. Miga, F. E. Kennedy, P. J. Hoopes, A. Hartov, and D. W. Roberts, 'A computational model for tracking subsurface tissue deformation during stereotactic neurosurgery', *IEEE Transactions on Biomedical Engineering*, (submitted), (1997).

11. G. T. Fallenstein, and V. D. Huke, 'Dynamic mechanical properties of brain tissue', *J. Biomech.*, vol. 2, pp. 217-226, 1969.

12. C. Ljung, 'A model for brain deformation due to rotation of the skull', *J. Biomechanics*, vol. 8, pp. 263-274, 1975.

13. E. K. Walsh, and A. Schettini, 'A pressure-displacement transducer for measuring brain tissue properties in vivo', *J. Appl. Physiol.*, 38, 187-189, (1975).

14. E. K. Walsh, W. Furniss and A. Schettini, 'On measurement of brain elastic response in vivo', *Am. J. Physiol.*, vol. 232, pp. R27-R30, 1977.

15. E. K. Walsh, and A. Schettini, 'Calculation of brain elastic parameters in vivo', *Am. J. Physiol.*, 247, R693-R700, (1984).

16. R. Mathupillai, P. J. Rossman, D. J. Lomas, J. F. Greenleaf, S. J. Riederer, and R. L. Ehman, 'Magnetic resonance elastography by direct visualization of propagating acoustic strain waves', *Science*, vol. 269, pp. 1854-1857, (1995).

17. R. Mathupillai, P. J. Rossman, D. J. Lomas, J. F. Greenleaf, S. J. Riederer, and R. L. Ehman, 'Magnetic Resonance Imaging of Transverse Strain Waves', *Magnetic Resonance in Medicine*, vol. 36, pp. 266-274, (1996).

18. T. A. Shugar, and M. G. Katona, 'Development of a finite element head injury model', *ASCE J. Eng. Mech. Div.*, EM3:101, E173, pp. 223-239, 1975.

19. C. C. Ward, and R. B. Thompson, 'The development of a detailed finite element brain model', *Proc. 19th Stapp Car Crash Conf.*, pp. 641-674, 1975.

20. T. B. Khalil, and R. P. Hubbard, 'Parametric study of head response by finite element modeling', *J. Biomech*, vol. 10, pp. 119-132, 1977.

21. J. A. Ruan, T. B. Khalil, and A. I. King, 'Human head dynamic response to side impact by finite element modeling', *ASME J. Biomech. Eng.*, vol. 113, pp. 276-283, 1991.

22. T. Nagashima, T. Shirakuni, and SI. Rapoport, 'A two-dimensional, finite element analysis of vasogenic brain edema,' *Neurol. Med. Chir.*, vol. 30, pp. 1-9, 1990.

23. T. Nagashima, Y. Tada, S. Hamano, M. Skakakura, K. Masaoka, N. Tamaki, and S. Matsumoto, 'The finite element analysis of brain oedema associated with intracranial meningiomas', *Acta. Neurochir. Suppl.*, vol. 51, pp. 155-7, 1990.

24. T. Nagashima, N. Tamaki, M. Takada, and Y. Tada, 'Formation and resolution of brain edema associated with brain tumors. A comprehensive theoretical model and clinical analysis', *Acta Neurochir Suppl*, vol. 60, pp. 165-167, 1994.

25. Y. Tada, and T. Nagashima, 'Modeling and simulation of brain lesions by the finite-element method', *IEEE Eng. Med. Bio.*, pp. 497-503, 1994.

26. H. Takizawa, K. Sugiura, M. Baba, C. Kudou, S. Endo, M. Nakabayashi, and R. Fukuya, 'Deformation of brain and stress distribution caused by putaminal hemorrhage–numerical computer simulation by finite element method', *No To Shinkei*, vol. 43, pp. 1035-1039, 1991.

27. H. Takizawa, K. Sugiura, M. Baba, and J. D. Miller, 'Analysis of intracerebral hematoma shapes by numerical computer simulation using the finite element method', *Neurol Med Chir*, vol. 34, pp. 65-69, 1994.

28. M. Biot, 'General theory of three dimensional consolidation', *J. Appl. Phys.*, vol. 12, pp. 155-164, 1941.

29. D.G. Taylor, J.L. Bert, and B.D. Bowen, 'A mathematical model of interstitial transport. I. Theory', *Microvasc Res*, vol. 39, pp. 253-278, 1990.

30. D.G. Taylor, J.L. Bert, and B.D. Bowen, 'A mathematical model of interstitial transport. II. Microvasculature exchange in the mesentery', *Microvasc Res*, vol. 39, pp. 279-306, 1990.

31. P. J. Basser, 'Interstitial pressure, volume, and flow during infusion into brain tissue', *Microvasc. Res.*, vol. 44, pp. 143-165, 1992.

32. K. K. Mendis, R. L. Stalnaker, and S. H. Advani, 'A constitutive relationship for large deformation finite element modeling of brain tissue', *J Biomech Eng*, vol. 117, pp. 279-285, 1995.

33. R. L. Spilker, and J. K. Suh. 'Formulation and evaluation of a finite element model for the biphasic model of hydrated soft tissue', *Comp. Struct.*, vol. 35, no. 4, pp. 425-439, 1990.

34. R. L. Spilker, and T. A. Maxian. 'A mixed-penalty finite element formulation of the linear biphasic theory for soft tissues', *Int. J. Numer. Methods Eng.*, vol. 30, pp. 1063-1082, 1990.

35. J.P. Laible, D. Pflaster, B. R. Simon, M. H. Krag, M. Pope, and L. D. Haugh, 'A dynamic material parameter estimation procedure for soft tissue using a poroelastic finite element model', *J Biomech Eng*, vol. 116, pp. 19-29, 1994.

36. M. I. Miga, K. D. Paulsen, F. E. Kennedy, 'Von Neumann stability analysis of Biot's general two-dimensional theory of consolidation', *Int. J. of Num. Methods in Eng.*, (submitted), (1997).

37. J. M. Sullivan Jr., G. Charron, and K. D. Paulsen, 'A three dimensional mesh generator for arbitrary multiple material domains, *Finite Element Analysis and Design*, vol. 25, pp. 219-241, 1997.

38. C. E. Wolfla, T. G. Luerssen, R. M. Bowman, and T. K. Putty, 'Brain tissue pressure gradients created by expanding frontal epidural mass lesion', *J. Neurosurg.*, vol. 84, pp. 642-647, 1996.

39. C. E. Wolfla, T. G. Luerssen, and R. M. Bowman, 'Regional brain tissue pressure gradients created by expanding extradural temporal mass legion', *J. Neurosurg*, vol. 86, pp. 505-510, 1997.

Addendum

The following papers were announced for publication in this proceedings but have been withdrawn or are unavailable.

[3254-05] **Immune modulation using photosensitizers and light***
J. G. Levy, M. Obochi, D. W. Hunt, J. Tao, QLT PhotoTherapeutics Inc. (Canada)

[3254-16] **Computer simulations of the effect of pulse length on laser-tattoo interaction**
D. Ho, R. A. London, M. E. Glinsky, D. A. Young, Lawrence Livermore National Lab.

[3254-30] **Effects of the ArF excimer laser on hard tissue: ablation, pressure wave generation, cleaning, and sterilization**
A. D. Karoutis, Univ. of Crete (Greece); A. Nikoloudakis, Univ. Hospital of Crete (Greece); J. Skoulas, Venizelion Hospital (Greece); S. Nikolopoulos, Univ. of Crete (Greece); A. P. Sviridov, Research Ctr. for Technological Lasers (Russia); A. G. Doukas, Wellman Labs. of Photomedicine, Massachusetts General Hospital, and Harvard Medical School; E. S. Helidonis, Univ. of Crete (Greece) and Univ. Hospital of Crete (Greece)

[3254-37] **Two-dimensional vapor bubble simulations for medical applications**
P. A. Amendt, D. S. Bailey, R. A. London, D. J. Maitland, Lawrence Livermore National Lab.; M. Strauss, Nuclear Research Ctr.–Negev (Israel)

[3254-44] **Laser-induced straining of a biologic material analyzed using a polariscopic imaging technique**
J. T. Walsh, Jr., Northwestern Univ.; G. P. Delacrétaz, D. Beghuin, Ecole Polytechnique Fédérale de Lausanne (Switzerland)

*Published as **Interleukin-12 reverses the inhibitory impact of photodynamic therapy (PDT) on the murine contact hypersensitivity response**, in *Optical Methods for Tumor Treatment and Detections: Mechanisms and Techniques in Photodynamic Therapy VII*, Thomas J. Dougherty, Editor, Proceedings of SPIE Vol. 3247, pp. 89-97 (1998).

Author Index